CARDIOLOGY SECRETS

2nd Edition

OLIVIA VYNN ADAIR, MD

Assistant Professor
Department of Medicine
Faculty
Department of Family Medicine Residency Program
University of Colorado Health Sciences Center
Denver, Colorado
   and
Cardiologist
Swedish Medical Center
Englewood
Porter Adventist Hospital
Denver, Colorado

HANLEY & BELFUS, INC. / Philadelphia

Publisher: HANLEY & BELFUS, INC.
                    Medical Publishers
                    210 South 13th Street
                    Philadelphia, PA 19107
                    (215) 546-7293; 800-962-1892
                    FAX (215) 790-9330
                    Web site: http://www.hanleyandbelfus.com

Note to the reader: Although the information in this book has been carefully reviewed for correctness of dosage and indications, neither the authors nor the editor nor the publisher can accept any legal responsibility for any errors or omissions that may be made. Neither the publisher nor the editors make any warranty, expressed or implied, with respect to the material contained herein. Before prescribing any drug, the reader must review the manufacturer's current product information (package inserts) for accepted indications, absolute dosage recommendations, and other information pertinent to the safe and effective use of the product described.

Library of Congress Cataloging-in-Publication Data

Cardiology Secrets / edited by Olivia Vynn Adair.—2nd ed.
      p. ; cm.—(The Secrets Series®)
   Includes bibliographical references and index.
   ISBN 1-56053-420-6 (alk. paper)
    1. Cardiology—Miscellanea. I. Adair, Olivia Vynn, 1956- II. Series.
   [DNLM: 1. Heart Diseases—Examination Questions. WG 18.2 C2697 2000]
   RC682.C397 2001
   616.1'2'0076—dc21

                                                              00-058135

CARDIOLOGY SECRETS, 2ND ED.   ISBN 1-56053-420-6

Last digit is the print number: 9   8   7   6   5   4   3   2   1

CONTENTS

CONTRIBUTORS

William T. Abraham, MD, FACP, FACC
Professor of Medicine and Chief of Cardiovascular Medicine, Department of Internal Medicine, University of Kentucky, Lexington, Kentucky

Olivia Vynn Adair, MD
Assistant Professor, Department of Medicine, and Faculty, Department of Family Medicine Residency Program, University of Colorado Health Sciences Center, Denver; Cardiologist, Swedish Medical Center, Englewood, Colorado

Stuart W. Adler, MD
Department of Medicine, University of Minnesota Medical School, Minneapolis, Minnesota

Astrid Andreescu, MD
Clinical Instructor of Medicine, University of Vermont, Burlington, Vermont

David B. Badesch, MD
Division of Pulmonary Sciences and Critical Care Medicine, University of Colorado School of Medicine, Denver, Colorado

William M. Bailey, MD
Clinical Cardiac Electrophysiologist, Heart and Vascular Center, Lake Charles Memorial Hospital, Lake Charles, Louisiana

Rajesh Bhola, MD
Fellow, Department of Radiology, Division of Nuclear Medicine, University of Colorado Health Sciences Center, Denver, Colorado

Fernando Boccalandro, MD
Cardiology Fellow, Department of Internal Medicine, Division of Cardiology, University of Texas Medical School, Houston, Texas

Jennifer L. Calagan, MD
Formerly of Fitzsimons Army Medical Center, Aurora, Colorado

Robert W. Cameron, MD
Formerly of Fitzsimons Army Medical Center, Aurora, Colorado

Mohamed Chebaclo, MD
Department of Medicine, State University of New York Health Sciences Center, Brooklyn; Catheterization Laboratory, Brooklyn VA Medical Center, Brooklyn, New York

Luther T. Clark, MD
Department of Medicine, State University of New York Health Science Center, Brooklyn, New York

David Harris Collier, MD
Associate Professor, Department of Medicine, University of Colorado Health Sciences Center, Denver, Colorado

Karen Cooper, MD
Private Practice, Hematology/Oncology, Kingston, Pennsylvania

Stephen T. Crowley, MD
Division of Cardiology, University of Colorado School of Medicine, Denver, Colorado

Talley F. Culclasure, MD
Formerly of Fitzsimons Army Medical Center, Aurora, Colorado

Ira M. Dauber, MD
Associate Clinical Professor, Department of Medicine, University of Colorado Health Sciences Center, Denver; Attending Cardiologist, Porter Hospital and Swedish Medical Center, Englewood, Colorado

Richard C. Davis, MD, PhD
Formerly of Fitzsimons Army Medical Center, Aurora, Colorado

Mark E. Dorogy, MD
Formerly of Fitzsimons Army Medical Center, Aurora, Colorado

James E. Ehrlich, MD
Medical Director, Colorado Heart Imaging; Medical Co-Director, HeartScan Houston and HeartScan Washington DC; Clinical Assistant Professor, Department of Anesthesiology, University of Colorado School of Medicine, Denver, Colorado

Arnold Einhorn, MD, FACC
Department of Medicine, Division of Cardiology, University of Florida, Gainesville, Florida

Ashraf ElSakr, MD
Division of Cardiology, State University of New York Health Sciences Center, Brooklyn, New York

Richard W. Erickson, MD
Department of Medicine, Division of Rheumatology, University of Colorado School of Medicine, Denver, Colorado

Karen A. Fagan, MD
Assistant Professor of Medicine, Department of Pulmonary Science and Critical Care Medicine, University of Colorado Health Sciences Center, Denver, Colorado

James J. Fenton, MD, FCCP
Medical Director, Porter Adventist Hospital, Denver, Colorado

Charles E. Fuenzalida, MD, FACC, FACP
Assistant Clinical Professor, Department of Cardiology, University of Colorado Health Sciences Center, Denver, Colorado; Staff Cardiologist, Presbyterian/Columbia Hospital and Aurora Medical Center

Edward Gill, MD
Associate Professor of Medicine, Division of Cardiology, University of Washington School of Medicine, Seattle; Director of Echocardiography, Harborview Medical Center, Seattle, Washington; University of Colorado, Denver, Colorado

Gregory R. Giugliano, MD
Cardiology Fellow, Department of Cardiology, University of Colorado Health Sciences Center, Denver, Colorado

Javier Mauricio Gonzalez, MD
Cardiology Fellow, Department of Cardiology, The Brooklyn Hospital Center, Brooklyn, New York

Michael E. Hanley, MD
Associate Professor of Medicine, Department of Pulmonary and Critical Care Medicine, University of Colorado Health Sciences Center, Denver, Colorado

Edward P. Havranek, MD
Associate Professor of Medicine, University of Colorado School of Medicine, Denver; Staff Cardiologist, Denver Health Medical Center, Denver, Colorado

William T. Highfill, MD
Formerly of Fitzsimons Army Medical Center, Aurora, Colorado

Fred D. Hofeldt, MD
Department of Medicine, University of Colorado School of Medicine, Denver, Colorado

Ali R. Homayuni, MD, FACC, FCCP
Division of Cardiology, Mt. Sinai School of Medicine, New York, New York

Evelyn Hutt, MD
Assistant Professor, Division of Geriatrics, Department of Medicine, University of Colorado Health Sciences Center, Denver, Colorado

David A. Kaminsky, MD
Division of Pulmonary and Critical Care Medicine, Department of Medicine, University of Colorado School of Medicine, Denver, Colorado

Christopher M. Kozlowski, MD
Formerly of Fitzsimons Army Medical Center, Aurora, Colorado

Norman Krasnow, MD
Clinical Professor, Department of Medicine, College of Physicians and Surgeons, New York; Senior Attending Physician, St. Luke's-Roosevelt Hospital, New York, New York

Mitchel Kruger, MD
Formerly of Fitzsimons Army Medical Center, Aurora, Colorado

James C. Lafferty, MD, FACC
Downstate Medical Center, Brooklyn, and Staten Island University Hospital, Staten Island, New York

Sumant Lamba, MD
Assistant Professor, Department of Internal Medicine, University of Kentucky, Lexington, Kentucky

Peter Levitt, MD
Cardiologist, Porter Adventist Hospital, Denver, and Swedish Medical Center, Englewood, Colorado

JoAnn Lindenfeld, MD
Department of Medicine, University of Colorado School of Medicine, Denver, Colorado

Catalin Loghin, MD
Chief Medical Resident and Clinical Instructor, Department of Internal Medicine, University of Texas Health Sciences Center, Houston, Texas

Brian D. Lowes, MD
Department of Medicine, University of Colorado School of Medicine, Denver, Colorado

John T. Madonna, MD
Formerly of Fitzsimons Army Medical Center, Aurora, Colorado

Mark Malyak, MD
Department of Medicine, Division of Rheumatology, University of Colorado School of Medicine, Denver, Colorado

Donald A. McCord, MD, FACC
Assistant Clinical Professor of Medicine, Downstate Medical Center, Brooklyn, and Staten Island University Hospital, Staten Island, New York

Querubin P. Mendoza, MD
Coronary Care Unit, William Beaumont Army Medical Center, El Paso, Texas

Raul Mendoza, MD
Private Practice, Lawrence, New York

William P. Miller, MD
Department of Medicine, University of Wisconsin Medical School, Madison, Wisconsin

George M. Pachello, M.D.
Interventional Cardiology, Porter Memorial Hospital, Swedish Medical Center, Denver, Colorado

Mark A. Perea, MD
Department of Family Medicine, Aurora Medical Center, Aurora, Colorado

Jeffrey Pickard, MD
Department of Medicine, University of Colorado School of Medicine, Denver, Colorado

Robert A. Quaife, MD
Associate Professor, Departments of Medicine and Radiology, University of Colorado Health Sciences Center, Denver, Colorado

Jane Reusch, MD
Department of Medicine, Division of Endocrinology, Metabolism, and Diabetes, University of Colorado School of Medicine, Denver, Colorado

Roy W. Robertson, MD
Fellow in Cardiovascular Medicine, Department of Cardiology, University of Wisconsin Medical School, Madison, Wisconsin

David T. Schachter, MD
Formerly of Fitzsimons Army Medical Center, Aurora, Colorado

Kimberly Anne Schleman, MD
Fellow, Department of Cardiology, University of Colorado Health Sciences Center, Denver, Colorado

June Yi Scott, MD
Clinical Instructor, Department of Renal Diseases and Hypertension, University of Colorado Health Sciences Center, Denver, Colorado

Paul D. Sherry, MD
Formerly of Fitzsimons Army Medical Center, Aurora, Colorado

Harmeet Singh, MD
Department of Medicine, Division of Renal Disease and Hypertension, University of Colorado School of Medicine, Denver, Colorado

Michael Staab, MD
Cardiologist, South Denver Cardiology, Denver, Colorado

Richard A. Stein, MD
Professor, Department of Medicine, State University of New York Health Science Center, Brooklyn; Chief of Cardiology, The Brooklyn Hospital Center, Brooklyn, New York

David Tanaka, MD
Department of Medicine, University of Colorado School of Medicine, Denver, Colorado

Nelson P. Trujillo, MD
Cardiologist, Rocky Mountain Cardiology, P.C., Boulder, Colorado

David C. Van Pelt, MD
Hospital Internist, Department of Internal Medicine, Swedish Medical Center, Englewood, Colorado

Gumpanart Veerakul, MD, FSCAI
Chief, Cardiology Division, and Director, Cardiovascular Intervention and Research Laboratory, Bhumibol Adulyadej Hospital, The Royal Thai Air Force, Bangkok, Thailand

Douglas Paul Voorhees, RRT
Chief Executive Officer, Ultra Imaging, Denver, Colorado

Donald L. Warkentin, MD
Department of Medicine, University of Colorado School of Medicine, Denver, Colorado

Mary L. Warner, MD
South Denver Pulmonary Associates, PC, Englewood, Colorado

Howard D. Weinberger, MD, FACC
Assistant Professor, Division of Cardiology, Department of Medicine, University of Colorado Health Sciences Center, Denver; Director of Cardiology Service, Cardiology Consultant, and Staff Physician, National Jewish Medical and Research Center, Denver, Colorado

Eric S. Weinstein, MD
Cardiologist, Colorado Cardiovascular Surgical Associates, P.C., and Porter Adventist Hospital, Denver; Swedish Medical Center, Englewood, Colorado

Madeline Jean White, MD
Clinical Associate Professor, Department of Medicine, Denver Health Medical Center, Denver, Colorado

Phillip S. Wolf, MD
Professor of Medicine, Division of Cardiology, University of Colorado Health Sciences Center, Denver, Colorado

Richard E. Wolfe, MD
Chief, Department of Emergency Medicine, Beth Israel Deaconess Medical Center, Boston, Massachusetts

Marie Wood, MD
Assistant Professor of Medicine, University of Vermont, Burlington, Vermont

Robert A. Zaloom, MD, FACC
Department of Cardiology, Lutheran Medical Center and St. Vincent's Hospital Medical Center, New York, New York

Dedication

In loving memory of my parents, Eunice and Lucky Adair, for all their support, encouragement, and never faltering confidence; and a special thanks for the patience of Lisa and Matthew.

PREFACE TO THE FIRST EDITION

There is no faster growing subspecialty than cardiology. All aspects of medicine require basic knowledge in cardiology no matter if you're in the emergency department, on the medical wards, or conducting your daily office patient visits. We hope this volume of *Cardiology Secrets* will make the acquisition of knowledge exciting, fun, and easy. It should serve as a basic review for the cardiologist and a primary fund of knowledge and references for other health professionals as well as medical students. We hope the reader will be stimulated to learn more and pass on the knowledge to the novice, as the question/answer format is ideal for teaching.

Special acknowledgment to Patricia Ross for her exceptional organizational and secretarial skills, making this book possible. Also special thanks to all the authors who took the time from their busy lives and professional schedules to prepare their chapters.

Olivia V. Adair, M.D.
Edward P. Havranek, M.D.

PREFACE TO THE SECOND EDITION

This second edition of *Cardiology Secrets* came with many challenges, including the incredibly expanding field of cardiology and the fast pace of subspecialty generation. As with the first edition, my hope was to present as much material as possible in the exciting and stimulating Secrets format to provide current and fundamental knowledge useful in everyday practice. The authors have also reviewed the updated literature, and many new techniques and therapies are presented herein.

A project such as this requires many hours from the authors' very busy schedules, as well as numerous interactions between the publisher's staff and myself to produce a finished product. A special thanks for the dedication to teaching exhibited by those willing to make this effort to share and pass on the knowledge. A special thanks to Jessica Jaquez for her organizational and secretarial skills.

Enjoy!

Olivia V. Adair, M.D.

I. General Examination

1. CARDIOVASCULAR PHYSICAL DIAGNOSIS

Phillip S. Wolf, M.D., and Gregory R. Giugliano, M.D.

1. List clues that may be evident on general inspection.

Begin the general inspection as soon as you enter the room. You may note numerous clues to the disease process you are about to encounter. Here are some examples:

- Blue sclera—osteogenesis imperfecta, which is associated with aortic or mitral regurgitation
- Ankylosing spondylitis—aortic regurgitation or heart block
- Exophthalmus and tremor—thyrotoxicosis leading to high output heart failure
- Deep voice and puffy eyelids—hypothyroidism and congestive heart failure (CHF)
- Cyanosis and clubbing—congenital heart disease with right to left shunting
- Head bob—aortic regurgitation
- Highly arched palate/arachnodactyly/tall stature—aortic regurgitation and aortic aneurysms (Marfan's syndrome)
- Violaceous cheeks of carcinoid—pulmonic systolic murmur

2. What is the proper position for examining the patient? How should I perform auscultation?

Place yourself on the patient's right side. Both you and the patient should be comfortable, and your hands should be warm. The surroundings must be quiet, and all conversation should cease. Before using the stethoscope, inspect the precordium and palpate for abnormal impulses.

Ideally, perform auscultation in the same manner each time, e.g., the stethoscope bell placed at the cardiac apex, then "inched" along to the lower left sternal border, then up to the left and right base. Because the bell records the difficult-to-hear, low-pitched sounds best, it is used first. The diaphragm is useful for registering high-pitched breath sounds, murmurs of aortic and pulmonic valve insufficiency, and splitting of the heart sounds.

3. What is meant by "grading" of heart murmurs?

The grading classification system was developed 60 years ago by Dr. Samuel Levine and is useful for following the course of a murmur in an individual. Murmurs are graded on a scale of 1 to 6:

GRADE	PHYSICAL FINDINGS
1	Barely audible
2	Soft but readily heard
3	Prominent but not loud
4	Loud
5	Audible with stethoscope partially off chest
6	Extremely loud; audible with stethoscope removed from chest

Grades 5 and 6 are uncommon. Using this system, you would list a soft murmur as grade 2 over 6 (2/6).

4. What are the characteristics of an innocent (functional) murmur?

Innocent murmurs are commonly of two types. One, heard in children and young adults, is best heard at the second left intercostal space and is thought to originate from vibrations within the main pulmonary artery. The other, audible between the apex and lower sternal edge, is apt to have a buzzing or vibrating quality and is thought to originate from vibrations of normal pulmonary leaflets. Both murmurs are midsystolic, usually no louder than grade 2/6 or 3/6, and common in young, healthy people.

Associated findings help in distinguishing an innocent from a pathologic murmur. For example, wide splitting of the second heart sound in conjunction with a basal systolic murmur favors the diagnosis of atrial septal defect or congenital pulmonary valve stenosis. A sharp, early systolic clicking sound (ejection sound) at the left second interspace suggests pulmonic stenosis. A similar click at the cardiac apex indicates congenital aortic stenosis. Single or multiple clicks that occur in mid or late systole are common with mitral valve prolapse and are best heard at the cardiac apex.

5. Are diastolic murmurs ever "innocent"?

In contrast to systolic murmurs, diastolic murmurs are seldom innocent. The most common diastolic murmurs are due to very mild degrees of regurgitation across the aortic or pulmonic valves, when they are high-pitched and decrescendo in shape. Mitral stenosis, heard precisely over the cardiac apex, has a low-frequency, rumbling characteristic. It is best heard using the stethoscope bell applied with very light pressure, with the patient reclining to the left. On rare occasions, an atrial tumor or clot produces a noise in diastole. Extracardiac diastolic bruits, on the other hand, may represent normal events. Examples include a venous hum, almost universally present in young people, and best heard over the anterior cervical fossa with the patient sitting and taking a deep breath. A mammary souffle audible over the breast of a nursing mother may occur as a continuous murmur (systole through diastole).

6. What are the cardivascular findings in normal pregnancy?

Plasma volume increases by 40–50% as pregnancy progresses. The elevated diaphragm and increased blood volume displace the apical impulse upward and laterally. Innocent midsystolic murmurs are common, best heard at the upper left sternal border. Splitting of the second heart sound is normal. Occasionally, a systolic-diastolic bruit is audible over the breast or over the gravid uterus, signifying flow through a functional arteriovenous shunt. Blood pressure (especially diastolic) tends to fall in early pregnancy and rise to prepregnancy levels toward term.

7. How can pulmonary hypertension be detected on examination?

Place the palm of your hand just left of the sternal margin. A diffuse heaving impulse in this region indicates right ventricular enlargement. Prior to listening to the heart, check for an elevation in jugular venous pressure. Typically, the "a-wave" is prominent and the overall level of pressure increased. With right ventricular failure, tricuspid regurgitation develops and the "v-wave" becomes predominant (see Question 17). Auscultation provides some valuable clues. The second sound tends to be narrowly split, and—with concentration—you will note an increase in the second (pulmonic) component. Finally, an audible S3 or S4 at the lower left sternal margin that increases on inspiration provides additional support for the diagnosis.

8. What is a paradoxical pulse?

Pulsus paradoxus is a misnomer, hallowed by decades of misuse. There is neither a pulse nor paradox involved. The term refers to an exaggeration of the normal slight decrease in blood pressure associated with inspiration. With paradoxical pulse, quiet inspiration produces a drop in systolic and diastolic pressure of at least 10 mmHg.

To elicit this finding, sit comfortably to observe for both the Korotkoff sounds and the patient's respiratory excursions. Slowly deflate the pneumatic cuff, approximately 2 to 3 mm with each quiet breath. With paradox, the initial systolic beats become audible with expiration and disappear on inspiration. Deflate the cuff until sounds are audible through all phases of respiration. The difference between these two pressures, measured in mmHg, is recorded as the level of "paradox."

9. What causes a paradoxical pulse?

The abnormality in pericardial tamponade is thought to occur when, with inspiration, intrathoracic pressure becomes increasingly negative and venous return to the right heart increases. The heart distends, but the abrupt rise in volume meets an elevated pressure in the taut pericardial sac, and the right ventricle quickly reaches its limit of expansion. The increased volume in the right ventricle displaces the ventricular septum to the left. This decreases left ventricular (LV) volume and, therefore, LV stroke output over the next few beats. This reduction in cardiac output accounts for a reduction in systolic pressure with inspiration.

Expiration reverses this process. The pulmonary blood volume enters the left heart chambers, restoring the septum to its usual position and raising LV volume. Systolic pressure rises.

Other conditions that abruptly raise right heart volume, such as acute pulmonary embolism, may share this same pathophysiologic process, since the acutely dilated right ventricle may distend against a relatively unyielding pericardial sac and produce septal displacement to the left.

10. How is coarctation of the aorta detected?

This important, reversible cause of hypertension is simple to diagnose, and every new case of hypertension should be screened for it. The most reliable diagnostic technique is to place the thumb of one hand on the brachial pulse and the other on the femoral pulse, and assess them simultaneously. Normally, these pulses are equal in volume and timing. A delay in the femoral impulse, or a reduction or absence of this pulse in a young person, strongly supports the diagnosis of coarctation.

Other suggestive features include a vigorous pulsation in the suprasternal notch and a systolic murmur under the left clavicle. Occasionally, a continuous murmur can be heard between the scapulae, signifying collateral circulation via intercostal arteries.

11. I am having difficulty measuring blood pressure in the arm. How can I improve the technique?

Blood pressure (Korotkoff) sounds may be difficult to hear in some patients. An obese or muscular arm, arterial obstruction from previous surgical cutdown or atherosclerosis, or simply repeating blood pressure measurements too quickly in succession may make the readings difficult. Emptying the venous circulation in the arm helps. Have the patient elevate his or her arm above the head, and then open and close the fist several times in succession. The pressure readings will appear much more distinct on subsequent measurement.

12. Which bedside maneuvers are useful in diagnosing murmurs?

The simplest and most readily available maneuver is **exercise**, which increases blood flow and may bring out indistinct murmurs, such as the low-frequency rumble of mitral stenosis. Have the patient perform sit-ups or straight leg raising while recumbent, and listen immediately afterward to the area of interest.

Respiratory maneuvers also are useful. Inspiration accentuates all murmurs as well as heart sounds that are of right-sided origin; thus, murmurs of tricuspid or pulmonic disease are brought out by deep inhalation. Similarly, expiration magnifies murmurs and heart sounds of left-sided origin.

Another helpful maneuver is the **Valsalva**. Instruct the patient to exhale and strain, while you listen during and immediately after release of the straining maneuver. Demonstrate this by placing the palm of your hand against the patient's abdomen and having the patient strain against it. This technique reduces LV volume; those murmurs that increase are due to a relatively empty left ventricle (e.g., murmurs of mitral valve prolapse and hypertrophic cardiomyopathy).

Likewise, **changing body position** accentuates or diminishes some murmurs. Having the patient squat (while you listen to the precordium) increases LV volume by raising systemic vascular resistance and increasing venous return. Murmurs of mitral prolapse and hypertrophic cardiomyopathy will lessen. Standing from the squatting position reverses the volume shift and accentuates these murmurs.

Another useful technique that augments the murmur of mitral stenosis is to listen at the cardiac apex when the patient turns from the recumbent to the left lateral position. This position is also useful for detecting faint left-sided "gallops" (S3 and S4). Having the patient cough vigorously three or four times further accentuates these findings.

13. What is the significance of an S4?

This heart sound represents atrial contraction (the late filling phase of diastole). It becomes more forceful and therefore more easily audible when LV filling is impaired. Causes of impairment include aortic stenosis, hypertension, myocardial ischemia, and almost all instances of acute myocardial infarction. The S4 is common, especially in people over the age of 60. It is best heard, as are all low-frequency sounds, with the stethoscope bell applied with very light pressure to the chest wall.

The S4 is often confused with a split S1. The following points favor an S4:
- The S4 tends to be softer and of lower frequency than a split S1.
- The S4 of left-sided origin is best heard at the cardiac apex and is accentuated by expiration.
- When the S4 derives from increased right ventricular "stiffness," it is accentuated on inspiration.
- Obvious splitting at the apex suggests an S4, whereas splitting of S1 is best heard at the lower sternal border.

14. What is the significance of an S3?

The S3 is a relatively rare heart sound. It is heard in early diastole as blood rushes to the LV apex from the base of the heart. Except for young, healthy adults, in whom an S3 often normally occurs, its presence denotes more advanced heart disease with cardiac dilatation and congestive failure. It is best heard at the apex and is more easily appreciated with the stethoscope bell and with the patient rolled onto the left side.

15. What are the common abnormalities to consider in evaluating a systolic murmur? How are they differentiated?

Statistically, most murmurs are innocent, especially in young, healthy people. The most common murmurs of pathologic origin include mitral and tricuspid regurgitation, aortic stenosis, and hypertrophic cardiomyopathy with outflow tract obstruction. Less common but important considerations in younger people include atrial or ventricular septal defects.

Systolic Murmurs

LESION	QUALITY OF MURMUR	SITE BEST HEARD	COMMENTS
Aortic stenosis (AS)	Harsh, often noisy murmur, especially when severe	Right upper sternal border	Increases in loudness as systole progresses Late peaking and duration of murmur correlate with severity of stenosis In severe AS, murmur may carry through S_2, which may be muffled or absent In LV failure, murmur may be soft or inaudible, but associated with late-rising and feeble arterial pulse
Mitral regurgitation	Evenly pitched sound, "blowing"	Cardiac apex; may radiate to left axilla and sometimes, when very loud, to the back	Continues through all or part of systole

(Table continued on next page.)

Systolic Murmurs (cont.)

LESION	QUALITY OF MURMUR	SITE BEST HEARD	COMMENTS
Tricuspid regurgitation	Evenly pitched sound, "blowing"	Lower left sternal border	Continues through all or part of systole Increases with inspiration Signs of elevated venous pressure present
Hypertrophic cardiomyopathy	Similar to AS	Mid-left sternal border or in path between sternum and cardiac apex	Increases with Valsalva or standing Increases in beat following premature ventricular contraction
Atrial septal defect	Widely split and fixed S_2 that does not vary with respiration; not very loud or harsh	Upper 2nd left interspace	Vigorous pulsation at upper left sternal border Right ventricular enlargement always present
Ventricular septal defect (VSD)	Loud, harsh murmur, especially when defect is small	Left sternal border at 3rd or 4th interspace	Holosystolic Cardiac exam otherwise normal if VSD is small

16. Describe the other sounds that might be heard besides murmurs.

Ejection sounds—There are two types: aortic and pulmonic. These are best heard with the stethoscope diaphragm placed over the respective listening area. The sound is heard just after the first heart sound. *Aortic ejection sounds* are usually noted with bicuspid valves prior to calcification and are due to "buckling" of the aortic leaflets. *Pulmonic ejection sounds* are noted with pulmonic stenosis and are also due to valve buckling.

Mid-systolic clicks—This high-pitched sound is best heard with the diaphragm over the apex, and may be produced by prolapse of the mitral valve with subsequent chordal snapping. This occurs earlier in systole, when the patient moves from a sitting to standing position.

Opening snap—Also best heard with the diaphragm placed at the apex. The sound occurs immediately after the second heart sound and represents the opening sound of a stenotic mitral valve. The higher the left atrial pressure, the closer the opening snap occurs to the second heart sound. Following this opening snap is the low-pitched rumble of mitral stenosis.

Tumor plop—Left atrial myxomas drop into the mitral orifice during diastole, producing a low-pitched sound after the second heart sound. It is often mistaken for an S3 gallop.

Pericardial knock—Also heard best with the diaphragm at the apex. It is caused by a rush of blood into a left ventricle that is not very compliant, as seen in constrictive pericarditis.

Pericardial friction rub—Best heard with the diaphragm at the left sternal border or apex. Classically, the rub is a three-component sound occuring when the atria contract, during ventricular systole, and during early diastole. The rub often disappears when a substantial amount of fluid builds up in the pericardial sac.

17. What is the significance of jugular venous waves?

Two positive waves are seen (see figure). The **a-wave** originates from right atrial contraction. It precedes the carotid pulse, i.e., it occurs in late diastole. It increases in amplitude as the vigor of atrial contraction increases. Increased right ventricular end-diastolic pressure from pulmonary hypertension is the usual cause. Occasionally, a giant a-wave, called a *cannon wave* is seen when atrial and ventricular contraction are out of phase and the atrium contracts against a closed tricuspid valve. This occurs in cardiac rhythm disorders such as complete heart block.

The **v-wave** begins during ventricular systole just after the carotid pulse. When increased, it signifies tricuspid regurgitation. In this circumstance, the right ventricle ejects some of its volume retrogradely into the atrium. The resultant v wave has a slow and undulatory form and is accentuated with deep inspiration.

The **x descent** follows the a wave. When prominent, it suggests pericardial constriction. The **y descent** follows the v wave. Abnormalities include a rapid descent as seen in constrictive pericarditis and a slow decline with tricuspid stenosis.

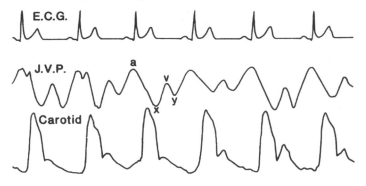

18. How do I measure venous pressure at the bedside?

This technique, with a little practice, is one of the most valuable features of the cardiac examination. It is preferable to examine the internal jugular vein, which lies in the carotid sheath just anterior to the sternocleidomastoid muscle. The patient should be placed in a semi-sitting position with the trunk elevated 30–45°. (The exact position is unimportant—what matters is that it allows you to observe the top of the oscillating venous column.) The neck should be relaxed so that the sternocleidomastoid muscle is not tensed. With a tongue blade and centimeter ruler, measure the distance between the top of the venous column and the sternal angle (the manubriosternal joint) (see figure). The sternal angle rests approximately 5 cm above the center of the right atrium. In the illustration, the venous pressure measurement is 2 cm above the sternal angle, so that the total venous pressure is 2 + 5 cm, or 7 cm. With the patient's trunk positioned at 30–45°, the venous pulse is ordinarily not visible more than 2 cm above the clavicle.

19. How is the venous jugular pulse differentiated from the carotid arterial pulse?

The most common error in assessing the jugular venous pressure, even for experienced observers, is to mistake the venous for the carotid arterial pulse. The following hints help identify the venous pulse:

- It varies with respiration, normally falling with inspiration and rising with expiration.
- It is easily obliterated by gentle finger pressure at the base of the neck.
- It is amplified, especially when pressure is elevated, by gentle pressure over the abdomen (hepatojugular reflux).
- Multiple waveforms are seen in contrast to the single carotid beat.

BIBLIOGRAPHY

1. Bruns DL: A general theory of the causes of murmurs in the cardiovascular system. Am J Med 27:360–374, 1959.
2. Chizner MA: Classic Teachings in Clinical Cardiology: A Tribute to W. Proctor Harvey, M.D. Cedar Grove, NJ, Laennec Publishing, Inc., 1996.
3. Craige E: Gallop rhythm. Prog Cardiovasc Dis 10:246, 1967.
4. Hurst JW: The examination of the heart: The importance of initial screening. Emory Univ J Med 5(3), 1991.
5. Leatham A: Auscultation of the heart. Lancet 2:703, 757, 1958.
6. Leatham A: The second heart sound: Key to auscultation of the heart. Acta Cardiol 19:395, 1964.
7. Lembo NJ, Dell'Italia LJ, Crawford MH, O'Rourke RA: Bedside diagnosis of systolic murmurs. N Engl J Med 318:1572, 1988.
8. Patel R, Bushnell DL, Sobotka PA: Implications of an audible third heart sound in evaluating cardiac function. West J Med 158:606–609, 1993.

2. MURMURS AND HEART SOUNDS

Mark A. Perea, M.D.

1. What are the effects of the Valsalva maneuver, standing, squatting, handgrip, and amyl nitrate on murmurs?

	PHYSIOLOGIC EFFECTS	EFFECT ON MURMURS
Valsalva maneuver	Decreases venous return	Most murmurs decrease in intensity except for those of hypertrophic obstructive cardiomyopathy and mitral valve prolapse, which increase.
Standing	Decreases venous return	Most murmurs decrease in intensity, except those of hypertrophic obstructive cardiomyopathy and mitral valve prolapse, which increase.
Squatting	Increases venous return, stroke volume, and systemic resistance	Most murmurs increase in intensity, except those of hypertrophic obstructive cardiomyopathy and mitral valve prolapse, which decrease.
Handgrip	Increases systemic vascular resistance and cardiac output	Most murmurs across normal or obstructed valves increase; mitral regurgitation, ventricular septal defect, and aortic regurgitation murmurs also intensify. The murmur of hypertrophic obstructive cardiomyopathy decreases, and the murmur of mitral valve prolapse occurs later.
Amyl nitrate	Potent vasodilator	The murmurs of hypertrophic obstructive cardiomyopathy and aortic stenosis increase, whereas the murmurs of mitral regurgitation, ventricular septal defect, and aortic regurgitation decrease.

2. Explain physiologic splitting of the second heart sound.

The second heart sound consists of the closing of the aortic and pulmonary valves. Splitting of an S_2 into two distinct, aortic (A_2) and pulmonic (P_2), components occurs normally with inspiration. Increased right heart filling occurs during inspiration due to increased blood volume returning via the vena cava. Because of this, the right ventricle takes slightly longer to empty, causing a delay in closure of the pulmonic valve. Therefore, the aortic valve closes before the pulmonic valve. This is termed **physiologic splitting**.

3. Differentiate fixed, persistent, and paradoxical splitting of the second heart sound.

Fixed splitting is defined as a split S_2 that does not vary with respirations. This can occur in an atrial septal defect or right ventricular failure.

Persistent splitting refers to a split that is heard during both inspiration and expiration. Though it is persistent it will vary unlike a fixed split. Persistent splitting can be caused by pulmonic stenosis or a RBBB (right bundle branch block).

Paradoxical splitting applies to an S_2 that is heard during expiration rather than during inspiration. This is due to a delayed closure of the aortic valve. Therefore, during expiration the A_2

component follows the P_2 component. The usual delay of P_2 during inspiration abates the usual split. Thus splitting is audible during expiration and disappears on inspiration. The most common cause of this, also termed *reverse splitting*, is a left bundle branch block (LBBB) (see Figure).

Second heart sound variations.

4. What are the five innocent systolic murmurs of childhood?

1. **Still's murmur**. The most common innocent murmur in children is the vibratory (Still's) murmur. It is usually audible between the ages of 3 and 6 years but can be heard at an earlier age and as late as adolescence. Its maximal intensity is at the lower left sternal border. The characteristic feature is its musical component, which is often described as "vibratory," "groaning," and "twanging."

2. **Pulmonary flow murmur**. This murmur is best heard at the second or third intercostal space at the left sternal border. It is described as an early to midsystolic, crescendo-decrescendo murmur, grade 2 or 3. These types of murmurs may be difficult to distinguish from the ejection murmur heard in an atrial septal defect (ASD). However, a fixed split S_2 will help to differentiate an ASD from an innocent pulmonary flow murmur.

3. **Neonatal physiologic peripheral pulmonary artery stenosis murmur**. This type, heard frequently in newborns, begins in early to midsystole and radiates to the infraclavicular areas, axilla, back, and up or down the left sternal border. This particular murmur subsides within the first year of life.

4. **Aortic systolic murmur**. This murmur is described as an innocent systolic ejection flow murmur heard maximally in the aortic area; often an S_3 is present. This type of murmur may be confused with the murmur of hypertrophic obstructive cardiomyopathy (HOCM). However, a murmur of HOCM should become louder with the Valsalva maneuver or upon standing. Although difficult at times, distinguishing the two is important and further investigations may be necessary.

5. **Supraclavicular systolic murmur**. This is a low-pitched systolic murmur heard in children and young adults. It is maximally audible above the clavicles and radiates to the neck bilaterally.

5. Is the usual murmur of an ASD caused by the low velocity across the defect?

Actually, the usual murmur associated with an ASD is caused by the increased flow across the normal tricuspid and pulmonary valve. Therefore, in addition to a split S_2, a soft systolic murmur in the left upper sternal border and a mid-diastolic murmur are often heard on physical examination.

6. Describe the auscultative findings in a mitral valve prolapse.

A murmur may not always be present in a mitral valve prolapse. Often a mid systolic click may be the only finding. This click is caused by sudden tensing of the redundant chordae or leaflets of the valve. If mitral regurgitation is present, a midsystolic murmur may be heard just after the click. The murmur is heard best at the apex and may radiate to the axilla. In severe cases the murmur may be holosystolic. The murmur of mitral regurgitation intensifies and commences earlier upon standing, with the Valsalva maneuver, and after administration of amyl nitrite.

7. Describe the physical findings of mitral stenosis.

Findings on physical examination include a loud S_1, an opening snap at the left sternal border near the left third or fourth intercostal space, and a low-pitched diastolic murmur. The murmur may be accentuated with the patient in the left sternal lateral decubitus position.

8. Name the clinical findings in acute pericarditis.

The classic finding is a precordial friction rub. The rub is described as a scratching, high-pitched sound that consists of one to three components. The rub is generated by abnormal visceral and parietal pericardial surfaces "rubbing" against each other. The rub can be intermittent and often varies in intensity. The rub may increase when the patient leans slightly forward or is resting on his or her elbows and knees.

9. What is Hamman's sign?

Hamman's sign, also known as mediastinal crunch sign, occurs when air is present in the mediastinum. Sounds are described as scratchy and occur most frequently during systole. This is commonly due to a pneumothorax or following cardiac surgery.

10. What is Kussmaul's sign?

Kussmaul's sign is an increase in the jugular venous pressure with inspiration. Normally during inspiration, the negative intrathoracic pressure causes a fall in systemic venous pressure and therefore a drop in the jugular venous pressure. However, in patients with constrictive pericarditis, the thickened pericardium causes the transmission of intrathoracic pressure to the chambers of the heart to fail; thus the venous pressure does not decrease.

11. How does the Müller maneuver differ from the Valsalva maneuver?

The seldomly used Müller maneuver has the opposite effect of the Valsalva maneuver. The patients holds the nose closed while inspiring forcibly through the firmly sealed mouth. This exaggerates the inspiratory phase, which increases right-sided heart filling. Thus, this maneuver will widen the split S_2 and accentuate murmurs originating in the right side of the heart.

12. What is an Austin Flint murmur?

The Austin Flint murmur is a low-pitched mid to late diastolic murmur that is associated with aortic regurgitation. The murmur is best heard at the apex and is due to intermixing of the regurgitant blood flow from the abnormal aortic valve and the flow across the normal mitral valve. The Austin Flint murmur may be difficult to differentiate from a murmur caused by mitral stenosis, but the presence of an opening snap and a loud S_1 in mitral stenosis are helpful clues.

13. What are the physical findings in aortic stenosis?

In aortic stenosis, a crescendo-decrescendo murmur heard maximally at the base of the heart and that radiates into both the carotid arteries is the most frequent finding. In severe cases a left ventricular thrill may be present, there may be a diminished or absent second heart sound, or paradoxical splitting of the second heart sound may be present. The most common cause of aortic stenosis is a congenital bicuspid aortic valve.

14. Describe a Graham Steell murmur.

This murmur, which is typical in pulmonic valve regurgitation, is described as an early diastolic murmur heard over the pulmonic valve with radiation along the left sternal border. Often it is heard after a loud pulmonic closure (P_2). It can be described as a high-pitched decrescendo murmur particularly if pulmonary hypertension is present.

15. What is the differential diagnosis of a continuous murmur?

A continuous murmur is one that is heard in both systole and diastole without interruption. It is generated by flow from a zone of high resistance to one of low resistance. All of the following can cause a continuous murmur:

Patent ductus arteriosis
Coronary atrioventricular (AV) fistula
Ruptured aneurysm of sinus of Valsalva
ASD
Cervical venous hum
Anomalous left coronary artery
Proximal coronary artery stenosis
Mammary souffle
Pulmonary artery branch stenosis
Bronchial collateral circulation
Small ASD with mitral stenosis
Intercostal AV fistula

BIBLIOGRAPHY

1. Bates B, Hoekelman RA, Bickley LS, Thompson JE: A Guide to Physical Examination and History Taking, 6th ed. Philadelphia, J.B. Lippincott, 1995.
2. Braunwald E (ed): Heart Disease, 5th ed. Philadelphia, W.B. Saunders, 1997.
3. Choudhry NK, Etchells EE: Does this patient have aortic regurgitation? JAMA 23:2231–2238, 1999.
4. Fauci AS, et al (eds): Harrison's Principles of Internal Medicine, 14th ed. New York, McGraw-Hill, 1998.
5. Leonard JJ, Shaver JA, Leon DF, et al: Examination of the Heart: Part IV. Auscultation of the Heart. Dallas, American Heart Association, 1990.
6. Pelech AN: The cardiac murmur: When to refer? Pediatr Clin North Am 45:107–122, 1998.

3. CHEST X-RAY

*James J. Fenton, M.D., FCCP**

1. Name cardiovascular problems that can be suggested or diagnosed by a chest x-ray.

CHF/pulmonary edema	Valvular heart disease
Pleural effusion	Calcific constrictive pericarditis
Severe pulmonary hypertension	Large pericardial effusions
Congenital malformations	Pericardial cyst
Left to right shunt	Cardiomyopathy

A chest x-ray is also valuable in diagnosing conditions that may mimic cardiac disease, such as pneumonia, pneumothorax, or pneumomediastinum.

2. Which cardiovascular problems cannot be readily diagnosed by a chest x-ray?

Acute MI	Small pericardial effusions
CAD	Aortic dissection
Systemic hypertension	Arrhythmias
Early pulmonary hypertension	Pulmonary embolism
Mild valvular heart disease	

3. Describe a systematic approach to interpreting a chest x-ray.

A common recommendation is to begin with general characteristics such as the age, gender, size, and position of the patient. Next, examine the periphery of the film, including the bones, soft tissue, and pleura. Look for rib fractures, rib notching, bony metastases, shoulder dislocation, soft tissue masses, and pleural thickening. Then evaluate the lung, looking for infiltrates, pulmonary nodules, and pleural effusions. Finally, concentrate on the heart size and contour, mediastinal structures, hilum, and great vessels. Also note the presence of pacemakers and sternal wires.

4. What additional items should I review when interpreting a chest x-ray from the intensive care unit?

On portable ICU radiographs, particular attention should be paid to the placement of the endotracheal tube, central lines, pulmonary arterial catheter, pacing wires, defibrillator pads, intra-aortic balloon pump, feeding tubes, and chest tubes.

5. Identify the major cardiovascular structures that form the silhouette of the mediastinum.

Right side: Ascending aorta, right pulmonary artery, right atrium, right ventricle
Left side: Aortic knob, left pulmonary artery, left atrial appendage, left ventricle
(*see figures, next page*)

6. What are the most common cardiovascular findings on an adult chest x-ray? What do they signify?

Mild enlargement of the left ventricle and aortic knob, and calcification of the aortic wall represent atherosclerotic heart disease and/or systemic hypertension.

7. How is heart size measured on a chest x-ray?

Identification of cardiomegaly on chest x-ray is subjective, but if the heart size is equal to or greater than twice the size of the hemithorax, then it is enlarged. Remember that a film taken during expiration, in a supine position, or by a portable AP technique will make the heart appear larger.

* The author acknowledges Marsha Heinig, M.D., Ph.D., whose text from the first edition is incorporated in this chapter.

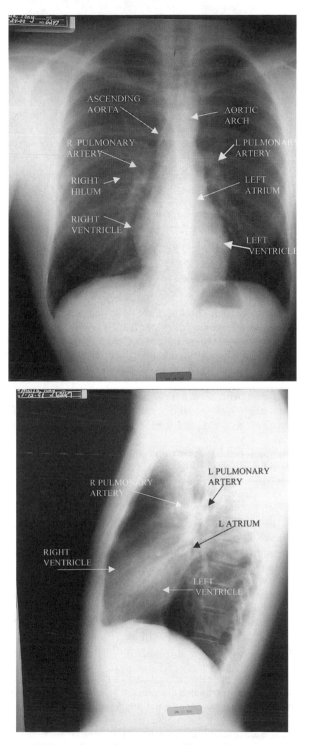

Major cardiovascular structures evident on chest x-ray.

8. What factors can affect heart size on the chest x-ray?
- Size of the patient—Obesity decreases lung volumes and enlarges the appearance of the heart.
- Degree of inspiration—Poor inspiration can make the heart appear larger.
- Emphysema—Hyperinflation changes the configuration of the heart, making it appear smaller.
- Contractility—Systole or diastole can make up to a 1.5 cm difference in heart size. In addition, low heart rate and increased cardiac output leads to increased ventricular filling.
- Chest configuration—pectus excavatum can compress the heart and make it appear larger.
- Patient positioning—The heart appears larger if the film is taken in a supine position.
- Type of exam—On an AP projection, the heart is further away from the film and closer to the camera. This creates greater beam divergence and the appearance of an increased heart size.

9. What are the causes of cardiac enlargement on a chest x-ray?
Cardiomyopathy (multiple etiologies)
Pericardial effusion
Aortic regurgitation
Mitral regurgitation
Cor pulmonale

10. How do I know which cardiac chambers are enlarged?
Ventricular enlargement—usually displaces the lower heart border to the left and posteriorly. Distinguishing RV from LV enlargement requires evaluation of the outflow tracts. In RV enlargement the pulmonary arteries are often prominent and the aorta is diminutive. In LV enlargement, the aorta is prominent and the pulmonary arteries are normal.

Left atrial enlargement—creates a convexity between the left pulmonary artery and the left ventricle on the frontal view. Also, a "double density" may be seen inferior to the carina. On the lateral view, LA enlargement displaces the descending left lower lobe bronchus posteriorly.

Right atrial enlargement—causes the lower right heart border to bulge outward to the right.

11. What are the common radiographic signs of congestive heart failure?
Enlarged cardiac silhouette
Left atrial enlargement
Hilar fullness
Vascular redistribution
Linear interstitial opacities (Kerley's lines)
Bilateral alveolar infiltrates
Pleural effusions (right > left)

12. What is vascular redistribution? When does it occur in congestive heart failure?
Vascular redistribution occurs when the upper-lobe pulmonary arteries and veins become larger than the vessels in the lower lobes. The sign is most accurate if the upper lobe vessels are increased in diameter greater than 3 mm in the first intercostal interspace. It usually occurs at a pulmonary capillary occlusion pressure of 12–19 mmHg. As the PAOP rises above 19 mmHg, interstitial edema develops with bronchial cuffing, Kerley's B lines, and thickening of the lung fissures.

Vascular redistribution is probably most consistently seen in patients with chronic pulmonary venous hypertension (mitral valve disease, left venticular dysfunction) due to the body's attempt to maintain more normal blood flow and oxygenation in the upper lungs. Some authors believe that this is a cardinal feature of congestive heart failure, but it may be a particularly unhelpful sign in the ICU patient with acute congestive failure. In these patients, all the pulmonary arteries look enlarged, making it difficult to assess upper and lower vessel size. In addition, the film is often taken supine, which can enlarge the upper lobe pulmonary vessels because of stasis of blood flow and not true redistribution.

13. What are the cardiogenic causes of pleural effusions?
- LV dysfunction causes increased hydrostatic pressures, which lead to interstitial edema and pleural effusions. Right pleural effusions are more common than left pleural effusions, but the majority are bilateral.
- RV dysfunction leads to system *venous* hypertension, which inhibits normal reabsorption of pleural fluid into the parietal pleural lymphatics.
- Pericardial disease causes tamponade and pericarditis.

Note: The subpulmonic space can hide up to 300 cc of pleural fluid. Decubitous radiographs not only help to diagnosis small pleural effusions, but often show that they are bilateral.

14. What is post-cardiac injury syndrome? What is the most common chest x-ray manifestation?
Post-cardiac injury syndrome (Dressler's syndrome) occurs following a variety of injuries to the heart. Most typically it occurs days to weeks following cardiac surgery or an acute MI and is characterized by pericarditis with chest pain, fever, and a pericardial effusion. The most common radiographic manifestation is a pleural effusion, which occurs in up to 80% of patients.

15. How helpful is the chest x-ray at identifying and characterizing a pericardial effusion?
The chest x-ray is not sensitive for the detection of a pericardial effusion, nor is it very helpful in determining the extent of the effusion. It is often difficult to distinguish pericardial fluid from chamber enlargement. Occasionally, the lateral chest x-ray will show the outline of the effusion anterior to the heart shadow between the epicardial and pericardial fat layers.

16. What are the characteristic radiographic findings of significant pulmonary hypertension?
Enlargement of the central pulmonary arteries with rapid tapering of the vessels is a characteristic finding in patients with pulmonary hypertension. If the right descending pulmonary artery is > 17 mm in transverse diameter, it is considered enlarged. Other findings of pulmonary hypertension include cardiac enlargement (particularly the right ventricle) and calcification of the pulmonary arteries. Pulmonary arterial calcification follows atheroma formation in the artery and represents a rare, but specific radiographic finding of severe pulmonary hypertension. In patients with pulmonary embolism, oligemia of the lung beyond the occluded vessel is called **Westermark's sign**.

17. What are the causes of pulmonary artery hypertension?
The best way to classify pulmonary hypertension is to identify the area of increased pulmonary arterial resistance.

• Resistance to pulmonary venous drainage, (post-capillary pulmonary hypertension)	LV dysfunction Mitral stenosis Constrictive pericarditis Pulmonary veno-occlusion
• Resistance due to abnormal pulmonary arteries	Primary pulmonary hypertension Pulmonary thromboemboli Pulmonary vasculitis Drug-induced injury

	Chronic lung diseases/chronic hypoxia
	    COPD, interstitial lung disease, high altitude
	    Kyphoscoliosis, obstructive sleep apnea

• Resistance from increased pulmonary flow (pre-capillary pulmonary hypertension)	Left to right shunts
	    Atrial septal defect
	    Ventricular septal defect
	    Patent ductus arteriosus

18. A right-sided aortic arch is evident on an adult patient's chest x-ray, but no other signs of cardiovascular disease. What other abnormality does this patient almost certainly have?

Aberrant left subclavian artery. Patients with "mirror-image" branching of a right sided aortic arch have a 95% chance of having congenital heart disease.

19. What congenital cardiovascular malformations may be seen on an adult chest x-ray?

- Anomalies of the aortic arch and   Right aortic arch
    great vessels   Aberrant subclavian arteries
                                   Coarctation of the aorta
                                   Aortic stenosis
- Mild shunts   Atrial septal defect
- Mild right-sided outflow obstruction   Pulmonic stenosis
                                   Ebstein's anomaly
- Partial anomalous venous return
- Corrected transposition of the great vessels

20. What acquired valvular diseases are most commonly demonstrated on chest x-ray? What are the radiographic findings?

- Mitral stenosis—enlarged left atrium and upper-lobe pulmonary vessels
- Mitral regurgitation—enlarged left atrium, ventricle, and pulmonary arteries
- Aortic stenosis—bulging left ventricular apex and enlarged ascending aorta

CONTROVERSIES

21. What is the best test for evaluating aortic dissection?

Several imaging methods have advantages and disadvantages, and all have claimed superiority. **CT scan** is probably the easiest test to do in the acute situation and is readily available and reliable (90% accuracy). True and false lumens can usually be readily demonstrated, as can the intimal flap in the ascending aorta if it is involved. Imaging before, during, and after contrast administration increases sensitivity.

The multiplanar imaging capability of **MRI** makes it an ideal method to image the aorta. Dissections are especially well demonstrated if the false lumen is partially clotted or if there is a dramatic difference in rate of blood flow between true and false lumens. However, because of pulsatile motion in the aorta, a thin intimal flap may be missed. MRI is also nearly impossible to perform in the critically ill patient.

Transesophageal echocardiography has been claimed to be quite sensitive for type B (descending) aortic dissection, but it is operator-dependent. A multiplane, or omniplane, scope is now available which visualizes the ascending aorta with accuracy.

Aortography images only contrast flowing in a lumen. If the false lumen is clotted, dissection may be only indirectly diagnosed by aortography as narrowing of the lumen of the aorta or thickening of the wall. Aortography is useful, however, in evaluating the origins of the great vessels in type A aortic dissection, as well as in evaluating associated aortic regurgitation.

22. What is the value of electron beam computed tomography (EBCT) in heart disease?

EBCT is a noninvasive method to diagnose subclinical coronary artery disease by quantitating the amount of calcium in the coronary arteries of asymptomatic patients. The amount of calcium accumulation correlates with the extent of atheromatous plaques in the arteries and permits risk stratification for future coronary events. If image quality is adequate, it may also be useful to detect or rule out high-grade coronary artery stenoses and occlusions.

BIBLIOGRAPHY

1. Achenbach S, et al: Value of electron-beam computed tomography for the noninvasive detection of high-grade coronary-artery stenoses and occlusions. N Engl J Med 333(27):1964–1971, 1998.

2. Armstrong P, et al: Imaging of Diseases of the Chest. St. Louis, Mosby, 1990.
3. Baron MG: Plain film diagnosis of common cardiac anomalies in the adult. Radiol Clin North Am 37:401–420, 1999.
4. Gross GW, Steiner RM: Radiographic manifestations of congenital heart disease in the adult patient. Radiol Clin North Am 29:293–317, 1991.
5. Matthay RA, Shub C: Imaging techniques for assessing pulmonary artery hypertension and right ventricular performance with special reference to COPD. J Thorac Imag 5:47–67, 1990.
6. Meholic A, et al: Fundamentals of Chest Radiology. Philadelphia, W.B. Saunders, 1996.
7. Newell J (ed): Diseases of the thoracic aorta: A symposium. J Thorac Imag 5:1–48, 1990.
8. Rumberger JA, et al: Electron beam computed tomographic coronary calcium scanning: A review and guidelines for use in asymptomatic persons. Mayo Clin Proc 74(3):243–252, 1999.

4. BEDSIDE HEMODYNAMIC MONITORING

Edward P. Havranek, M.D., and Mary Laird Warner, M.D.

1. What is a Swan-Ganz catheter?

A Swan-Ganz catheter is a relatively soft, flexible, right heart catheter with an inflatable balloon at its tip. This balloon allows the catheter to "float" with the flow of blood from the great veins through the right heart chambers and into the pulmonary artery, before "wedging" in a distal radicle of the pulmonary artery.

2. How is a Swan-Ganz catheter constructed?

The basic Swan-Ganz catheter in current clinical use has four lumens. One is connected to the distal port of the catheter, allowing for measurement of the pulmonary artery pressure when the balloon is deflated, and the pulmonary artery wedge pressure (PAWP) when the balloon is inflated. The second lumen is attached to a temperature-sensing thermocouple 5 cm proximal to the catheter tip and is used for measurement of cardiac output (CO) by thermodilution. The third lumen is connected to a port 15 cm proximal to the catheter tip, allowing for measurement of pressure in the right atrium and for infusion of drugs or fluids into the central circulation. The fourth lumen is used to inflate the balloon with air; when initially floating the catheter into position; and later to reinflate the balloon with air for intermittent measurement of PAWP. (Note that the balloon must be left deflated between measurements to avoid complications, such as pulmonary artery infarction.) Many catheters contain an additional proximal port for infusion of fluids and drugs.

Newer-generation Swan-Ganz catheters have fiberoptics for measuring continuous mixed venous oxyhemoglobin saturation (SvO_2), a heating filament for measuring near continuous thermodilution CO, and advanced software to calculate right ventricular (RV) ejection fraction and end-diastolic pressures and volumes. Some catheters have an additional lumen through which a temporary pacing electrode can be passed into the apex of the right ventricle for internal cardiac pacing.

3. How is a Swan-Ganz catheter inserted?

An 8.5 French introducer sheath is inserted into the internal jugular or subclavian vein using the Seldinger technique. (In rare clinical situations, the antecubital or femoral vein is used.) Next, a 7.5 French Swan-Ganz catheter is passed through the introducer sheath and advanced approximately 15 cm to exit the sheath into the central vein. Then, the balloon is inflated with 1.5 cc air, and the catheter advanced slowly, allowing the balloon to float through the right atrium, right ventricle, and pulmonary artery, before wedging into a distal branch of the pulmonary artery that is smaller in diameter than the balloon itself. Wedging usually occurs when the catheter has advanced a total of 35 to 55 cm, depending on which central vein is cannulated.

As the catheter is advanced, continuous monitoring of pressure tracings from the distal port and simultaneous EKG tracings allow the operator to determine the catheter's position and to detect any arrhythmias caused by the catheter, as it passes through the right ventricle.

4. Describe the pressure waveforms along the path of an advancing Swan-Ganz catheter.

They have a characteristic profile:

The **a wave** is produced by atrial contraction and follows the electrical P wave on EKG.

The **x descent** reflects atrial relaxation and sudden downward movement of the atrioventricular junction.

The **c wave** indicates the onset of ventricular systole as the tricuspid and mitral valves begin to close.

The **v wave** is caused by venous filling of the atria during ventricular systole, when the tricuspid and mitral valves are closed. This follows the electrical T wave.

The **y descent** is produced by rapid atrial emptying, when the tricuspid and mitral valves open at the onset of diastole.

Abnormal waveforms, particularly of the PAWP tracing, suggest pathology (see Question 9).

PULMONARY ARTERY WEDGE

Representative normal pressure tracing from the right side of the heart.

5. What information can be gained from a Swan-Ganz catheter?

Direct measurements obtained from the catheter include vascular pressures in the thorax, CO, and when available, SvO_2. Pressures are measured at various points along the catheter and include right atrial pressure, RV pressure, pulmonary artery pressure, pulmonary artery mean pressure, and PAWP.

PAWP is obtained by inflating the balloon while the catheter is positioned in the left or right main pulmonary artery. Blood flow then carries the catheter distally until it wedges in a distal arterial branch. With the balloon shielding the catheter tip from the pressure in the pulmonary artery proximally, the pressure transducer measures pressure distally in the pulmonary arterioles. This pressure closely approximates left atrial pressure, which in turn approximates left ventricular (LV) preload.

Cardiac output is measured by the thermodilution method. Five cc of normal saline is injected via the proximal port into the right atrium, while the temperature of the blood in the pulmonary artery is measured continuously by a thermocouple near the catheter tip. The brief dip in the blood's temperature with time is integrated to calculate CO.

SvO_2 is measured by two fiberoptic bundles in the catheter, which transmit and receive narrow wavebands of light that reflect off hemoglobin. The relative fraction of total hemoglobin that is oxygenated is the oxyhemoglobin saturation. When measured from the tip of the Swan-Ganz catheter in the pulmonary artery, this is the mixed venous oxygen saturation.

Hemodynamic parameters are obtained by calculations that integrate the measured intravascular pressures and CO. These parameters include the cardiac index, stroke volume index, LV and RV stroke work indices, systemic and pulmonary vascular resistances, oxygen consumption and delivery, and oxygen extraction ratio. All of these variables are indexed to the body surface area of the patient to enable comparison to normal values.

Measured Intravascular Pressures

PRESSURE	NORMAL VALUES (mmHg)
Right atrium	0–4
Right ventricle	15–30/0–4
Pulmonary artery	15–30/6–12
Pulmonary artery mean	10–18
Pulmonary artery wedge	6–12

Derived Hemodynamic Parameters

PARAMETER	NORMAL VALUE	UNITS
Cardiac index	2–4	1/min/m2
Stroke volume index	36–48	ml/beat/m2
RV stroke work index	7–10	gm-m/m2
LV stroke work index	44–56	gm-m/m2
Pulmonary vascular resistance index	80–240	dyne-sec/cm5/m2
Systemic vascular resistance index	1200–2500	dyne-sec/cm5/m2
Oxygen delivery	500–600	ml/min/m2
Oxygen uptake	110–160	ml/min/m2
Oxygen extraction ratio	22–32	—

6. What does the PAWP signify?

Inflating the balloon at the tip of the Swan-Ganz catheter creates a static column of blood between the catheter tip and the left atrium, such that pressures along the blood column equilibrate. Thus, the PAWP approximates the left atrial pressure. Assuming there is no obstruction between the left atrium and left ventricle, the PAWP in turn approximates the LV end-diastolic pressure (LVEDP). LVEDP is used as a clinical measure of preload on the left ventricle, i.e., the force stretching the ventricle at rest. (Technically, LV end-diastolic *volume* determines preload, but this parameter is very difficult to measure at the bedside, so LVEDP is used as a surrogate.)

7. Why are cardiac output and LV preload important?

CO and LV preload are important physiologic parameters because knowing them allows the clinician to apply Starling's law, which states that an increase in preload produces an increase in CO at any given level of myocardial contractility. For instance, in a patient with a low CO and a low PAWP, IV fluid infusion would be expected to improve CO.

However, some critics argue that PAWP is a misleading predictor of which critically ill patients will respond to a fluid challenge. This is because PAWP is a reliable index of preload *only* when myocardial contractility is normal and stable. Conditions such as myocardial ischemia, ventricular hypertrophy, and pericardial tamponade all decrease contractility and in turn elevate PAWP. In these instances, PAWP is elevated when preload is normal or even low. Instead, critics argue, RV end-diastolic volume index, which can be measured by newer-generation catheters, is a more accurate measure of preload and should be used clinically to monitor a patient's volume status.

8. When is placing a Swan-Ganz catheter clinically indicated?

Whenever knowledge of CO or PAWP would change management, a Swan-Ganz catheter is useful, because clinical data are unreliable for predicting these parameters. Catheters typically are used to:

- Differentiate between cardiogenic and non-cardiogenic pulmonary edema.
- Diagnose and manage patients in shock.
- Manage congestive heart failure refractory to traditional treatment, especially in the setting of acute myocardial infarction.
- Manage high-risk surgical patients in the perioperative period, including cardiac surgery, aortic surgery, and peripheral vascular surgery.
- Manage patients with large shifts in intravascular fluid volume, such as following extensive burns or trauma.

9. What diagnoses can the catheter help make?

The characteristic waveform of the Swan-Ganz catheter is altered in several disease states. In atrial fibrillation, the *a* wave disappears from the right atrial pressure tracing, while in atrial flutter, mechanical flutter waves occur at a rate of 300/min. "Cannon" *a* waves occur when the atria contract against closed valves due to atrioventricular dissociation. Irregular cannon *a* waves during a wide-complex tachycardia strongly suggest ventricular tachycardia. Complications of myocardial infarction can be detected on the PAWP tracing, such as giant *v* waves seen with acute mitral insufficiency, and the "dip and plateau" pattern of the RV pressure tracing seen with RV infarction. In addition, constrictive pericarditis and pericardial tamponade have distinctive pressure waveforms detectable with the catheter.

Hemodynamic profiles can also assist in diagnosis. Equalization of diastolic pressure is across the right atrium, right ventricle, and pulmonary artery suggests pericardial tamponade. A low PAWP in the setting of a high CO can be seen in septic shock, while a high PAWP with a low CO can occur in cardiogenic shock. A low PAWP with a low CO can develop in hemorrhagic shock.

Likewise, changes in oxygen delivery (DO_2), oxygen uptake (VO_2), and oxygen extraction ratio (O_2ER) are valuable in the diagnosis and management of shock. In hemorrhagic shock, DO_2 and VO_2 are low, while O_2ER is high. Conversely, in septic shock, DO_2 and VO_2 are high, while O_2ER is low.

Simultaneous sampling of blood from the right atrium via the proximal port and from the pulmonary artery via the distal port can detect the pathognomic "step up" in oxygen saturation caused by an acute ventricular septal defect.

10. What complications are associated with use of a Swan-Ganz catheter?
- All complications of central venous cannulation
- Right bundle branch block (especially in patients with pre-existing left bundle branch block)
- Ventricular tachyarrhythymias
- Pulmonary infarction, if the tip migrates into a permanently wedged position
- Pulmonary artery rupture, if the balloon is overinflated
- Catheter knotting from careless insertion

11. How can complications be minimized?
Think twice about the need to insert a pulmonary artery in the first place. Consider removing the catheter after the first set of data is obtained. Try to leave the catheter in place no more than 48 hours. Minimize use of the introducer side arm for infusion of medications. Use fluoroscopy for placement of the catheter.

12. The wedge tracing is abnormal. What do I do?
- Check a chest x-ray for proper catheter position. The tip should lie in lung zone 3, below the level of the left atrium.
- Aspirate and flush the catheter to remove clots and bubbles.
- Check all connecting lines and stopcocks.
- Confirm that the pressure transducers are zeroed to the level of the right atrium.
- Check that the balloon is not overinflated; try letting out the air and refilling it slowly.
- Consider the possibility that the tracing really is a wedge tracing with a giant *v* wave, as is seen in acute mitral insufficiency and several other conditions.

13. The cardiac output doesn't make sense. What is wrong?
- Check that at least three values were averaged and that the range of these values is no greater than 20% of the mean.
- Check the chest x-ray: is the distal tip of the catheter in the pulmonary artery and the proximal port in the right atrium?
- Check to see if the computer is calibrated to the proper temperatures.
- If the computer can display the time vs. temperature curve, check that the curve is shaped properly.

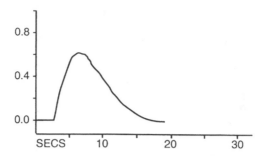

Typical time versus fall-in-temperature curve obtained from a thermodilution cardiac output computer. The curve rises steeply, then falls slowly. The downsloping limb of the curve is not perfectly concave, indicating some early recirculation of the indicator (cold saline). This tracing was obtained from a patient with heart failure; the recirculation is probably the result of tricuspid regurgitation, and does not affect the accuracy of the cardiac output determination.

14. Do Swan-Ganz catheters benefit all patients?

Despite widespread use of these devices in intensive care units, few if any studies have shown their use to decrease mortality, and randomized studies have not been performed. However, many studies have shown that clinical data predict PAWP and CO poorly and that insertion of the catheter frequently changes patient management. The truth lies somewhere in between.

A recent pulmonary artery catheter consensus conference (see ref. no. 4) examined published literature to grade the number and quality of studies supporting use of the catheter in different clinical situations.

BIBLIOGRAPHY

1. Gore JM, Godlberg RJ, Spodick DH, et al: A community-wide assessment of the use of pulmonary artery catheters in patients with acute myocardial infarction. Chest 92:721–731, 1987.
2. Leatherman JW, Marini JJ: Clinical use of the pulmonary artery catheter. In Principles of Critical Care, 2nd ed. New York, McGraw-Hill, 1998.
3. Nelson LD: The new pulmonary arterial catheters: Right ventricular ejection fraction and continuous cardiac output. Crit Care Clin 12(4):795–818, 1996.
4. Pulmonary Artery Catheter Consensus Conference Participants: Pulmonary artery catheter consensus conference: Consensus statement. Crit Care Med 25(6):910–925, 1997.
5. Robin ED: The cult of the Swan-Ganz catheter. Ann Intern Med 103:445–449, 1985.
6. Sharkey SW: Beyond the wedge: Clinical physiology and the Swan Ganz catheter. Am J Med 83:111–122, 1987.
7. Sise MJ, Hollingsworth P, Brimm JE, et al: Complications of the flow-directed pulmonary-artery catheter: A prospective analysis of 219 patients. Crit Care Med 9:315–318, 1981.
8. Walston A, Kendall ME: Comparison of pulmonary wedge and left atrial pressure in man. Am Heart J 86:159–164, 1973.

II. Diagnostic Procedures

5. ELECTROCARDIOGRAM

Donald L. Warkentin, M.D., and Olivia V. Adair, M.D.

1. Can the ECG offer useful information about supraventricular tachycardia (SVT)?

Ordinarily, identifying the various types of SVT from the standard ECG is difficult. In many cases, electrophysiologic intracardiac testing is required. Of the major types of SVT—sinus node reentry, intra-atrial reentry, accelerated conduction syndromes with narrow QRS complex, and atrioventricular (AV) nodal reentry—the latter condition makes up about 60% of the total. If the P waves are inverted in the inferior leads, and when they are present before or immediately after the QRS complex, they allow accurate diagnosis. Unfortunately, many times, the P waves are superimposed in the QRS complex and prevent easy diagnosis. Thus, the standard ECG is only occasionally helpful. Sinus node reentry and AV nodal reentry usually can be terminated by carotid sinus massage.

2. How does the signal-averaged electrocardiogram aid clinical decision-making?

The signal-averaged ECG (SAECG) amplifies exceedingly weak electrical signals generated by the heart and passes them through an electronic filter. The remaining signals from many cardiac cycles are averaged by a computer and printed out as a single QRS complex. Of particular importance are low-amplitude potentials (usually < 40 μV) occurring late in the QRS complex. To a lesser extent, the magnitude of the QRS vector and the total duration of the QRS complex are also important.

Abnormal SAECG findings have been recorded in many patients with episodes of sustained ventricular tachycardia and may indicate which of those patients, as well as those with unexplained syncope, might benefit from electrophysiologic testing. A potential application of SAECG is in risk stratification of patients after myocardial infarction; there is a high correlation between late potentials and inducible ventricular tachycardia, and the test may pinpoint individuals at high risk of sudden death.

3. What are the criteria for ventricular hypertrophy?

In **left ventricular hypertrophy** (LVH), the increased muscle mass generates increased QRS voltage, often with secondary changes in ST and T waves. Because some of these changes are subtle, numerous (at least 25) specific ECG criteria have been proposed to aid the diagnosis of LVH. Voltage criteria appear to be the most helpful:

   Limb lead: R amplitude in aVL > 11 mm
   R wave in aVF > 20 mm
   R wave in lead I plus S wave in lead III > 25 mm
   Precordial lead: R wave in V_5 or V_6 > 26 mm
   R wave in V_{5-6} plus S wave in V_1 > 35 mm

Most cases of LVH can be diagnosed by these criteria. Note, however, that the sensitivity of ECG for LVH is low compared to echocardiography.

In **right ventricular hypertrophy** (RVH), diagnosis also depends on voltage amplitude. In RVH, however, frontal plane axis deviation is also helpful. Among the important criteria of RVH are:

Right axis deviation of $\geq 110°$

R wave in V1 ≥ 7 mm

R/S ratio in $V_1 > 1$

qR patterns in V_1 and rSR' in V_1 with R' ≥ 10 mm

When both RVH and LVH occur in the same patient, most bets are off because the forces counterbalance each other.

4. Is non–Q-wave infarction an ECG diagnosis?

The short answer is no! For positive diagnosis of non–Q-wave infarction, confirmatory evidence (such as elevated cardiac muscle enzyme levels) must accompany these highly suspicious ECG findings. Q waves have long been recognized as a hallmark in transmural infarct, but experience shows that using that criteria alone will result in missing a large number of acute infarctions. It is also true that Q waves occasionally will be recorded in nontransmural infarcts.

The ECG changes that occur with non–Q-wave infarctions are those involving the ST segment and T waves. Both ST-segment elevation and depression may be recorded, although depression numerically outnumbers elevation. A particularly striking ECG finding, and one that should raise a high level of suspicion for infarction, is the exceedingly deep symmetric inversion of the precordial T waves. Indeed, the presence of ST segment depression and the above T-wave changes is almost always a result of nontransmural infarction. It is clinically important to diagnose non–Q-wave infarction accurately because this subset of patients has a high risk of further ischemic events.

Note that the terms "transmural" and "nontransmural" have been largely dropped at this time. Most current clinical trials divide infarctions into Q-wave and non–Q-wave.

5. What is torsade de pointes?

By definition, torsade de pointes is an intermediate arrhythmia between ventricular tachycardia and ventricular fibrillation. The term was coined by Dessertenne to describe cycles of tachyarrhythmia with alternating peaks of QRS amplitude appearing to twist around the isoelectric line. That said, torsade de pointes is a strident alarm to alert clinicians to underlying pathophysiology and the possibility of sudden death.

The basic prerequisite for this condition is thought to be a prolonged QT interval, but any condition or drug affecting the QT interval may spark the arrhythmia. Quinidine is the most common cause, but other class I antiarrhythmics also have been implicated. Discontinuing any possible offending drugs is of paramount importance. Electrolyte imbalance, intrinsic heart disease, marked bradycardia, and the prolonged QT syndrome also can stimulate the disorder. When the ECG finding occurs, immediate efforts must be made to determine the underlying cause of QT lengthening, lest the arrhythmia become irreversible.

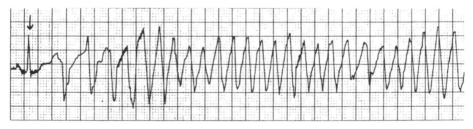

Torsades de pointes. A single sinus beat (arrow) is followed by ventricular tachycardia with an oscillating or swinging pattern of the QRS complexes. (From Seelig CB: Simplified EKG Analysis. Philadelphia, Hanley & Belfus, 1992, p 75, with permission.)

6. What are the ECG features of bradycardia-tachycardia syndrome?

Bradycardia-tachycardia syndrome is a particular manifestation of the sick sinus syndrome in which the sinus node is faulty either in its impulse formation or in the transmittal of the impulse to the atrium. In such cases, it is often associated with episodes of supraventricular tachycardia.

Detection of the bradycardia-tachycardia syndrome usually requires ambulatory monitoring. Sinus pauses of > 2 seconds are generally considered abnormal, particularly if symptoms accompany the rhythm disturbances. Between one-half and three-quarters of patients with the sick sinus node syndrome have episodes of tachycardia and may develop syncope when there is prolonged asystole following a run of supraventricular tachycardia. Many patients with this syndrome also have additional conduction defects, such as AV block, intraventricular condition defect, and/or bundle branch block. One confounding feature of the syndrome is its intermittent nature. Repeat episodes of ambulatory monitoring may be required to document the diagnosis.

7. Why are there three degrees of heart block?

Heart block, or AV block, is either complete or incomplete. The term **third-degree AV block**, or complete heart block, is applied when there is no relationship between the atrial and ventricular beats and the atrial rate is faster than the ventricular. Incomplete AV block is divided into first-degree, second-degree, and advanced AV block. By definition, **first-degree AV block** occurs when the PR interval is > 0.20 seconds and each atrial beat is followed by a ventricular complex. **Second-degree AV block** results in intermittent failure of atrial impulses to be conducted to the ventricles and is divided into two basic types: **Type I** or Wenckebach (also called Mobitz I) shows progressive lengthening of the PR interval from beat to beat until an atrial complex is not conducted. Because of these periodic pauses, "grouped beating" occurs and, when present, aids in the diagnosis of Mobitz I block. It may be seen transiently in acute inferior wall myocardial infarction. **Type II** AV block (advanced or Mobitz II) shows intermittent blocked P waves where the PR intervals of the conducted beats are constant. In these situations, the block is usually below the His bundle and may be accompanied by an associated bundle branch block.

Mobitz II is usually considered more serious than Mobitz I and may require artificial pacemaker treatment. In third-degree block, pacemaker cells in the AV node or in the His-Purkinje system may initiate ventricular contraction. Except for some cases of congenital third-degree AV block, this condition usually requires an artificial pacemaker.

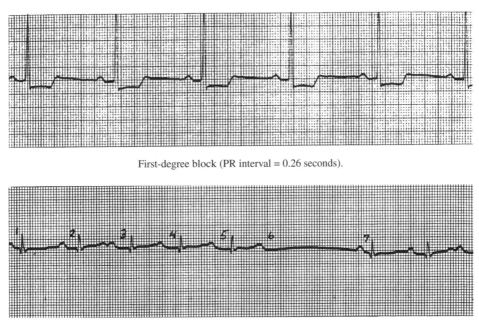

First-degree block (PR interval = 0.26 seconds).

Mobitz type I second-degree AV block (Wenckebach). Note the gradual prolongation of the PR interval (1–5), the missing QRS complex after the sixth P wave, and the return of the PR interval to its shortest duration (7).

Mobitz type II second-degree AV block. Note that when beats are conducted, the PR interval is unvarying.

Third-degree AV block with a ventricular escape rhythm at 32 bpm. P-wave activity is somewhat irregular.

(Figures from Seelig CB: Simplified EKG Analysis. Philadelphia, Hanley & Belfus, 1992, pp 77–80, with permission.)

8. What is the power spectrum of the ECG?

Recent interest in autonomic nervous system dysfunction and its effect on mortality from cardiac events has led to power spectrum ECG measurements. There seems to be a significant relationship between decreased heart rate variability and mortality in ECGs recorded from patients following myocardial infarction. Further autonomic nervous system activity in patients can be evaluated by spectral frequency analysis of the ECG. This analysis is divided into ultra low, very low, low, and high frequencies. Such analysis demonstrates a marked decrease in variability in all four frequency categories in postmyocardial infarct patients. It is postulated that high-frequency power and heart rate variability are modulated by the parasympathetic nervous system, whereas low-frequency power is modulated by both the sympathetic and parasympathetic nervous systems. This effect appears to last for at least 12 months following infarction. The recovery of normal heart rate variability and the declining rate of mortality following infarction appear to occur nearly simultaneously, although further analysis is needed to rule out a coincidental finding.

9. How important are the signs of atrial abnormality?

Because atrial hypertrophy is usually of a minor degree, the ECG findings of atrial abnormality are more dependent on the duration of atrial contraction than on its amplitude. Likewise, the common increase in P-wave amplitude suggestive of right atrial hypertrophy or dilation (P pulmonale) often correlates poorly with clinical and anatomic findings—hence, the descriptive term *atrial abnormality*. Prolongation and notching of P waves often indicate enlargement or delayed conduction within the atria, and these signs are helpful, but not diagnostic, in those conditions. Therefore, most electrocardiographers use the finding of atrial abnormality as an adjunct to the diagnosis of other conditions, such as rheumatic heart disease and left or right ventricular hypertrophy. Atrial enlargement may result in numerous arrhythmias, the most common being atrial fibrillation. There is some correlation between the amplitude of the fibrillatory waves and atrial size. Overall, the signs of atrial abnormality seem less important than the other ECG criteria of abnormal size or function.

10. Can right ventricular infarction be determined on the ECG?

Myocardial infarction involving the right ventricular wall is rarely isolated. Pathologic studies have revealed that right ventricular infarction is present in 14–36% of patients with inferior wall infarction. It is <u>not</u> seen in hearts with isolated anterior infarction. Because the right ventricular muscle mass is small in comparison to the left ventricle, the ECG diagnosis depends on the finding of acute inferior or inferoposterior myocardial infarction plus ST-segment elevation of 1 mm or more of the right precordial leads. Of significant help is the finding of ST-segment elevation in leads V_3R and V_4R. Thus, in patients with inferior infarcts, these leads should be included with the standard 12-lead ECG. When anterior infarction is present, the diagnosis of right ventricular infarction is difficult. Right ventricular infarction can clinically mimic severe left heart failure, and because current treatment for the two conditions is quite different, the importance of proper diagnosis is evident.

11. What are the common causes of ST-segment elevation?

The most dramatic and worrisome ST segment elevations occur as a result of severe coronary ischemia resulting in acute injury. The elevation occurring with transmural myocardial infarction is the best known and may be the earliest ECG finding during the acute process. Less frequent, but still a result of coronary ischemia, is the elevation seen in a small percentage of treadmill exercise tests and in patients with Prinzmetal's variant angina. Usually, the ST segment must be > 1 mm above baseline to merit attention. Adding spice to the evaluation is the fact that a goodly proportion of normal ECGs will have significant ST elevation. This is attributed to the early repolarization phenomenon and can be seen in healthy individuals. Of help in differentiating normal from abnormal elevations is the shape of the initial portion of the segment. In normals, it has an upward concavity, whereas in severe ischemia it usually has an upward convexity. The normal is often accompanied by a notched J point and prominent T wave.

12. How helpful is the ECG in "wide complex" tachycardia?

With the advent of surgical and ablation therapy for tachycardias, it becomes imperative to discern the correct type and site of origin of the arrhythmia. A regular tachycardia of 120–200 beats per minute (bpm) and a QRS duration of ≥ 0.12 seconds may be either ventricular or supraventricular. Unfortunately, definitive diagnosis may require invasive electrophysiologic studies. Wide complexes appear with supraventricular tachycardia if there is preexisting bundle branch block, anterograde conduction through bypass tracts, or aberrant ventricular conduction. Ventricular tachycardia is more likely if there is AV dissociation, right bundle branch block with QRS duration > 0.14 seconds or left bundle branch block with QRS duration > 0.16 seconds, QRS axis in right upper quadrant (–90° to +180°), positive QRS deflections in all precordial leads (V_1–V_6), captive or fusion beats, or a QRS pattern identical to that of premature ventricular beats during sinus rhythm.

13. Can the ECG diagnose electrolyte abnormalities?

ECG abnormalities due to electrolyte imbalance, particularly potassium and calcium, have been evident for years. However, because multiple electrolyte may be involved and because of the patient's underlying disease or even drug effects, the ECG should not be used in lieu of direct laboratory electrolyte determination. When an abnormality has been identified, the ECG may be used as a guide to the effectiveness of therapy.

The classic ECG changes of hyperkalemia are tall, narrow, peaked T waves, intraventricular conduction defect, decreased amplitude or absence of P waves, bradyarrhythmias, and AV blocks (see Figure). Hypokalemia causes ST-segment depression, decreased T amplitude, prominent U waves, cardiac arrhythmias, and rarely QRS prolongation. Serum calcium primarily alters the QT interval, with calcium excess causing shortening and deficiency causing prolongation. Currently, serum magnesium levels are assuming importance, but unfortunately are unlikely to be detected by the ECG.

Mild hyperkalemia. Note the tall, peaked T waves, most prominent in V_2–V_5. (From Seelig CB: Simplified EKG Analysis. Philadelphia, Hanley & Belfus, 1992, pp 107–110, with permission.)

14. What are the ECG signs of "drug effect"?

Although many drugs and substances can affect the ECG, most do so subtly. Certain compounds, however, leave a characteristic mark. Digitalis causes classic depression and coving of the ST segment. Toxic doses primarily affect AV conduction, resulting in various degrees of heart block. Many class I antiarrhythmics cause classic QT-interval prolongation. Toxic quantities of these and other antiarrhythmics can cause intraventricular conduction abnormalities and QRS prolongation. Some substances, such as cocaine, cause shortening of both the PR and QT intervals, and their adrenergic effect results in sinus tachycardia. Toxic doses of cocaine can result in ventricular tachycardia and/or fibrillation. Conversely, beta adrenergic blockers, such as propranolol, cause sinus bradycardia as a most common ECG side effect.

15. When is ambulatory ECG monitoring most useful?

Holter (ambulatory) monitoring initially was used to detect cardiac arrhythmia. It is also possible to detect ST-segment changes indicative of myocardial ischemia. Programs are also available to detect abnormal changes in the circadian variability of cardiac rate. At present, Holter monitoring is used both in detection of arrhythmia and in monitoring efficacy of treatment. Overt and silent myocardial ischemic episodes in patients can be detected and are powerful predictors of future serious illness. The predictive value of heart rate variability is less certain. The highest return of information comes from monitoring patients at highest risk of disease—i.e., those with coronary artery disease, unexplained syncope, or known cardiac arrhythmias. It should be noted that 24-hour monitoring may not be sufficient to truly detect disease and that ambulatory recordings should always be correlated with the standard ECG.

16. Are ECG findings of arrhythmias common in otherwise healthy patients?

Many studies have evaluated the occurrence of various arrhythmias in normal individuals of all ages, and a high incidence of both atrial and ventricular arrhythmias have been seen. Sobotika et al. studied 50 healthy women ranging in age from 20 to 28 years. Heart rates ranged between 37 and 189 bpm (37–59 bpm at sleep), 64% had premature atrial contraction (PAC), 54% had premature ventricular contraction (PVC), 4% had periods of second-degree heart block, and 2%

had 3-beat runs of ventricular tachycardia. In a study of healthy 80-year-olds, supraventricular arrhythmias were found in 100% of patients, and more than 10 PVCs per hour were recorded in 32% of patients (18% had multifocal PVCs).

17. How common is atrial flutter compared to atrial fibrillation in adults?
    Atrial flutter is less common, occurring about one twentieth as often as atrial fibrillation. Atrial flutter occurs more often with ischemic heart disease but is rarely seen in mitral valve disease, which is commonly associated with atrial fibrillation. Atrial flutter often occurs after cardiac surgery but usually is transient. The atrial rate in flutter is usually 300 and with fibrillation 300 or greater. The conducted ventricular rate in flutter is higher, however (180–200 than that conducted by fibrillation [70–150]). Digoxin seldom decreases atrial flutter atrioventricular conduction, but it usually does in atrial fibrillation.

0:00:53

Atrial flutter with variable block.

18. You are called to the emergency department concerning a 32-year-old who experienced syncope while jogging. The ECG is abnormal with deep inverted T waves, V_2–V_6, and I,aVL. The patient remembers no chest pain or shortness of breath. What test should you recommend?
    This is a classic ECG of hypertrophic cardiomyopathy, which is inherited in an autosomal dominant pattern in about 50% of cases. Echocardiogram with Doppler to evaluate for left ventricular outflow obstruction would be the test of choice initially. Recent studies show no direct relation between gradient and sudden cardiac death (SCD), and SCD may occur without a high gradient. SCD is often the first clinical symptom and is common in families with a history of multiple deaths at young ages. The histology of hypertrophic cardiomyopathy is gross disorganization of muscle bundles and a characteristic whorled pattern. One may have this pattern and be at high risk of SCD without significant hypertrophy but with inherited genetic make up (see figure, next page).

BIBLIOGRAPHY

  1. Abildskov JA: The atrial complex of the electrocardiogram. Am Heart J 57:930–941, 1959.
  2. Bigger JT Jr, Fleiss JL, Rolinski LM, et al: Time course of recovery of heart period variability after myocardial infarction. J Am Coll Cardiol 18:1643–1649, 1991.
  3. Braat S, Brugada P, DeZwaan C, et al: Value of electrocardiogram in diagnosing right ventricular involvement in patients with an acute inferior wall myocardial infarction. Br Heart J 49:368–372, 1983.

ECG of hypertrophic cardiomyopathy.

4. Chou T: Electrocardiography in Clinical Practice, 3rd ed. Philadelphia, W.B. Saunders, 1991.
5. Clark AL, Coats AJ: Screening for hypertrophic cardiomyopathy. Br Med J 306:409–410, 1993.
6. Damato AN, Law SH, Helfant R: A study of heart block in man using His bundle recordings. Circulation 39:297–305, 1969.
7. Gersh BJ: Lone atrial fibrillation: Epidemiology and natural history. Am Heart J 137:592–595, 1999.
8. Goldberg RJ, Gore JM, Alpert JS, Dalen JE: Non-Q wave myocardial infarction: Recent changes in occurrence and prognosis: A community-wide perspective. Am Heart J 113:273–279, 1987.
9. Josephson ME, Koster JA: Supraventricular tachycardia: Mechanisms and management. Ann Intern Med 87:346–358, 1977.
10. Kennedy HL, Wiens RD: Ambulatory (Holter) electrocardiography and myocardial ischemia. Am Heart J 117:164–167, 1989.
11. Lansdown LM: Signal-averaged electrocardiograms. Heart Lung 19:329–336, 1990.
12. Rubenstein JJ, Schulman CL, Yurchak PM, et al: Clinical spectrum of the sick sinus syndrome. Circulation 46:5–13, 1972.
13. Scardi S, Mazzone C, Pandullo C, et al: Lone atrial fibrillation: Prognostic differences between paroxysmal and chronic forms after 10 years of follow-up. Am Heart J 137:686–691, 1999.
14. Scott RC: Ventricular hypertrophy. Cardiovasc Clin 5:220–253, 1973.
15. Surawicz B: Electrophysiologic substrate of torsade de pointes: Depression of repolarization or early afterdepolarization? J Am Coll Cardiol 14:172–184, 1989.
16. Zimetbaum PJ, Schreckengost VE, Cohen DJ, et al: Evaluation of outpatient initiation of antiarrhythmic drug therapy in patients reverting to sinus rhythm after an episode of atrial fibrillation. Am J Cardiol 83:450–452, 1999.

6. HOLTER MONITORING AND SIGNAL-AVERAGED ELECTROCARDIOGRAPHY

Olivia V. Adair, M.D.

1. What symptoms lead to suspicion of arrhythmia?

Symptoms that commonly lead to suspicion of arrhythmia are palpitations, syncope, presyncope, or congestive heart failure. The physician must evaluate the patient's overall status, rather than the rhythm disturbance in isolation.

2. What are the major indications for Holter monitors?
- Detection of a suspected rhythm disturbance
- Syncope work-up
- Evaluation after myocardial infarction (MI)
- Evaluation of high-risk cardiac patient
- Risk stratification
- Evaluation after cardiac surgery
- Diagnosis of silent ischemia
- Diagnosis of suspected myocardial ischemia
- Evaluation of therapy, i.e., antiarrhythmic drugs, pacemaker function, cardiac ablation
- Evaluation of heart-rate variability

3. Should tests for patients with established or suspected arrhythmia be done in a particular order?

The clinical setting has as great a significance as the arrhythmia on choice of work-up and possible risk to the patient. Some arrhythmias are potentially fatal *regardless* of the clinical setting, whereas others are potentially dangerous *because of* the clinical setting. The usual progression is from the less expensive, simpler, noninvasive tests to tests that are more complex and invasive. Certain clinical circumstances, however, necessitate a more complex initial study (e.g., electrophysiology test).

In the usual circumstance, **Holter monitor** and **signal-averaged electrocardiogram** (SA-EKG) are the first tests. SA-EKG is especially appropriate if ventricular arrhythmias are expected. Individualize the type of Holter monitor to the patient, depending on associated symptoms as well as frequency and awareness of arrhythmia. An important consideration in the work-up of rhythm disturbance is underlying heart disease (e.g., valve disease, cardiomyopathy, MI). A **resting EKG** and **echocardiogram** may answer any questions and help to categorize the patient as high risk (e.g., low ejection fraction) or low risk (a normal ejection fraction and normal EKG). If the rhythm disturbance is associated with ischemia, an **exercise stress test** may be appropriate. If the data are positive, or if a diagnosis is not established but symptoms or potentially fatal arrhythmias recur, order an **electrophysiology test**.

4. Is there a particular subset of patients post MI who should be evaluated via Holter monitor before discharge?

The complete patient situation must be considered for appropriate risk stratification. Most patients post MI can be risk stratified without Holter monitoring. However, patients with certain high-risk clinical situations should be considered for Holter monitoring after MI:
- Patients with an anterior infarction and bundle-branch block are at high risk for arrhythmia. Up to 35% have late ventricular fibrillation (VF) in the hospital, and the risk persists for 6 weeks after infarction.

- In addition, atrioventricular (AV) block and intraventricular conduction abnormalities were found in 90% of patients who had recurrent VF during hospitalization and prehospital resuscitation for cardiac arrest.
- Patients with frequent ventricular ectopy after approximately 48 hours post MI; high-grade heart block 48–72 hours following an acute MI; and persistance of marked bradycardia 48–72 hours after MI should be evaluated with Holter monitoring before discharge.
- Finally, patients at risk for sudden death (e.g., low ejection fraction) may be considered for predischarge Holter monitoring.

Note that, at this time, any indication for Holter monitoring post-MI is in the class IIb category, and there is still some controversy involving its use.

5. Should patients with suspected arrhythmias undergo Holter monitoring and exercise tolerance testing (ETT)?

During ETT about one-third of patients with normal hearts develop ventricular ectopy, usually occasional monomorphic pairs or even 3- to 6-beat nonsustained runs. Ectopy may occur in older patients with no coronary artery or other heart disease and is not a predictor of increased mortality or morbidity. Although ETT is more sensitive than a resting, standard 12-lead EKG in detecting ventricular arrhythmias, a Holter monitor is more sensitive than ETT. However, because each may uncover serious arrhythmias that the other does not detect, both tests may be indicated in selected patients, such as those with known or suspected coronary artery disease (CAD).

6. What types of monitoring devices are available for long-term recording of the EKG?

Traditional Holter monitors record on 2 or 3 EKG channels for 24 hours. Recorders are currently available in four types:

- Continuous recorders, with every beat recorded and available for analysis
- Patient-activated recorders, which are especially useful when a patient can predict symptoms of the arrhythmias and activate the recorder
- Arrhythmia-activated recorders, in which the monitor turns on when a rhythm disturbance begins and off when it terminates (accuracy depends on the arrhythmia-detection algorithm)
- Transmitters for on-line or stored transtelephonic sending of EKG signals during a detected arrhythmia or during symptoms (especially helpful with infrequent but predicted symptoms; not indicated for arrhythmias associated with syncope).

Event monitors, continuous or transmitted, have the disadvantage of requiring patient perception of the arrhythmias. Many patients are unaware of significant or serious bradyarrhythmias or tachyarrhythmias, but are able to detect others. Therefore, incorrect treatment strategies employed.

Each system has advantages and disadvantages; selection must be tailored to the individual. With any system, however, patients must record in some fashion (e.g., diary) symptoms and activities during the monitored period.

Holter monitor strip with two-channel recording shows 5-beat run of ventricular tachycardia.

7. What percentage of patients have symptoms during the monitoring? What percentage of such symptoms occur with a rhythm disturbance?

Approximately 25–50% of patients experience a complaint or symptom during a 24-hour recording. Of such symptoms, only 2–15% correlate with or are believed to be caused by arrhythmia.

8. In general, when is a Holter monitor considered positive?

It is rather uncommon for healthy, young persons to have significant rhythm disturbances; in fact, several arrhythmias are not necessarily abnormal, including sinus bradycardias (35–40 beats/minute), sinus arrhythmias (with pauses up to 3 seconds), sinoatrial exit block, Wenckenbach block (second-degree AV block type I), wandering atrial pacemaker, junctional escape complexes, and premature atrial or ventricular contractions.

Of concern are frequent and complex atrial and ventricular rhythm disturbances that are less commonly observed in normal subjects, including second-degree AV block type II, sinus pauses > 3 seconds, and brady- or tachyarrhythmias associated with symptoms. Results of the Holter monitor need to be analyzed with the diary to correlate specific symptoms to the rhythm and rate recorded.

9. What is the role of the Holter monitor in patients with known ischemic heart disease?

Patients post MI and those with other forms of ischemic heart disease frequently have premature ventricular contractions (PVCs). After MI the frequency of PVCs increases for several weeks and then declines after 6 months. The frequency and complexity of PVCs are independent markers for sudden death or acute cardiac event; risk may be increased 2–5 times. Patients with symptoms and known ischemic heart disease are in a higher-risk group and should be evaluated with both a Holter monitor and SA-EKG.

10. Can Holter monitors assist in the diagnosis of suspected ischemic heart disease?

Yes. Transient ST-segment depressions ≥ 0.1 mV for less than 30 seconds are rare in normal subjects and correlate strongly with myocardial perfusion scans that show regional ischemia.

11. What have Holter monitors demonstrated about angina and its pattern of occurrence?

Holter monitoring has shown that the majority of ischemic episodes that occur during normal daily activities are silent (asymptomatic), and that symptomatic and silent episodes of ST-segment depression exhibit a circadian rhythm, with ischemic ST-changes more common in the morning. Studies also have shown that nocturnal ST-segment changes are almost always an indicator of two- or three-vessel CAD or left mainstem stenosis.

12. Do certain groups of patients benefit from Holter monitoring for detection of silent ischemia?

The answer depends on the clinical picture, but patients with an "anginal equivalent" and risk factors for CAD (e.g., exertional shortness of breath) are also at high risk for ischemia. Patients with type II diabetes mellitus also have a greater incidence of asymptomatic ischemia as well as silent MIs, and may benefit from Holter evaluation for silent ischemia.

13. What is heart-rate variability?

Holter monitor recordings can be used to assess heart-rate variability as a measurement of the standard deviation of the sinus rhythm cycle length (or fluctuation around the mean RR interval). Heart-rate variability reflects the parasympathetic and sympathetic balance of the autonomic nervous system and therefore offers insight into the risk for sudden cardiac death.

14. What is the clinical significance of heart-rate variability?

Recent studies show that analysis of heart-rate variability is important in evaluation of postinfarction and diabetic patients. In both groups decreased heart-rate variability is associated with an increased risk of sudden cardiac death. Lower heart-rate variability is also recorded with acute

MI. Here a predominance of sympathetic activity and reduction in parasympathetic cardiac control result in increased sympathetic activity, which decreases the fibrillation threshold and predisposes to ventricular fibrillation. In addition, anterior-wall MI results in a more profound reduction in heart-rate variability than inferior-wall infarction.

15. What is signal-averaged electrocardiography (SA-EKG)?

SA-EKG is a method of recording the EKG in which amplifiers and filters record cardiac signals with amplitudes of only a few microvolts. Electrical potentials corresponding to delayed and fragmental conduction in the ventricle are recorded in microvolts and waveforms continuous with the QRS complex. Three criteria are of importance: (1) QRS duration, (2) low-voltage signals in the last 40 msec of the QRS, and (3) low-frequency waveforms lasting > 30 msec after the terminal QRS complex.

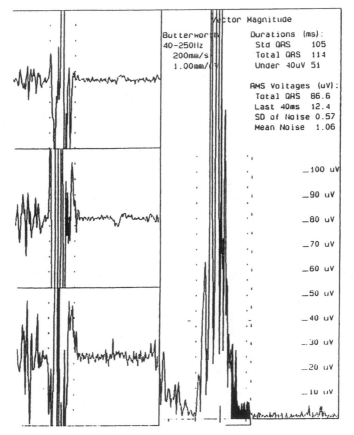

Positive SA-EKG with late potentials highlighted at the end of the QRS complex between 150 and 190 ms. The low amplitude signals (< 25 mV) exceed the voltage for noise at the terminal 40 ms. The QRS duration is normal (114 ms). QRS 114 ms (NL < 120 ms) LA S - 51 ns. RMS 40 12.5 mv.

16. How is the SA-EKG used clinically?

Late potentials have been detected in 73–92% of patients with sustained and inducible ventricular tachycardia after MI. Late potentials also have been identified in patients with nonischemic heart disease and ventricular tachycardia, such as those with dilated cardiomyopathy. Early use of thrombolytic agents reduces the prevalence of late potentials after coronary occlusion and therefore the risk of sudden death, ventricular fibrillation, and tachycardia.

Late potentials after MI are an independent marker of patients at high risk for ventricular tachycardia. SA-EKG results combined with other noninvasive data (e.g., Holter, ETT, ejection fraction) provide a highly sensitive and highly specific method of identifying patients at risk for ventricular tachycardia or sudden death.

17. Aside from providing information about ventricular arrhythmias, how is Holter monitoring helpful in predicting sudden cardiac death in patients with chronic heart failure (CHF)?

Though it remains difficult to predict sudden cardiac death in CHF patients, the prediction must be attempted, because defibrillation treatment is increasingly available. Galinier et al. looked at time and frequency domain measures of heart rate variability in 190 CHF patients, mean ejection fraction 28%, class II (189 points) and class III or IV (81 points). In follow-up (22 months), 55 deaths had occurred, of which 21 were sudden cardiac death. In data analysis, depressed heart rate variability was an independent prognostic value.

18. A 52-year-old man presents for the fourth time in 18 months with palpitations, dizziness, and one episode of syncope. Extensive cardiac and neurologic evaluation were performed previously; no etiology was found. On this visit, the patient is hospitalized for approximately 40 hours on telemetry. There are no arrhythmias and no symptoms. What are the diagnostic options at this point?

An implantable loop recorder (ILR) allows correlation of symptoms and rhythm abnormalities in many patients where these are infrequent or unexpected. The device is small (61mm X 19 mm; 8 mm thick) and easy to implant with a single chamber lead. It provides up to 14 months of continuous monitoring (see figure below) and has shown a high diagnostic yield (up to 94%). The Metronic Reveal ILR may reduce cost and inconvenience of repeated testing and hospital visits (see figure next page).

```
Reveal(tm) Model 9525                              22:26  10/12/1998
Gain: x4 (+/- 0.4 mV)                    Programmer 9790 9802E01
Storage Mode: A - 1 event (20 min. pre / 1 min. post)   (c) Medtronic, Inc. 1997
| Event 1 of 1 recorded 02/19/1997     070197A                Page 3 of 4 |
12.5 mm/sec, 12.5 mm/mV
```

EKG event recording of sinus arrest and inadequate ventricular response.

Insertable loop recorder Medtronic Reveal.

BIBLIOGRAPHY

1. Cohen TJ, Ibrahim B, Sassower MJ: Revealing data retrieved from an implantable loop recorder. J Invasive Cardiol 12(3):174–175, 2000.
2. DiMarco JP, Philbrick JT: Use of ambulatory electrocardiographic (Holter) monitoring. Ann Intern Med 113:53–68, 1990.
3. Galinier M, Pathak A, et al: Depressed low-frequency power of heart rate variability as an independent predictor of sudden death in chronic heart failure. Eur Heart J 21(6):475–482, 2000.
4. Kennedy HL: Long-term (Holter) electrocardiogram recordings. In Zipes DP, Jalife J (eds): Cardiac Electrophysiology: From Cell to Bedside. Philadelphia, W.B. Saunders, 1990, p 791.
5. Langer A, Freeman MR, Josse RG, et al: Detection of silent myocardial ischemia in diabetes mellitus. Am J Cardiol 67:1073, 1991.
6. Lazzeri C, LaVilla G, et al: 24-hour heart rate variability in patients with vasovagal syncope. Pacing Clin Electrophysiol 23 (4 Part 1):463–468, 2000.
7. Van Ravenswaaij-Arts MA, Kollee AA, Hopman JC, et al: Heart rate variability. Ann Intern Med 118:436–447, 1993.
8. Yeung AC, Barry J, Orav J, et al: Effects of asymptomatic ischemia on long-term prognosis in chronic stable coronary disease. Circulation 83:1598, 1991.

7. ECHOCARDIOGRAPHY AND DOPPLER/COLOR-FLOW IMAGING

Olivia V. Adair, M.D.

1. **Why has echocardiography become so popular in assessment of cardiovascular diagnosis?**
Echocardiography has become the most common imaging and hemodynamic modality because:
   • It allows high-quality imaging.
   • As a biologically safe modality, with no cumulative effects, it lends itself to serial studies as well as use in children and pregnant women.
   • It is painless.
   • No preparation is required (except for transesophageal echocardiography).
   • It is mobile and quick, and allows on-line interpretation.
   • Doppler imaging provides anatomic as well as hemodynamic data.
   • It can be used as an early screening test.

2. **What are the major anatomic data obtained with echocardiography?**
   Although the number of possible cross-sectional planes through which the heart can be viewed is almost infinite, standard sections are based on the transducer position—parasternal, apical, subcostal, and suprasternal—whereas the planes are long-axis, short-axis, four-chamber, and two-chamber (see figure). Chamber size and function are well imaged, as are the mitral, aortic, tricuspid and pulmonic valves. The thickness of the walls is easily evaluated as well as the septum; wall motion is evaluated by segments in each view (inferior, posterior, anterior, and lateral walls). The aorta and sometimes even coronary arteries are visualized. The pericardium can be evaluated as well as the pulmonary artery and right ventricular (RV) outflow tract. The left atrial appendage is occasionally seen on transthoracic echocardiography.

A, Parasternal long-axis view of left ventricles, left atrium, aortic valve, and mitral valve. *B*, Short-axis view of left ventricle. *C*, Four-chamber view. *D*, Two-chamber view of left ventricle, mitral valves, and left atrium.

3. Is Doppler/color-flow imaging a separate imaging technique from echocardiography?

Doppler imaging uses the direction and velocity of blood flow to evaluate cardiovascular hemodynamics, and color-flow imaging (CFI) provides real-time, two-dimensional imaging of blood flow. Echocardiography, Doppler imaging, and CFI are complementary rather than competitive; the best studies integrate the three techniques.

4. What are the major hemodynamic measurements and clinical applications of Doppler echocardiography?

Multiple hemodynamic measurements and analyses are possible with Doppler acquisition, but the major categories of application are ventricular performance, valvular function, and shunt lesions.

- **Stroke volume** can be obtained with measurements of the LV outflow tract, blood flow into the ascending aorta, and flow velocities.
- Doppler evaluation of pulmonary artery flow allows measurement of **RV output**.
- Measurement of time intervals aids in the evaluation of **systolic and diastolic ventricular function**.
- The differences in flow volumes can be used to calculate **intracardiac shunts** and **regurgitant flows**.
- One of the most valuable uses of Doppler is to evaluate **valve function**, especially pressure gradients, which can be used to calculate the area of the stenotic valve and maximal velocity across the valve.
- Flow disturbances (turbulence) are used to diagnose **valvular regurgitation** and evaluate its severity.

5. Describe the limitations of echocardiography and Doppler imaging.

The major limitation is the lack of anatomic quantitative measurements in echocardiography, which necessitates technical skill in performance and interpretation. Another limitation is the acquisition of total cardiac anatomic information, which is achieved in 80–90% of studies. Moreover, the complexity of anatomic and hemodynamic information often leads to incorrect or incomplete interpretations by examiners who are not well versed or adequately experienced. In transesophageal echocardiography the images are frequently clear, but should be interpreted only by an experienced cardiologist. Misinterpretation also may be due to technical limitations, misreading of artifacts, or extraneous echoes.

6. What are the clinically useful recommendations for echocardiography and Doppler imaging?

- Evaluating ventricular systolic and diastolic performance
- Estimating right-sided heart hemodynamics
- Measuring pressure gradients and valvular orifice areas in stenotic valves or other discrete narrowings
- Detecting valvular regurgitation and estimating its hemodynamic significance
- Evaluating function of valvular prostheses
- Establishing the presence and determining the significance of intracardiac shunts

7. What is contrast echocardiography?

Contrast echocardiography is used to delineate structures not readily seen (superior and inferior vena cava, descending aorta, RV outflow tract, pulmonary arteries) as well as to evaluate intracardiac shunts, regurgitant lesions, and complex congenital heart problems. The technique uses microbubbles from agitating approximately 8 cc of saline between two 10-ml syringes connected to a three-way stopcock and an intravenous line (see figure, next page). The agitated saline is injected with extreme force into the intravenous line while recording in the four-chamber view or focusing on the suspected site. Apical or subcostal four-chamber views allow visualization of a small number of microbubbles crossing a right-to-left shunt as well as a negative jet of left-to-right flow that causes a defect in the otherwise bubble-filled right chamber.

Normal contrast echocardiography. Four-chamber view shows complete filling of right atrium and ventricle (to left) with microbubbles and no bubbles in left atrium or ventricle (to right).

8. How is contrast echocardiography performed?

If a large shunt is suspected, the number of injections and amount of contrast should be limited. An appropriate routine is first to inject 3 cc , record, and evaluate; if a large shunt is not present, 8–10 cc are then injected. If the study is negative at this point, reinjection, with the patient coughing when the right atrium is filled, increases right-sided pressure and allows even the smallest shunt to be identified.

9. How is contrast echocardiography applied clinically?

This technique is extremely sensitive and specific for shunt diagnosis, which can be confirmed with only a few microbubbles; it is even more sensitive than oximetry and dye dilation and can detect shunts as small as 3%. It is also sensitive enough to evaluate patency of the foramen ovale or surgical repairs of shunts. Some institutions use contrast in the echocardiographic evaluation of all patients with stroke or transient ischemic attacks.

10. What about contrast echocardiography of the *left* ventricle?

Questions 7–9 addressed contrast produced by agitated saline. Agitated saline only allows imaging of the right heart, unless intracardiac shunting exists. This is advantageous for the diagnosis of shunts, but disadvantageous for imaging of the left heart. Agitated saline typically does not cross the pulmonary circuit and flow into the left ventricle. Newer contrast agents are now available that do cross the pulmonary circuit and allow optimal imaging of the left ventricle.

11. How is left ventricular contrast being developed?

Optison, made by Mallinckrodt, is the prototype and currently the only FDA-approved agent, although others are likely to be released in the foreseeable future. These agents allow left ventricular opacification and enhancement of the endocardial borders. The use of contrast improves quality of images, especially those in obese patients and in patients with lung disease, who account for approximately 10–20% of echocardiographic examinations. Also, contrast can markedly improve image acquisition in stress echocardiography: delineation of regional wall motion abnormality at peak exercise is enhanced, and there is more time available for imaging with contrast enhancement.

Optison was developed as human albumin microspheres in which octafluororpropane replaces air. This provides a slow gas diffusion giving longer contrast effect, up to several minutes. In a study of 85 patients, contrast allowed diagnostic study of 58%, in whom plain stress echocardiography produced nondiagnostic results due to noninterpretable segments, and allowed study of 75% in a technically difficult subset of patients. Contrast echo also has the potential to demonstrate normal and abnormal myocardial perfusion, much the same way that current nuclear myocardial perfusion does.

12. Describe the role of echocardiography plus Doppler imaging in the evaluation of a patient with suspected ischemic heart disease (IHD).

Echocardiography is useful in evaluating possible IHD, chest pain syndromes, and LV function and in establishing risk stratification and complications of acute myocardial infarction (MI). Assessment of regional wall motion and absence of systolic thickening of the myocardium may implicate coronary artery disease (CAD). Serial studies can be evaluated in side-by-side formats to compare wall motion abnormalities or to evaluate myocardial remodeling.

Also, exercise echocardiography adds sensitivity and specificity to routine stress electrocardiography and has been advocated as especially useful in diagnosing CAD in women, with a sensitivity and specificity comparable to radionuclear stress studies. Whereas only 50% of ECGs are diagnostic for acute MI, the detection of regional wall motion abnormalities is much more sensitive (though less specific). A negative echocardiogram during chest pain predicts a very low risk of ischemia.

Another advantage of using echocardiography with chest pain syndromes is the additional diagnostic information about other causes of chest pain, such as aortic stenosis, aortic dissection, mitral valve prolapse, pericardial effusions, or hypertrophic cardiomyopathy.

13. Why is echocardiography the imaging technique of choice for valvular disease?

It is the best choice because it provides hemodynamic, structural, and functional data as well as assesses the severity of valvular disease, its possible etiology, and prognosis. Evaluation of the valve may include information about leaflet calcification (see figure, top of next page), pliability, and mobility; any coexisting pathology also can be assessed along with LV function and thrombi. Because echocardiography and Doppler imaging are safe for serial studies, they can be used to follow the patient or to evaluate interventions and management. Doppler imaging and CFI enable more accurate location of the lesion as well as better assessment of pressure gradient, valve areas, and regurgitant flows.

14. What are the applications for stress echocardiography? How is it performed?

Stress echocardiography is an important imaging technique for evaluating ventricular function, global ejection fraction, regional wall motion, and myocardial thickening and for assessing hemodynamic or cardiac function at baseline as well as at maximal stress or point of symptoms. Among the most common clinical applications is hemodynamic assessment of mitral stenosis in symptomatic patients in whom resting hemodynamic status is insufficient for a clinical decision.

In addition, other dynamic lesions are better assessed with stress, including hypertrophic cardiomyopathy, coarctation of the aorta, and dysfunction of prosthetic valves. The most common use is diagnosis of IHD with an immediate post-exercise echocardiogram to evaluate wall motion.

The test is relatively inexpensive and is as sensitive and specific as single-photon emission computed tomography (SPECT) with thallium during exercise for assessment of IHD. For patients who cannot do conventional treadmill stress tests, dobutamine or dipyridamole can be used.

15. Describe the role of echocardiography in patients with acute MI.

Electrocardiography is not always diagnostic for acute infarction, but echocardiography is easily used to detect **wall motion abnormalities**. Immediate evaluation of ischemia and the amount of myocardium at risk is especially important for decisions about early intervention, such as use of thrombolytic agents or angioplasty. Echocardiography also assesses patients with infarction

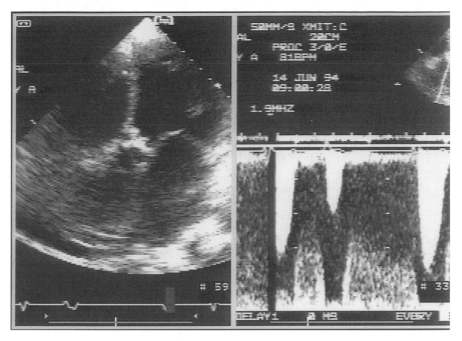

Left, Aortic stenosis with thickened and calcified aortic valve. *Right*, With Doppler imaging, aortic stenosis velocity is demonstrated by the white envelope, flow direction away from transducer (downward), maximal velocity of 3.5 m/s, and peak gradient of 49 mmHg.

for complications such as severity of ischemic mitral regurgitation, post-infarction ventricular septal defect, aneurysm (true vs. false), and right-sided pressures. Serial studies can evaluate reperfusion. Because the most powerful prognostic indicator after infarction is LV function, the larger the infarct, the higher the risk for subsequent cardiac events; echocardiography and Doppler imaging are essential in risk stratification and prognostic evaluation, both of which help to determine the management plan.

16. What are the indications for transesophageal echocardiography (TEE)?

TEE has increased imaging abilities tremendously through multiplane windows from the stomach and esophagus that provide high-resolution tomographic imaging views. TEE is used both in the awake patient and intraoperatively. A study of TEEs done at the Mayo Clinic over 5 years shows three major indications: (1) source of emboli, (2) native and prosthetic valve disease, and (3) endocarditis (see figure, top of next page).

For the intraoperative patient the most frequent applications are monitoring of cardiac function, intraoperative diagnosis, and assessment of postoperative results. Victims of trauma often are best evaluated with TEE because of its mobility, speed, and capacity for on-line interpretation.

17. What are the risks in TEE? How invasive is TEE?

TEE is a low-risk procedure that provides a tremendous amount of clinically important data. It should be performed only by trained echocardiographers who are fully aware not only of the diagnostic interpretation, but also of technique, potential complications, and contraindications. Two large studies reported only 1 death each (0.02%): in one study the cause of death was unclear; in the other, a malignant lung tumor infiltrating the esophagus was lacerated during probe introduction and caused massive hemorrhage and subsequent death. The Mayo Clinic reported a complication rate of 0.18–0.5% over 5000 procedures (see figure, middle of next page). Most complications are minor and easily treatable.

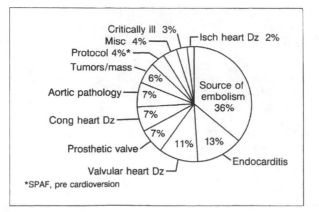

Indications for TEE examination at the Mayo Clinic from November 1987 to November 1992 (5,441 procedures). Three major indications are source of embolism, native and prosthetic valve disease, and endocarditis. SPAF = Stroke Prevention in Atrial Fibrillation trial, Isch = ischemic, Cong = congestive, Dz = disease. (From Freeman WK, et al (eds): Transesophageal Echocardiography. Boston, Little, Brown. © 1994 by Mayo Foundation, Rochester, Minnesota. Used with permission.)

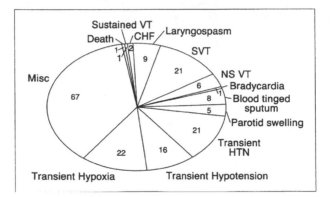

Classification of 180 complications (3.3%) of TEE examinations encountered in the Mayo Clinic experience with 5,441 procedures between November 1987 and November 1992. Major complications included laryngospasm, sustained ventricular tachycardia (VT), acute congestive heart failure (CHF), and one death. SVT = supraventricular tachycardia, NS = nonsustained, HTN = hypertension. (From Freeman WK, et al (eds): Transesophageal Echocardiography. Boston, Little, Brown. © 1994 by Mayo Foundation, Rochester, Minnesota. Used with permission.)

Overall, TEE is a safe procedure and is used to complement transthoracic echocardiography in approximately 10% of patients. The physician should be aware of contraindications to avoid complications.

Contraindications to TEE

ABSOLUTE CONTRAINDICATIONS	RELATIVE CONTRAINDICATIONS
Esophageal obstruction (stricture, neoplasm)	Recent gastroesophageal operation
Esophageal fistula, laceration, or perforation	Esophageal varices
Esophageal diverticulum	Upper gastrointestinal bleeding
Cervical spine instability	Atlantoaxial arthritis
	Unexplained symptoms of dysphasia or odynophagia

18. How should a patient with a prosthetic valve be evaluated and followed?

Patients with a prosthetic valve are best managed by using the patient as his or her own control and obtaining early postoperative echocardiography and Doppler evaluations, which can be compared with follow-up evaluations. This approach is helpful because the gradients of prosthetic valves are inherently higher than the gradients of native valves and may vary with positioning.

The transthoracic (TTE) approach in echocardiography, and less so in Doppler imaging, is limited by acoustic shadowing, whereas TEE circumvents many of these imaging problems. Assessment of mitral valve prostheses is especially difficult with TTE, but TEE sensitively detects and quantitates regurgitation, valvular or perivalvular leaks, abnormal morphology, vegetation, thrombi, abscess, and leaflet tear. Although aortic valve prostheses are easier to view via TTE, TEE is much superior in evaluating vegetation or abscess cavities, especially when a mitral prosthesis is also present. Certainly TEE should be considered strongly for any patient with suspected or proven prosthetic valve endocarditis because of its high sensitivity and ability to detect complications.

Serial echocardiography and Doppler imaging have replaced cardiac catheterization as the procedure of choice for hemodynamic and morphologic evaluation.

19. How useful is TEE in the diagnosis of infectious endocarditis? How does it help in the management of patients?

TEE has been shown in several large studies to have higher sensitivity than TTE for native valves (94–100% vs. 44–63%) and prosthetic valves (75% vs. 25%); both have high specificity (91–98%). TTE detection of vegetation depends largely on the extent of the vegetation, whereas TEE can detect much smaller vegetations. TEE also has an effect on patient management, because it detects complications such as abscesses, chordal rupture, and secondary valve involvement. Because mortality is higher and prognosis is worse with such complications, identification of affected patients should prompt consideration of early interventions.

20. What are the echocardiographic findings in patients with hypertrophic obstructive cardiomyopathy (HOCM)?

Two-dimensional echocardiographic images show asymmetric septal hypertrophy and systolic anterior motion of the mitral valve, two classic signs of hypertrophic cardiomyopathy. *A*, Long-axis view, diastole. *B*, Long-axis view, systole. *C*, Short-axis view. S = septum; LA = left atrium; LV = left ventricle. (From Pandian NG, Simonetti J: Echocardiography in hypertrophic cardiomyopathy. Cardiovasc Rev Rep Oct 1988, p 60, with permission.)

Echocardiography is the best method of diagnosing HOCM and is extremely sensitive. The classic finding is asymmetric septal hypertrophy, but symmetric hypertrophy may be seen, as well as other varieties (e.g., apical or midventricular hypertrophy). Echocardiography also assesses systolic anterior motion of the mitral valve and contact of the anterior leaflet and the septum. The aortic valve closes early in mid-systole, either partially (notch) or completely. The LV cavity is usually decreased, whereas the left atrium is dilated.

21. What is the imaging technique of choice to evaluate the aorta?

TEE has become the modality of choice in patients with suspected aortic dissection, especially with the involvement of the descending aorta, which is poorly visualized by TTE. TEE also can be used for evaluations of other aortic abnormalities, such as plaque, aneurysm, or thrombus. The reported sensitivity for aortic dissection is 97–100%; the reported specificity, 98–100%. (See also Chapter 24, Aortic Dissection.)

22. What is tissue Doppler imaging? How is it used?

Tissue Doppler imaging is a Doppler echocardiography technique that selectively measures the velocity of the myocardium. This is accomplished by using conventional pulsed or color Doppler and filtering out the higher velocity signals created by blood flow, allowing detection of the much slower myocardial velocities. The technique has been available commercially since 1994, but the most useful clinical application is still under debate. It has been evaluated in hypertrophic cardiomyopathy, heart transplant, and arrhythmology. However, tissue Doppler is emerging as one of the best methods of evaluating diastolic function. It has the distinct advantage over conventional pulsed Doppler of mitral and pulmonary venous inflow of being relatively preload independent.

23. Has three-dimensional echocardiography developed for clinical use?

Three-dimensional (3-D) reconstruction of the heart using echocardiography has been in development since the 1970s, when two-dimensional (2-D) techniques were new. Several methods have been explored, but currently the most common approach uses rotational scanning with acquisition of multiple 2-D cross-sectional images of the heart. Each moving 2-D image encompasses the entire cardiac cycle and hence has a range of 9–16 frames of data from each cardiac cycle, depending on the heart rate. The 3-D image (really four dimensions if motion is included) is reconstructed using all of the 2-D moving images. The 3-D data set, when reconstructed, allows the user—in theory—to view the heart from any imaginable cross-sectional cut.

To date, the most clinically useful application of 3-D echo is evaluation of ventricular volumes, with accuracy similar to MRI. Other possible and developing applications include measurement of valve areas, intracardiac masses, evaluation of valve lesions, particularly mitral valve prolapse, and complex congenital heart disease. Three-dimensional echocardiography awaits further advances in computer technology and documentation of clinical outcomes for widespread clinical use.

24. Scuba diving is a popular recreational sport. A recent study showed RV alteration. Are there clinical implications in this finding?

A recent study of 50 recreational divers compared to age/sex-matched controls showed that recreational scuba divers had increased occurrence of RV dilatation and electrocardiographic signs of RV hypertrophy, sinus bradycardia, and sinus arrhythmia. This may be related to the findings of Knauth, presented at the Radiological Society of North American meeting in Chicago in 1999, which showed MRI evidence of brain lesions and increased susceptibility to decompression sickness in divers with patent foramen ovale (PFO). Though the long-term effect of the brain lesions is still unclear, and though PFO is a rather common heart defect occurring in approximately 25% of the general population, the implications are certainly provoking. It is possible that PFO leads to arterialization of venous gas bubbles which would normally be "filtered" to the lungs, whereas in the clinical situation of PFO, these present as brain lesions. Prospective scuba divers may need screening to evaluate for PFO before certification. (See figure, top of next page.)

Contrast bubble study displays a bubble-filled right atrium (RA) and a group of bubbles passing into the left atrium with a cough via a patent foramen ovale (PFO).

BIBLIOGRAPHY

1. Cardim N, Morais H, et al: Tissue Doppler imaging: Clinical topics for the new millennium. Rev Port Cardiol 19(4):449–458, 2000.
2. deSimone G, Schillazi G, Palmieri V, et al: Should all patients with hypertension have echocardiography? J Hum Hypertens 14(7):417–421, 2000.
3. Felner JM, Martin RP: The echocardiogram. In Schlant R, Alexander R (eds): The Heart Arteries and Veins, 8th ed. New York, McGraw-Hill, 1994.
4. Freeman WK, Seward JB, Khandheria BK, Tajik AJ: Transesophageal Echocardiography. Boston, Little, Brown, 1994.
5. Meissner G, Whisnant JP, et al: Prevalent and potential risk factors for stroke-assisted by transesophageal echocardiogram and carotid ultrasonography: The SPARC study. Mayo Clin Proc 74:862–869, 1999.
6. Mukerji B, Alpert MA, Mukerji V: Right ventricular alteration in scuba divers: Findings on electrocardiography and echocardiography. South Med J 93(7):673–667, 2000.
7. Pearlman AS: Technique of Doppler and color flow Doppler in the evaluation of cardiac disorders and function. In Schlant R, Alexander R (eds): The Heart Arteries and Veins, 8th ed. New York, McGraw-Hill, 1994.
8. Pearson AC: Transthoracic echocardiography versus transesophageal echocardiography in detecting cardiac source of embolism. Echocardiography 10:397–403, 1993.
9. Plein S, Williams GJ: Developments in cardiac ultrasound. Hosp Med 61(4):240–245, 2000.
10. Salustri A, Roelandt JR: Three-dimensional echocardiography: Where we are, where we are going. Ital Heart J 1(1):26–32, 2000.

8. ECHOCARDIOGRAPHY IN THE CRITICALLY ILL PATIENT

Olivia V. Adair, M.D., and Douglas Paul Voorhees, R.R.T.

1. Why has echocardiography emerged as such an important diagnostic tool in critically ill patients?

Critically ill patients need urgent diagnostic evaluation and expedient, appropriate intervention to improve the course of disease and chance of survival. Often their clinical condition and medical environment (e.g., respirator, multiple intravenous lines, cardiac monitoring) limit diagnostic options, because transport involves major effort and risk. Echocardiography offers: (**1**) bedside mobility, (**2**) high-quality imaging, (**3**) noninvasive nature, (**4**) immediate on-line image analysis, and (**5**) extensive yield of data, including structural, functional, and hemodynamic information. In addition, **transesophageal echocardiography (TEE)** has increased the quality of studies in patients on respirators, with chest injuries requiring chest tubes, or with surgical wounds of the chest, all of which limit the transthoracic windows.

2. How important is an echocardiography study in a critically ill patient?

The bedside echocardiography study gives **immediate data** to direct management strategies. The extensive differential diagnosis of hemodynamic instability includes critical valve disease, intracardiac shunt, cardiomyopathy, and tamponade—all of which are easily diagnosed with echocardiography and require different management despite similar clinical presentations. Pulmonary embolism presents similarly, but is not as easily diagnosed by echocardiography; however, the secondary findings of right ventricular failure often are seen. Therefore, emergent echocardiography is important to help eliminate several of the possible etiologies and either to make the diagnosis or to establish a foundation for initial management.

3. Are different risks or procedural problems involved in the use of TEE in critically ill patients?

TEE is semi-invasive. Passing the probe into the stomach of critically ill patients requires more experience and manual guidance. The patient may be agitated, unable to cooperate, and confined to the supine position. Adequate sedation in patients with prosthetic valves is necessary before passage of the probe. Problems with hemodynamically unstable and critically ill patients are uncommon, except in the presence of extensive neck and facial trauma. A laryngoscope can be helpful if the procedure proves difficult. Although patients are often hemodynamically unstable, clinically significant complications are rare. TEE should be performed by a cardiologist ready to manage hemodynamic deterioration, fully trained in endoscopic intubation procedures, and experienced in TEE interpretation.

4. What are the common indications for TEE in the intensive care unit?

The primary reason for TEE in critically ill patients is hemodynamic instability, which may result from hypotension, pulmonary edema, acute myocardial infarction, endocarditis, tamponade, trauma, or cardiogenic shock. Patients frequently present with shock syndrome that requires prompt intervention. Several reports show favorable results from the use of TEE in such patients.

For example, of 44 patients with shock syndrome, only 48% were partially diagnosed by transthoracic echocardiography (TTE), whereas 100% were diagnosed by TEE. Critical information was obtained in 68%, with 30% undergoing urgent cardiac surgery (including mitral valve replacement, tamponade relief, correction of postinfarction ventricular septal rupture and aortic rupture, and closure of patent foramen ovale). Of the 4 patients with normal TEEs, all had a noncardiovascular cause of hemodynamic compromise, as established by other investigations.

Pearson et al. reported similar success with different indications (aortic dissection, 29%; source of emboli, 26%; postinfarction complications, 10%); critically important clinical information, not seen on TTE, was obtained in 44%.

5. What is the best diagnostic procedure when aortic dissection is suspected?
Although magnetic resonance imaging permits visualization of the thoracic aorta in multiple planes with high sensitivity, delay and transport of patients often pose problems. Moreover, multiple support systems, such as intravenous pumps, respirators, and monitors, make transport impossible or involve an unacceptably high risk. Newer-generation computed tomography also has 95% accuracy, but involves similar problems of transport and time for acquisition. Transthoracic echocardiography has a sensitivity of 75–85%; sensitivity is lower for distal dissection. **TEE**, however, is portable and quick, providing on-line interpretation, and has sensitivity and specifity of 98%.

TEE is also useful for detecting extracardiac complications of dissection, such as pericardial effusion (seen in about 25%) and coronary artery dissection, as well as conditions that mimic dissection. Traumatic rupture of the aorta and contained intimal disruption with thrombus also are diagnosed by TEE, especially with multi-plane imaging, with high sensitivity and specificity. Furthermore, TEE has the advantage of providing added diagnostic information, particularly in patients with chest trauma (e.g., from automobile accidents) that may result in pericardial effusions or hematomas, contusion, and infarction.

Intravascular ultrasound also has gained popularity in diagnosing aortic dissection, especially in victims of trauma, but requires an invasive test and specialized training and equipment; it also lacks the advantage of additional echocardiographic data. More studies are needed to make direct comparisons among these options.

6. How common is trauma to the heart? When should it be suspected and evaluated?
Accidental or intentional trauma is the leading cause of death and hospitalization, especially in young people, among whom violent injuries are increasing. Cardiac and great-vessel injuries are major contributors to mortality and morbidity secondary to penetrating and nonpenetrating trauma.

Any penetrating injuries to the precordium, chest, neck, or upper abdomen should prompt investigation for cardiac trauma; such injuries usually involve knife or gunshot wounds. Of special concern are signs of tamponade or hemothorax. Over 50% of victims with penetrating cardiac trauma die immediately; in the others, who survive for varying lengths of time, immediate evaluation is essential. TEE is an important procedure, because small-caliber bullets and tears can be missed on TTE. The majority of nonpenetrating injuries are due to automobile accidents (50% involve fatal or severe chest injuries); contact sports, falls, and altercations also result in such injuries. TEE is the procedure of choice to evaluate patients for pericardial, myocardial, valvular, coronary artery, and aortic injury.

7. What role should TEE play in the evaluation of potential cardiac donors?
TEE should be considered an important part of donor evaluation. Many donors are victims of motor vehicle accidents or violent crimes and have suffered significant cardiac or chest trauma. Such injuries may cause ventricular contusion (right or left), coronary thrombus, regional wall motion abnormalities, tricuspid valve disruption and regurgitation, or aortic dissection. Affected patients may not be easily imaged by transthoracic echocardiography. Notably, 50% of the significant findings in potential donors on TEE often are *not* diagnosed by TTE. Donor candidates, therefore, should undergo TEE before cardiac status is established. Consider surgical repair of detected lesions, especially if the recipient has an urgent need.

8. Other than intracardiac thrombus and septal defects, what findings might be seen in a TEE evaluation of a stroke patient?
Atherosclerosis of the thoracic aorta is recognized as a source of both systemic and cerebral embolization. In addition, characteristics of aortic plaque morphology have prognostic and therapeutic significance. For example, an **ulcerated plaque** associated with a **large, mobile thrombus** should be evaluated closely. A recent study shows less recurrent stroke and increased

mortality with anticoagulation, as compared to aspirin, when an aortic atheroma is found. Also, thoracic aorta evaluation for atherosclerosis is important when aortic manipulation is to be undertaken in surgical procedures that could produce perioperative neurological complications.

A plaque ≥ 4 mm in size, especially with a superimposed thrombus, predicts a high risk (12%) of recurrent stroke within 1 year and a 33% risk of peripheral embolization.

Aortic thrombi seen on TEE predict an approximately 12% risk of stroke during heart surgery requiring cardiopulmonary bypass (this represents a six-fold increase in intraoperative stroke).

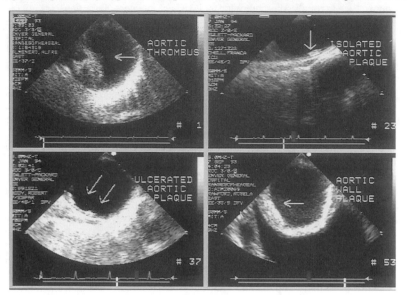

TEE findings of thrombus, plaque, ulcerated plaque, and wall plaque.

9. A 19-year-old male is brought to the emergency department (ED) after sustaining blunt trauma to his chest from a steering wheel. He was unstable in the field, with hypotension, chest pain, and dyspnea. In the ED, he appears acutely ill, with hypertension, cool extremities, and tachycardia. There are no other significant physical findings. What is an important diagnostic step at this point?

A bedside TEE is critical to evaluate for effusion, tamponade, contusion, pericardial hematoma, and possible aortic dissection—all of which would be immediate and could cause severe hemodynamic compromise. This patient had a more unusual finding, however: the aortic valve was flail, and there was severe aortic regurgitation. Because you need clear visualization of the aorta and valve, a transesophageal echo is a better choice than transthoracic, as it can be performed and read simultaneously at the bedside. (See Figures, top of next page.)

10. When should a TEE be performed in acute stroke? Can it help direct therapy?

A recent review by Kapral and colleagues demonstrated high sensitivity and specificity of both TEE and TTE, but TEE was found to be superior in evaluating patients with stroke and was recommended as the initial screening test. TTE detected intracardiac mass in 13% of patients, versus 19% by TEE.

Stroke continues to be the third leading cause of mortality in the U.S. (approximately 500,000 deaths per year). Identification of the source and mechanism of stroke is critical in secondary and primary prevention strategies. It is not enough to start patients on anticoagulants or aspirin and send them on their way. Conservative estimates indicate a cardiovascular etiology for more than one-third of strokes, but the problem with assessment of cause is that data is being ascertained from patients who have already experienced an end-point stroke.

A, Flail aortic valve leaflets associated with, *B*, severe aortic regurgitation.

11. Is it safe to perform TEE in a patient with acute MI? What situations may direct such testing?

TEE can be done without causing hemodynamic problems of significant stress, and without provoking ischemia. A small amount of conscious sedation may be required if the patient is intubated; this too, does not prevent a TEE from being performed with good results, and in fact ensures better imaging quality.

Several complications of MI may be evaluated with TEE in a patient not responding well to standard therapy. For example, in cardiogenic shock, severe pulmonary edema/changed murmur may be the prompt to proceed to a TEE. Findings may drastically direct the treatment for the critical evaluation of the patient. For example, patients with left ventricular aneurysm, pseudoaneurysm, or flail mitral valve with ruptured papillary muscle may present as nonresponders to what was expected to be appropriate therapy.

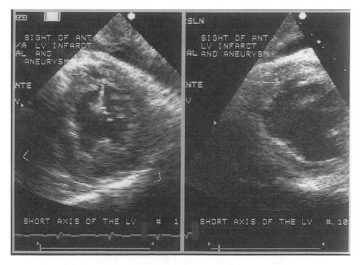

TEE revealed a left ventricular aneurysm at the site of an acute anterior wall MI. The patient tolerated the procedure, which was done within 1 hour of presenting to the hospital with the acute MI and a murmur not identified with TTE.

BIBLIOGRAPHY

1. Brathwaite CEM, Weiss RL, Baldino WA, et al: Multichamber gunshot wounds of the heart: The utility of transesophageal echocardiography. Chest 101:287–288, 1992.
2. Brooks SW, Young JC, Cmolik B, et al: The use of transesophageal echocardiography in the evaluation of chest trauma. J Trauma. 32:761–766, 1992.
3. Davis GA, Sauerisen S, Chandrassekaran K, et al: Subclinical traumatic aortic injury diagnosed by transesophageal echocardiography. Am Heart J 123:534–536, 1992.
4. Ferrari E, Vidal R, et al: Atherosclerosis of the thoracic aorta and aortic debris: A marker of poor benefit of oral anticoagulation. J Am Coll Cardiol 33:1317–1322, 1999.
5. Font VE, Obarski TP, Klein AL, et al: Transesophageal echocardiography in the critical care unit. Cleve Clin J Med 58:315–322, 1991.
6. Foster E, Schiller NB: The role of transesophageal echocardiography in critical care: UCSF experience. J Am Soc Echocardiogr 5:368–374, 1992.
7. Freeman WK, Seward JB, Khandheria BK, Tajik AJ: Transesophageal Echocardiography. Boston, Little, Brown, 1994.
8. Kapral MK, Silver FL: Preventive health care, 1999 update: 2. Echocardiography for the detection of cardiac source of embolism in patients with stroke. CMAJ 19:161:989–996, 1999.
9. Nienaber CA, von Kodolitsch Y, Nicolas V, et al: The diagnosis of thoracic aortic dissection by noninvasive imaging procedures. N Engl J Med 328:1–9, 1993.
10. Tunick PA, Kronzon I: Atheromas of the thoracic aorta: Clinical and therapeutic update. J Am Coll Cardiol 1:35(3):545–554, 2000.
11. Willens HJ, Kessler KM: Transesophageal echocardiography in the thoracic aorta. Chest 117(1):233–243, 2000.

9. EXERCISE STRESS TESTING

Fernando Boccalandro, M.D.

1. Describe the different types of exercise stress tests.

Exercise stress tests (ESTs) can be static (isometric) or dynamic (isotonic). *Static* stress tests are performed with little muscle shortening, but with a higher pressor response using a hand dynamometer. This type of stress test is not used in clinical practice since the intensity of exercise is usually not enough to generate an ischemic response.

Dynamic ESTs are routinely performed to assess cardiovascular and pulmonary reserve. They are accomplished with a treadmill, a bicycle ergometer, or an arm ergometer, and may involve ventilatory gas analysis (the latter is called a cardiopulmonary stress test [see Question 15]). Different protocols of progressive cardiovascular work have been developed specifically for stress testing (e.g., Bruce, Cornell, Balke-Ware, ACIP, mAICP, Naughton, Weber).

ESTs may involve only EKG monitoring to assess for ischemia, or may employ echocardiography or nuclear cardiology techniques to help localize the distribution of the ischemic myocardium.

2. What parameters are monitored during an exercise stress test?

During an EST, three principal parameters are monitored:
- Clinical response of the patient to exercise (e.g., shortness of breath, dizziness, chest pain, angina pectoris, Borg Scale [see Question 13])
- Hemodynamic response (e.g., heart rate, blood pressure response, double product, peak workload)
- EKG changes that occur during stress (e.g., rhythm, ST and T changes) and recovery phase.

3. What are the indications for an exercise stress test?

Clear indications:
- When diagnosing obstructive coronary artery disease (CAD), for risk stratification, functional class assessment, and prognosis in patients with suspected CAD based on age, gender and clinical presentation
- When evaluating patients with known CAD who witnessed a significant change in their clinical status
- After a myocardial infarction (MI) for prognosis assessment, physical activity prescription, or evaluation of current medical treatment
- When treating patients who underwent a coronary revascularization procedure with recurrent symptoms
- When evaluating the proper settings in patients who received rate-responsive pacemakers

Relative indications:
- When caring for patients with vasospastic angina
- When evaluating patients who have undergone a coronary revascularization procedure after an MI (e.g., angioplasty or bypass surgery)
- To evaluate the exercise capacity of non-critical valvular heart disease.
- When treating asymptomatic adults with multiple risk factors for CAD who plan to start a vigorous exercise program or who are involved in occupations involving public safety.
- When investigating patients with known or suspected exercise-induced arrythmias.

4. List the contraindications for an exercise stress test.

Acute MI (less than 48–72 hours)	Decompensated arrhythmias
Acute pulmonary embolism	Uncontrolled hypertension

Acute myocarditis
Acute pericarditis
Acute aortic dissection
Unstable angina
Left main disease
Decompensated heart failure

Severe aortic stenosis
Significant electrolyte imbalances
Outflow tract obstruction including hyper-
    trophic cardiomyopathy
Mental or physical impairment leading
    to inability to exercise

5. What is the difference between a maximal and submaximal exercise stress test?

A *maximal* stress test is performed when attempting to achieve a maximal tolerated exercise capacity. A *submaximal* EST is performed when the goal is lower than the maximum exercise capacity. Reasonable goals are 70% of the maximum predicted heart rate, 120 bpm or 5–6 METs. This test is also ordered for patients early after they experience an acute MI.

6. What is an adequate heart rate to illicit an ischemic response?

When significant coronary artery stenosis exists, a heart rate of 85% of the maximal predicted heart rate for the age of the patient is enough to elicit an ischemic response and is considered an adequate heart rate for exercise stress testing.

7. How do I calculate the predicted maximal heart rate?

The maximum predicted heart (MPHR) rate can be estimated with the following formula: MPHR = 220 – Age.

8. When can an exercise stress test be performed after an acute myocardial infarction?

A submaximal EST is recommended after an MI and can be done as early as 4 days after the acute event. This submaximal EST should be followed by a late (3–6 weeks), symptom-limited EST. It is recommended that physicians conduct an early (14–21 days) symptom-limited EST after an MI if a submaximal EST was not done before discharge. Exercise stress testing in this circumstance assists in formulating a prognosis, determining activity levels, assessing medical therapy, and planning cardiac rehabilitation.

It is unclear if asymptomatic patients who undergo an acute MI with a consequent revascularization procedure benefit from further exercise stress testing.

9. What factors interfere with the interpretation of an exercise stress test EKG?

Complete left bundle branch block
Ventricular pacing
≥ 1 mm baseline ST depression
Left ventricular hypertrophy with > 1 mm ST depression
Use of digoxin with or without resting abnormalities
Pre-excitation syndromes (Wolf-Parkinson-White syndrome)

10. How helpful is an exercise stress test in the diagnosis of coronary artery disease?

Multiple studies have been undertaken to compare the accuracy of exercise stress testing with coronary angiography. However, different criteria have been used for coronary stenosis, and this lack of standardization has clouded the issue. A meta-analysis of 24,074 patients reported a mean sensitivity of 68% and a mean specificity of 77%. The sensitivity increases to 81% and the specificity decreases to 66% for multi-vessel disease, and to 86% and 53%, respectively, for left main or three-vessel disease.

The diagnostic power of an EST can be improved by adding imaging techniques during peak exercises and at rest; ecochardiography or perfusion imaging can be used with the traditional EKG. In both techniques, the heart at rest is compared with its performance at peak exercise. With **perfusion techniques**, the relative distribution of a radiotracer is compared in the different parts of the myocardium. In the ischemic regions, there is a relative decrease in the uptake of the nuclear tracer during exercise compared with the areas of no flow limitation. In **echocardiography**, the wall motion is used as a reference. In areas of critical stenosis, the walls become hypokinetic or dyskinetic when compared with normal myocardium.

11. List the markers associated with an adverse prognosis in an exercise stress test.
- Early onset of angina (less then 6 METs)
- Failure to increase systolic pressure > 120 mmHg or failure to sustain an increase of 10 mmHg above resting levels in systolic bood pressure
- ST segment depressions > 2 mm
- ST elevations
- Ischemic changes in more than five or more leads
- Reproducible sustained (> 30 seconds) or symptomatic ventricular tachycardia
- Persistence of EKG changes in recovery

12. What are the indications to stop an exercise stress test?
- Severe chest pain, ataxia, fatigue or shortness of breath
- Ischemic ST-segments depressions > 3 mm
- Ischemic ST segments elevations > 1 mm in a non-Q-wave lead
- Ventricular tachycardia
- Supraventricular tachycardia
- Progressive decrease in blood pressure
- Abnormal elevation of blood pressure
- Decrease in heart rate
- Technical problems with the EKG monitoring or blood pressure

13. What is the Borg Scale?
The Borg Scale is a numeric scale of perceived patient exertion. Usually it is placed in front of the patient during the EST to assess the patient's effort. Values of 7–9 reflect light work, 13–17 hard work, and a value above 18 is close to the maximum exercise capacity. Readings of 14–16 reach the anaerobic threshold.

14. What are the risks associated with exercise stress testing?
The risks are very low. In the general population, the mortality is < 0.01%, and the morbidity is < 0.05%. A survey of 151,944 patients 4 weeks after MI showed a slight increase to 0.03% and 0.09%, respectively. In a study of 1377 tests by Young et al., 2.2%of the patients required cardioversion, cardiopulmonary resucitation, or antiarrythmic drugs for ventricular tachycardia.

15. What is a cardiopulmonary exercise stress test?
During a cardiopulmonary EST, the patient's gas exchange is monitored in a closed circuit. It is a useful tool in assisting in the diagnosis of patients with cardiovascular and pulmonary disease. Measurements of gas exchange are obtained during this test (e.g., oxygen uptake, carbon dioxide output, minute ventilation, anaerobic threshold) with the standard parameters taken during a regular EST.

16. What are the indications for a cardiopulmonary exercise stress test?
A cardiopulmonary EST is indicated when it is clinically difficult to differentiate cardiac versus pulmonary cause of exercise-induced dyspnea or impaired exercise capacity. It is also used in the assesment and therapeutic follow-up of patients with heart failure who are candidates for heart transplantation.

17. Can I obtain a stress test if a patient cannot exercise?
Yes. If the patient is unable to exercise, pharmacologic methods can detect ischemia with the use of ecocardiography or perfusion imaging. Adenosine and Dypiridamole can be used to induce vasodilatation in the coronary circulation and unmask critical stenosis. Dobutamine can be used

to induced tachycardia, increase contractility and increase the demand in the myocardium. Both methods are equivalent to exercise, although they can not predict functional capacity.

BIBLIOGRAPHY

1. Ashley EA, Myers J, Froelicher V: Exercise testing in clinical medicine. Lancet 356(9241):1592–1597, 2000.
2. Borg G: Perceived exertion as an indicator of somatic stress. Scand J Rehab Med 2(3):92, 1972.
3. Carter H, Jones AM, Barstow TJ, et al: Oxygen uptake kinetics in treadmill running and cycle ergometry: A comparison. J Appl Physiol 89(3):899–907, 2000.
4. Chaitman BR: Exercise stress testing. Braunwald E (ed): Heart Disease: A Textbook of Cardiovascular Medicine, 5th ed. Vol 1. Philadelphia, WB Saunders, 1997, pp 153–176.
5. Detrano R, Gianrossi R, Mulvihill D, et al: Exercise-induced ST segment depression in the diagnosis of multivessel coronary disease: A meta-analysis. J Am Coll Cardiol 14(6):1501–1508, 1989.
6. Detrano R, Gianrossi R, Froelicher V: The diagnostic accuracy the exercise electrocardiogram: A meta-analysis of 22 years of research. Prog Cardiovasc Dis 32(3):173–206, 1989.
7. Fletcher FF, Schlant RC: The exercise test. In Hurst (ed): Hurst's The Heart, 9th ed. Volume 1. New York, McGraw-Hill, 1998, pp 519–536.
8. Franke A, Hoffmann R, Kühl HP, et al: Non-contrast second harmonic imaging improves interobserver agreement and accuracy of dobutamine stress echocardiography in patients with impaired image quality. Heart 83(2):133–140, 2000.
9. Gibbons RJ, Balady GJ, Beasley JW, et al: ACC/AHA guidelines for exercise testing: Executive summary. A report of the American College of Cardiology/American Heart Association Task Force on Practice Guidelines (Committee on Exercise Testing. Circulation 96(1):345–354, 1997.
10. Hamm LF, Crow RS, Stull GA, Hannan P: Safety and characteristics of exercise testing early after acute myocardial infarction. Am J Cardiol 63(17):1193–1197, 1989.
11. Jouven X, Zureik M, Desnos M, et al: Long-term outcome in asymptomatic men with exercise-induced premature ventricular depolarizations. N Engl J Med 343(12):826–833, 2000.
12. Morise AP: Are the American College of Cardiology/American Heart Association guidelines for exercise testing for suspected coronary artery disease correct? Chest 118(2):535–541, 2000.
13. Nishime EO, Cole CR, Blackstone EH, et al: Heart rate recovery and treadmill exercise score as predictors of mortality in patients referred for exercise ECG. JAMA 284(11):1392–1398, 2000.
14. Noonan V, Dean E: Submaximal exercise testing: Clinical application and interpretation. Phys Ther 80(8):782–807, 2000.
15. Reybrouck T: Gas exchange kinetics in patients with cardiovascular disease. Chest 118(2):285–286, 2000.
16. Stuart RJ Jr, Ellestad MH: National survey of exercise stress testing facilities. Chest 77(1):94–97, 1980.
17. Vanzetto G, Ormezzano O, Fagret D, et al: Long-term additive prognostic value of thallium-201 myocardial perfusion imaging over clinical and exercise stress test in low to intermediate risk patients : Study in 1137 patients with 6-year follow-up. Circulation 100(14):1521–1527, 1999.
18. Young DZ, Lampert S, Graboys TB, Lown B: Safety of maximal exercise testing in patients at high risk for ventricular arrhythmia. Circulation 70(2):184–191, 1984.

10. NUCLEAR CARDIOLOGY, MAGNETIC RESONANCE IMAGING, AND COMPUTED TOMOGRAPHY

Rajesh Bhola, M.D., and Robert A. Quaife, M.D.

1. What is myocardial perfusion imaging?

Myocardial perfusion imaging (MPI) is a noninvasive method to assess regional myocardial blood flow and the cellular integrity of myocytes. This technique uses radiotracers such as thallium-201, technetium sestamibi, and tetrofosmin as blood flow markers. Since they cross the myocyte cellular membrane and are trapped intracellularly, these perfusion agents are distributed in normally perfused and viable myocardial tissue. Therefore, tissue supplied by normal coronary blood flow will possess normal regional myocardial tracer uptake, and regions supplied by stenosed coronary vessel will have lower coronary blood flow and less relative myocardial uptake.

When cardiac tissue faces increased metabolic demand, as during exercise, the relative difference in blood flow between normal and stenotic vascular distribution is disparate. Despite maximal coronary vasodilatation beyond a point of coronary narrowing, the resultant improvement of blood flow during exercise is minimal, producing a relative reduction in blood flow and a perfusion defect between normal and ischemic myocardium. This **difference between normal and stenotic vascular territories** during stress forms the basis for MPI.

2. Differentiate reversible and fixed perfusion defects.

Myocardial stress testing enhances the blood flow difference between normal and underperfused myocardium and magnifies the relative perfusion differences between the two regions. Stress-induced perfusion defects are used to define myocardium at risk for an ischemic or infarction event. A perfusion defect induced by stress that later demonstrates normal perfusion on delayed rest images is termed *reversible perfusion defect*. A perfusion defect that demonstrates no change between stress and rest images is termed *fixed defect*.

Fixed perfusion defects in general define irreversibly damaged or infarcted tissue. However, 25–30% of these defects may possess viable or living tissue that is severely ischemic even at rest. Such tissue is considered to be "hibernating." Hibernating myocardium possesses cellular metabolism that is altered to conserve energy at the expense of reduced or absent contractile function. This phenomenon is probably the result of severe resting ischemia and episodic ischemia.

3. What diagnostic questions are addressed by myocardial perfusion imaging?

- MPI is primarily used in the diagnosis of coronary artery disease (CAD).
- Stress perfusion imaging is used to define the severity of physiologic significance of a stenosed vessel already identified by coronary angiography.
- MPI is also used for preoperative risk assessment. Dipyridamole perfusion imaging with perfusion tracers is highly predictive of either perioperative or postoperative cardiac-related death or myocardial infarction (MI) in patients with reversible perfusion defects. These reversible perfusion defects are equivalent to ischemic tissue or myocardium at risk of infarction, and therefore the extent and severity is directly related to the risk of a perioperative cardiac event.
- MPI has been used to evaluate and define prognosis following acute MI. Areas of fixed defect as well as reversible perfusion abnormalities in vascular distribution other than the original infarct region are risk factors for subsequent myocardial events. Early dipyridamole thallium 201 perfusion imaging following acute myocardial imaging (within 48–96 hrs) may be useful for identifying patients at greatest risk for subsequent myocardial

events. This technique is superior to pre-discharge submaximal exercise treadmill testing as a predictor of cardiac events.
- MPI with thallium-201 and sestamibi have been used to identify myocardial tissue that has potential to recover function following resupply of normal coronary blood flow (i.e., viable myocardium). Following successful coronary revascularization with either angioplasty or coronary artery bypass surgery, regional coronary flow improves, resulting in reversal of regional wall motion abnormalities and, in many cases, recovery of global systolic function (improved LV ejection fraction).

4. List the different perfusion agents used in myocardial perfusion imaging.
   Thallium-201. Thallium is a potassium analog used extensively for MPI. Initial regional distribution of thallium in the myocardium is a function of regional coronary blood flow and tracer extraction by the myocardium. Thallium enters myocardium largely by active transport of a membrane-bound $Na^+K^+ATPase$.

Advantages and Disadvantages of Thallium-201 (T-201) for Myocardial Perfusion Imaging

ADVANTAGES	DISADVANTAGES
1. Rapid myocardial extraction	1. Low energy emission attenuated by overlying
2. Minimal uptake by abdominal organ during exercise	soft tissue, i.e., diaphragm and left breast.
3. Thallium redistribution permits differentiation of myocardial ischemia from a single injection.	2. Long physical half-life. Limited use in serial studies.
4. Diagnostic and prognostic value of T-201 lung uptake.	3. Cyclotron produced and requires shipment.
	4. Slow course of T-201 redistribution results in long imaging sequence.

Technetium 99m–based agents. Potential advantages of Tc 99m in comparison to T-201:
- 140 keV gamma ray emission is ideal for imaging on standard gamma camera.
- Less attenuated by soft tissue as compared to 69 and 83keV lower energy emission of T-201.
- Shorter half-life (6h) of Tc 99m as compared to 73 hrs half life of T-201 permits larger dose administration.
- Tc 99m is produced by generator or onsite, and therefore is more readily available.

First-Generation Agents
   - Tc 99m sestamibi—hexakis-2-methoxyisobutyl isonitrile (Cardiolite)
   - Tc 99m teboroxime—a boronic acid derivative (Cardiotech)
   Tc 99m sestamibi is a cationic compound that is distributed by myocardial blood flow and traverses the cell membrane to concentrate within the mitochondrial wall. It is comparable to thallium in perfusion properties, although it possesses improved imaging characteristics resulting from greater γ-photon energy emission (140keV).
   Tc-teboroxime is a boronic acid derivative with neutral valency which functions as a pure myocardial blood flow tracer. Because of rapid clearance of ^{99}Tc-teboroxime from the myocardium, imaging was required within 5–10 minutes after injection either at rest or exercise and is complicated by rapid myocardial washout.
   Both thallium and technetium-based agents have same sensitivity for detecting CAD, although Tc-MIBI has a slightly higher specificity due to its improved image quality. Technetium-based agents allow analysis methods that simultaneously assess myocardial perfusion and systolic function from the same study.

Second-Generation Agents
   - Tc 99m furifosmin (Q12)
   - Tc 99m tetrofosmin (Myoview)
   The principal clinical advantage of Tc 99m tetrofosmin relates to its more rapid hepatic clearance following both exercise and rest injection. Rapid hepatic clearance of tracer may permit rapid imaging protocols.

Tc 99 tetrofosmin is concentrated in myocardial mitochondria similar to Tc 99m sestamibi. Tc 99 furifosmin has similar properties to that of Tc 99m tetrofosmin but is not currently FDA approved.

Third-Generation Agents
 • Tc 99m-NOET

Tc 99m-NOET is a newer investigational myocardial perfusion agent that has similar physical and imaging properties to that of other Tc 99m–based agents and appears to have favorable redistribution properties similar to T-201.

5. Describe exercise stress testing.

Exercise stress testing is validated extensively as a form of stress for evaluation of known or suspected CAD. It increases myocardial blood flow and metabolic demand. Techniques include:
 • Treadmill stress testing
 • Erect bicycle testing
 • Alternative forms of exercise (i.e., supine bicycle, dynamic arm, and isometric handgrip)

Exercise testing is indicated in physically active patients. It provides functional capacity as well as cardiac stress information about the patient.

6. Are there alternatives to exercise-induced stress?

Yes. Alternative methods that simulate the effects of exercise include:
 • Atrial pacing
 • Cold pressor stimulation test
 • Dobutamine and arbutamine (inotropic) stress test

These agents or methods increase the cardiac workload by increasing the heart rate. Inotropic stress has been shown to be comparable to exercise/pharmacologic coronary vasodilatation. Dobutamine and arbutamine (inotropic agents) are used when vasodilators are contraindicated or when patients are taking xanthine derivatives or have reactive airways disease. Side effects include chest pain, ventricular arrhythmias, and hypotension.

7. True or false: Pharmacologic coronary vasodilatation increases coronary blood flow independently of changes in myocardial metabolic demand.

True. The two vasodilators currently used are adenosine and dipyridamole. The active vasodilator of both agents is adenosine, whether exogenously administered (adenosine) or endogenously increased by inhibited degradation, as with dipyridamole.

Pharmacologic stress testing is indicated in patients with inability to ambulate (e.g., obesity, degenerative joint diseases, peripheral vascular diseases, peripheral neuropathy, spinal cord disorders, and underlying medical and surgical disorders that impair adequate exercise). Dipyridamole and adenosine are contraindicated in patients with history of chronic obstructive pulmonary disease and bronchospastic airway disease. Caffeine and theophylline are both competitive inhibitors of dipyridamole and adenosine and block their vasodilating effects. Current recommendations suggest that caffeine be withheld 24 hrs and theophylline 72 hrs before the study. Side effects of dipyridamole and adenosine injections are nausea, vomiting, headache, dizziness, flushing, chest pain, tachycardia, and AV-conduction abnormalities.

8. Is it possible to assess both myocardial perfusion and left ventricular (LV) function from the same myocardial study?

Yes. Technetium-based agents allow administration of larger radiotracer doses and provide improved imaging characteristics. Therefore, a bolus injection of the radiotracer can be used to assess LV performance at peak stress using a "first pass" LV imaging technique. Second, gated perfusion imaging using single photon emission computed tomography (SPECT) 3-D analysis may quantify LV-end diastolic and end-systolic relative volumes and LV ejection fraction (see figure).

Gating is a method of stopping cardiac motion and allows assessment of the phases of the cardiac cycle. This triggering of the imaging camera at the onset of R-wave over multiple cardiac cycles provides an 8- or 16-frame average of multiple cardiac beats—necessary for assessing cardiac motion and wall thickening. Assessment of wall thickening also improves the specificity for interpreting Tc 99m–based perfusion images.

Left: Myocardial perfusion at stress (*top*) and rest (*bottom*). Note large anterior, septal, and apical area of stress-induced hypoperfusion that is reversible at rest, consistent with myocardial ischemia. *Right:* Perfusion maps demonstrate the large area of anterior-apical ischemia. Note that end-diastolic and end-systolic volumes and ejection fraction are also quantitated.

9. What is the role of electron beam computed tomography (EBCT) in the risk assessment of CAD?

The presence and amount of coronary calcification determined by EBCT is a method for assessing patients at risk of premature CAD or those patients with nondiagnostic chest pain syndromes but also cardiac disease risk factors.

Agatston and colleagues developed a calcium scoring algorithm for EBCT images that is now being used in research and clinical practice. The calcium scoring is a product of the area of calcification per tomographic segment and a factor rated 1 through 4 dictated by maximal calcium density within the segment (Hounsfield units). Calcium scoring has been correlated with atherosclerotic heart disease and luminal coronary artery stenoses.

Recommended EBCT Calcium Score Guidelines

EBCT CALCIUM SCORE	PLAQUE BURDEN	PROBABILITY OF SIGNIFICANT CAD	CV RISK	RECOMMENDATION
0	No identifiable plaque	Very low < 5%	Very low	Reassure the patient and discuss the guidelines for prevention of CV diseases

(Table continued on next page.)

Recommended EBCT Calcium Score Guidelines (cont.)

EBCT CALCIUM SCORE	PLAQUE BURDEN	PROBABILITY OF SIGNIFICANT CAD	CV RISK	RECOMMENDATION
1–10	Minimal identifiable plaque burden	< 10%	Low	Discuss the guidelines for primary prevention of CV diseases.
11–100	Definite, at least mild atherosclerotic plaque	Mild or minimal coronary stenoses	Moderate	Counsel about risk factor modification and strict adherence with NCEP primary prevention cholesterol guidelines and daily ASA.
101–400	Definite, at least moderate atherosclerotic plaque burden	Nonobstructive CAD, although obstructive diseases	Moderately high	Risk factor modification and secondary prevention guidelines. Consider exercise testing for further risk stratification.
> 400	Extensive atherosclerotic plaque burden	High likelihood (> 90%) of at least 1 significant stenoses	High	Institute aggressive risk factor modification. Consider exercise or pharmacologic testing to evaluate for ischemia.

From Electron beam computed tomographic coronary calcium scanning: A review and guidelines for use in asymptomatic persons. Mayo Clin Proc 74:243–252, 1999; with permission.

The EBCT calcium score correlates with increased calcified plaque burden score (see figure), especially when values are stratified by quartile depending upon age and gender. A low calcium score cannot exclude the presence of coronary atherosclerosis, but suggests a lower likelihood of fixed obstructive coronary lesion. A higher calcium score is associated with advanced plaque burden and often with at least one obstructive lesion.

A single 3-mm slice from an EBCT set of images is shown in this axial projection. Note the central and right areas of increased intensity (just posterior to the large circular structures; aorta [left] and pulmonary artery [right]), which demonstrate left main and left anterior descending coronary artery calcification.

10. In which patients should EBCT be considered?

EBCT can be useful in an asymptomatic person with multiple risk factors, including early familial CAD or death from cardiac events, in whom a decision to start cholesterol lowering therapy is not clear. The results of EBCT may be helpful in defining potential risk. The higher the calcium score, the more compelling the rationale for drug therapy in patients with mild to moderate hypercholesteremia in whom the need for drug therapy based on conventional risk assessment is uncertain.

11. What is the role of positron emission tomography (PET) in the assessment of myocardial tissue viability in ischemic heart disease?

Several PET perfusion tracers, such as ^{15}O water, ^{13}N ammonia, and rubidium-^{82}Rb, are used to quantitate absolute and relative regional myocardial blood flow. ^{18}Fluorodeoxyglucose (18-FDG), ^{11}C palmitate, and ^{11}C acetate are some of the metabolic agents used as substrate analogs for assessing metabolic activity in the myocardium. ^{15}O water and ^{13}N ammonia require onsite cyclotron for production of radiotracer. Rubidium-82 is generator-produced, but is a cost-effective agent only in a high-volume nuclear cardiology laboratory since the life of one rubidium generator is approximately 1 month and the cost is approximately $27 thousand/month.

Regional blood flow is quantified by using PET perfusion tracers. In most PET laboratories, perfusion images are performed before metabolic imaging. Perfusion is assessed in both normal and pharmacologic coronary vasodilatation. Metabolic activity of myocardium can be assessed in different physiologic states using radiotracers as substrate analogs, such as FDG for glucose metabolism and acetate for fatty acid metabolism.

Viable myocardium may be identified by PET on the basis of myocardial blood flow and preserved or enhanced substrate utilization. Combined imaging with ^{13}N ammonia or rubidium perfusion and metabolic imaging with 18-FDG is the gold standard for assessment of myocardial viability. Most assessments of viability begin in the regional myocardial segments with impaired contraction. Then relative blood flow to the region is assessed, followed by determination of the regional metabolic activity.

Definition and Interpretation of 18-FDG and Blood-Flow Relationship in PET Imaging

REGIONAL WALL MOTION	BLOOD FLOW	FDG-UPTAKE	DIAGNOSIS
Normal	Normal	Normal	Normal metabolically acting myocardium
Depressed	Normal	Normal	Stunned myocardium
	Abnormal	Normal	Hibernating myocardium (resting ischemia)
	Abnormal	Reduced	Scar tissue infarction

12. Functional assessment of cardiac performance is determined using which nuclear cardiology techniques?

Standard LV performance may be assessed in two ways: A **first-pass bolus technique** quantitates individual end-systolic and end-diastolic relative volumes as the bolus passes through the right heart into the lungs and through the LV. Regions of interest are manually determined around the LV at end-diastolic and end-systolic to provide the counts necessary for calculation of LV ejection fraction (EF) (end-diastolic volume minus end-systolic volume divided by end-diastolic volume).

Alternatively, **gated equilibrium blood pool imaging** (multiple gated acquisition, MUGA) of the left and right ventricles may be performed to assess myocardial performance. An aliquot of the patient's red blood cells is labeled with sodium pertechnetate and reinjected for subsequent imaging in three planar images. The camera is triggered at the onset of each R-wave for each cardiac cycle; the R-R interval is divided into 16 frames and is compiled into summed images. These average data in image format are subsequently processed and displayed as a continuous cinematic loop to simulate cardiac motion during the cardiac cycle. From this display, a region of interest is identified around LV end-diastolic and end-systolic volumes again to calculate LVEF. Also from the display, regional myocardial wall motion may be determined for each LV segment.

13. How important is assessment of LVEF in radionuclide techniques?

- Overall, the LVEF is one of the most powerful predictors of future cardiac events and sudden death in patients with CAD. Its predictive value in CAD is probably related to global LV dysfunction manifested as the combination of poor myocardial perfusion and the presence of underlying scar tissue from previous MIs. This ischemia/scar tissue is the substrate for future ischemic events or life-threatening cardiac arrhythmias.
- LVEF is important in evaluating valvular heart disease, as baseline LVEF suggests already-compromised LV function and is a poor prognostic sign when considering surgical intervention.
- Exercise LVEF may be useful in the early detection of compromised LV systolic performance. When semi-erect or supine bicycle testing is used, the lack of increase in LVEF with exercise may predict loss of LV reserve, signaling the need for early intervention.
- Both hypertrophic and dilated cardiomyopathy patients may benefit from diagnostic and prognostic information gained from determinations of LV systolic and diastolic performance. From idiopathic dilated cardiomyopathy to doxorubicin-induced cardiomyopathy, reduced LVEF is one of the greatest predictors of subsequent severe CHF and death.

14. When is computed tomography (CT) important for the diagnosis of cardiac or cardiac-related diseases?

Standard state-of-the-art CT imaging systems, much faster than their earlier counterparts, still have limited temporal resolution for the beating heart. Therefore, investigations of intracardiac structures—except within the atria, pericardial space, or aorta—are limited. CT has been useful for evaluating suspected constrictive pericarditis or other pericardial diseases (determining pericardial thickness) and intracardiac thrombi (usually in the pulmonary arteries or atria, where there are less cardiac motion artifacts). In many centers, CT has become the first-line assessment for abnormalities of the ascending and descending aorta, especially in suspected aortic dissection.

15. What are the limitations of standard CT imaging?

Cardiac evaluation by CT is primarily limited by **insufficient temporal resolution** to allow stop-frame assessment of cardiac structures, therefore limiting evaluations of LV chamber thickness, contraction, and intracardiac structures. Additionally, this technique requires administration of an **iodinated contrast agent** to opacify the intravascular regions and to identify abnormalities within these structures. These contrast agents can provoke adverse reactions.

Recently, the introduction of ultrafast CT (Imitron, Inc.) has allowed assessment of multiple cardiac slides within 10–20 cardiac beats at a temporal resolution of approximately 50 ms. Unlike standard CT, this modality has high resolution for intracardiac structures and masses. It also allows bolus contrast injections to study intracardiac transit times and coronary artery bypass graft flow. Unfortunately, ultrafast CT imaging is not widely available and is of limited general use except in thoracic pathology. Another new technique, "multidetection" CT, has imaging speeds approaching those of ultrafast CT.

16. How does CT compare to other imaging modalities for the diagnosis of aortic dissection?

A recent comparison of aortic dissection detected by multiple imaging modalities found that, overall, CT had a 93% sensitivity and 87% specificity for detecting dissecting aortic aneurysm. The difficulty in defining a second lumen and the potential false-positive of artifacts resulting from the streaming of contrast and other issues reduced the sensitivity of standard CT. Overall, the sensitivity and specificity are acceptable for a screening test for aortic dissection. Spiral acquisition techniques also enhance CT assessment.

Additionally, CT allows assessment of the ascending aorta as well as aortic arch and descending aorta; however, this evaluation requires administration of intravenous contrast. This potentially renal toxic contrast, when combined with either total ischemic time or cardiopulmonary bypass pump use at surgical dissection repair, can induce acute and prolonged renal failure postoperatively.

17. What are the advantages of magnetic resonance imaging (MRI) over standard imaging techniques?

MRI employs inherent physiologic properties of tissues to create images of body structures. It provides a **wide field of view** for assessing structures within the thoracic cage, specifically for cardiac imaging. The ability to orient images in **multiple planes** and off-axis planes is key to the technique's diagnostic utility and allows images to be oriented within specific oblique or perpendicular views for careful inspection of cardiac structures and/or the great vessels.

Additionally, **gating or triggering** of the MRI scanner based on the R wave of the patient's ECG for each cardiac cycle allows stop-frame imaging of the heart and great vessels. The inherent characteristics of flowing blood result in contrast enhancement of vascular structures without the administration of iodinated contrast agents. Major uses include the assessment of congenital heart disease (adult and pediatric), intracardiac structures, and the great vessels.

Unlike other imaging modalities, such as CT or planar blood pool imaging, MRI provides 3-D assessment of myocardial structures. Its advantages, including image resolution and field of view, outweigh some of its limitations, such as placing the patient within a closed area, potential difficulties with cardiac gating, and increased cost.

18. What role does MRI play in diagnosing aortic aneurysm and dissection?

MRI provides full field-of-view assessment of the ascending aorta, aortic arch, and descending aorta. With use of turbo spin-echo techniques, static views of the cardiac structures and great vessels are assessed in a multi-slice format. Spin-echo MRI has high sensitivity for detecting false lumens and intramural flaps associated with dissection, identifying areas of intraluminal thrombosis, and assessing potential rupture of dissecting aortic aneurysms into visceral spaces of pericardium. Contrast enhancement using special imaging sequences provides evaluation of the site of aortic tear into the intima and potential flow within the false lumen of the aortic dissection free of iodinated contrast.

Aortic insufficiency may also be assessed as one of the associated markers of aortic dissection, and the reported sensitivity and specificity of MRI for detecting aortic dissection were 98% for both type A and B dissection. In a comparison of transthoracic and transesophageal echocardiography, CT, and MRI for the diagnosis of aortic dissection, the primary limitations of MRI were: (1) inability to image significantly unstable patients, and (2) limited availability in emergency situations at all centers. Therefore, CT or transesophageal echocardiography may be indicated for evaluating aortic dissection, depending on the availability and expertise within specific hospitals.

19. Elaborate on the use of MRI in the cardiac patient.

Tissue characterizations resulting from MRI-induced physical properties allow the assessment of *intracardiac* masses, with the greatest sensitivity in the atria and great vessels. There is somewhat less sensitivity, although greater specificity, for detecting *intramural* cardiac masses, due to the similar image intensity between tumors and myocardial tissues. MRI provides assessment of pericardial and pleural spaces and localization of masses extending into or arising from these structures. MRI and echocardiography are probably the two most sensitive techniques for determining the extent of intracardiac masses.

Additionally, new methods using **gadolinium DTPA** as a contrast agent have allowed assessment of myocardial perfusion. This includes assessment of regional coronary artery vasodilator reserve as a marker of CAD and assessment of myocardial viability using delayed contrast enhancement of viable tissue.

New methods of **image acquisition** have also been developed to assess regional and global LV contractile function. The *tagging method* assesses regional torsional and conformational changes of the LV during systole, to assess LV wall strain and stress as well as regional thickening. Without contrast enhancement (Gd DTPA), this method may better identify infarcted myocardium versus myocardial tissue without retained regional contractility and function.

20. What is the diagnostic accuracy of MRI for congenital heart disease?

Congenital heart disease imaging with MRI is significantly enhanced by the simultaneous evaluation of visceral, vascular, and cardiac structures. Complex congenital heart disease often involves not only cardiac abnormalities but also abnormalities of the associated vascular structures or visceral organs. With MRI, the wide field of view provides associated information important for correct diagnosis. For example, transposition of the great vessels is easily evaluated by MRI, since the orientation of the aorta, pulmonary artery, and cardiac chambers is visualized together rather than separately (see figure).

A single phase and slice from a breath-hold, cine-gated MRI study is shown in sagittal oblique format. Note the anterior origin of the aorta and aortic arch with the posterior origin of the pulmonary artery. This finding is diagnostic of congenital transposition of the great vessels. Using this technique, blood flow is bright and provides clear images of the vessels without the administration of contrast agents.

Recently, the increased survival of patients with congenital heart disease into adulthood has supported diagnostic-niche MRI. Many of these patients receive surgical shunts or vascular procedures that are not well studied or investigated by standard imaging techniques, but flow, size of vessels, and physiologic function of these shunts may be assessed using the multiple orientations of MRI.

21. True or false: A prosthetic valve is a contraindication to MRI.

False. In general, prosthetic valves are not a contraindication to MRI (except for the early Starr-Edwards 1200 series ball-cage valves). However, assessment of structures in the region of prosthetic heart valves is limited due to absorption of imaging signal by metallic structures within the heart.

BIBLIOGRAPHY

1. Achenbach S, Moshage W, Roper D, et al: Value of electron-beam computed tomography for the non-invasive detection of high grade coronary artery stenoses and occlusions. N Engl J Med 339:1964–71, 1998.
2. Agatston AS, Janowitz WR, Hildner FJ, et al: Quantification of coronary artery calcium using ultrafast computed tomography. J Am Coll Card 15:827–832, 1990.
3. Axel L, Goncalves RC, Bloomgarden D: Regional heart wall motion two-dimensional analysis and functional imaging with MR imaging. Radiology 183(3):745–50, 1992.
4. Beller GA: Evaluation of myocardial viability using thallium 201. Cardiol Rev 1(2):78–86, 1996.
5. Budoff MJ, Georgiou D, Brody A: Ultrafast computed tomography as a diagnostic modality in the detection of coronary artery diseases: A multicenter study. Circulation 93:898–904, 1996.

6. Chien D, Merboldt KD: Advances in cardiac applications of subsecond FLASH MRI. Magn Reson Imaging 8:829–836, 1990.
7. Dilsizian V, Rocco TP, Friedman NMT, et al: Enhanced detection of ischemic but viable myocardium by reinjection of thallium after-redistribution imaging. New Engl J Med 323:141–146, 1990.
8. Kim RJ, Fieno DS: Relationship of MRI delayed contrast enhancement to irreversible injury, infarct age, and contractile function. Circulation 100:1992–2002, 1999.
9. Klingenbeck K, Schaller S, Flohr T, et al: Sub-second multi-slice computed tomography: Basics and application. Eur J Radiol 31(2), 1997.
10. Manning WJ, Li W, Edelman RR: A preliminary report comparing magnetic resonance coronary angiography with conventional angiography. New Engl J Med 328:828–832, 1993.
11. Mohiaddin RH, Longmore DB: Functional aspect of cardiovascular nuclear magnetic resonance imaging. Circulation 88:264, 1993.
12. Nienabar CA, Kodolitsch Y, Nicolas V, et al: The diagnosis of thoracic aortic dissection by noninvasive imaging procedure. NEJM 328:1, 1993.
13. Rumberger JA, Brundage BH, Rader DJ, George K: Electron beam computed tomographic coronary calcium scanning. Mayo Clinic Proceding 74:243–252, 1999.
14. Sakuma H, Takeda K, Higgins CB: Fast magnetic resonance imaging of the heart. Eur J Radiol 29:101–133, 1999.

11. CARDIAC CATHETERIZATION AND ANGIOGRAPHY

Roy W. Robertson, M.D., and William P. Miller, M.D.

1. What are the general indications for performing cardiac catheterization?
Assessment of patients with:
1. Known or suspected coronary artery disease
2. Valvular heart disease
3. Congenital heart disease
4. Cardiomyopathy
5. Sudden cardiac death
6. Pericardial constriction or tamponade
7. Cardiac transplantation

2. What are the indications for coronary angiography in patients with known or suspected coronary artery disease?
In order of most to least agreed-upon indications:
1. Exercise test predictive of left main and/or multivessel coronary artery disease
2. Limiting angina pectoris
    a. In patients who have failed medical therapy
    b. Most patients with unstable angina
3. Myocardial infarction (MI). Primary coronary intervention is the treatment of choice in many patients with acute MI.
    a. Cardiogenic shock
    b. Clinically failed thrombolysis
    c. Postinfarction angina
    d. Assessment of acute mechanical complications (e.g., ventricular septal defect)
    e. Failed low-level predischarge exercise stress test
    f. Following most non-Q-wave myocardial infarctions
4. Positive exercise and/or pharmacologic stress test
5. Diagnostic evaluation and assessment of "atypical" chest pain and/or suspected coronary spasm
6. Evaluation of high-risk patients prior to a major noncardiac surgical procedure
7. Asymptomatic patients at increased risk for coronary artery disease
    a. Occupational status (e.g., pilot)
    b. Significant cardiovascular risk factors (diabetes mellitus, hyperlipidemia, hypertension)
    c. Abnormal resting electrocardiogram

3. What predisposing factors place patients at high risk for complications from cardiac catheterization?
1. Age (< 1 year or > 60 years of age)
2. Functional class: Patients classified as New York Heart Association class IV are at 10 times higher risk than patients in class I or II.
3. Severity of coronary atherosclerosis: Left main occlusive stenosis poses a 10 times higher risk than single-vessel occlusive coronary disease.
4. Valvular heart disease
5. Left ventricular dysfunction: Mortality rate is 10 times higher for patients with ejection fraction < 30% compared to those with ejection fraction > 50%.
6. Severe noncardiac disease (e.g., diabetes mellitus, renal insufficiency, peripheral vascular disease, chronic lung disease).

4. List some of the potential complications from a diagnostic cardiac catheterization and their frequencies.

Major Complications of Cardiac Catheterization

Death	0.1–0.2%
Myocardial infarction	0.1–0.3%
Cerebrovascular accident	0.1–0.3%

Minor, Transient, or Reversible Complications of Cardiac Catheterization

Vasovagal reactions	1.5–2.5%
Local vascular complications at access site	1–3%
Serious arrhythmias	0.3–0.5%
Allergic reaction to contrast agent	< 2%
Infection	< 0.5%
Nephropathy	< 0.5%

Complication rates depend on operator experience, equipment, and patient characteristics.

5. Describe the most common sites of vascular access for cardiac catheterization.

Catheterization can be accomplished by introduction of catheters into the brachial, radial, or femoral artery and brachiocephalic or femoral vein. Whereas brachial artery cutdown and arteriotomy (Sones) was the original approach, the percutaneous femoral (Judkins) approach is now used most commonly. The transradial percutaneous approach has become popular in recent years. Choice of access site depends on preference and experience of the operator and the extent of peripheral vascular disease in the patient.

6. What are the major components of routine left and right cardiac catheterization?

Initially, pressures are measured in the aorta, right heart, and left heart. Right heart pressures include pulmonary capillary wedge pressure, pulmonary artery pressures, right ventricular pressures, and right atrial pressure. Left heart pressures are the left ventricular systolic, early diastolic, and end-diastolic pressures. Pressure measurement is followed by determination of cardiac output. Contrast opacification of the left ventricular chamber (left ventricular cineangiography) and other chambers if clinically indicated is also included—e.g., contrast opacification of the left atrium in the assessment of an atrial septal defect. Selective angiography of the coronary arteries follows.

7. How is cardiac output measured?

Cardiac output is commonly measured by dilutional techniques (e.g., thermodilution) or by the Fick method. In the Fick method, cardiac output (CO) = oxygen consumption (VO_2)/arteriovenous oxygen difference ($AVO_2\Delta$). Oxygen consumption is measured directly by a mask that fits over the patient's mouth or face, and blood is sampled from the pulmonary artery and femoral artery to compute $AVO_2\Delta$.

8. What are the normal values for intracardiac chamber pressures in the human heart?

Recalling this information is made easy by applying the "**rule of fives**": all pressures are estimated as multiples of five. The right atrial pressure (central venous pressure) is normally ~5 mmHg. The right ventricular systolic pressure is –25 mmHg with an end-diastolic pressure of ~5 mmHg. The left atrial pressure (estimated by the pulmonary capillary wedge pressure) is ~10 mmHg. The left ventricular systolic pressure is normally –125 mmHg with a left ventricular end-diastolic pressure of 10 mmHg.

9. What information is obtained from the left ventricular cineangiogram?

Left ventricular (LV) volumes can be measured using quantitative ventriculography. The LV ejection fraction provides a measure of LV systolic function. Regional systolic wall motion is assessed by grading each segment of the left ventricle as hyperkinetic, normal, hypokinetic, akinetic, or dyskinetic. Space-occupying lesions might also be identified, if present, within the LV chamber (e.g., thrombus). Stroke volume is determined by subtracting the end-systolic LV chamber volume from the end-diastolic LV chamber volume. Ejection fraction (EF) is the stroke volume divided by the end-diastolic LV volume. Finally, an assessment of mitral valve competence is made. Mitral incompetence (regurgitation) is graded as mild (1+), moderate (2+), moderately severe (3+), or severe (4+).

10. Typically the left ventriculogram is obtained in one or, ideally, two projections to assess ventricular function. What LV wall segments are assessed in each of the views and how are they graded?

Each segment is graded as hyperkinetic, normal, hypokinetic, akinetic, or dyskinetic.

Right anterior oblique (RAO) projection:
1 = Anterobasal
2 = Anterolateral
3 = Apical
4 = Diaphragmatic
5 = Posterobasal

Left anterior oblique (LAO) projection:
6 = Septal
7 = Posterolateral

11. Define coronary dominance.

The nomenclature that describes the coronary artery as dominant can be misleading. It is not simply the degree of importance, but instead identifies the coronary artery that crosses the crux of the heart (junction of the posterior atrioventricular groove with the posterior interventricular groove) and therefore generally supplies the basal posterior interventricular septum of the left ventricle. This same artery commonly gives rise to the atrioventricular nodal artery in the region of, or just beyond, the crux. In approximately 85% of humans, the right coronary artery is dominant. In most of the remaining 15%, the left circumflex artery is dominant; however, "codominance" does occur.

12. How is the degree of coronary artery stenosis assessed on a coronary angiogram?

For routine clinical evaluation of coronary angiograms, an experienced angiographer qualitatively estimates the degree of stenosis visually. Multiple views of the regions of interest are obtained over a range of projection angles to best define the three-dimensional geometry of the lesions. The result is generally reported as a percent of reduction in lumen diameter (e.g., a 75% stenosis is a lesion that narrows the lumen diameter by approximately 75%). Quantitative coronary angiography can be performed using digital image processing algorithms that are now generally available in modern cardiac catheterization laboratories. Quantitative angiography is routinely used as a research tool in clinical trials.

13. Name the coronary arteries and their major branches as they are commonly identified by coronary angiography.

This drawing depicts right-dominant coronary anatomy:

LMC = left main coronary artery	AC = atrial circumflex
LAD = left anterior descending	PL = posterolateral branch
D = diagonal branch	RCA = right coronary artery
S = septal perforator	SA = sinus node branch
CX = circumflex	RV = right ventricular branch
RI = ramus intermedius	AM = acute marginal branch
OM = obtuse marginal	PDA = posterior descending artery

14. How do angiographers commonly categorize the severity of coronary artery stenoses?

A grading system of reduction in percent lumen diameter has been designed that incorporates the limitations of the qualitative nature of assessing the significance of coronary artery disease. Coronary atherosclerosis is graded as absent (normal), intimal, 25%, 50%, 75%, 90%, 99% (subtotal occlusion), and 100% (occluded). A ≥ 75% reduction in luminal diameter is considered to be a "significant" stenosis in that a lesion of this severity will affect that artery's ability to increase coronary blood flow as needed during increased demand. The left main coronary artery is "unique" in that a ≥ 50% stenosis is prognostically significant. Lesion characteristics such as presence of calcium, length of stenosis, location within the coronary artery tree, concentric vs. eccentric morphology, presence of an ulcerated plaque, and intraluminal thrombus are also important and should be described.

15. How does the degree of coronary artery stenosis affect coronary blood flow both at rest and with maximal vasodilatation?

Under resting conditions, progressive reduction of vessel luminal diameter does not reduce resting coronary blood flow until the vessel luminal diameter is approximately 90% stenosed. A normal distal coronary artery bed is able to dilate and increase coronary blood flow to about four to five times its resting value. This is a normal coronary flow reserve and can be achieved during maximal vasodilation, such as occurs with maximal exercise and pharmacologic stress (e.g., IV adenosine or dipyridamole). A 50% reduction in luminal diameter will prevent a coronary vessel from achieving this normal four- to fivefold increase in coronary blood flow during maximal vasodilation. For this reason, a ≥ 75% reduction in coronary luminal diameter is considered "significant."

16. Additional procedures in the cardiac catheterization laboratory are performed in select clinical conditions. List several procedures and their indications.

PROCEDURE	INDICATION
Serial blood sampling to measure percent oxygenation at different points in the circulation	Determination of cardiac output (Fick method) Assessment of intracardiac shunting
Measurement of oxygen consumption	Determination of pulmonary and systemic cardiac output by the Fick method
Right ventricular endomyocardial biopsy	Monitoring of antirejection therapy in patients with heart or heart-lung transplantation
Pericardiocentesis	Treatment of cardiac tamponade Diagnostic evaluation of pericardial effusion
Aortography	Assessment of aortic valve competence Assessment of suspected aortic dissection Evaluation of aortic root dilatation Localization of reverse saphenous vein bypass grafts
Coronary artery bypass angiography	Assessment of coronary artery bypass graft patency
Hemodynamic assessment during exercise or pharmacologic intervention	Assessment of valvular heart disease Determination of "reversibility" of pulmonary hypertension

BIBLIOGRAPHY

1. Baims DS, Grossman (eds): Cardiac Catheterization, Angiography, and Interventions, 5th ed. Baltimore, Williams & Wilkins, 1996.

2. Bittl JA, Levin DC: Coronary angiography. In Braunwald E (ed): Heart Disease: A Textbook of Cardiovascular Medicine, 5th ed. Philadelphia, W.B. Saunders, 1997, pp 240–272.
3. Davidson CJ, Fishman RF, Bonow RO: Cardiac catheterization. In Braunwald E (ed): Heart Disease: A Textbook of Cardiovascular Medicine, 5th ed. Philadelphia, W.B. Saunders, 1997, pp 177–203.
4. Franch RH, King SB III, Douglas JS Jr: Techniques of cardiac catheterization including coronary arteriography. In Schlant RC, Alexander RW (eds): Hurst's The Heart, 8th ed. New York, McGraw-Hill, 1994, pp 2381–2418.
5. Gould KL, Kirkeeide RL, Buchi M: Coronary flow reserve as a physiologic measure of stenosis severity. J Am Coll Cardiol 15:459–474, 1990.
6. Hillis DL, Lange RA: Cardiac catheterization. Cardiovasc Rev Rep 11(1):56–74, 1990.
7. Johnson LW, Lozner EC, Johnson S, et al: Coronary arteriography 1984–1987: A report of the Registry of the Society for Cardiac Angiography and Interventions: I. Results and complications. Cathet Cardiovasc Diagn 17:5–10, 1989.
8. Lozner EC, Johnson LW, Johnson S, et al: Coronary arteriography 1984–1987: A report of the Registry of the Society for Cardiac Angiography and Interventions: II. An analysis of 218 deaths related to coronary arteriography. Cathet Cardiovasc Diagn 17:11–14, 1989.
9. Ross J Jr, Brandenburg RO, Dinsmore RE, et al: Guidelines for coronary angiography: A report of the American College of Cardiology/American Heart Association Task Force on assessment of diagnostic and therapeutic cardiovascular procedures (Subcommittee on Coronary Angiography). J Am Coll Cardiol 10:935–950, 1987.

12. PERCUTANEOUS TRANSLUMINAL CORONARY ANGIOPLASTY AND OTHER INTERVENTIONS

Peter Levitt, M.D., and Robert Zaloom, M.D.

1. What are the current indications for coronary angioplasty in single-vessel disease?

Percutaneous transluminal coronary angioplasty (PTCA) is well accepted as an effective nonsurgical treatment for coronary artery disease (CAD). The American College of Cardiology/American Heart Association (ACC/AHA) Task Force on Assessment of Diagnostic and Therapeutic Cardiovascular Procedures has provided guidelines for performing PTCA. In **symptomatic patients** with a significant lesion in a major vessel supplying a large area of viable myocardium, PTCA is indicated if any of the following exist:

- Inducible ischemia on stress testing done on medical therapy
- Intolerance to medical therapy
- Continued anginal symptoms despite medical therapy

In **asymptomatic patients**, PTCA is indicated for single-vessel disease affecting a large area of myocardium if any of the following are present:

- Significant inducible ischemia on stress testing
- Survivor of a near-death episode without a myocardial infarction (MI)
- History of MI with an ischemic stress test
- Planned high-risk noncardiac surgery with objective evidence of ischemia present

2. What are the current indications for coronary angioplasty in multivessel disease?

For **symptomatic patients**, significant lesions should involve each of two major arteries, both supplying moderate areas of viable myocardium, before considering PTCA. Furthermore, there should be objective evidence for ischemia on stress testing, angina unresponsive to maximal medical therapy, and/or intolerance to medications. Lesion characteristics should suggest a moderate to high success rate, and patients should be in a low-risk group for morbidity and mortality from PTCA.

Selection of **asymptomatic patients** with multivessel disease generally depends on the presence of the same conditions for PTCA in asymptomatic patients with single-vessel disease (see Question 1). However, there is the stipulation that a large area of myocardium must be at risk from the diseased vessel. Additional lesions supply small or nonviable regions.

3. How does the AHA/ACC classify lesion-specific characteristics?

Note that with stents, all lesions have a 90–95% success rate. **Type A lesions** are low risk. Their characteristics include:

Discrete lesions (< 10 mm length)	Smooth contour and without calcification
Concentric lesions	Not involving major branches
Readily accessible to angioplasty	Not ostial
Nonangulated	No thrombus present

Type B lesions are moderate risk. Their properties include:

Tubular lesions (10–20 mm in length)	Ostial location
Eccentric lesions	Recent total occlusion (< 3 months)
Moderate angulation	At points of bifurcation (often requiring
Irregular contour	two wires)
Moderate tortuosity of proximal segment to the lesion	Moderately heavy calcification
	Some thrombus present

Type C lesions are high risk. Their characteristics include:

Diffuse lesions (> 2 cm in length)   Chronic total occlusions (> 3 months)
Excess tortuosity of proximal segment   Extremely angulated
Inability to protect major branches   Vein grafts with friable lesions

4. What is the success rate for elective angioplasty?

The primary success rate for elective PTCA now exceeds 90% for most cases. What previously were considered to be risk factors for adverse outcome (i.e., female gender, distal lesions, or anatomy such as circumflex lesions) may no longer be so. Rather, success is more affected by the presence of significant calcification, severe stenosis, and/or thrombus.

5. List the major acute complications of PTCA.

Ischemia, acute coronary artery closure, MI, and death. All of these complications are fairly uncommon now. Their incidence relates to patient selection, lesion type, operator skill, and technology.

6. What causes these complications? How are they managed?

The more common causes of **ischemia** during PTCA are coronary artery dissection and intracoronary artery thrombus. When dissection occurs and ischemia is present, repeat dilation with longer inflations may result in an adequate result.

Repeated **reclosure** should be treated with bailout catheters and surgical revascularization. Newer techniques including intracoronary stenting are useful in this setting to obviate the need for surgery.

Thrombus is a more difficult complication to deal with. Use of IIb/IIIc agents is most promising. Otherwise, bypass surgery may be the preferred treatment, particularly when infarction is likely to ensue.

The risk of death is greatest in the above settings when acute arterial closure occurs and a significant amount of myocardium is at risk. In various studies, mortality from acute closure is greatest with:

Multivessel disease
Female gender
Elderly patients over 70 years old
History of congestive heart failure
Left ventricular dysfunction (ejection fraction < 30%)

7. How often does restenosis occur following angioplasty?

In general, the restenosis rate is approximately 20–30% (12–20% with stenting), and it can be even greater in complex lesions. This process depends on a number of factors which together can cause restenosis. The most important factor is probably elastic recoil of the vessel at the site of the PTCA, which is aided by platelet adhesion and aggregation, as well as thrombus formation. Platelets release factors that aggregate more platelets, activate the clotting system, and cause vasoconstriction. Smooth muscle proliferation at the site of injury also plays a role.

8. List lesion-specific characteristics that promote restenosis after angioplasty.

- Ostial lesions
- Left anterior descending artery lesions over circumflex and right coronary artery lesions
- Saphenous vein graft lesions
- Multivessel disease
- Totally occluded vessels
- Multilesion disease
- Post-PTCA residual stenosis
- Lesions located on bends
- Lesions at points of bifurcation

- Lengthy lesions
- Calcified lesions

9. What are the proposed pathophysiologic mechanisms of PTCA?

The original explanation given by Andreas Gruentzig for enlargement of a vessel lumen by PTCA was compression of plaque, but we now know that this is a minor effect. Also contributing minimally is extrusion of some liquid components from a soft plaque. More important, however, is that PTCA leads to cracking of the intimal plaque with resultant stretching of media and adventitia and expansion of the outer diameter of the vessel. This is apparent on postmortem histologic examination of these vessels.

10. How is PTCA performed when disease occurs at points of bifurcation?

When both branches of a bifurcation of a coronary artery are diseased, angioplasty of one lesion may cause shifting of plaque to the other lesion, resulting in worsening stenosis or occlusion. Thus, to avoid this problem, the operator uses two steerable guidewires simultaneously. The wires are positioned down each limb of the bifurcation and then dilated one at a time. In some instances, two balloons are used and inflated simultaneously. This prevents shifting of plaque from one branch to the other and is known as the ``kissing balloon technique.''

11. Describe the patient risk factors for restenosis following angioplasty.

The restenosis rates are fairly similar for men and women, but slightly higher for men. Other traditional risk factors for atherogenesis seem to be operative after angioplasty as well. Diabetes promotes restenosis, as demonstrated in various studies. Hypertension, however, has not been proved sufficiently to cause restenosis. Continued smoking following PTCA is clearly a major risk factor due to its vasoconstricting effects and platelet-stimulating properties. Variable results have been reported regarding hypercholesterolemia and restenosis, but it does not seem to be a major risk factor. Unstable angina at the time of PTCA is an independent risk factor for restenosis when compared to those with stable symptoms.

12. Name some of the minor complications associated with angioplasty.

- Embolization of plaque constituents, thrombi, calcium, and others (fortunately rare)
- Ventricular fibrillation (usually due to ischemia)
- Loss of branch vessels during PTCA of a main vessel
- Hypotension from bleeding, tamponade, medications, hypovolemia
- Femoral artery complications, e.g., hematoma, pseudoaneurysms, arteriovenous fistulas
- Coronary artery aneurysm at the site of PTCA (rare)

13. Describe interventional devices that can overcome some of the problems of conventional PTCA.

When conventional PTCA results in abrupt closure or restenosis or suboptimal results, these interventional techniques may be preferred:

Intravascular stents are endovascular "splints" used to maintain vascular patency. Different types of stents have been used, but now the balloon expandable ones are preferred. They are useful for reversal of abrupt closure when due to dissection. The most important complication of balloon expandable stents is thrombosis, which is prevented by a vigorous antithrombotic regimen.

Directional coronary atherectomy enlarges the coronary lumen by actually removing plaque by high-speed rotation. It is useful in cases of restenosis, vein graft disease, ulcerated plaque, eccentric lesions, or ostial lesions.

Laser balloon angioplasty applies both heat and pressure to the arterial wall in an attempt to dilate the lumen. This combination may result in desiccation of the thrombus and decreased elastic recoil. *Note:* There is a high restenosis rate with this technique, and it is rarely used.

BIBLIOGRAPHY

1. American College of Cardiology/American Heart Association Ad Hoc Task Force on Cardiac Catheterization: ACC/AHA guidelines for cardiac catheterization and cardiac catheterization laboratories. J Am Coll Cardiol 81:1149–1182, 1998.
2. Ellis SG, De Cesare NB, Pinkerton CA, et al: Relation of stenosis morphology and clinical presentation to the procedural results of directional coronary atherectomy.Circulation 84:644–653, 1991.
3. George B, et al: Multicenter investigation of coronary stenting to treat acute or threatened closure after percutaneous transluminal coronary angioplasty: Clinical and angiographic outcomes. J Am Coll Cardiol 22:135–143, 1993.
4. Gibbons RJ, Holmes DR, Reeder GS, et al: Immediate angioplasty compared with the administration of a thrombolytic agent followed by conservative treatment for myocardial infarction. N Engl J Med. 328:685–691, 1993.
5. Grines CI, Browne KF, Marco J, et al: A comparison of immediate angioplasty what thrombolytic therapy for acute myocardial infarction. N Engl J Med 328:673–679, 1993.
6. Grossman W, Baim DS (eds): Cardiac Catheterization, Angiography, and Intervention. Philadelphia, Lea & Febiger, 1992.
7. National Heart, Lung, and Blood Institute Balloon Valvuloplasty Registry Participants: Multicenter experience with balloon mitral commissurotomy: NHLBI Balloon Valvuloplasty Registry report on immediate and 30-day follow-up results. Circulation 85:448–461, 1992.
8. Zijlestra F, De Boer MJ, Hoorntje KCA, et al: A comparison of immediate coronary angioplasty with intravenous streptokinase in acute myocardial infarction. N Engl J Med 328:680–684, 1993.

13. ELECTRON BEAM TOMOGRAPHY

James E. Ehrlich, M.D.

1. What is electron beam tomography (EBT) scanning technology? What are its applications in cardiology?

EBT (also called electron beam computed tomography [EBCT] or ultrafast CT) employs a 5th generation CT scanner with ultrafast acquisition speeds specifically designed for cardiac imaging. Electronically gated for cardiac studies, large 3D data sets can be acquired during a single breath-hold with high temporal and spatial resolution (see figure). The most frequent applications of EBT include the **coronary artery scan** for individual risk assessment in asymptomatic individuals and **electron beam angiography** (intravenous, noninvasive CT coronary angiography) in patients with symptoms. In addition, the technology can be used for intracardiac structural and functional analysis, including myocardial perfusion imaging, wall thickness determinations, valvular imaging, and coronary "fly-through" examinations.

Left, Electron beam angiography of a saphenous vein coronary bypass graft. *Right,* Conventional (invasive) angiography of the same graft. (Images courtesy of Dr. Achenbach, University of Erlangen, Germany)

2. What is the essential purpose of coronary imaging in preventive cardiology?

The noninvasive EBT coronary artery scan represents the only extensively validated noninvasive method to identify and quantify **coronary calcium**, a recognized marker for preclinical coronary atherosclerosis. Clinicians integrate this measure of **plaque burden** with conventional risk factor assessment to influence the need and aggressiveness of cardioprotective therapies in a primary prevention setting. The procedure is used to detect early plaque and mildly obstructive coronary disease, a far more prevalent precursor to acute coronary events than the "significantly" stenotic lesions detectable by stress tests. An asymptomatic individual with a high coronary artery calcium score (CACS) has evidence of substantial subclinical coronary disease and should be considered for intense risk factor modification—therapy usually reserved for survivors of previous cardiac events (i.e., secondary National Cholesterol Education Program guidelines). *See Case #1,* top of next page.

3. What is the significance of coronary calcium and the coronary artery calcium score?

Coronary calcium deposition appears to be an actively regulated process, similar to bone formation, that occurs in many phases of coronary atherosclerosis. It may represent an attempt to stabilize plaque. **Histopathologic studies** prove that it tracks atherosclerosis consistently, generally comprising about 20% of total plaque burden. Calcium typically appears first in the walls of

Case #1: Family history of premature CAD in asymptomatic male

45-year-old, active, asymptomatic male. Father deceased at age 53, ant. MI. No other risk factors. Total cholesterol = 200, LDL = 140, HDL = 34. Patient does not meet NCEP guidelines for drug therapy.

Coronary artery scan by EBCT:

Reveals 3-vessel (LAD, RCA, circumflex) coronary calcification with a CACS = 530

Assessment:

Extensive multivessel preclinical atherosclerosis, high risk for premature symptomatic CAD. Moderate risk for underlying coronary obstruction.

Plan:

a) Further lipid characterization (Lp(a), homocyst., small dense LDL, etc.)

b) Plaque stabilization (2° guidelines) with stains +/or niacin depending on lipoprotein profile; ASA Rx.

c) Stress imaging for further risk stratification and to rule out occult ischemia

d) Recommend siblings for EBCT

e) Re-check EBCT in 2 years for evidence of plaque stabilization/regression

coronary arteries, years or decades before angiographic lumenal changes are discernible. Therefore, correlations with invasive intravascular ultrasound (depicting both wall and lumen abnormalities) are close.

With progressively higher CACSs (see figure, next page), the likelihood of obstructive coronary artery disease (CAD) also increases non-linearly, and the stronger correlations with invasive **angiography** can be appreciated best by examining calcium "cutpoints." Impressively, outcome studies depicting the **prognostic significance** of a high absolute coronary score (and a high percentage score relative to age/sex) demonstrate a very powerful predictive capability of the calcium score compared to any conventional risk factor. This is consistent with previous analyses by Gofman demonstrating that events increase appreciably as the magnitude of atherosclerosis exceeds certain thresholds.

4. Why do an expensive test? Can't the astute clinician predict who is at risk in his/her practice?

Approximately 50% of heart attacks occur in persons with no prior history of coronary disease. A total cholesterol of < 200 occurs in 35% of people who have sustained MIs. Traditional risk factor assessment is suitable for population analysis but frequently mischaracterizes the **individual**, accounting for only one-third of the clinical variability in risk. Millions will develop clinical

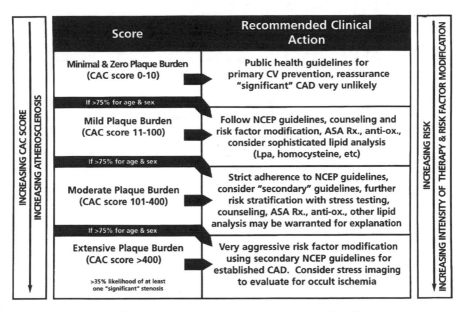

Score	Recommended Clinical Action
Minimal & Zero Plaque Burden (CAC score 0-10)	**Public health guidelines for primary CV prevention, reassurance "significant" CAD very unlikely**
If >75% for age & sex	
Mild Plaque Burden (CAC score 11-100)	**Follow NCEP guidelines, counseling and risk factor modification, ASA Rx., anti-ox., consider sophisticated lipid analysis (Lpa, homocysteine, etc)**
If >75% for age & sex	
Moderate Plaque Burden (CAC score 101-400)	**Strict adherence to NCEP guidelines, consider "secondary" guidelines, further risk stratification with stress testing, counseling, ASA Rx., anti-ox., other lipid analysis may be warranted for explanation**
If >75% for age & sex	
Extensive Plaque Burden (CAC score >400) *>35% likelihood of at least one "significant" stenosis*	**Very aggressive risk factor modification using secondary NCEP guidelines for established CAD. Consider stress imaging to evaluate for occult ischemia**

INCREASING CAC SCORE / INCREASING ATHEROSCLEROSIS

INCREASING RISK / INCREASING INTENSITY OF THERAPY & RISK FACTOR MODIFICATION

Matching the intensity of preventive therapy to the cardiac risk.

coronary disease with an insufficient number of risk factors (e.g., only a family history, as in Case #1) to meet NCEP guideline criteria for directed therapy. Others will be identified by guidelines as suitable candidates for lifelong statin therapy, but in fact, have no evidence of plaque to stabilize. EBT scanning more precisely stratifies the at-risk individual.

5. Won't a stress test detect the high-risk, asymptomatic individual?

Occasionally. Stress tests become positive when there is a significant obstruction to coronary blood flow (ischemia). However, it is now known that **68% of MIs occur from lesions that are not significantly obstructive**. This accounts for the common observation that sudden coronary events occur after a normal treadmill test. Stress tests are more helpful in symptomatic patients and can be useful for functional and exercise assessments in the asymptomatic.

6. Lots of patients have positive EBT tests, while other cardiac exams (e.g., stress, angiograms) are normal. Are false positives common?

A coronary artery scan is a very sensitive and specific (almost 100%) measure of calcified plaque and is only moderately specific (depending on score and number of vessels) for obstructive disease determined by stress testing and angiography. There are virtually no false positives for plaque itself, which is the lesion of interest in asymptomatics. Plaque burden by EBT has been shown to reflect the angiographic extent of disease better than stress tests. However, it has been established that many individuals can accomodate substantial amounts of plaque without showing significant obstruction (Glagov phenomenon of compensatory vessel enlargement). To a cardiologist who equates "real" coronary disease with significant obstruction detected by traditional tests, coronary scores by EBT will frequently appear to be false positives.

7. How predictive is the coronary artery calcium score by EBT?

The CACS should be examined in terms of prediction (or an odds ratio) of future coronary events, currrent angiographic obstruction, and presence of silent ischemia demonstrated by stress imaging modalities. There is some disagreement about the magnitude of the incremental "event-predictive" capabilities of an EBT-derived calcium score beyond risk factors in various populations. However, it has become clear that the presence and amount of calcium (by absolute and relative scores) is more highly predictive of future events among apparently healthy individuals than are risk factors. In addition, up to 45% of asymptomatic individuals with extensive plaque (CACS > 400) can be demonstrated to have a positive SPECT thallium test (silent ischemia). Finally, EBT coronary scanning offers improved discrimination over risk factors for the presence of angiographically demonstrated coronary disease.

8. **What are the major controversies and misconceptions surrounding coronary imaging?**
   • **Stable vs. unstable plaque:** EBT imaging detects the calcified portion of plaque, which may, in fact, commonly represent stable plaque. Proponents of the technology have advanced the concept that the calcified portion merely represents the atherosclerotic "tip of the iceberg," raising concern for the unstable "company it keeps" statistically. The higher the amounts of calcified plaque, the more total (stable and unstable) plaque is likely to be present. Outcome studies bear out the premise that EBT can identify the vulnerable patient, regardless of its inability to directly measure vulnerable plaque.
   • **Events can occur in patients with zero scores:** Detractors of EBT correctly point out that an MI can occur in a patient with no evidence of coronary calcium. Coronary disease is complex, as some events may arise predominantly from a thrombogenic mechanism with purely soft plaque present. However, as the overwhelming majority of events occur in patients with coronary calcium (especially above average amounts), the presence of substantial calcium is regarded as an opportunity to direct clinical interventions to confirmed high-risk individuals.
   • **Coronary exams as a screen for self-referreds:** There is widespread concern about whether the individual should be able to undergo a cardiac screening test independent of the recommendation of a physician. In addition, advertising such availability is controversial nationwide. Proponents of self-referral believe that the purpose of screening is to protect middle-aged individuals who are unexpectedly at risk for the nation's number one killer. Marketing of protective screening reflects a belief that preventive testing is often neglected by physicians in a managed care environment.
   • **Coronary scanning inevitably leads to unnecessary further testing:** There is currently no evidence for this claim, which has been levied by some cardiologists without personal experience in the field. As the roles and limitations of all cardiac tests are more widely appreciated, it will become clear that the test leads to a more rational use of other cardiac modalities. For example, asymptomatics with very high scores will need to undergo a stress test to determine the physiologic significance of the disease . . . some will be determined to have ischemia. On the other hand, a coronary scan has been shown to be a very cost-effective first test for patients with "atypical" chest symptoms, because the absence of calcium on EBT weighs strongly against further expensive testing.

9. **Other than for risk stratification, is it worth identifying people with early non-obstructive atherosclerosis?**
   Large lipid intervention trials have convincingly demonstrated the value of aggressive risk-factor modification even for **populations** with relatively normal cholesterol (as was proven by the AFCAPS/TexCAPS study). Atherosclerosis can be slowed, stopped, or even reversed with aggressive medical strategies, but the challenge has been a more cost-effective targeting of expensive medications to the **individuals** at "true risk." Statins lower event rates by mechanisms that include plaque stabilization. For the asymptomatic person, the test helps the clinician decide whether simple public health strategies (lifestyle choices) are adequate or if a clinical approach (medications, etc.) is necessary. For patients with high plaque burden and no conventional risk factor explanation, sophisticated blood testing is often advised in a search for more novel causes of occult coronary disease. Recent studies have verified that statins applied to individuals with EBT-proven plaque results in an overall decrease in progression of the disease (with frequent cases of reversal), leading to optimism that EBT imaging can be used as a surrogate for monitoring the success of therapeutic interventions.

10. How can EBT imaging be used in the symptomatic patient?

EBT is a cost-effective first test in symptomatic patients who have a low to moderate "pretest" likelihood for coronary obstruction (e.g., atypical chest pain). Because the test is so sensitive for plaque, a zero (or minimal) calcium plaque burden implies a low likelihood for significant fixed obstruction and may quickly prompt the clinician to consider non-coronary causes of chest symptoms. However, the test should be regarded as only one piece of the diagnostic puzzle; it does not substitute for a complete examination. A patient with classic angina should undergo more traditional testing directly, without an EBT exam. Because of its high negative predictive value for obstruction, a zero calcium score in a patient with an equivocal stress test may signal a false-positive stress test, whereas a very high score may prompt further investigation, including angiography. Intelligent use of EBT imaging can avoid unnecessary angiography for some, and allow confident expectation of abnormal findings in others. *See Case #2*.

Case #2: Low-risk symptomatic female with chest pain history

52-year-old, anxious female with two episodes of chest pain, considered to be panic attacks by her physician. Lab testing and EKG normal. Previous admission to hospital to rule out MI was unrevealing of heart disease. Stress testing has been equivocal. Patient is being considered for a stress echo.

Coronary artery scan by EBCT:

CACS = 0

Assessment:

No evidence of calcified coronary atherosclerosis. Chest pain episodes unlikely to represent fixed coronary obstructive disease.

Plan:

Search for noncardiac causes, including panic reaction.

---

11. Which patients should be considered for a coronary scan?

- **Asymptomatic**, middle-aged men and women with one or more additional risk factors to help the clinician make a decision about the intensity of risk factor modification or provide advice and reassurance. Serial exams to examine progression at suitable intervals.
- **Symptomatic** patients with atypical presentations or who have a low to moderate pretest likelihood for ischemia, to help decide whether a coronary origin is likely.
- **Screening** of middle-aged consumers with few if any risk factors, to look for unexpected disease or for reassurance (not cost-effective, normally self-pay).

Indications-Patient Groups	Goals of Testing
1. Screen in low-moderate risk asymptomatics (Male 35-65, female 45-70)	1. Detect occult atherosclerosis. Decide upon clinical (pharmacologic) risk reduction vs. public health approach
2. Targeted decision making in high risk asymptomatic (e.g., diabetic, or elevated cholesterol)	2. Verify need for aggressive therapy
3. Family members of pt. with premature CAD	3. Determine which 1st degree relatives need preventive therapy and counseling. Search for novel risk factors in family
4. Preop. assessment in high risk pt. undergoing noncardiac surgery	4. Determine appropriateness of surgery, need for cardioprotective medicine perioperatively and need for advanced monitoring
5. Pt. with chest pain or symptoms with low to moderate pretest likelihood for ischemia	5. R/O CAD vs. noncardiac causes. Guide to further testing
6. Pt. with equivocal stress test result	6. Help establish true vs. false positive. Reduce rate of unnecessary angiography
7. Pt. with known systemic disease with potential coronary effects (e.g. hypertension, diabetes)	7. Risk stratification, influence intensity of therapy and risk factor modification – monitor progression
8. Pt. treated with cholesterol lowering drug	8. Monitor progression vs. regression of atherosclerosis to determine drug efficacy
9. Pt. with established CAD (MI, hx of CABG or angioplasty)	9. Under guidance of doctor, serial EBCT to determine if disease is progressing on therapy. Not useful as single scan to establish diagnosis of CAD
10. Pt. with cardiomyopathy - cause unknown	10. Help determine ischemic vs. nonischemic etiology simply and safely
11. Post-menopausal asymptomatic female	11. Help in decisions concerning hormone therapy

Patient selection for EBT.

12. What are the limitations of the test? In which groups is the EBT scan of coronary arteries of less value?

A simple coronary scan can determine anatomy—the amount and distribution of coronary calcium, pericardial abnormalities, etc.—but cannot directly determine coronary blockage, nor the physiologic effects of such blockage. There are also groups in which the test could be misleading or may not add incremental value such as:

• **Young adults**, unless there is a family history of early CAD or the patient has, for example, diabetes or significant familial hypercholesterolemia. Few young adults show coronary calcification yet, so the absence of calcium could be falsely reassuring.
• **Older senior citizens**, unless a physician is specifically planning to make a clinical decision based upon the score (e.g., patient prefers not to be treated with statins, and the clinician would like to confirm a suitably low plaque burden). The prevalence of atherosclerosis is high in this group, and the test rarely changes management.
• Most patients with **established coronary disease** (history of MI, angioplasty, bypass). The coronary scan will confirm the presence of plaque, a finding that should be expected. The value of serial scans in determining disease progression in vessels is unclear.
• Very high-risk patients, when the clinician has decided to treat aggressively, regardless of a coronary score. For example, some physicians routinely treat all diabetics as having a "CAD-equivalent," and use secondary NCEP guidelines.

13. What is electron beam angiography (EBA)? What are its best uses?

CT coronary angiography or EBA is a relatively noninvasive approach to cardiac testing approved in November 1999. By injecting contrast dye in an antecubital vein and following specific scanning protocols, images of the coronary arteries and lumens are obtained after 3D reconstruction with an advanced workstation. EBA shows great promise as an alternative to invasive cardiac catheterizations in diagnostic situations where the likelihood for surgical intervention is low. In addition, many centers are performing post-CABG and post-angioplasty EBA assessments in patients with symptoms after their revascularizations.

BIBLIOGRAPHY

1. Achenbach S, Moshage W, Bachmann K: Noninvasive coronary angiography by contrast-enhanced electron beam computed tomography. Clin Cardiology 21:323–330, 1998.
2. Arad Y, Guerci AD, et al: Predictive value of electron beam computed tomography of the coronary arteries: 19 month follow-up of 1173 asymptomatic subjects. Circulation 93:1951–1953, 1996.
3. Baumgart D, Schmermund A, et al: Comparison of electron beam computed tomography with intracoronary ultrasound and coronary angiography for detection of coronary atherosclerosis. J Am Coll Cardiol 30:57–64, 1997.
4. Budoff MJ, Georgiou D, Brody AS, et al: Ultrafast computed tomography as a diagnostic modality in the detection of coronary artery disease: a multicenter study. Circulation 93:898–904, 1996.
5. Callister TQ, Raggi P, et al: Effect of HMG-CoA reductase inhibitors on coronary artery disease as assessed by electron beam computed tomography. New Engl J Med 339:1972–1978, 1998.
6. He, Zuo-Xiang, Roberts R, Mahmarian JJ, et al: Severity of coronary calcification by electron beam computed tomography predicts silent myocardial ischemia. Circulation 101:244–251, 2000.
7. Janowitz W, Agatston AS, Kaplan G, Viamonte M Jr: Differences in prevalence and extent of coronary artery calcium detected by ultrafast computed tomography in asymptomatic men and women. Am J Cardiol 72:247–254, 1993.
8. Kaufman R, Sheedy PF, Maher JE, et al: Quantity of coronary artery calcium detected by electron beam computed tomography in asymptomatic patients and angiographically studied patients. Mayo Clinic Proc 70:223–232, 1995.
9. Laudon DA, Rumberger JA, Sheedy PF, et al: Use of electron beam computed tomography in the evaluation of chest pain patients in the emergency department. Ann Emerg Med 33:15–21, 1999.
10. Mautner GC, Mautner SL, Froehlich J, et al: Coronary artery calcification: assessment with electron beam CT and histomorphometric correlation. Radiology 192:619–623, 1994.
11. Raggi P, Callister TQ, et al: Evaluation of chest pain in patients with low to intermediate pretest probability of coronary artery disease by electron beam computed tomography. Am J Cardiol 85:283–288, 2000.
12. Raggi P, Callister TQ, et al: Identification of patients at increased risk of first unheralded acute myocardial infarction by electron beam computed tomography. Circulation 101:850–855, 2000.
13. Rumberger JA, Behrenbeck T, Breen JF, Sheedy PF: Coronary calcification by electron beam computed tomography and obstructive coronary disease: A model for costs and effectiveness of diagnosis as compared with conventional cardiac testing methods. J Am Coll Cardiol 33:453–462, 1999.
14. Rumberger JA, Brundage BH, Rader DJ, Kondos G: Electron beam computed tomographic coronary calcium scanning: A review and guidelines for use in asymptomatic persons. Mayo Clinic Proc 74:243–252, 1999.
15. Rumberger JA, Sheedy PF, Breen JF, Schwartz RA: Electron beam computed tomographic coronary calcium cutpoints and severity of associated lumen stenosis. J Am Coll Cardiol 29:1542–1548, 1997.
16. Shavelle DM, Budoff MJ, Brundage BH, et al: Exercise testing and electron beam computed tomography in the evaluation of coronary artery disease. J Am Coll Cardiol 36:32–38, 2000.

III. Arrhythmias

14. SUPRAVENTRICULAR TACHYCARDIAS

Kimberly A. Schleman, M.D., and Stuart W. Adler, M.D.

1. What is the most common supraventricular arrhythmia?

Excluding simple atrial premature depolarizations, atrial fibrillation (AF) is the most commonly encountered supraventricular arrhythmia. Its incidence rises with increasing age for men and women, with an estimated prevalence of 5% at age 75 and 15% at age 85. As many as 1–2 million Americans are estimated to have AF.

2. List the routine evaluations to be done in patients newly diagnosed with AF.

Look for a precipitating cause, such as thyrotoxicosis, valvular disease, pulmonary emboli, pericarditis, coronary ischemia, or recent alcohol abuse. For most patients, obtain an echocardiogram and TSH levels. Cardiac enzymes can be assessed and a V/Q scan done if clinically indicated.

3. What cardiovascular diseases are likely to coexist in patients with AF?

Hypertensive heart disease is the most common pre-existing condition. However, congestive heart failure (CHF), rheumatic heart disease, nonrheumatic valvular heart disease, chronic lung disease, coronary artery disease, and thyrotoxicosis are other strong risk factors. Patients without identifiable cardiovascular disease or other conditions associated with AF—an estimated 3–25% of all patients with chronic AF—are said to have "lone atrial fibrillation."

4. Which agents are effective in slowing the ventricular response in acute AF?

Although frequently used as a first-line drug, **digoxin** is much less effective in acute rate control than other drugs. The onset of action for digoxin is slow, and it exerts its acute rate-slowing effects largely by an indirect vagotonic activity. Although digoxin may provide adequate rate control for elderly, sedentary patients, its effect is minimal in patients who are active and increase their circulating catecholamine levels with exercise throughout the day. Digoxin continues to be a first-line agent for rate control in patients with CHF or impaired left ventricular (LV) function.

In contrast to digoxin, intravenous **diltiazem** (bolus of 10–20 mg and maintenance of 5–15 mg/hr) has an onset of action within minutes. Intravenous **beta blockers** (esmolol drip or IV lopressor 2.5–5 mg IV followed by oral dosing) are also effective and are the treatment of choice in AF associated with elevated catecholamine levels (i.e., postoperative patients). Note, however, that beta blockers and calcium channel blockers may precipitate hypotension or CHF—use caution in patients with LV dysfunction. IV diltiazem tends to be less associated with hypotension than IV verapamil, another calcium channel blocker.

5. What techniques are used to evaluate heart rate in patients with chronic AF?

It's important to assess the efficacy of long-term rate control therapy. The use of **24-hour Holter monitoring** allows for the assessment of ventricular response during the activities of daily living. The formal, graded **exercise treadmill test** yields information about the rate of rise for the ventricular response as well as peak heart rate at maximal exercise. Both forms of evaluation are helpful in establishing the efficacy of chronic medical therapy.

6. Can thromboembolic risk in patients with AF be predicted from clinical variables? Echocardiographic variables?

Yes, and yes. The risk of stroke in patients with chronic AF (nonvalvular) is approximately 4–5% per year. The Stroke Prevention in Atrial Fibrillation (SPAF) trial, as well as earlier studies (Copenhagen Atrial Fibrillation Trial; Canadian Atrial Fibrillation Anticoagulation Study; and Boston Area Anticoagulation Trial in Atrial Fibrillation [BAATAF]) suggest that a history of hypertension, CHF, and previous stroke all are significant clinical predictors of stroke in patients with chronic AF. Additional clinical risk factors may include age > 65 years and diabetes.

The echocardiographic findings in BAATAF and SPAF and in the Veterans Affairs atrial fibrillation study identified LV dysfunction as the single most important predictor of stroke. The SPAF study also showed that left atrial size predicted the combined endpoint of stroke and systemic emboli. Additionally, mitral stenosis, a prosthetic mitral valve, and rheumatic heart disease all appear to be associated with increased risk of stroke.

7. Are warfarin and aspirin effective in reducing the risk of systemic embolism?

Many randomized studies have addressed this question. These studies have all demonstrated efficacy of warfarin therapy, with stroke risk reduction of approximately 60% in treated patients. The level of anticoagulation varied (target international normalized ratio [INR] was 1.5–4.2), and no increased benefit appeared when more aggressive anticoagulation was used. In two studies, aspirin (80 or 325 mg/day) reduced the risk of thromboembolism by approximately 35%. Warfarin is also superior to low-dose warfarin (INR 1.2–1.5) with aspirin.

In patients with lone AF (see Question 3), i.e., those who have no history of hypertension, diabetes, or cardiac structural abnormality, who are under the age of 65, the risk of stroke is low enough (1–2% per year) that aspirin is the treatment of choice.

8. In patients with chronic AF, does the benefit of anticoagulation outweigh the risk of bleeding?

Yes. The risk of a serious bleeding complication while on warfarin therapy (with an INR goal of 2–3) is 1.3–2.5% per year. Although the elderly (older than 74 years) were shown to have a greater risk of bleeding (4.2% per year in the SPAF II trial), they also carry a greater risk of stroke, and therefore benefited the most from warfarin therapy in terms of stroke reduction.

9. Does paroxysmal AF (intermittent) carry the same risk of thromboembolism as chronic AF?

Yes. The BAATAF study showed similar rates of thromboembolism with both types of AF. Both types should be anticoagulated long term. Note, however, that this issue remains controversial.

10. When should cardioversion be considered to convert a patient from AF to sinus rhythm?

When the patient has new-onset AF that is < 48 hours in duration. If the duration is > 48 hours or unknown, the patient needs to be anticoagulated 3 weeks before and 4 weeks after cardioversion to prevent thromboembolism. Or, a patient can undergo transesophageal echocardiography to rule out left atrial thrombus and, if negative, proceed with cardioversion.

11. When should antiarrhythmic therapy be used to maintain sinus rhythm long term and prevent AF recurrence?

Whether it is preferable to treat AF long term with rate-controlling medications or with antiarrhythmic therapy to maintain sinus rhythm is still an unanswered question. The Atrial Fibrillation Follow-up Investigation of Rhythm Management (AFFIRM) trial that is currently underway will address this. Patients with heart failure or rapid ventricular rates not easily controlled by medications can substantially improve their systolic function when kept in sinus rhythm, since they have the addition of an "atrial kick" and a slower heart rate—both of which contribute to improved cardiac output.

The antiarrhythmics most commonly used have been Class III (e.g., sotalol, amiodarone), Class Ic such as propafenone, and Class Ia (e.g., quinidine, procainamide). Quinidine and procainamide have fallen out of favor because of safety concerns. Two studies have suggested increased mortality, potentially due to sudden death in patients treated with quinidine specifically or class Ia agents generally. The Class Ic (e.g., propafenone) and Class III drugs also have a rate control effect when the patient is in AF.

12. What is a paroxysmal supraventricular tachycardia (PSVT)?

PSVT is a broad label that encompasses arrhythmias of several different causes. The most common is **AV node reentry tachycardia**, which manifests as a regular, narrow QRS complex tachycardia with heart rates that vary widely, but usually run between 160–180 bpm. Typically, the P wave is "buried" within the QRS complex and not readily visible. If it *is* visible, the P wave vector is negative in the inferior leads, and it usually follows the QRS complex by < 80 msec. P waves that follow the QRS by > 80 msec typically are seen in reentry tachycardias using a bypass tract.

The second most common form of PSVT is **AV reentry tachycardia**, which is due to an accessory connection between the atrium and ventricle. **Wolff-Parkinson-White syndrome** is an example of this. The accessory connection allows for a reentrant circuit, which uses the AV node for one limb and the accessory pathway for the other limb.

13. What maneuvers and medications are effective in terminating regular, narrow QRS complex PSVT?

Vagal stimulation (Valsalva maneuver or carotid sinus massage) may affect the tachycardia and, in some cases, bring about termination. These maneuvers can slow or transiently interrupt conduction through the AV node, thereby disturbing the reentry circuit and stopping the tachycardia.

Several intravenous medications also can be used to terminate sustained supraventricular tachycardias by achieving the same result in the AV node. Intravenous adenosine (6–12 mg), verapamil (5–10 mg), diltiazem (20–25 mg), and esmolol (0.5 mg/kg) are all effective in slowing and/or blocking AV node conduction and thereby terminating the tachycardia. It is useful to record the rhythm during these maneuvers or drug administration, as the tracings can provide insight into the tachycardia mechanism.

14. What is the delta wave in patients with the Wolff-Parkinson-White (WPW) syndrome?

The delta wave represents the portion of ventricular muscle that is activated before normal ventricular activation via the His-Purkinje system. Depending on the location of the accessory connection and the conduction of the AV node at a given time, the delta wave may be more or less apparent. Patients with WPW can have a normal EKG without visible delta waves.

The delta wave is manifest in the first portion of the QRS, and the vector may be positive (upright), negative (pseudo-Q wave), or isoelectric (inapparent), depending on the location of the accessory connection. The delta wave vector on the 12-lead EKG is frequently helpful in making a first approximation of the accessory connection location.

15. Is there a treatment of choice for patients with WPW syndrome who present in AF?

These patients typically have a bizarre-looking EKG, with an irregularly irregular wide complex tachycardia. The QRS width varies, depending on how much of the impulse travels down the AV node versus the accessory pathway. In these patients, any drugs that slow conduction through the AV node (calcium channel blockers, adenosine, beta blockers, digoxin) *must be avoided*. These drugs paradoxically accelerate the ventricular response by increasing the conduction down the accessory pathway, thereby making a stable patient become unstable. Furthermore, drug-induced hypotension may result in increased catecholamine release, which can enhance accessory pathway conduction. This is the clinical setting in which ventricular fibrillation is most likely to occur.

If the patient is hemodynamically stable, intravenous procainamide is the drug of choice, as it slows accessory pathway conduction and may also convert the atrial fibrillation to sinus rhythm. Unstable patients require immediate direct-current cardioversion.

16. What about long-term management of WPW?

If a patient has evidence of pre-excitation on EKG, i.e., delta waves, but no history of tachyarrhythmias, then no electrophysiologic study or treatment is necessary. If a patient has had tachyarrhythmias, then either pharmacologic therapy should be initiated or radiofrequency ablation performed.

For long-term management, beta blockers and calcium channel blockers *can* be used. They prolong conduction time and increase refractoriness in the AV node. This should prevent the tachycardia from achieving rapid ventricular rates, and may even prevent the tachycardia from continuing indefinitely. Digoxin should not be used, as it has variable effects on the accessory pathway conduction.

Ablation should be performed in patients that fail drug therapy or present with a hemodynamically unstable tachycardia.

17. How is SVT with aberrancy distinguished from ventricular tachycardia (VT)?

When a patient presents with a wide-complex tachycardia, try to obtain a 12-lead EKG to help distinguish between different types of SVT and VT. Patients with SVT with aberrant conduction typically have a wide QRS complex that manifests as either a right or left bundle branch block pattern, with typical characteristics for bundle branch block seen on EKG. If AV dissociation is seen, (P waves march through at a constant rate with variable relationship to the QRS complex), the rhythm is VT.

A good rule of thumb: if the patient is known to have LV dysfunction or a history of myocardial infarction (MI), the rhythm is VT until proven otherwise.

18. Do vital signs or symptoms help distinguish between SVT and VT?

Definitely not. Patients with SVT can be very hypotensive and have syncope, while patients with VT can have only minimal symptoms. Again, if an elderly patient presents with wide complex tachycardia and had a prior MI and an ejection fraction $\leq 40\%$, but looks comfortable, do not assume it is SVT.

19. Does the patient with PSVT require treatment once an episode is terminated?

Except for patients with WPW syndrome in whom there is very rapid conduction over their accessory connection (manifest during AF or electrophysiologic study), most episodes of PSVT are not life-threatening. The frequency of arrhythmia recurrence and the need for medical intervention to terminate episodes influence the decision to treat individual patients. Medical therapies (digoxin, calcium channel blockers, beta blockers, and antiarrhythmic agents) are all associated with relatively high failure rates (often 40% in the first year). Patients with frequent arrhythmia recurrence despite medical therapy should be evaluated by a cardiac electrophysiologist for possible ablation.

20. What is radiofrequency ablation?

Radiofrequency ablation is the delivery of energy (400–500 Hz) via a catheter to create small, discrete burn lesions. Before ablation, the electrophysiologist performs a diagnostic electrophysiologic study to determine the tachycardia mechanism. Then mapping catheters are used to precisely locate the patient's abnormal electrical connection (i.e., the accessory connection in patients with WPW syndrome). The success rate for curing WPW and AV node reentry tachycardia is > 90%.

21. Is there a simple algorithm I can use to figure out the type of SVT?

Yes. Note that this algorithm includes only the most common types of SVT. (See algorithm, next page.)

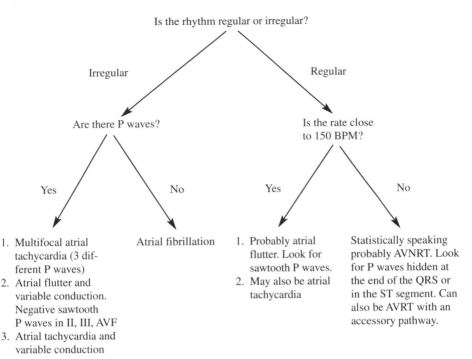

Is the rhythm regular or irregular?

Irregular

Regular

Are there P waves?

Is the rate close
to 150 BPM?

Yes

No

Yes

No

1. Multifocal atrial
tachycardia (3 dif-
ferent P waves)
2. Atrial flutter and
variable conduction.
Negative sawtooth
P waves in II, III, AVF
3. Atrial tachycardia and
variable conduction

Atrial fibrillation

1. Probably atrial
flutter. Look for
sawtooth P waves.
2. May also be atrial
tachycardia

Statistically speaking
probably AVNRT. Look
for P waves hidden at
the end of the QRS or
in the ST segment. Can
also be AVRT with an
accessory pathway.

AVNRT = AV node reentry tachycardia

BIBLIOGRAPHY

1. Antman EM, Beamer AD, Cantillon C, et al: Therapy of refractory symptomatic AF and atrial flutter: A staged care approach with new antiarrhythmic drugs. J Am Coll Cardiol 15:698, 1990.
2. The Atrial Fibrillation Investigators: Echocardiographic Predictors of Stroke in Patients with Atrial Fibrillation: A Prospective Study of 1066 Patients From 3 Clinical Trials. Arch Intern Med 158:1316, 1998.
3. The Boston Area Anticoagulation Trial for AF Investigators: The effect of low-dose warfarin on the risk of stroke in patients with nonrheumatic AF. N Engl J Med 323:1505, 1990.
4. Connelly SJ, Laupacis A, Gent M, et al: Canadian AF Study (CAFA). J Am Coll Cardiol 18:349, 1991.
4a. Ezekowitz MD, Bridgers SL, James KE: Warfarin in the prevention of stroke associated with non-rheumatic atrial fibrillation. Veterans Affairs Stroke Prevention in Nonrheumatic Atrial Fibrillation Investigation. N Engl J Med 327(20):1406–1412, 1992.
5. Falk RH, Podrid PJ (eds): AF: Mechanisms and Management. New York, Raven Press, 1992.
6. Jackman WM, Wang X, Friday KJ, et al: Catheter ablation of accessory atrioventricular pathways (Wolff-Parkinson-White syndrome) by radiofrequency current. N Engl J Med 324:1605, 1991.
7. Jackman WM, Beckman KJ, McClelland JH, et al: Treatment of supraventricular tachycardia due to atri-oventricular nodal reentry by radiofrequency catheter ablation of slow pathway conduction. N Engl J Med 327:313, 1992.
8. Kay GN, Chong F, Epstein AE, et al: Radiofrequency ablation for treatment of primary atrial tachycar-dias. J Am Coll Cardiol 21:901, 1993.
9. Pritchett E: Management of atrial fibrillation. N Engl J Med 326:1264, 1992.
10. Scheinman MM, Olgin JE: Comparison of high energy direct current and radiofrequency catheter abla-tion of the atrioventricular junction. J Am Coll Cardiol 21:557, 1993.
11. The Stroke Prevention in Atrial Fibrillation Investigators: Predictors of thromboembolism in atrial fibril-lation: I. Clinical features of patients at risk. Ann Intern Med 116:1, 1992.
12. The Stroke Prevention in AF Investigators: Predictors of thromboembolism in atrial fibrillation: II. Echocardiographic features of patients at risk. Ann Intern Med 116:6, 1992.
13. The Stroke Prevention in Atrial Fibrillation Investigators: Warfarin versus aspirin for prevention of thromboembolism in atrial fibrillation: Stroke Prevention in Atrial Fibrillation, Study II. Lancet 343:687, 1994.

15. VENTRICULAR TACHYCARDIA

William Bailey, M.D.

1. What is the differential diagnosis of a wide complex tachycardia?
Ventricular tachycardia
Supraventricular tachycardia with aberration
Supraventricular tachycardia using an accessory pathway (Wolff-Parkinson-White syndrome)
Hyperkalemia

2. What are the clinical characteristics of patients with ventricular tachycardia?
The majority of patients with recurrent sustained ventricular tachycardia have a history of ischemic coronary artery disease associated with previous infarction and aneurysm. The next largest group of patients have an underlying congestive or hypertrophic cardiomyopathy. The remainder have a primary electrical disorder (with or without a normal structural heart), valvular disorder, congenital heart disease (repaired or nonrepaired), metabolic disorder, or drug toxicity.

3. What presenting symptoms and features on physical exam may help to make the diagnosis of ventricular tachycardia?
The presenting symptoms of ventricular tachycardia in large part depend on the rate of the rhythm and the extent of underlying cardiac disease. The presenting symptoms can be modulated by coronary artery narrowing, carotid and peripheral vascular disease, ejection fraction, and even relative hydration of the patient. Concomitant medications also may play a role in the initial symptoms. Symptoms vary from minor palpitations, chest heaviness, and light-headedness to frank syncope and cardiac arrest; most patients experience a constellation of symptoms between the two extremes.

The classic findings on physical exam depend on the interrelationship between atrial and ventricular contraction. If the patient is not capable of conducting an electrical impulse retrograde from the ventricle to the atrium, the classic findings of atrioventricular (AV) dissociation are present: variable intensity of the first heart sound, inconsistent relationship between the jugular a wave and the v wave, and occasional cannon a waves when the atrium and the ventricle contract simultaneously. Retrograde conduction is associated with a regularity to the cannon a waves, and the signs of AV dissociation are absent.

4. What three features of the rhythm strip of a wide complex tachycardia establish it as ventricular tachycardia?
The three classic features are fusion beats, capture beats, and AV dissociation. **Fusion beats** are an intermediate form between the wide complex rhythm and the narrow rhythm of sinus and represent simultaneous depolarization of the ventricle by both a supraventricular impulse and an impulse originating in the ventricle. This is best understood by mentally combining the wide ventricular beat with the narrow sinus beat. **Capture beats** are interspersed narrow complex beats that generally occur at a shorter interval than the tachycardia. P waves identical to P waves seen during sinus rhythm may precede. **AV dissociation** is the finding of independent atrial and ventricular activity at differing rates. Careful measurement with calipers shows differing rates for ventricular and atrial rhythms. These findings are uncommon but highly specific. AV dissociation is present in about 25% of patients with ventricular tachycardia, whereas fusion beats and capture beats are found in about 5%.

5. Which electrocardiographic characteristics help to differentiate ventricular tachycardia from supraventricular tachycardia with aberration?

Although rate has been proposed as a potential way to differentiate the two rhythms, it is highly unreliable in individual patients. A QRS width of greater than 140 msec strongly favors ventricular tachycardia, especially in the setting of a normal QRS during sinus rhythm. A leftward QRS axis strongly favors ventricular tachycardia. Concordance (identical QRS direction) in the precordial leads (V_1–V_6), especially negative concordance, is highly specific for the diagnosis of ventricular tachycardia. Certain QRS morphologic features also may be helpful. An atypical right bundle pattern (R > R'; in classic right bundle-branch block, R < R'), a monophasic or biphasic QRS in lead V_1, and a small R wave coupled with a large deep S wave or a Q-S complex in V_6 support the diagnosis of ventricular tachycardia of right bundle branch block morphology. The presence in V_1 of an R wave of > 30 msec, notching of the downstroke of the S wave, a time > 60 msec from the onset of the R wave to the bottom of the S wave, and in lead V_6 the presence of any small Q wave with a large R wave strongly favor the diagnosis of ventricular tachycardia with left bundle branch block morphology. The longest R-S interval also may be measured. The finding of a longest R-S interval in any precordial lead of > 100 msec is highly specific for the diagnosis of ventricular tachycardia.

Slowing or termination of a rhythm with vagal maneuvers strongly supports the diagnosis of supraventricular tachycardia with aberrancy. Clear linkage of the atrial and ventricular rhythm, presence of a classic bundle branch pattern, and a very short R to P interval (time from the onset of the QRS to the next P wave) characterize supraventricular tachycardia with aberrancy.

6. What critical decisions must be made in the management of ventricular tachycardia?

The critical decision in the management of a patient with sustained ventricular tachycardia is the urgency with which to treat the rhythm. In a patient who is hemodynamically stable, treatment should be delayed until a 12-lead electrocardiogram has been obtained. During the delay, a brief medical history and baseline laboratory values can be obtained. Specific attention should be paid to a history of myocardial infarction and potentially proarrhythmic drugs. If you are not sure about a drug, look it up. Levels of potassium and magnesium and appropriate drugs must be checked. Toxicologic screens should be obtained immediately on arrival in the emergency department.

7. Why is it important to obtain a 12-lead electrocardiogram?

The axis and morphology help to make the diagnosis of ventricular tachycardia, as well as shed light on the potential mechanism and origin of the rhythm. For example, a rhythm with a right bundle branch block morphology generally originates from the left ventricle and implies that the rhythm is secondary to ischemic heart disease with scar formation and/or aneurysm. Rhythms with left bundle branch block morphology generally originate from the right ventricle. Once the initial electrocardiographic data are obtained, a decision has to be made about the best way to terminate the rhythm. If there is any question about the patient's stability or if the clinical situation deteriorates, it is best to terminate the rhythm by cardioversion.

8. After the baseline data have been obtained, what method is used to terminate the rhythm?

With any question of hemodynamic instability, termination should be done immediately with synchronized DC electrical cardioversion. Hemodynamic instability is defined as hypotension resulting in shock, congestive heart failure, myocardial ischemia (infarction or angina), or signs or symptoms of inadequate cerebral perfusion. It is important to ensure that the energy is delivered in a synchronized fashion before cardioversion. Failure to do so may introduce the energy in a vulnerable period (into the T wave—late phase 3 in repolarization) and accelerate the rhythm or induce ventricular fibrillation.

Energy levels as low as 10 watt-seconds may be successful, but at the risk of ventricular fibrillation due to incomplete defibrillation of a critical mass of the myocardium sufficient to extinguish the rhythm. It is therefore wise to begin at a level of 100 watt-seconds. If the patient is conscious, adequate intravenous sedation should always be provided.

9. How is hemodynamically stable ventricular tachycardia terminated?

Termination of hemodynamically stable ventricular tachycardia may be attempted medically. Treatment is begun with intravenous lidocaine or procainamide, followed by a maintenance infusion if the drug is successful. Levels of the drug should be checked and used to guide maintenance infusion rates.

Amiodarone may now be administered via intravenous infusion for the termination and prevention of the recurrence of ventricular arrhythmias. Another intravenous drug, ibutilide, is also available but is not approved for use in ventricular arrhythmias.

10. How is medically unresponsive ventricular tachycardia treated?

Stable medically refractory ventricular tachycardia may be terminated by insertion of a temporary transvenous pacing wire and ventricular pacing. This method is most useful for patients who have frequent recurrences of a hemodynamically stable ventricular rhythm. There is a small risk (about 5%) of acceleration of the rhythm and/or inducing ventricular fibrillation. Provisions for immediate defibrillation should be in place when attempting pace termination. Pace termination should be done only by physicians with adequate training and experience. There is inadequate experience with transcutaneous pacing to recommend its use to terminate sustained ventricular tachycardia. Rhythms that are refractory to medical therapy also may be electrically cardioverted with synchronized direct current (DC) shock and appropriate patient sedation.

11. Once the acute episode is terminated, how is recurrence prevented?

Any potentially reversible cause should be sought and treated—specifically, ischemia or electrolyte abnormalities. Antiarrhythmic drugs have been the mainstay of preventive therapy. Appropriate drug therapy has been guided by Holter monitor or electrophysiologic testing. When single-drug therapy has failed, combination regimens have been tried. The long-term clinical success of medical regimens is low. Sotalol and amiodarone are the most effective medications.

Recent technologic advances have given patients the option of an implantable antitachycardia cardioverter-defibrillator. Such devices are capable of sensing the rhythm continuously and responding with an appropriate algorithm (either pacing or defibrillation), as previously programmed by the physician. The success rate for rhythm termination is high. Studies have been published that show improved long-term survival with these devices. Additional options include ablation of the arrhythmia focus either with catheter or surgical ablation. Ablation and device therapy demand specialized training on the part of the physician.

12. What is the evidence to support the use of the implantable cardioverter defibrillator (ICD) in patients presenting with ventricular tachycardia?

Long-term survival benefit has now been shown in a randomized trial comparing ICD with antiarrhythmic drug therapy. The Antiarrhythmics Versus Implantable Defibrillators (AVID) trial enrolled patients who were survivors of cardiac arrest, had symptomatic sustained ventricular tachycardia, or had ventricular tachycardia with low ejection fraction (< 40%). Just over 1000 patients were randomized to receive ICD, empiric amiodarone, or electrophysiologic guided sotalol. There was a significant reduction in the number of deaths in the ICD group compared to the drug-treated group. This study lends strong support to the use of ICD as first-line therapy for treatment of patients who were fortunate enough to have survived a life-threatening arrhythmia.

13. Is it possible to identify and treat patients at high risk of sudden death from a ventricular arrhythmia?

The Multicenter Automatic Defibrillator Implantation Trial (MADIT) demonstrated that prophylactic implantation of an implantable defibrillator resulted in improved survival in high-risk patients compared to conventional antiarrhythmic therapy. Individuals were screened for further risk by electrophysiology study and were identified by three features: history of myocardial infarction, ejection fraction ≤ 35%, and a documented episode of asymptomatic nonsustained ventricular tachycardia. Individuals who met these three criteria underwent further electrophysiologic testing. Patients who were found to have inducible but nonsuppressible ventricular arrhythmia were deemed to be at high risk. The implantable defibrillator resulted in a 62% reduction in mortality compared to antiarrhythmic drugs (primarily amiodarone).

BIBLIOGRAPHY

1. AVID Investigators: A comparison of antiarrhythmic drug therapy with implantable defibrillators in patients resuscitated from near fatal ventricular arrhythmias. N Engl J Med 337:1576–1583, 1997.
2. Echt D, Liebson P, Mitchell B, et al: Mortality and morbidity in patients receiving encainide, flecanide, or placebo. N Engl J Med 324:781–788, 1991.
3. Fogel RI, Prystowsky EN: Management of malignant ventricular arrhythmias and cardiac arrest. Crit Care Med 28(10 Suppl):N165–169, 2000.
4. Mason J, ESVEM investigators: A comparison of electrophysiologic testing with Holter monitoring to predict antiarrhythmic-drug efficacy for ventricular tachyarrhythmias. N Engl J Med 329:445–451, 1993.
5. Moss AJ, Hall WJ, Cannom DS, et al: Improved survival with an implanted defibrillator in patients with prior myocardial infarction, low ejection fraction, and asymptomatic non-sustained ventricular tachycardia. N Engl J Med 335:1933–1940, 1996.
6. Pavia S, Wilkoff BL: Preventing sudden death in coronary cardiomyopathy: Implantable defibrillators lead the way. Cleve Clin J Med 68(2):113–129, 2001.
7. Shensa M, Borggrefe M, Haverkamp W, et al: Ventricular tachycardia. Lancet 341:1512–1519, 1993.
8. Zipes DP, Wellens HJ: What have we learned about arrhythmias? Circulation 102(20 Suppl 4):IV52–57, 2000.

16. CARDIAC PACING IN ATRIOVENTRICULAR BLOCK

William Bailey, M.D.

This chapter deals with the indications for pacing in the setting of atrioventricular (AV) block. Decisions about pacing arise in one of three settings: (1) acquired AV block, (2) AV block associated with myocardial infarction, and (3) bifascicular and trifascicular block. The indications presented are those for which there is widespread agreement that pacing is indicated and for which survival benefit is expected. Indications for which there is not a consensus are excluded.

1. What are the three types of acquired AV block?
There are three degrees of AV block: first, second, and third (complete). This classification is based on the electrocardiogram.

First-degree block refers to prolongation of the PR interval to > 200 msec and represents delay in conduction in the AV node. There are no accepted indications for pacing in isolated first-degree block.

Second-degree block is divided into two types. Type I (Wenckebach) exhibits progressive prolongation of the PR interval before an impulse fails to stimulate the ventricle. Anatomically, this form of block occurs above the bundle of His in the AV node. Type II exhibits no prolongation of the PR interval before a dropped beat and anatomically occurs at the level of the bundle of His. This rhythm may be associated with a wide QRS complex. Advanced second-degree block refers to the block of two or more consecutive P waves.

Third-degree or **complete block** refers to complete dissociation of the atrial and ventricular rhythms, with a ventricular rate less than the atrial rate. The width and rate of the ventricular rhythm help to identify an anatomic location for the block: narrow QRS results in minimal slowing of the rate, generally at the AV node, and wide QRS results in considerable slowing of rate at or below the bundle of His.

2. What is the most important clinical feature that establishes the need for cardiac pacing?
The most important clinical feature consists of symptoms clearly associated with bradycardia secondary to AV block. Reversible causes such as digoxin or beta blockers should be sought, and, when possible, the offending agents should be discontinued. This is not always possible, especially if a medication is necessary for the control of tachyrhythmia. Symptomatic bradycardia is the cardinal feature in the placement of a permanent pacemaker in acquired AV block in adults. The clinical manifestations of symptomatic bradycardia include light-headedness, dizziness, near syncope, frank syncope, manifestations of cerebral ischemia, dyspnea on exertion, decreased exercise tolerance, and even congestive heart failure.

3. In what clinical settings is placement of a pacemaker indicated in acquired AV block?
Pacing is indicated for third-degree (complete) block that is either permanent or paroxysmal when it is associated with symptoms that are clearly related to (1) bradycardia, (2) congestive heart failure, (3) treatment to suppress other rhythms or to control medical conditions (e.g., digitalis for congestive heart failure with agents that suppress automaticity of pacemaker tissue), (4) an escape rhythm < 40 beats/min or asystole for > 3.0 seconds (may be symptom free), (5) mental cloudiness that clearly resolves with temporary pacing, (6) ablation of the AV node, and (7) myotonic dystrophy.

Pacing is indicated in second-degree block, regardless of the site, when symptoms are clearly related to heart block.

Pacing is also indicated in the setting of atrial fibrillation or flutter when it is associated with complete third-degree block or advanced second-degree block resulting in bradycardia and any of the seven symptoms listed above.

4. Does pacing in the setting of AV block and myocardial infarction require the presence of symptoms?

No. Symptoms related to the form of block are not a requirement. The indications in large part are to treat the intraventricular conduction defects that result from infarction. The prognosis of patients requiring pacing is influenced more by the extent of the infarction than by symptoms. Pacing in the setting of an acute myocardial infarction may be temporary rather than long-term or permanent.

5. What are the indications for pacing after myocardial infarction?

Indications in this setting do not require the presence of symptoms. Pacing is indicated in the setting of acute myocardial infarction for (1) complete third-degree block or advanced second-degree block that is associated with block in the His-Purkinje system (wide complex ventricular rhythm) and (2) transient advanced (second- or third-degree) AV block with a new bundle-branch block.

6. What is the anatomic location of bifascicular or trifascicular block?

Bifascicular or trifascicular block is located below the AV node and involves a combination of either two or three of the fascicles of the right or left bundle (divided into the left anterior and left posterior fascicle).

7. Are symptoms required for permanent pacing in the setting of bifascicular and trifascicular block?

Yes. Symptoms must be present in the setting of bifascicular and trifascicular block, just as in acquired AV block.

8. What are the indications for permanent pacing in bifascicular and trifascicular block?

Pacing is indicated when bifascicular or trifascicular block is associated with (1) complete block and symptomatic bradycardia or (2) intermittent type II second-degree block with or without related symptoms.

BIBLIOGRAPHY

1. Dreifus LS, Fisch C, Griffin JC, et al: Guidelines for implantation of cardiac pacemakers and antiarrhythmic devices. A Report of the American College of Cardiology/American Heart Association Task Force on Assessment of Diagnostic and Therapeutic Cardiovascular Procedures (Committee on Pacemaker Implantation). J Am Coll Cardiol 18:1–16, 1991.
2. Frye RL, Collins JJ, DeSanctis RW, et al: Guidelines for permanent cardiac pacemaker implantation. May 1984. A Report of the Joint American College of Cardiology/American Heart Association Task Force on Assessment of Cardiovascular Procedures (Subcommittee on Pacemaker Implantation). Circulation 70:331A–339A, 1984.
3. Gregoratos G, Cheitlin MD, Conill A, et al: ACC/AHA guidelines for implantation of cardiac pacemakers and antiarrhythmic devices. A report of the American College of Cardiology/American Heart Association Task Force on Practice Guidelines (Committee on Pacemaker Implantation). J Am Coll Cardiol 31:1175–1209, 1998.
4. Mitrani RD, Simmons JD, Interian A, et al: Cardiac pacemakers: Current and future status. Curr Probl Cardiol 24(6):341–420, 1999.
5. Wolbrette DL, Naccarelli GV: Emerging indications for permanent pacing. Curr Cardiol Rep 2(4):353–360, 2000.

IV. Symptoms and Disease States

17. CHEST PAIN

Howard D. Weinberger, M.D., FACC

1. What is angina and what causes it?

Angina is a discomfort in the chest or adjacent area that is associated with myocardial ischemia without myocardial necrosis. Angina is due to an imbalance in myocardial oxygen supply and demand.

2. What factors contribute to myocardial oxygen supply and demand?

Myocardial oxygen supply may be decreased by hypoxia, coronary arterial vasoconstriction, atherosclerotic narrowing of one or more coronary arteries, a nonocclusive intracoronary thrombus, or a combination of two or more of these conditions. Myocardial oxygen demand may be increased by physical exertion, eating (by shunting blood to the gut for digestion), emotional stress (by increasing sympathetic stimulation), and increased metabolic demands (e.g., fever, tachycardia, thyrotoxicosis). Cold weather increases myocardial oxygen demand by increasing peripheral vascular resistance, causing the heart to work harder to maintain adequate peripheral perfusion.

3. Can the history provide any helpful clues in establishing the diagnosis of angina?

Yes. With a careful history and physical examination, the etiology of the patient's symptoms can be determined most of the time. The key features of the history that can help in making the diagnosis of angina are:
- Character and quality of the chest pain
- Location and radiation (if any) of the chest pain
- Precipitating, exacerbating, and relieving factors
- Duration of the chest pain
- Associated symptoms

4. What conditions increase the likelihood of a patient's chest pain being angina?

There are five major risk factors for coronary artery disease. The more risk factors present, the greater the likelihood that any one patient's symptoms may be due to myocardial ischemia (angina). The risk factors are:
1. Smoking cigarettes
2. Hypertension
3. Elevated cholesterol
4. Diabetes mellitus
5. Family history of premature coronary artery disease (before age 55 in men and 65 in women)

Not only are these factors important in helping to establish the diagnosis of angina (and therefore coronary artery disease), but all except family history can be modified to reduce the chances of developing (or of having progression of currently existent) coronary artery disease.

5. Besides myocardial ischemia, are there other conditions that cause angina-like chest pain?

Yes. Many entities may cause chest pain, several of which may produce symptoms similar to angina. The differential diagnosis of angina-like chest pain includes, but is not limited to:

Angina   Acute pulmonary embolus
Myocardial infarction   Esophageal spasm
Pericarditis   Chest wall pain
Aortic dissection   Peptic ulcer disease
Mitral valve prolapse   Pancreatitis
Pulmonary hypertension   Myocarditis

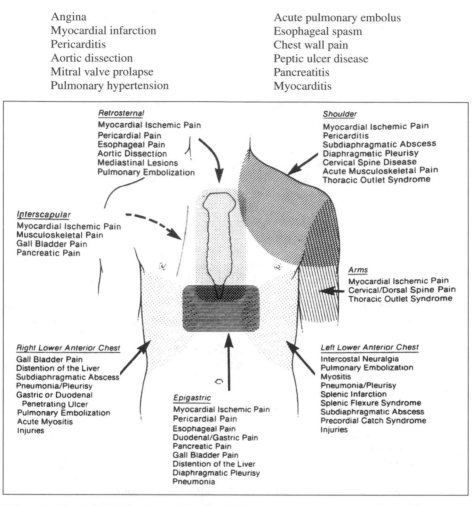

Differential diagnosis of chest pain according to location where pain starts. (From Miller AJ: Diagnosis of Chest Pain. New York, Raven Press, 1988, p 175; with permission.)

6. How do patients describe anginal chest pain?

Patients may not refer to their symptoms as "pain." They may describe a deep discomfort or unpleasant sensation that is hard to define, often as a pressure sensation, tightness, squeezing, or "weight on the chest." Angina is rarely pleuritic and not positional.

7. How long does an episode of angina last?

Angina may last from 2–5 minutes after cessation of exercise or taking nitroglycerin. If symptoms last longer than 20 minutes, they are usually due to myocardial necrosis (myocardial infarction) or are noncardiac in etiology. Brief, fleeting pains are rarely cardiac in origin.

8. What factors may induce or exacerbate angina, and what may relieve it?

Anything that increases cardiac work (myocardial oxygen demand) and/or decreases myocardial oxygen supply may precipitate or worsen angina. Rest, by decreasing myocardial work and oxygen demand, often relieves angina. Nitroglycerin, which dilates coronary arteries, allowing increased blood flow and oxygen delivery to the myocardium, also relieves angina.

9. Where is anginal pain felt and where may it radiate?

Anginal chest pain may occur anywhere between the diaphragm and mandible, but it is most often retrosternal or on the left side of the chest. It tends to be diffuse and not localized to a small discrete area. It may radiate to the neck, throat, mandible, shoulder, or arm (usually the inner aspect of the arm and more commonly the left arm).

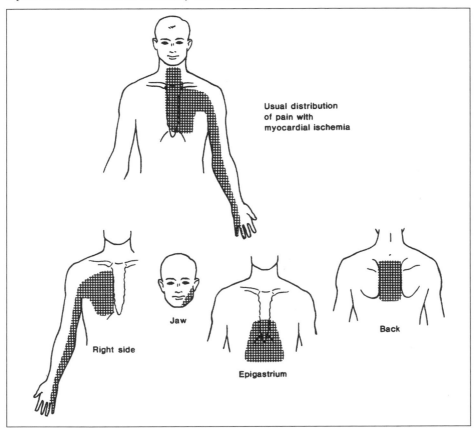

Usual distribution
of pain with
myocardial ischemia

Jaw

Right side

Back

Epigastrium

Pain patterns with myocardial ischemia. (From Horwitz LD: Chest pain. In Horwitz LD, Groves BM (eds): Signs and Symptoms in Cardiology. Philadelphia, J.B. Lippincott, 1985, p 9; with permission.)

10. What are the classic associated symptoms for myocardial ischemia?

In addition to typical anginal chest pain, one or more of the following may be observed:
- Shortness of breath
- Diaphoresis
- Nausea and emesis

11. What findings on the physical examination may be seen with myocardial ischemia?

The physical findings may be normal. An **S$_4$ gallop** (4th heart sound) is due to atrial contraction against a stiff or noncompliant ventricle. If an S$_4$ gallop is heard with symptoms and disappears as the symptoms resolve, this suggests transient ventricular noncompliance (from ischemia) and is strong evidence for myocardial ischemia. An S$_4$ gallop may be present before symptoms develop (and then will likely be present after symptoms resolve) due to other causes of ventricular noncompliance (e.g., left ventricular hypertrophy, hypertension, aortic stenosis, previous myocardial infarction). Evidence of **congestive heart failure** may exist (elevated jugular

Differential Diagnosis of Episodic Chest Pain Resembling Angina

	DURATION	QUALITY	PROVOCATION	RELIEF	LOCATION	COMMENT
Effort angina	5–15 min	Visceral (pressure)	Effort or emotion	Rest, nitroglycerin	Substernal, radiates	First episode vivid
Rest angina	5–15 min	Visceral (pressure)	Spontaneous (? with exercise)	Nitroglycerin	Substernal, radiates	Often nocturnal
Mitral prolapse	Minutes to hours	Superficial (rarely visceral)	Spontaneous (no pattern)	Time	Left anterior	No pattern, variable character
Esophageal reflux	10 min to 1 hr	Visceral	Recumbency, lack of food	Food, antacid	Substernal, epigastric	Rarely radiates
Esophageal spasm	5–60 min	Visceral	Spontaneous, cold liquids, exercise	Nitroglycerin	Substernal, radiates	Mimics angina
Peptic ulcer	Hours	Visceral, burning	Lack of food, "acid" foods	Foods, antacids	Epigastric, substernal	—
Biliary disease	Hours	Visceral (waxes and wanes)	Spontaneous, food	Time, analgesia	Epigastric, ? radiates	Colic
Cervical disc	Variable (gradually subsides)	Superficial	Head and neck movement, palpation	Time, analgesia	Arm, neck	Not relieved by rest
Hyperventilation	2–3 min	Visceral	Emotion, tachypnea	Stimulus removal	Substernal	Facial paresthesia
Musculoskeletal	Variable	Superficial	Movement, palpation	Time, analgesia	Multiple	Tenderness
Pulmonary	30 min +	Visceral (pressure)	Often spontaneous	Rest, time, bronchodilator	Substernal	Dyspneic

From Christie LG Jr, Conti CR: Systematic approach to the evaluation of angina-like chest pain. Am Heart J 102:897, 1981; with permission.

venous pressure, pulmonary rales, S_3 gallop). There may be a visible and/or palpable **dyskinetic bulge** of the chest wall during active ischemia or infarction. **Murmurs**, especially if new, may suggest ischemic-related processes. Papillary muscle ischemia may lead to mitral regurgitation. Rupture of the interventricular septum will produce a ventricular septal defect and its associated murmur. Aortic stenosis and hypertrophic obstructive cardiomyopathy have characteristic murmurs and can cause myocardial ischemia and symptoms of angina.

12. What changes on the 12-lead electrocardiogram (ECG) may be seen with myocardial ischemia?

The classic ECG changes of myocardial ischemia are horizontal ST-segment depression in leads corresponding to the anatomic regions of the heart. ST depression is neither 100% sensitive (there can be myocardial ischemia and angina without ST depression) nor 100% specific (not all ST depression represents myocardial ischemia). ECG changes associated with symptoms that resolve as the symptoms resolve more strongly suggest myocardial ischemia.

13. How do you differentiate between angina and myocardial infarction?

The symptoms of an acute myocardial infarction are usually more intense, longer in duration (1–8 hours), and more often associated with shortness of breath, diaphoresis, nausea, and emesis. In addition, the 12-lead ECG shows ST-segment elevation rather than depression and may show T-wave inversion and/or pathologic Q waves.

BIBLIOGRAPHY

1. Braunwald E (ed): Heart Disease: A Textbook of Cardiovascular Medicine, 5th ed. Philadelphia, W.B. Saunders, 1997.
2. Donat WE: Chest pain: Cardiac and noncardiac causes. Clin Chest Med 8:241–252, 1987.
3. Hammermeister KE: Cardiac and aortic pain. In Bonica JJ (ed): The Management of Pain. Philadelphia, Lea & Febiger, 1990, pp 1001–1042.
4. Hill B, Geraci SA: A diagnostic approach to chest pain based on history and ancillary evaluation. Nurse Practitioner 23:20–24, 29–30, 33–34, 1998.
5. Lee MG, Sullivan SN, Watson WC, Melendez LJ: Chest pain—esophageal, cardiac, or both? Am J Gastroenterol 80:320–324, 1985.
6. Mayou R: Chest pain, palpitations and panic. J Psychosomat Res 44:53–70, 1998.
7. Nevens F, Janssens J, Piessens J, et al: Prospective study on prevalence of esophageal chest pain in patients referred on an elective basis to a cardiac unit for suspected myocardial ischemia. Dig Dis Sci 36:229–235, 1991.

18. ANGINA

Michael Staab, M.D., and Stephen T. Crowley, M.D.

1. What are the characteristic features of angina?

Angina is chest pain discomfort associated with myocardial ischemia. Typically, it is described as substernal discomfort, pressure, heaviness, or a weight-like sensation that often radiates across the mid-thorax, into the left arm (ulnar aspect), neck, or jaw. It is also associated with shortness of breath, diaphoresis, and nausea. Angina is often related to precipitating causes, the most common of which is exertion. Other precipitating factors include stress or emotion and secondary conditions such as anemia, tachycardia, and aortic stenosis. Angina discomfort usually occurs for at least 30 seconds and < 15 minutes and is typically relieved with rest or nitroglycerin. Because angina is a visceral sensation, it is poorly localized, and patients therefore rarely point to the location of their discomfort with one finger.

2. What is the differential diagnosis of a patient presenting with chest pain?

Differential Diagnosis of Chest Pain

CONDITION	QUALITY OF PAIN
Cardiac causes	
Aortic stenosis	Angina-like chest pain
Hypertrophic cardiomyopathy	Angina-like chest pain associated with dyspnea
Acute periocarditis	Sharper in quality; lasts for hours; not affected by effort; positional
Aortic aneurysm	Localized; radiates to back; severe
Mitral valve prolapse	Variable in character
Syndrome X	Angina-like chest pain
Noncardiac causes	
Esophageal disorders (reflux or spasm)	Often spontaneous; rarely radiates; relieved by food or antacids
Peptic ulcer or gastritis	More epigastric; lasts for hours; related to food ingestion
Costochondritis and musculoskeletal syndromes	Exacerbated with inspiration, movement, or palpation; superficial
Pulmonary hypertension	Frequently spontaneous and associated with dyspnea

3. What is the relationship between clinical presentation and coronary anatomy in patients with chest pain?

Patients who present with chest pain can be divided into three subsets:
- Typical angina
- Atypical angina
- Nonanginal chest pain

The incidence of coronary artery disease in these patients is approximately 90%, 50%, and 16%, respectively. In many instances, the clinical-pathologic correlation is poor, such as in patients with advanced coronary artery disease who have silent ischemia or those with Prinzmetal's angina (vasospastic) who have severe angina but usually minimal or no coronary atherosclerosis.

4. Compare underlying pathophysiologic mechanisms in angina and unstable angina.

Stable angina is most commonly related to an increase in myocardial oxygen demand triggered by physical activity. Invariably, a fixed coronary artery obstruction is present, which limits oxygen delivery during times of increased metabolic demands. The severity of the obstruction determines the threshold for cardiac ischemia.

Angina also can be caused by transient decreases in oxygen delivery due to coronary vasoconstriction. Nonocclusive intracoronary thrombi are usually present in patients with **unstable angina** and cause acute impairment in oxygen delivery. Intracoronary thrombi and platelet aggregation occur in unstable or "ruptured" coronary artery plaques. The local release of vasoactive compounds, such as serotonin and thromboxane A_2, is thought to mediate acute vasoconstriction in patients with unstable angina.

5. What role does exercise ECG have in the diagnosis of coronary artery disease (CAD)?

In patients with a chest pain syndrome of uncertain etiology and a normal resting ECG, a standard exercise test is useful in the diagnosis of CAD.

1. Exercise ECG testing adds little in detecting the presence or absence of CAD in patients with a high pretest probability of CAD (i.e., history of typical angina with one or more risk factors). A positive test confirms the clinical impression, but a negative test with a high clinical suspicion cannot rule out CAD.

2. Exercise testing is most valuable in confirming or excluding the diagnosis of CAD in patients with an intermediate pretest probability of CAD. Typically, these are patients with some atypical anginal features and a normal ECG, who may or may not have risk factors for CAD. In such patients, if typical anginal discomfort occurs during exercise and is associated with $\geq$ 1-mm ST-segment depression (horizontal or downsloping in nature), the predictive value for the diagnosis of CAD is > 90%. If a $\geq$ 2-mm ST-segment depression occurs with typical angina, this finding is virtually diagnostic of CAD. An exercise ECG test associated with a hypotensive blood pressure response carries an 80% predictive value for significant CAD.

A negative exercise test in a patient with a low pretest probability of CAD is highly reliable in excluding the diagnosis of significant CAD, but a positive test is still more likely to be false-positive.

6. How is prognosis assessed in patients with angina?

Prognosis can be assessed initially with clinical characteristics, including prolonged rest pain, pulmonary edema, dynamic ST changes, and hypotension.

Exercise testing can further stratify risk by evaluating exercise capacity, symptoms, ECG changes, and exertional hemodynamics. This can be calculated with the Duke treadmill score:

$$\text{Exercise time minutes} - (5 \times \text{maximum ST deviation}) - (4 \times \text{angina index})$$

The angina index = 0 if there is no angina, 1 if angina is present, and 2 if angina was the cause of stopping exercise. Patients with lower scores (< –10) had significantly worse survival rates.

Additional parameters, such as exertional hypotension, also indicate a high-risk subgroup. Noninvasive imaging may also contribute to risk assessment. Depressed left ventricular function, exertional regional wall motion abnormalities on stress echocardiography, or multiple ischemic segments on nuclear perfusion imaging suggests multivessel CAD.

7. How effective is risk factor modification in improving the prognosis of patients with angina?

Risk factor modification is effective in reducing risk for cardiac events in patients who are asymptomatic or do not carry a diagnosis of CAD. Once symptoms of angina have appeared, risk factor modification should be intensified.

- Control of **hyperlipidemia** in patients with prior myocardial infarction have a reduced risk of death when treated with 3-hydroxy-3-methylglutaryl coenzyme A (HMG CoA) reductase inhibitors. Fewer recurrent coronary events can be expected in patients with average lipid levels.
- **Smoking** increases the relative risk for myocardial infarction 2.8-fold, and this risk is substantially reduced after patients quit smoking. Cessation of smoking after coronary artery bypass grafting also improves graft patency and prognosis.

- How effective **blood pressure control** is at preventing subsequent cardiac mortality in patients with known CAD has not been well studied. Reduction in first myocardial infarctions may be achieved with hypertension control, particularly in diabetics.

8. What is the optimal medical management for patients with angina?

Aspirin has been shown to reduce the risk of myocardial infarction by 87% during a 5-year follow-up in men with chronic stable angina. It should be given to all patients with angina who are without contraindications to the drug.

Aspirin and **beta-blockers** have both been shown to improve survival in patients with prior myocardial infarction and to reduce the incidence of reinfarction. If tolerated, beta-blockers should be used in these patients. A meta-analysis has shown a mortality benefit for beta-blockers.

Nitroglycerin administered sublingually is the drug of choice for treatment of acute angina episodes. Sublingual nitroglycerin is also very effective as a prophylactic to prevent an anticipated angina attack.

Because of problems with marked variations in plasma concentration and tolerance, long-acting oral **nitrates** are often used as secondary therapy. A mortality benefit has not been shown for nitrate therapy.

In patients with variable-threshold angina, in whom anginal episodes can occur due to increased oxygen demand or concomitant coronary vasoconstriction, a calcium channel blocker is the treatment of choice. Such patients have anginal patterns that vary considerably due to presumed vasoconstriction acting on a fixed obstructive lesion. Calcium channel blockers are also preferable in patients with variant or Prinzmetal's angina. Beta-blockers and verapamil should be avoided in patients with overt congestive heart failure and a left ventricular ejection fraction of < 30% (although carefully initiated low-dose beta-blockade is beneficial in selected patients).

9. Define unstable angina.

Unstable angina is a poorly defined syndrome but includes patients with one of the following: (1) crescendo angina (more severe or frequent) superimposed on chronic stable angina, (2) angina at rest or with minimal activity, or (3) new-onset angina (within 1 month) that is brought on by minimal exertion. Unstable angina describes a very heterogenous population with single or multivessel disease, with or without prior myocardial infarction, and an uncertain outcome. Unstable angina can be classified according to severity (accelerating angina versus angina at rest, acute), clinical circumstances (secondary to other extrinsic conditions or primary), and intensity of treatment.

10. What is the approach to management in patients with unstable angina?

Unstable angina is a potentially dangerous condition, and management should be tailored to prevent adverse outcomes. Patients with high-risk features should be admitted to the cardiac care until, placed at bedrest, and begun on antianginal therapy with either β-blockers or calcium channel blockers, aspirin, heparin, and intravenous nitrates. Aspirin also decreases recurrent ischemia and infarctions in patients with unstable angina, although neither aspirin nor heparin taken as sole therapy appears to be better than the other. Long-term aspirin therapy should be given to all patients with unstable angina without contraindications, because it reduces the incidence of nonfatal myocardial infarction and death. Most patients with unstable angina will stabilize on this regimen of medical therapy.

A small percentage of patients will develop medically refractory rest angina. Treatment with intra-aortic balloon counterpulsation is usually effective in stabilizing patients with refractory symptoms or poor hemodynamic profiles. This technique is useful to stabilize patients before and during cardiac catheterization.

Although most patients with unstable angina have nonocclusive intracoronary thrombi, to date the use of thrombolytic agents has not demonstrated a benefit in recurrent ischemia, myocardial infarction, or mortality when compared to heparin or aspirin. Glycoprotein IIb/IIIa inhibitors (see question 16) are an additional tool in the treatment of high-risk unstable angina patients.

11. When is the term "acute coronary syndrome" used instead of unstable angina?

At the time of initial presentation, cardiac enzymes may be negative, and therefore it will be unclear whether a chest pain episode represents unstable angina or myocardial infarction. The term acute coronary syndrome denotes that the physician does believe a coronary event is occurring and that it should be treated as such.

12. How useful is the resting ECG in evaluating patients with angina?

A resting ECG should be obtained in all patients who complain of chest discomfort. In patients with chronic stable angina, the ECG is normal in one-third of patients and, if abnormal, most often shows nonspecific ST-T changes without evidence for myocardial infarction.

The presence of left bundle branch block in patients with angina is often associated with significant left ventricular dysfunction and may reflect multivessel CAD. The presence of Q waves is usually a specific but insensitive indicator of myocardial infarction. Ischemic ST-segment deviations (depressions or elevations) and/or T-wave inversions occur commonly in patients with unstable angina; these changes usually resolve with relief of pain. New persistent symmetric T-wave inversion in the anterior precordial leads is a marker for high-grade left anterior descending or left main artery disease, and it should be recognized that these patients are at increased risk for infarction. Persistence of ST and T-wave changes may also suggest a non–Q wave infarction.

There is a fairly close correlation between ischemic ECG lead abnormalities and the anatomic site of coronary obstruction. Ischemic changes in the inferior leads (II, III, aVF) indicate right coronary or circumflex artery disease. Abnormal changes in the anterior precordial leads suggest left anterior descending artery disease, and changes in the left lateral (V_2–V_4) or high lateral leads (I, aVL) imply either diagonal or circumflex artery disease.

13. What are the indications for cardiac catheterization in patients with angina?

Cardiac catheterization and coronary angiography should be performed if the diagnosis of CAD cannot be reliably made by noninvasive diagnostic tests. Whether all patients with unstable angina need catheterization is controversial. Clearly, those patients with unstable angina who carry high-risk clinical markers need coronary angiography. An aggressive approach (early catheterization) has been shown to be beneficial in the TACTICS (TIMI 18) trial for patients with unstable coronary syndromes, especially those with elevated troponin I levels. An argument can be made to assess those patients with low-risk clinical profiles and who respond quickly to medical therapy with a noninvasive test such as a stress thallium scan. Catheterization is indicated for patients with chronic stable angina who begin to "break through" or fail medical therapy. Patient age, in itself, is not a contraindication to catheterization, but patients who are not candidates for either angioplasty or bypass grafting and who have another life-threatening illness usually do not need cardiac catheterization.

14. When are serum troponins used in the evaluation of chest pain?

Serum troponin I and T are sensitive indicators of myocardial cell injury and may be elevated when creatine kinase (CK)-MB is not. At what point an elevated serum troponin indicates a myocardial infarction is debatable, and troponin elevation at low levels is not 100% specific for coronary disease. However, elevated troponin levels in unstable angina identify a higher risk group with an increased risk of subsequent coronary events. Higher levels of troponin elevation usually confirm elevations in CK and isoenzyme MB.

15. What does low–molecular-weight heparin add to the treatment of unstable angina?

Low–molecular-weight heparin has improved pharmacokinetic properties compared to unfractionated heparin so it allows for more rapid and complete anticoagulation. This has translated into modest reductions in ischemic end points but not in mortality.

16. What are glycoprotein IIb/IIIa inhibitors?

The glycoprotein IIb/IIIa platelet receptor is an integral part of platelet aggregation when bound to fibrinogen, leading to initiation of an arterial thrombus. Blockade of these receptors has shown improved outcomes in treatment of high-risk patients with unstable angina and in percutaneous coronary revascularization.

BIBLIOGRAPHY

1. Braunwald E: Unstable angina: A classification. Circulation 80:410–414, 1989.
2. Braunwald E, Jones RH, Mark DB, et al: Diagnosing and managing unstable angina. Circulation 90:613–622, 1994.
3. Cohen M, Demers C, Gurfinkel EP, et al: A comparison of low–molecular-weight heparin with unfractionated heparin for unstable coronary artery disease. N Engl J Med 337:447–452, 1997.
4. Hamm CW, Ravkilde J, Gerhardt W, et al: The prognostic value of serum toponin T in unstable angina. N Engl J Med 327:146–150, 1992.
5. Hansson L, Zanchetti A, Carruthers SG, et al: Effects of intensive blood-pressure lowering and low-dose aspirin in patients with hypertension: Principal results of the Hypertension Optimal Treatment (HOT) randomised trial. Lancet 351:1755–1762, 1998.
6. Mark DB, Shaw L, Harrell FE, et al: Prognostic value of a treadmill exercise score in outpatients with suspected coronary artery disease. N Engl J Med 325:849–853, 1991.
7. Platelet Receptor Inhibition in Ischemic Syndrome Management in Patients Limited by Unstable Signs and Symptoms (PRISM-PLUS) Study Investigators: Inhibition of the platelet glycoprotein IIb/IIIa receptor with tirofiban in unstable angina and non-Q-wave myocardial infarction. N Engl J Med 338:1488–1497, 1998.
8. Ridker PM, Manson JE, Gaziano JM, et al: Low dose aspirin therapy for chronic stable angina: A randomized, placebo-controlled clinical trial. Ann Intern Med 114:835–839, 1991.
9. Sacks FM, Pfeffer MA, Moye LA, et al: The effect of pravastatin on coronary events after myocardial infarction in patients with average cholesterol levels. N Engl J Med 335:1001–1009, 1996.
10. Scandinavian Simvastatin Survival Study Group: Randomised trial of cholesterol lowering in 4444 patients with coronary heart disease: The Scandinavian Simvastatin Survival Study (4S). Lancet 344:1383–1389, 1994.
11. Vane JR, Anggard EE, Botting RM: Regulatory functions of the vascular endothelium. N Engl J Med 323:27–36, 1990.
12. Yasue H, Takizawa A, Nagao M, et al: Long-term prognosis for patients with variant angina and influential factors. Circulation 78:1–9, 1988.
13. Yehgiazarians Y, Braunstein JB, Askari A, Stone PH: Unstable angina pectoris. N Engl J Med 342:101–114, 2000.

19. MYOCARDIAL INFARCTION

Nelson P. Trujillo, M.D., and JoAnn Lindenfeld, M.D.

1. What are the known risk factors for coronary artery disease?

- Dyslipidemias (total cholesterol > 200 mg/dl, low density lipoprotein cholesterol > 160 mg/dl, increased triglycerides, and high density lipoprotein cholesterol < 35 mg/dl)
- Age
- Male sex
- Tobacco use
- Hypertension
- Sedentary lifestyle
- Obesity
- Family history (first myocardial infarction in a first-degree relative at < 55 years of age)
- Diabetes mellitus

Other, more controversial risk factors include elevated lipoprotein (a), alcohol use, stress, hyperinsulinemia, elevated fibrinogen levels, left ventricular (LV) hypertrophy, angiotensin-converting enzyme (ACE) genotype, and cocaine use. Data also suggest that elevated homocysteine levels may be a marker of increased cardiovascular risk. C-reactive protein levels, a marker of inflammation, may predict cardiovascular events.

2. What is the pathophysiology of acute myocardial infarction (MI)?

The pathophysiology of acute MI is currently based on observations made in 1912 by Herrick and reconfirmed in 1980 by Dewood. They described occlusion of stenotic coronary arteries by thrombus in the setting of acute MI. Thrombus formation most often results in the setting of a ruptured atherosclerotic plaque. The degree of obstruction and thrombus is variable and due to multiple factors, including dysfunctional coronary endothelium, extent of obstruction, platelet aggregation, and altered vasomotor tone. These mechanisms are believed to be responsible for at least 85% of all MIs.

Other mechanisms of MI include coronary artery vasculitis, embolic phenomena, coronary artery spasm, congenital abnormalities, and increased blood viscosity. Cocaine-induced MI is thought to be multifactorial since severe vasospasm and acute thrombus have been described in both stenotic and normal coronary arteries.

In most patients, no precipitating cause for ruptured plaques resulting in MI can be found. A modest relationship to heavy exercise, emotional stress, trauma, and neurologic disturbances has been described. Early-morning predilection for acute MI has also been demonstrated; this may be related to circadian rises in catecholamines and platelet aggregation. Infection with *Chlamydia pneumoniae*, *Helicobacter pylori*, and other infectious agents has been linked to acute plaque rupture and MI.

3. Describe the typical signs and symptoms of acute myocardial infarction.

The classic symptoms of MI include dull substernal chest pain, dyspnea, nausea, diaphoresis, palpitations, and/or sense of impending doom. The chest pain typically lasts at least 15–30 minutes and may radiate into the arms, jaw, or back. The elderly often have atypical presentations, such as dyspnea, confusion, vertigo, syncope, and abdominal pain. Approximately 25% of MIs are either asymptomatic or unrecognized, and are termed "silent."

General examination findings include pallor, diaphoresis, and anxiety. Abnormalities in blood pressure, heart rate, and respiratory rate are variable, depending on the type and extent of MI. A low-grade fever may be present. A fourth heart sound is almost always present. Jugular venous distention and a third sound may occur, again depending on the site and extent of MI. Precordial friction rubs and peripheral edema may be present later, but are not usually present in the first few hours after MI. In the setting of papillary muscle dysfunction or rupture, the murmur of mitral regurgitation may occur, although it is often much shorter and softer than expected.

4. How is the diagnosis of acute myocardial infarction made?

The diagnosis of MI is made on the basis of clinical presentation, electrocardiographic (ECG) findings, and elevated serum enzymes.

5. Describe the ECG findings that can help make the diagnosis.

Classic ECG findings of acute **Q-wave MI** initially include hyperacute T waves and ST-segment elevation. T-wave inversion and the development of Q waves follow over hours to days. In **nontransmural infarction**, ECG findings are less specific and include T-wave inversion and ST-segment depression. Note that the ECG is normal in 20% of acute MIs. **Right ventricular infarction** can be diagnosed using right-sided precordial ECG leads. ST elevation of 0.5 mm or more in V3R–V6R is diagnostic. Precordial lead V4R is the most sensitive. Right-sided ECG leads should be obtained routinely in the setting of inferior ischemia.

6. Which serum enzymes can be indicative of an acute MI?

Creatinine kinase, troponin I, troponin T, lactate dehydrogenase, and serum glutamic oxaloacetic transferase are enzymes used in making the diagnosis of infarction. **Creatinine kinase** (CK) rises within 6–8 hours of infarction, peaks at 24 hours, and normalizes by 48–96 hours. CK-MB is an isoenzyme of CK found almost exclusively in myocardium, and is the cornerstone of enzymatic diagnosis. Elevations in CK-MB have also been reported with myocarditis, cardiac defibrillation, cardiac surgery, cardiac contusions, and prolonged ischemia without infarction. It may be falsely elevated in renal failure and hypothyroidism.

Troponin I and T rise within 3 hours of myocardial injury. Elevation in these cardiac enzymes predicts not only MI, but also increased cardiovascular mortality in the absence of MI.

Lactate dehydrogenase (LDH) and its isoenzymes also rise in MI, beginning at 24–48 hours, peaking in 3–5 days, and normalizing in 7–10 days. A ratio of isoenzymes LDH1/LDH2 of > 1.0 is sensitive for MI. LDH has been largely replaced by CK and troponin I measurements.

Serum glutamic oxaloacetic transferase levels usually peak in 48–72 hours, although this enzyme is not specific for MI and has been replaced by CK measurements.

7. True or false: Echocardiography plays no role in the diagnosis of acute MI.

False. Echocardiography may have a limited role by demonstrating new wall-motion abnormalities when the ECG is nondiagnostic. This tool is essential in diagnosing mechanical complications (see Question 21).

8. What are the differences between Q-wave and non-Q-wave MI?

Q-wave infarction (once called "transmural" infarction) represents 60–70% of all acute MIs and generally occurs when the ECG initially shows ST elevation and there is no intervention. Non-Q-wave infarction (once referred to as "subendocardial" infarction) represents 30–40% of all acute MIs. Pathologically, non-Q-wave infarctions may exhibit complete transmural involvement. Thus, the terms transmural and subendocardial infarction have been replaced by the terms Q-wave and non-Q-wave infarction as defined by the development of Q waves postinfarction.

NON-Q-WAVE INFARCTION	Q-WAVE INFARCTION
Nonspecific ST or T-wave changes or ST depression	ST-segment elevation
10–20% early total occlusion rate in infarct-related vessels	90% early total occlusion rate in infarct-related vessels
Lower CK peaks	Higher CK peaks
Higher ejection fractions	Lower ejection fractions
Less wall-motion abnormalities	Wall-motion abnormalities more frequent
Higher early reinfarction rate (40%)	Higher early morbidity (1.5–2 times increased)

The 3-year mortality is the same in the two groups. Up to 60% of patients with non-Q-wave MI have significant two- or three-vessel coronary artery disease. In light of this, many physicians suggest early angiography to stratify the risk in these patients. Calcium channel blockers may affect the short-term reinfarction rate in non-Q-wave infarction but have not been shown to improve mortality. In non-Q-wave infarction, the benefit of routine acute therapy with thrombolytic agents or percutaneous transluminal angioplasty has not been definitively proven.

9. What is the initial management of acute myocardial infarction?

The cornerstone of management of acute MI is prompt emergency care. Initial therapy in the field should include oxygen, nitroglycerin, morphine (if hypotension is not present), rapid transport to an emergency department, and evaluation for reperfusion therapy.

On arrival at the hospital, assessment should focus on hemodynamic stability and eligibility for thrombolytic therapy or emergency angioplasty. All patients should be given aspirin if there are no contraindications.

10. What forms of therapy can result in reperfusion?

• Prompt use of thrombolytic agents
• Percutaneous transluminal coronary angioplasty
• Coronary artery bypass surgery

11. Explain the recommendations for thrombolytic therapy.

Reperfusion therapy should be considered in all patients with presumed acute MI and ST elevation or new left bundle branch block. The benefit of thrombolytic therapy in these patients has been demonstrated in numerous studies, where it routinely decreased mortality, improved LV function, was associated with fewer arrhythmias, and improved long-term survival. Thrombolytic therapy accelerates the conversion of plasminogen to plasmin, an enzyme which dissolves fibrin clots, enhancing endogenous fibrinolysis. Nearly 80% of thrombosed arteries can be opened with thrombolytic therapy; however, there is a 15–20% reocclusion rate.

12. How do I choose thrombolytic agents?

The choice of thrombolytic agents is controversial. There are several approved agents and regimes (see table). *Timely use of thrombolytic therapy seems to be the most important factor in predicting who will benefit.* Therapy within 6 hours of presentation confers the most survival benefit, although effectiveness has been shown up to 12 hours. Accelerated tPA may provide some survival benefit over other regimens. Combination therapy with glycoprotein IIb/IIIa inhibitors and tPa has shown increased reperfusion rates and may improve outcomes with thrombolytic therapy.

Adjunctive therapy for thrombolysis includes aspirin and heparin to prevent reocclusion. Heparin is necessary in conjunction with tPA, but is probably not necessary with streptokinase or APSAC. More specific anticoagulants, including thrombin-specific inhibitors (hirudin) and other platelet inhibitors, are being developed.

Thrombolytic Regimens for Acute Myocardial Infarction

Streptokinase	1.5 million units IV over 1 hr
APSAC*	30 units IV over 2–5 min
Tissue-plasminogen activator (tPA)[†]	
Standard	IV: 10 mg bolus, 50 mg in first hour, 20 mg each in second and third hours (+ heparin)
Accelerated	IV: 15-mg bolus, 0.75 mg/kg over 30 min up to 50 mg, then 0.5 mg/kg up to 35 mg over the next 1 hr (+ heparin)
Reteplase	10 units over 2 min, followed at 30 min by second 10-unit bolus

* APSAC = anisoylated plasminogen-streptokinase activator complex.
[†] Heparin is generally recommended for both tPA regimens as a 5000-U bolus, followed by an IV (intravenous infusion of 1000 U/hr (1200 U/hr in patients > 80 kg), with dose adjustments to raise the activated partial thromboplastin time (aPTT) to 60–85 seconds.

13. Are there contraindications to thrombolytic therapy?
- Absolute contraindications
  Active bleeding
  Puncture of a noncompressible vessel
  Possible aortic dissection
  Active intracranial malignancy
  Recent major surgery (< 1 wk)
  Acute pericarditis
  Previous drug allergy (to streptokinase or APSAC)
- Relative contraindications
  Major trauma or surgery in last 6–8 wk
  Severe uncontrolled hypertension
  Recent stroke or brain tumor
  Pregnancy
  Prolonged cardiopulmonary resuscitation
  History of bleeding diathesis
  History of peptic ulcer disease
  Cancer
  Diabetic retinopathy
  Severe hepatic dysfunction

14. What are the possible complications of thrombolytic therapy?
Both minor and major complications have been reported. Allergic reactions have been described with streptokinase and APSAC secondary to streptokinase antibodies. Hypotension is more frequent with streptokinase than tPA. The major complications of thrombolytic therapy are directly related to impairment of hemostasis and are far more common in the presence of a vascular procedure. In the absence of a vascular procedure, major bleeding occurs in 0.1–0.3% of patients, and hemorrhagic cerebral infarctions occur in up to 0.6%.

15. How is thrombolytic therapy reversed?
Bleeding complications occur in 5% of patients receiving thrombolytic therapy and may be divided into major and minor events. Intracranial bleeding is the most severe and occurs in 0.2–0.6% of cases, with a 50–75% mortality. Fortunately, 70% of all bleeding complications occur at the site of an invasive procedure and can be controlled locally. Treatment of bleeding complications should be tailored to the individual.

In the initial evaluation of the bleeding patient, inspect all vascular sites and apply pressure as needed. Send blood for crossmatch testing. Discontinue heparin and any antiplatelet drugs therapies. If necessary, protamine may be given to reverse the heparin effect (1 mg protamine/100 U heparin not to exceed 50 mg in 10 min). For severe bleeding, give cryoprecipitate and fresh frozen plasma, especially if the fibrinogen level is < 100 mg/dl. Platelets can be given when the bleeding time is prolonged. If life-threatening bleeding continues, antifibrinolytic drugs may be considered.

16. What are the indications for primary and secondary use of percutaenous transluminal coronary angioplasty (PTCA)?
Primary PTCA is indicated in all patients with acute MI where the service is available. Outcomes depend on the experience of the operator and the center. PTCA should only be performed in high-volume centers with surgical backup, where mortality is expected to be better than that for standard thrombolytic therapy. Consider PTCA in all patients with contraindications to thrombolytic therapy, when lytic therapy has failed to achieve reperfusion, and in high-risk patients (age > 70 years, persistent sinus tachycardia, cardiogenic shock).

Primary PTCA for MI is associated with > 90% patency rates, lower rates of serious bleeding, decreased recurrent ischemia, and decreased mortality when compared to thrombolytic therapy.

In patients undergoing PTCA for acute MI, adjuvant use of glycoprotein IIb/IIIa inhibitors and coronary stents has led to improved clinical outcomes when compared to reperfusion therapy with thrombolytics.

The overall goal in patients with MI is safe, prompt restoration of brisk antegrade flow in the occluded artery—by whatever method is readily available. There is no role for early and/or routine PTCA in patients who have received successful thrombolytic therapy.

17. Is there a role for surgery in acute myocardial infarction?

Coronary artery bypass graft surgery (CABG) can be used in acute MI as both primary and secondary therapy. Patients with recurrent ischemia uncontrolled by medical therapy who are ineligible for PTCA may require emergent CABG. Operative mortality is increased in the peri-infarction period, primarily in patients with poor hemodynamics, congestive heart failure (CHF), and advanced age.

18. What arrhythmias occur in acute myocardial infarction?

Both supraventricular and ventricular arrhythmias are seen in acute MI. Of **supraventricular arrhythmias**, sinus bradycardia is present most commonly with inferior infarction and suggests a better prognosis. Sinus tachycardia (heart rate > 100 bpm) in acute MI may be caused by pain, anxiety, LV dysfunction, hypovolemia, pericarditis, or atrial infarction; it is a marker of poor prognosis because it generally signals a significant amount of LV dysfunction. Premature atrial contractions are also common, and may result from increased atrial pressure with CHF. Atrial fibrillation occurs in 15% of infarctions and is a marker of poor prognosis. Other supraventricular tachycardias are infrequent in MI, but should be treated promptly if symptomatic.

Ventricular arrhythmias are the leading cause of prehospital mortality in acute MI. Ventricular fibrillation (VF) is believed to be responsible for 60% of infarction-related prehospital mortality; it occurs predominantly in the first 12 hours. Primary VF (without heart failure) should be distinguished from secondary VF (with significant heart failure). *Primary* VF occurs predominantly in the first few hours after MI and rarely results in death if the patient is hospitalized and defibrillation is available early. *Secondary* VF may occur at any time during the hospitalization, and defibrillation is not always successful. Premature ventricular beats (PVCs) occur in 90% of patients with acute MI and do not predict VF. However, in the immediate post-infarction period, PVCs that occur frequently or in pairs or groups of three do predict risk of VF.

Although prophylactic lidocaine is no longer recommended for all patients with acute MI, it may be indicated in those with very frequent or complex ectopy in the first 24 hours post infarction. Treatment of chronic but asymptomatic PVCs with antiarrhythmic drugs in the late post-infarction period leads to higher mortality and is not recommended. Accelerated idioventricular rhythm is a nonspecific marker for myocardial reperfusion and should not be treated unless symptoms exist.

19. How is the risk for sudden death assessed in post-infarction patients?

The signal-averaged ECG may be useful in predicting risk for sudden death in post-infarction patients as well as for guiding medical management or placement of an automatic implantable defibrillator. Electrophysiologic studies can be helpful in assessing risk of late sudden death post-infarction; they are usually performed if the patient has an episode of ventricular tachycardia or VF after the first 48 hours of infarction or if the signal-averaged ECG is positive in patients with complex ventricular ectopy.

20. When are pacemakers useful in acute myocardial infarction?

Abnormalities of atrioventricular (AV) conduction occur in as many as 25% of patients MI. Often these progress to third-degree heart block and are associated with a 50% in acute mortality. In general, patients with inferior MI have block in the AV nodal area often a junctional escape rhythm with a rate of 40–60 beats per minute. These p have an associated right ventricular (RV) infarction. In patients with anterior infa occurs in the His-Purkinje system, and there is often an unreliable ventricular escape rhythm with a rate of < 40 beats per minute.

Temporary pacing is required whenever any bradyarrhythmia or conduction disturbance results in significant symptoms, hypotension, or shock. In asymptomatic patients with *inferior* MI, prophylactic pacing is rarely required. In asymptomatic patients with *anterior* MI, indications for prophylactic pacing are controversial, but generally include new bilateral (bifascicular) bundle branch block (BBB), i.e., right BBB with left anterior or posterior divisional block and alternating right and left BBB. First-degree AV block adds to this risk. However, isolated new block in only one of the three fascicles—even with P-R prolongation and preexisting bifascicular block and normal P-R interval—poses less risk and does not mandate pacing. Such patients should be closely monitored, with insertion of a temporary pacemaker performed only if higher-degree AV block develops.

The only absolute indication for **permanent pacing** in acute MI is high-degree AV block that persists. In patients with acute inferior MI, high-degree AV block almost always resolves within 2 weeks, and permanent pacing is not indicated. There is controversy surrounding the use of prophylactic permanent pacing in patients with first-degree AV block combined with fascicular blocks in whom high-degree AV block has resolved.

21. Explain the potential mechanisms for hypotension in acute MI.

The differential diagnosis for hypotension in the patient with MI is important because treatment depends on the etiology. **Cardiogenic shock** is categorized as hypotension (systolic blood pressure < 90 mmHg) with a cardiac index of < 1.8 L/min/m^2 and elevation of LV filling pressures (generally measured by the capillary wedge pressure). Clinical signs of hypoperfusion are also present, including oliguria, mental status changes, pulmonary edema, tachycardia, and pallor.

Commonly, massive LV myocardial damage (> 40% of LV myocardium) is the etiology of shock in acute MI. Another potential etiology of cardiogenic shock is RV infarction that occurs in an inferior infarction. In this situation, the right ventricle may not be able to pump sufficient blood through the pulmonary circulation to support cardiac output. Suspect this in patients with inferior infarction, hypotension, clear lung fields, and elevated neck veins with Kussmaul's sign. The diagnosis can be confirmed with right-sided ECG leads or echocardiography. Right atrial pressures will be elevated out of proportion to pulmonary capillary wedge pressure in this situation, and invasive monitoring may be indicated. Consider hypovolemia early in these patients, since fluid resuscitation alone may reverse the shock state. Also consider pulmonary emboli, sepsis, aortic dissection, and tamponade.

Symptomatic **mechanical complications** occur in < 1% of patients with MI and result from rupture of necrotic cardiac tissue. These complications usually occur during days 3–7 following acute MI and include rupture of the ventricular free wall (often seen in first transmural anterior infarctions in hypertensive women), ventricular septal rupture, and acute papillary muscle rupture causing acute mitral regurgitation. Patients with these complications often present with hypotension and shock, and approach 90% mortality if managed medically. *Surgical repair* of these mechanical complications is the only option if the patient can be stabilized using intra-aortic balloon pumping and vigorous vasodilator therapy. The diagnosis can be established with the use of echocardiography and invasive hemodynamic monitoring. Mild to moderate mitral regurgitation is common in acute MI and is managed medically.

22. What are the indications for invasive hemodynamic monitoring in acute MI?

Use of invasive hemodynamic monitoring should be reserved for those patients with clear indications, including diagnosis of suspected LV or RV failure with hypotension and pulmonary edema, acute mitral regurgitation, acute ventricular septal defects, or persistent oliguria and azotemia in the patient with unclear volume status. Invasive monitoring may also be useful when initiating treatment with inotropic or vasocactive agents.

23. What techniques are used to risk stratify patients with MI?

Post-infarction risk stratification and assessment of prognosis are important in planning ng-term therapy. In patients with post-infarction angina, heart failure, or late arrhythmias, perform urgent angiography to evaluate the need for PTCA or CABG. In patients with uncomplicated MI, noninvasive means may be used to assess ventricular function and residual ischemia, including a symptom-limited exercise test and assessment of LV function by echocardiography or gated blood pool scan.

Other tests available for special problems include exercise thallium testing, stress echocardiography, dipyridamole thallium scanning, positron emission tomography, and ambulatory Holter monitoring. These tests can be performed in most patients 1–4 weeks after MI to determine high- and low-risk groups. High-risk groups are identified by low exercise capacity, hypotension, ST-segment depression at low heart rates, and angina during traditional exercise testing. Evidence of ischemia in addition to the infarction visualized on echocardiography or radionuclide imaging may also be useful in assessing risk after MI.

These principles should be applied to those who have received thrombolytic therapy as well as those who have had a Non-Q-wave MI. There is controversy surrounding the use of noninvasive tests for risk stratification following non-Q-wave infarctions, and some recommend routine angiography in these patients.

24. What agents or interventions are used in secondary prevention of MI?
Secondary prevention of MI focuses on modification of risk factors.
- Encourage **smoking cessation**.
- **Lipid-lowering agents** in combination with **diet modification** in certain subsets of patients can reduce mortality by 20%.
- Encourage **exercise** and supplement it with a rehabilitation program.
- **Beta-blockers** have been extensively studied and, in the postinfarction patient with moderate to high risk, have been shown to reduce mortality and risk of reinfarction by as much as 33%.
- **Aspirin** decreases the rates of reinfarction and should be used in all post-infarction patients.
- **Calcium channel blockers** may have a role in secondary prevention of non-Q-wave infarctions, particularly reinfarction, but no mortality benefit has been shown.
- **ACE inhibitors** decrease reinfarction rates and incidence of sudden death and improve mortality; they should be standard in post-infarction patients with ejection fractions < 40%, especially those with symptoms of heart failure.

25. Is there a role for free radical scavengers?
In animal models, free radical scavengers have been shown to limit reperfusion injury in MI. Such drugs may have a role in the future, although currently none are approved for clinical use. Vitamin E may benefit patients in primary prevention of MI, but further study is necessary. Current evidence (the HOPE trial) does *not* demonstrate usefulness of vitamin E in this capacity.

26. What is ventricular remodeling?
Remodeling of the heart is defined as a change in the mass and shape of the heart in response to damage caused by MI. It is characterized by hypertrophy and progressive dilatation. Depending on the extent of damage, subsequent wall stress, and local tissue environment, remodeling may result in late pump failure, instability of electrical activity, and reinfarction. Factors that favorably modify this process include prevention of reinfarction, reperfusion, afterload reduction, and possibly prevention of reperfusion injury by free radicals. Therapy should aim to prevent complications of ventricular remodeling by ventricular unloading with ACE inhibitors and resolving chronic ischemia by PTCA or CABG.

27. A 55-year-old man is admitted for increased shortness of breath on minimal exercise and paroxysmal nocturnal dyspnea. He has a history of an MI 3 years ago. On physical examination, he is diaphoretic and in orthopnea, and his respiratory rate is 32 breaths/minute. He has a loud left ventricular gallop. EKG shows prominent Q waves in leads II, III, and aVF, which have been present since his previous infarction. No new EKG

Subendocardial infarction. The "delayed-hyperenhancement" MRI technique was applied to this patient with a previous MI. Gadolinium contrast enhancement identifies irreversibly damaged myocardium as white, and viable, undamaged myocardium as dark. Subendocardial infarction of the inferior wall is evident in this two-chamber, long-axis view of the left ventricle. (Image courtesy of S. Flamm, MD.)

changes are detected, and his myocardial enzymes are within normal limits. What is essential in evaluating this patient for possible coronary revascularization?

You must determine the size of the scar tissue from his previous infarct. Equally important, you should detect and quantify the presence of viable myocardium. Both issues can be addressed by MRI, which can be a most valuable tool in evaluating viable and scarred myocardium.

BIBLIOGRAPHY

1. ACC/AHA guidelines for the early management of patients with acute myocardial infarction. Circulation 82:664–707, 1990.
2. Falk E: Why do plaques rupture? Circulation Suppl 3:30–42, 1992.
3. Fuster V, Badiman L, Badiman JJ, Chesebro JH: The pathogenesis of coronary artery disease and the acute coronary syndromes. N Engl J Med 326:242–250, 310–318, 1992.
4. Grines CL, Brorone KF, Marco J, et al: A comparison of immediate angioplasty with thrombolytic therapy for acute myocardial infarction. N Engl J Med 328:673–679, 1993.
5. GUSTO Investigators: An international randomized trial comparing four thrombolytic strategies for acute myocardial infarction. N Engl J Med 329:673–682, 1993.
6. ISIS-2 (Second International Study of Infarct Survival) Collaborative Group: Randomized trial of intravenous streptokinase, oral aspirin, both, or neither among 17,187 cases of suspected acute myocardial infarction: ISIS-2. Lancet ii:349–360, 1988.
7. Schomig A, Kastrati A, et al: Coronary stenting plus platelet glycoprotein IIb/IIIa blockade compared with tissue plasminogen activator in acute myocardial infarction. N Engl J Med 343:385–391, 2000.
8. TIMI Study Group: Comparison of invasive and conservative strategies after treatment with intravenous tissue plasminogen activator in acute myocardial infarction. N Engl J Med 320:618–627, 1989.
9. Vatterott PJ, Hammill SC, Bailey KR, et al: Signal-averaged electrocardiography: A new non-invasive test to identify patients at risk for ventricular arrhythmias. Mayo Clin Proc 63:931–942, 1988.

20. COMPLICATIONS AND CARE FOLLOWING MYOCARDIAL INFARCTION

Raul Mendoza, M.D., and Nelson Trujillo, M.D.

1. What are the causes of a new pansystolic murmur following myocordial infarction?

The development of a new systolic murmur following myocardial infarction (MI) often is catastrophic due to the hemodynamic instability that usually accompanies this murmur. The etiologies include:

- Rupture and/or dysfunction of a left papillary muscle causing severe mitral regurgitation
- Rupture of the interventricular septum
- Right ventricular infarction and tricuspid regurgitation
- False aneurysm and rupture of the external wall

2. What is the clinical presentation of right ventricular infarction?

Right ventricular (RV) infarction is observed in 29–36% of patients presenting with acute inferoposterior or true posterior MI. Isolated RV infarctions are rare. Ischemia or infarction of the RV may lead a range of disorders, from minimal hemodynamic abnormalities to its most severe presentations, which include jugular venous distention, clear lung fields and hypotension, a positive Kussmaul's sign, and RV third and fourth sounds.

3. How is RV infarction diagnosed? What is its recommended management?

The electrocardiogram (ECG) demonstrates the features of acute inferior MI (direct posterior or lateral infarction also may be present) and ST elevation in leads V4R–V6R. Hemodynamic evaluations with a pulmonary artery catheter usually demonstrate an elevated right atrial or RV end-diastolic pressure, a normal or minimally elevated pulmonary artery pressure, and usually normal or low pulmonary capillary wedge pressure.

The mainstay of therapy is fluid administration to maintain a wedge pressure of 18–20 mmHg. Inotropic support may be needed and, rarely, intra-aortic balloon pump insertion is indicated in patients with refractory hypotension. Vasodilator drugs should be strictly avoided. Milrinone, a parenteral phosphodiesterase inhibitor, is an RV inotrope, and may be be helpful in cases of RV failure.

4. What is the difference between true and false aneurysms that develop after myocardial infarction?

A *true ventricular aneurysm* is a circumscribed, noncontractile outpouching of the left ventricle and develops in 8–14% of patients who survive MI. The wall of the true aneurysm usually is composed of fibrous tissue as well as necrotic and viable myocardium. In contrast, a *psuedoaneurysm* results from rupture of the left ventricle free wall and is concealed by the adjacent pericardium. The wall of the pseudoaneurysm is composed of fibrous tissue and no myocardial elements. Rupture is frequent with pseudoaneurysms, but rarely seen in true aneurysms.

5. Is mitral regurgitation following MI of clinical concern?

Murmurs of mitral regurgitation are common (55–80%), especially in the early phase of MI. However, they are transient and are related to the dynamic nature of the ischemic process. A more serious form of ischemic mitral regurgitation may develop post-MI, though fortunately with a low incidence (0.9–5.0%). This complication may lead to severe mitral regurgitation frequently associated with pulmonary edema, hypotension, and death. Three etiologies have been described: (1) papillary muscle dysfunction. (2) generalized left ventricular (LV) dilatation, and (3) papillary muscle rupture.

Complete transection of an LV papillary muscle is uniformly fatal because of sudden massive mitral regurgitation that is usually hemodynamically intolerable. Mitral regurgitation post-MI has a wide clinical spectrum, ranging from minimal hemodynamic consequences to a catastrophic syndrome, frequently fatal unless aggressive medical and surgical management is rapidly implemented.

6. Why does severe mitral regurgitation occur following MI?

Blood supply to the anterolateral papillary muscle is dual, with branches from both the left anterior descending and circumflex arteries. In contrast, the posteromedial papillary muscle has a single blood supply: either the posterior branches of the dominant right coronary artery or the dominant circumflex artery. Therefore, inferoposterior and posterolateral MIs are the ones most commonly associated with severe mitral regurgitation. Ischemic mitral regurgitation is seen mostly in women and the elderly. Its prognosis depends on the degree of rupture, severity of mitral regurgitation, and previous LV function.

7. How often does rupture of the interventricular septum occur?

This complication occurs in 1–3% of all infarctions and accounts for approximately 12% of all cardiac ruptures. It usually occurs early, 2–6 days after MI, with 66% occurring in the first 3 days. It is commonly seen in patients with hypertension and those with anteroseptal MI (60%); the rest occur usually in patients with inferior wall MI with rupture of the posterobasilar septum.

8. Is rupture of the ventricular free wall always fatal?

Rupture of the ventricular free wall is a most feared complication and accounts for 8–15% of all infarct deaths and up to 10% of hospital deaths post-MI. Most ruptures (84%) occur in the first week and 32% in the first day. The most common presentation is sudden hemodynamic collapse followed by rapid demise with or without clinical signs of tamponade.

This complication is more commonly seen in the anterior or lateral wall of the left ventricle and usually is preceded by infarct expansion. In some instances, rupture may be heralded by episodes of recurrent pericardial pain, at times with features of pericardial effusion, hypotension, and tamponade. If treatment is to be successful, diagnosis must be prompt and management aggressive. Interventions include infarctectomy, closure of viable myocardial wall, and bypass surgery.

9. Is surgical intervention required immediately in patients with papillary muscle rupture or interventricular septal rupture?

These two complications post-MI have an abrupt onset, with rapid development of a new systolic murmur, pulmonary edema, and shock. Prognosis depends on the degree of rupture, severity of mitral regurgitation, and previous LV function. Initial therapy usually consists of hemodynamic support, including inotropic and vasodilator therapy, guided arterial and pulmonary artery catheterization, and, on occasion, the use of an intra-aortic balloon pump. If hemodynamic stability is not achieved with these measures and if the patient remains hypotensive, then surgical intervention is required immediately. However, perioperative mortality is high (35–50%). In patients who achieve hemodynamic stability with medical therapy, surgery is usually delayed 6–12 weeks in an attempt to improve healing around the infarct margins, thus facilitating surgery as well as lowering the mortality rate.

10. What are the clinical and hemodynamic features of cardiogenic shock?

Cardiogenic shock is profound circulatory failure, usually due to cumulative myocardial loss of 40% or more. Cardiogenic shock is most often secondary to acute MI, but other etiologies that include primary myocardial disease (myocarditis or end-stage cardiomyopathy).

   Clinical findings
      Peak systolic blood pressure < 90 mmHg
      Peripheral vasoconstriction with cool, clammy, and often cyanotic skin

Oliguria or anuria

Altered mental status (confusion, lethargy, obtundation, coma)

Persistence of shock after correction of contributory factors (e.g., hypovolemia, drug side
    effect or toxicity, arrhythmias, acid-base imbalance)

Hemodynamic findings

Low cardiac index of < 1.8 L/min/m2

Blood pressure of < 90 mmHg systolic and 60 mmHg diastolic

Elevated pulmonary capillary wedge pressure of ≥ 18 mmHg

Tachycardia

Increased systemic vascular resistance

Low stroke volume index of < 20 ml/m2

11. Can cardiogenic shock be predicted?

Approximately 7–9% of patients admitted with acute MI develop cardiogenic shock. The
average time from admission to onset of this complication is 3.4 ± 0.8 days. The following factors, present at the time of admission, are related to the inhospital development of cardiogenic
shock:

Age > 65 years

Poor LV function (LV ejection fraction < 35%)

Large infarct size

History of diabetes mellitus

Previous MI

Female gender

The probability for development of cardiogenic shock depends on the number of these factors present: when three are present, there is an 18% probability of shock, and when five are present, it is 54%.

12. What other complications can develop in patients with cardiogenic shock?

Patients with cardiogenic shock have a significantly higher incidence of atrioventricular
block, intraventricular conduction defects, congestive heart failure (CHF), cardiac arrest, cardiac
arrhythmia, ventricular septal rupture, and significant mitral regurgitation. The inhospital mortality rate among these individuals is approximately 65%. In patients who have increased risk factors for cardiogenic shock, initiation of early aggressive therapy, including a specific invasive
intervention, may be warranted to prevent further myocardial damage.

13. Do all patients who develop hypotension post-MI require inotropic support or/and a pulmonary artery catheter?

Hypotension that develops post-MI has many causes and is not necessarily secondary to
LV dysfunction. RV infarction is a common cause of hypotension post-MI. Hypovolemia (absolute or relative) is frequent in the setting of acute MI; patients may be fluid-depleted due to
anorexia, vomiting, diaphoresis, or fever, as well as the common use of many drugs that have
hypotensive effects. These drugs include narcotic analgesics or tranquilizers, nitrates, diuretics, and most antianginal and antiarrhythmic drugs that tend to be used in patients with acute
MI. Recognition and treatment of these reversible causes of hypotension often improve the hemodynamic status of the patient without the need of inotropic drug support or invasive monitoring procedures.

14. Why do patients with complete heart block and acute MI have a higher mortality?

Acute heart block complicates MI in 5–8% of all cases. Most of the cases of complete heart
block occur with inferior wall MI; however, mortality is higher with anterior wall MI. This increased mortality is due to the fact that heart block developing during MI signifies increased infarct size, which explains the higher incidence of CHF, cardiogenic shock, and cardiac arrest in
this group of patients.

15. What is the clinical implication of LV mural thrombus formation post MI?

LV mural thrombi are common, occurring in 20–40% of patients with anterior infarcts; usually are well visualized by echocardiography; and are mainly seen in anteroseptal and apical MI. Unfortunately, embolism occurs in these patients with a highly variable incidence of 0–25%, usually in the first 10 days post-MI, although thrombus formation may persist during the first 1–3 months. Infarct size is directly related to the thromboembolic risk. The clinical problem is how to prevent emboli rather than how to treat "LV thrombus." It is not entirely clear whether heparinization or combined thrombolytic-heparin therapy prevents emboli. Recommendations for anticoagulation vary, but a reasonable approach is to recommend anticoagulation for 3–6 months with warfarin in patients with demonstrable mural thrombi, particularly if the thrombus is mobile, and in patients in whom an embolic event has already occurred.

16. Differentiate the kinds of pericarditis that develop post MI.

Two kinds of pericarditis occur in the post-MI period. **Early pericarditis** usually develops 24–72 hours after the onset of MI and is seen in patients with transmural MI and CHF. **Delayed pericarditis** (Dressler syndrome) is characterized by fever, persistent and recurrent pericarditis, and pericardial and pleural effusions and usually appears days to weeks after MI.

Early pericarditis is a marker of extensive myocardial damage and frequently is seen in anterior infarction that may be complicated by the development of atrial and ventricular arrhythmias. Despite a frequently stormy hospital course, patients with early pericarditis usually do not have increased early mortality; however, their 12-month mortality is higher than that of patients who do not develop this complication (18% vs 12%).

17. What are the indications for using an intra-aortic balloon pump post MI?

The intra-aortic balloon pump is used as adjunctive therapy in acute MI in patients who:
• have conditions that are hemodynamically unstable and in whom circulatory support is required to perform cardiac catheterization and assessment of potentially correctable lesions.
• have cardiogenic shock unresponsive to medical therapy, including those who develop mechanical complications (i.e., ventricular septal rupture or papillary muscle rupture).
• have persistent ischemic pain despite all medical therapy, including beta and calcium channel blockers, nitrates, full anticoagulation, and oxygen.

Note that intra-aortic balloon pumps are *contraindicated* in cases of significant aortic insufficiency, aortic dissection, and severe peripheral vascular disease.

18. Does temporary pacing improve survival in patients with conduction disturbances in MI?

Patients who develop significant conduction disturbances in acute MI usually have increased morbidity and mortality, mainly because this conduction defect occurs in larger MIs regardless of the coronary artery occluded. Temporary pacing will not improve prognosis in these patients despite the resumption of a physiologic heart rate, since the extent of the myocardial damage is directly related to mortality.

19. What are the indications for temporary and permanent pacing post MI?

Temporary pacing is recommended in patients with MI who have high-grade atrioventricular (AV) block (second or third degree) or are at risk of developing these conduction disturbances.

Indications for temporary pacing include:
• Second-degree Mobitz II block
• Second-degree Mobitz I block and hemodynamic instability
• Third-degree heart block
• New left bundle branch block
• New right bundle branch block with either left anterior or left posterior hemiblock
• Asystole

Pacing is rarely necessary with inferior MI unless associated with hemodynamic instability. The indications for permanent pacing post-MI remain controversial; the aim of this therapy is to prevent sudden death, but not all sudden deaths are due to high-grade AV block. Also, the timing for implantation of a permanent pacemaker is debatable.

Indications for permanent pacing include:
- Persistent advanced AV block (usually > 7–10 days duration), located at either the AV node or His-Purkinje system
- Transient advanced AV block in association with bundle branch block
- Paroxysmal AV block

20. Which diagnostic tests are helpful in diagnosing complications of MI?

Echocardiography, transesophageal and transthoracic, are the primary tests to diagnose complications of acute MI. Emergent left and right cardiac catherization may also be helpful.

BIBLIOGRAPHY

1. ACC/AHA Task Force Report: Guidelines for implantation of cardiac pacemakers and antiarrhythmia devices. J Am Coll Cardiol 18:1–13, 1991.
2. Berger PB, Ryan TJ: Inferior MI: High risk subgroups. Circulation 81:401–411, 1990.
3. Braunwald E (ed): Heart Disease: A Textbook of Cardiovascular Medicine, 4th ed. Philadelphia, W.B. Saunders, 1992, pp 1239–1291.
4. Goldstein TA: Right heart ischemia. Choices in Cardiology 7: 292–296, 1993.
5. Lehmann KG, et al: Mitral regurgitation in early myocardial infarction. Ann Intern Med 117:10–17, 1992.
6. Pappas DJ, et al. Ventricular free-wall rupture after myocardial infarction. Chest 99:892–895, 1991.
7. Tcheng JE, et al: Outcome of patients sustaining acute ischemic mitral regurgitation during myocardial infarction. Ann Intern Med 117:18–24, 1992.
8. Tcheng JE, et al: Managing myocardial infarction complicated by mitral regurgitation. Prim Cardiol 19(10):40–48, 1993.

21. CORONARY RISK FACTORS AND MODIFICATION

Gumpanart Veerakul, M.D., FSCAI

1. What is the purpose of identifying coronary risk factors in people with and without coronary artery disease (CAD)?

CAD is multifactorial in origin with a long latent period. Despite a 24% decline in its mortality since 1980, CAD remains a leading cause of death in Western society and has a high morbidity. In an attempt to prevent CAD and its related complications, epidemiologic data have verified a number of risk factors that are statistically associated with CAD development. Therefore, it is a primary concern to normalize all potential modifiable risk factors in order to postpone or regress well-established lesions in patients with preexisting CAD (**secondary prevention**) and to delay disease development in healthy individuals who are at high risk (**primary prevention**).

2. What characteristics put people at risk for developing CAD?

Owing to the multifactorial origin of CAD, its underlying mechanism is not completely understood. However, certain characteristics have been found to be independently related to the subsequent occurrence of CAD although they may not necessarily have a causal relationship (see Table).

Risk Factors for Coronary Artery Disease

MAJOR RISK FACTORS	MINOR RISK FACTORS
Nonmodifiable	
Increasing age	Obesity
Family history of CAD before age 55 in men or before age 65 in women	Physical inactivity
	Psychological stress
Male gender	Oral contraceptive use
Postmenopause (women)	Impaired glucose tolerance
Modifiable	
Hypertension	
Dyslipidemia (elevated LDL-C and Lp(a) and low HDL-C)	
Diabetes mellitus	
Cigarette smoking	

LDL-C = low-density lipoprotein cholesterol, TG = triglyceride, Lp(a) = lipoprotein (a), HDL-C = high-density lipoprotein cholesterol.

Combinations of those risk factors are synergistic and greatly increase the probability of CAD. For example, a 50-year-old, nonsmoking normotensive man with an elevated serum cholesterol (total cholesterol 7.0 mmol/L) will have an estimated 10% risk of developing CAD over the next 10 years. The risk doubles if he becomes a smoker and has hypertension. For proper assessment, all possible risk factors must be evaluated when approaching the population at risk.

3. Which groups of patients should be instructed in risk reduction measures?

- Patients with established CAD or other atherosclerotic diseases because they are at very high risk of developing further vascular complications

- Healthy individuals who are at high risk from having combinations of major risk factors including diabetes mellitus, smoking, hypertension, elevated low-density lipoprotein cholesterol (LDL-C) levels, and low high-density lipoprotein cholesterol (HDL-C) levels (< 35 mg/dl)
- Close relatives of patients with early onset of CAD and other atherosclerotic diseases

4. When should hypercholesterolemia be treated?

The suggested desirable value of total cholesterol (TC) is less than 190 mg/dl (4.9 mmol/L). The positive association between elevated TC and CAD is primarily due to the high level of LDL-C. Data from epidemiologic studies and recent clinical trials clearly confirm the role of LDL cholesterol (LDL-C) as a cause of atherosclerosis. In general, a 10% increase in LDL-C is associated with a 20% increase in the risk of CAD.

National Cholesterol Educational Program Guidelines for Treatment of LDL-C in Primary and Secondary Prevention

	LEVEL FOR DRUG CONSIDERATION		THERAPEUTIC GOAL	
	mg/dl	mmol/L	mg/dl	mmol/L
No CAD, < 2 risk factors	≥ 190	≥ 4.9	< 160	< 4.1
No CAD, ≥ 2 risk factors	≥ 160	≥ 4.1	< 130	< 3.4
Established CAD	≥ 130	≥ 3.4	≤ 100	≤ 2.6

LDL-C can be calculated from LDL-C = TC – HDL-C – 0.2 (triglyceride-C)

5. For primary prevention of CAD, is there a firm benefit of cholesterol reduction?

Evidence from five major randomized, placebo-controlled trials confirms the beneficial effects of cholesterol-lowering agents in reducing the risk of coronary events.

1. **World Health Organization Trial** (1978): Five years of treatment with clofibrate, 1.6 gm/day, reduced the incidence of ischemic events by 20% in the treated group compared to those in the control group.

2. **Lipid Research Clinics Coronary Primary Prevention Trial** (1984): The group of patients treated with cholestyramine (14–24 gm/day) exhibited a 19% reduction in coronary death and nonfatal myocardial infarction (MI) rates over a 7-year period. Roughly, reducing the cholesterol level by 1% resulted in a 2% reduction of CAD risk.

3. **Helsinki Heart Study** (1988): Treatment with **gemfibrozil**, 600 mg twice a day for 5 years, resulted in a 34% reduction of coronary events.

4. **West of Scotland Coronary Prevention Study** (WOSCOPS) (1995): This trial involved a total of 6595 men with hypercholesterolemia, most of whom had no prior CAD. After an average follow-up of 4.9 years, the incidence of major coronary events (nonfatal MI or coronary death) was 7.9% in the placebo-treated group and 5.5% in the group treated with pravastatin (40 mg/day). The risk reduction of major coronary events was 31% (p < 0.001), and the total mortality was also reduced by 22% (p = 0.051).

5. **Air Force/Texas Coronary Atherosclerosis Prevention Study** (AFCAPS/TexCAPS; 1998): The total of 6605 healthy men and women with average TC and LDL-C and low HDL-C level (mean 36 mg/dl) were randomized into a group receiving placebo and a group receiving lovastatin, 40 mg/day. After 5.2 years of treatment with lovastatin and a diet low in saturated fat and cholesterol, the treatment group's incidence of major acute coronary events (sudden death, fatal and nonfatal MI, and unstable angina) was reduced by 37% (p < 0.001), and the need for revascularization was reduced to 33% (p = 0.004). However, there was no significant difference in total mortality between the two groups.

6. What about the effect of cholesterol reduction in patients with known CAD?

The beneficial effects of secondary prevention seem to be confirmed by the convincing results of trials reported since 1994. Most studies show an average of 25% risk reduction in both major coronary events and total mortality in CAD patients after 5 years of treatment with 3-hydroxy-3-methylglutaryl coenzyme A (HMG Co-A) reductase inhibitors (statin) drugs.

1. **Coronary Drug Project:** Nicotinic acid effectively reduced LDL-C and very low density lipoprotein (VLDL-C) levels and increased HDL-C level in male heart attack victims, resulting in a 29% lower rate of MI recurrence than in those receiving placebo treatment. The overall mortality in this trial was not significant initially but later showed an 11% reduction at the end of 9 years.

2. **Stockholm Ischemic Heart Study:** A combination of clofibrate and nicotinic acid resulted in a 36% reduction of CAD-related mortality in most MI victims compared to those in the control group.

3. **Scandinavian Simvastatin Survival Study** (4S; 1994): A total of 4444 men and women with CAD were enrolled. After 5.4 years, treatment with simvastatin reduced the plasma TC by 25%, reduced the plasma LDL-C by 35%, and increased plasma HDL-C by 8%. The total mortality (primary end point) was 11.5% in the placebo group versus 8.2% in the simvastatin group (p = 0.0003). Although the non–cardiac death rates were similar, the relative risk of total mortality was decreased 30%, and the relative risk of coronary death was reduced by 42%. There was also a 34% reduction in major coronary events (p < 0.00001).

4. **Long-term Intervention with Pravastatin in Ischemic Disease** (LIPID; 1995): This study randomized a total of 9014 post-MI/unstable angina patients with modest cholesterol levels (TC 155–271 mg/dl) to placebo and pravastatin groups. At follow-up after a mean of 6 years, there was a 24% risk reduction in coronary death (p = 0.0004), a 29% reduction in total MI (p = 0.000006), and 23% reduction in total mortality (p = 0.00002) in the pravastatin-treated group compared to the placebo group.

5. **The Cholesterol and Recurrent Events** (CARE) **Trial** (1996) randomly divided a total of 4159 men and women with known CAD (age ranged from 65 to 75 years) and borderline plasma levels (mean TC 221 ± 21 mg/dl, mean LDL-C 150 ± 17 mg/dl) into pravastatin and placebo groups. After 5 years of treatment, pravastatin reduced total major coronary events by 24% (p = 0.002), and there was no significant difference in overall mortality or mortality from noncardiovascular causes.

7. Is there any excess in mortality occurring along with cholesterol reduction?

One trial in 1984 (the report of the Committee of Principal Investigators of the WHO Cooperative Trial on Primary Prevention of Ischemic Heart Disease with Clofibrate) showed an increase in noncardiovascular deaths in the treated group. Whether or not this trial requires a longer time and a larger sample size to show a reduction in total mortality remains unanswered. In fact, plotting the data from the prospective epidemiologic studies on a graph demonstrated the relationship of plasma TC and total mortality as a J-shaped figure. While the causes of death in people with a high level of plasma cholesterol are mainly from excess cardiovascular deaths, the mortality causes of the group with lower level of cholesterol are mostly from noncardiovascular etiologies such as cancers, violence, and trauma. However, the relationship between cholesterol reduction and noncardiovascular death is not seen in the recent clinical trials. No deaths from noncardiovascular causes have been recorded in cholesterol reduction groups from the WOSCOPS, 4S, and CARE studies.

8. What is the clinical impact of a high-density lipoprotein cholesterol?

Epidemiologic data has shown a strong but inverse association between HDL-C and the risk of CAD. People with low HDL-C (< 40 mg/dl) but have either elevated serum triglyceride (> 180 mg/dl) or elevated TC level (> 200 mg/dl) are considered at risk for CAD whereas those with high HDL-C (ratio of TC to HDL-C of < 4.5) achieved a protective effect against atherosclerosis. Although its exact role is not well understood, HDL-C is believed to protect the arterial wall by helping transportation of LDL-C back to the liver for further degradation or by inhibiting oxidation of LDL-C in the wall. HDL-C level is lowered by smoking, obesity, and physical inactivity. Increasing levels of HDL-C can be achieved by stopping smoking, reducing body weight (in obese persons), controlling elevated triglyceride, getting regular aerobic exercise, and taking estrogen supplements and nicotinic acid.

9. Is hypertriglyceridemia an independent risk factor of CAD?

The relationship between hypertriglyceridemia and atherosclerosis has been confusing for years. Only a small portion of triglyceride (TG) is found in LDL-C and HDL-C, but the most TG-rich particles, such as chylomicrons (from intestinal mucosa) and VLDL (from liver), are not atherogenic. Several case-control and prospective observational studies have identified elevated TG as a univariate predictor of CAD. However, the support from multivariate analyses is not convincing, especially after the HDL-C level was adjusted. Recently, increasing evidence has suggested that elevated TG is an important risk factor for CAD in selected population groups. In the Framingham Heart Study, after a 14-year follow-up, TG has been shown to be an independent risk factor in women between the ages of 50 and 69 years. In an 8-year follow-up of the Copenhagen Male Study, with adjusting HDL-C level, a high level of fasting TG is a strong and independent risk factor of CAD in middle-aged and elderly white man. A meta-analysis of 17 prospective studies also confirms that TG is an independent risk factor for CAD by revealing a 30% increase in cardiovascular risk in men and a 75% increase in similar risk in women.

Although it is difficult to show the benefit of reduction of only serum TG and coronary events without affecting other lipoproteins, recent studies report some interesting results. In the Stockholm Ischemic Heart Disease Prevention Study (SIHDPS), after 5 years of treatment with niacin and clofibrate, a reduction in total mortality, coronary death, and TG were observed but a reduction in TC was not. In the Bezafibrate Coronary Atherosclerosis Intervention Trial (BECAIT), the angiographic benefit observed was related to reduction in VLDL, reduction in fibrinogen, and elevation of HDL-C but not elevation of LDL-C level. Despite growing evidence to support the connection between elevated TG and the risk of CAD, the causal relationship in the absence of other risks, including HDL-C, remains to be proven.

10. What lifestyle changes should be recommended for people at risk of CAD?

Lifestyle changes should be strongly encouraged and supported in a professional way before any other intervention is undertaken. Physicians should recommend that patients:

- Stop smoking all forms of tobacco. This will reduce not only the risk of atherosclerosis but also the risk of thrombosis.
- Reduce total fat intake to < 30% of total daily calories, and limit intake of cholesterol to < 300 mg/dl. Replace saturated fats with mono- and polyunsaturated fats from vegetable and carbohydrates. Increase intake of fresh fruit, cereal, and greens.
- Reduce salt and alcohol intake, especially if hypertension exists and take medication regularly to keep blood pressure below 140/90 mmHg.
- Increase physical activity with regular aerobic exercise 4–5 times per week.
- Reduce body weight if body mass index is > 30 kg/m^2.

11. Is there a reduction in MI incidence when hypertension is under control?

A meta-analysis of 14 randomized trials showed that a reduction of 5–6 mmHg in diastolic pressure was associated with a 42% reduction in stroke incidence but only a 14% decrement in MI incidence. The reason for this difference is not known. Recent data from the Framingham study of patients treated for hypertension for 20 years have shown a reduction of absolute risk of cardiovascular mortality by 60% and a reduction of all-cause mortality of 30%. This result raises the possibility that controlling hypertension may require a longer follow-up time to reduce the CAD events.

12. To what degree does smoking cessation truly reduce CAD and major coronary events?

In general, ceasing to smoke results in a 50–70% reduction in CAD risk at the end of 5 years. When combined with lowering dietary cholesterol, as in the Oslo study, the incidence of MI (fatal and nonfatal) and CAD death was 47% and 55% lower, respectively, than those in the control group. Similar results were observed in the Multiple Risk Factor Intervention Trial (MRFIT), in which hypertensive treatment was combined with smoking cessation.

13. Are elevated homocysteine levels and low serum folate and B_6 levels associated with the risk of CAD?

Homocysteine is an intermediate amino acid resulting from the metabolism of methionine and is known to be toxic to vascular endothelium. Several case-control studies have shown that higher levels of homocysteine and lower levels of folic acid, B_6, and B_{12} are found more frequently in subjects with atherosclerotic diseases (such as myocardial infarction, stroke, peripheral vascular diseases) than in control subjects. However, the causal role of elevated homocysteine and the risk of atherosclerosis remain inconclusive:

1. Atherosclerotic patients may have a higher level of homocysteine because they have more advanced inflammatory disease, not because homocysteine caused their vascular diseases. Low levels of folic acid (essential for DNA synthesis), which has been proposed by retrospective study as an independent risk factor for fatal CAD, may reflect the repairing process in those patients.

2. Measuring this rapidly oxidized amino acid requires a standard technique that is not available in previous reports. For example, storing a blood sample at room temperature may cause falsely increased homocysteine levels resulting from red cell release. Homocysteine also increases in several conditions including after a meal and as a person ages and is higher in men than in women.

3. Epidemiologic studies show a significant correlation between homocysteine levels of $11-16$ μmol/L and cardiovascular disease, which is only 3 μmol/L higher than the level in the control group. In fact, the normal range of homocysteine is not well defined, although it is believed to be in the range of $5-15$ μmol/L. Therefore, it is probably too early to conclude that homocysteine causes CAD. Clinical trials with folate, B_6, and B_{12} supplement, correlating homocysteine level and CAD, are required in both primary and secondary prevention to prove this hypothesis.

14. Is there a link between chronic infection and CAD?

At least 50% of patients who develop acute MI have no identifiable risk factors, suggesting that many risks remain undiscovered. Recent serologic studies demonstrated an association between antibodies against certain organisms (i.e., *Chlamydia pneumoniae*, *Helicobactor pylori*, and cytomegalovirus) and human CAD. While the clinical and epidemiologic studies supporting *H. pylori* and cytomegalovirus remain weak and limited, stronger evidence exists for *C. pneumoniae*, a gram-negative bacteria causing respiratory tract infection. Detection of this microbe in human atheroma and in tissue macrophages suggests the possibility that inflammation is caused by this organism. Two small trials showed that eradicating this organism with macrolide antibiotics (azithromycin and roxithromycin) results in reduction of ischemic events. However, the detection of *C. pneumoniae* DNA in other sites such as stenotic aortic valve, hepatic vessels, and spleen suggests that this organism may be only an innocent bystander in the inflamed tissues. The causative role of chronic infection in CAD remains to be defined, but it leads to the hope of identifying another potentially treatable risk in the future.

BIBLIOGRAPHY

1. Downs GR, Clearfield M, Weiss S, et al: Primary prevention of acute coronary events with lovastatin in men and women with average cholesterol levels: Results of the Air Force/Texas Coronary Atherosclerosis Study. JAMA 279:1615–1622, 1998.
2. Farmer LA, Gotto AM: Risk factors for coronary artery disease. In American Heart Association: 1991 Heart and Stroke Facts. Dallas, American Heart Association, 1991.
3. Hokanson JE, Austin MA: Plasma triglyceride level is a risk factor for cardiovascular disease independent of high-density lipoprotein cholesterol level: A meta-analysis of population-based prospective studies. J Cardiovasc Risk 3:213–229, 1996.
4. Jeppesen J, et al: Triglyceride concentration and ischemic heart disease: An eight-year follow-up in the Copenhagen Male Study. Circulation 97:1029–1036, 1998.

5. Lipid Research Clinics Program: The Lipid Research Clinics' Coronary Primary Prevention Trial results: I. Reduction in incidence of coronary heart disease; II. The relationship of reduction in incidence of coronary heart disease to cholesterol lowering. JAMA 251:351–364, 1984.

6. LIPID Study Group: Design features and baseline characteristics of the Long-Term Intervention with Pravastatin in Ischemic Disease (LIPID) Study: A randomized trial in patients with previous acute myocardial infarction and/or unstable angina pectoris. Am J Cardiol 76:474–479, 1995.

7. Mannienn V, Elo MO, Frick L, et al: Lipid alterations and decline in the incidence of coronary heart disease in the Helsinki Heart Study. JAMA 260:641–651, 1988.

8. National Cholesterol Educational Program: Second report of the Expert Panel on Detection, Evaluation, and Treatment of High Blood Cholesterol in Adults (Adult Treatment Panel II). Circulation 89:1329–1345, 1994.

9. Scandinavian Simvastatin Survival Study Group (4S): Randomised trial of cholesterol lowering in 4444 patients with coronary heart disease. Lancet 344:1383–1389, 1994.

10. West of Scotland Coronary Prevention Study Group: Influence of pravastatin and plasma lipids on clinical events in the West of Scotland Coronary Prevention Study (WOSCOPS). Circulation 97:1440–1445, 1998.

22. CONGESTIVE HEART FAILURE

Edward P. Havranek, M.D., and Gregory R. Giugliano, M.D.

1. What is heart failure?
Believe it or not, heart failure is somewhat difficult to define. It is best thought of as a condition in which the heart cannot meet the demands of the peripheral circulation in all situations.

2. How is it diagnosed?
No single test is diagnostic for congestive heart failure (CHF). The diagnosis is usually not difficult to make and is based on an assessment of the history, physical examination, and chest x-ray. It is important to use these data to decide if the patient has **left ventricular failure**, **right ventricular failure**, or a combination of both, since the causes and treatments differ. Occasionally, it is necessary to call on more sophisticated testing to make the diagnosis.

3. What are the four determinants of cardiac output?
Afterload, preload, heart rate, and myocardial contractility.

4. Which of these is abnormal in heart failure?
Actually, all four are abnormal. In most cases of heart failure, the initial event is a decline in myocardial contractility from any one of a number of causes.

5. What happens to afterload?
In response to decreased peripheral perfusion caused by a decline in cardiac output, systemic vascular resistance rises. Although there are several mechanisms for this, the most important are a rise in circulating catecholamines and activation of the sympathetic nervous system. Initially, this rise in afterload helps to maintain organ perfusion. When more advanced, it can become counterproductive and lead to a further reduction in cardiac output.

6. What happens to preload?
In response to decreased renal perfusion, intravascular volume rises. Again, several mechanisms contribute. Activation of the renin-angiotensin system is the most important. The dilated, poorly contractile left ventricle becomes less compliant. This means that small increases in volume produce a relatively large increase in pressure. The net result is an increase in preload. Initially, this helps to maintain cardiac output via the Frank-Starling mechanism. As with the changes in afterload, more severe rises are counterproductive and cause pulmonary vascular congestion and edema.

7. What happens to heart rate?
It rises. With decreased stroke volume (SV) caused by decreased contractility, an increase in heart rate helps preserve cardiac output according to the formula $CO = HR \times SV$. The rise in heart rate is due in part to the increased sympathetic tone.

8. What are the symptoms of heart failure?
The hallmark of heart failure is **exercise intolerance**. This is most commonly experienced as dyspnea on exertion, but some patients report easy fatigue. When **left heart failure** is more severe, patients may complain of orthopnea or paroxysmal nocturnal dyspnea. With this latter symptom, patients are awakened by a severe sensation of shortness of breath, often described as a "smothering" feeling. It is relieved by sitting on the edge of the bed or walking around; some patients get relief from sitting by an open window.

With **right heart failure**, patients most frequently notice edema of the feet and ankles. Sometimes, they are aware only of their shoes getting tighter. When edema involves the liver and gut, they notice right upper quadrant discomfort and abdominal fullness.

9. What are the signs of heart failure?

The **precordial examination** is of key importance. Lateral displacement of the apical impulse indicates left ventricular enlargement. With systolic dysfunction, the impulse is enlarged, sustained, and not forceful. An atrial filling wave (corresponding to S4) or a late diastolic filling wave (corresponding to S3) is sometimes palpable. On auscultation, listen for S3 and S4. A soft holosystolic murmur from mitral or tricuspid insufficiency may be heard when the left or right ventricles are enlarged.

Jugular venous distention is the most specific indicator of right heart failure. The examination is most reproducible if patients are examined sitting upright. The jugular venous pressure can then be measured as the distance from the top of the pulsation to the clavicle or manubrium. In almost all patients, if the jugular pulsation cannot be seen above the clavicle, the jugular venous pressure is normal.

Rales are usually, but not universally, present in left heart failure. They are, however, nonspecific.

Hepatomegaly is common in right heart failure. The liver edge is soft to slightly firm and frequently tender. Sustained pressure on the liver may cause sustained elevation of the jugular venous pressure (hepatojugular reflux).

Pitting edema is present in dependent body parts, usually the feet and ankles. Edema should be graded by how deeply pitting is noted and by how far up the lower extremity it extends.

10. Are there other diagnoses I should consider?

Pulmonary disease and CHF share many signs and symptoms, and it can be difficult to differentiate the two disease states. Patients with pericardial tamponade frequently present with dyspnea, jugular venous distention, and an enlarged heart on x-ray. Constrictive pericarditis may mimic many conditions, including heart failure. Some forms of valvular heart disease or congenital heart disease may be confused with heart failure.

Differential Diagnosis of Congestive Heart Failure

ISOLATED RIGHT HEART FAILURE	LEFT OR BIVENTRICULAR FAILURE
Pulmonary embolus	Aortic stenosis
Tricuspid stenosis	Aortic insufficiency
Tricuspid regurgitation	Mitral stenosis
Right atrial tumor	Mitral regurgitation
Cardiac tamponade	Most cardiomyopathies
Constrictive pericarditis	Restrictive cardiomyopathy
Pulmonic insufficiency	Acute myocardial infarction (MI)
Right ventricular (RV) infarction	Myxoma
Intrinsic lung diseasE	Hypertensive heart disease
Ebstein's anomaly	Myocarditis
	Supraventricular arrhythmias
	Left ventricular (LV) aneurysm
	Cardiac shunts
	High cardiac output states (anemia, systemic fistulae, beriberi, Paget's disease, carcinoid, thyrotoxicosis, etc.)

11. What are the chest x-ray findings?

The chest x-ray is important in diagnosing left heart failure. The x-ray shows signs of interstitial edema or alveolar filling. The cardiac shadow is usually enlarged. A pleural effusion may be present.

12. Define pulmonary edema.

This term refers to the presence of extracellular fluid in the alveolar spaces. In heart failure, it occurs when pulmonary venous pressure rises acutely and hydrostatic forces push fluid out of capillaries faster than it can be removed by the lymphatic system. This fluid accumulates in the alveoli, and pulmonary edema is present.

13. What other studies are useful?

More specialized studies may help establish the diagnosis or assess the course of the disease. **Echocardiography** is the most useful test when there is diagnostic uncertainty, because it can exclude the cardiac diseases similar to heart failure, assess left ventricular contractility, and give physiologic data such as estimates of pulmonary artery pressure. The **radionuclide ventriculogram** is best at quantifying ejection fraction. **Right heart catheterization** is useful in assessing response to therapy in some situations and in confirming an elevated pulmonary capillary wedge pressure and decreased cardiac output.

An **exercise treadmill test**, particularly when combined with expired gas analysis, is a useful functional test for determining the degree of heart failure and response to therapy. In difficult cases, it can separate cardiac disease from pulmonary disease.

14. Define "diastolic heart failure."

The term diastolic heart failure refers to cardiac diastolic dysfunction that results from excessive stiffness of the heart, resulting in an inability of the heart to fill properly. It contrasts with systolic dysfunction, which is an impairment of contractility. By definition, diastolic heart failure can be diagnosed only when the systolic function is normal.

Diastolic dysfunction can cause CHF via two mechanisms: First, the noncompliant left ventricle develops a high pressure during diastole, causing an elevation in pulmonary capillary wedge pressure. Second, less blood fills the ventricle during diastole, reducing preload, which in turn reduces cardiac output. Heart failure from diastolic dysfunction is seen in a wide variety of cardiac diseases.

15. What are some causes of diastolic dysfunction?

- Familial hypertrophic obstructive cardiomyopathy (also known as asymmetric septal hypertrophy or idiopathic hypertrophic subaortic stenosis)
- Severe hypertrophy (as in hypertensive heart disease or aortic stenosis)
- Restrictive cardiomyopathies (such as amyloidosis or endomyocardial fibroelastosis)

Although not usually classified with diastolic heart failure, constrictive pericarditis represents the same pathophysiology. Occasionally, ischemic heart disease may cause intermittent heart failure in the absence of systolic dysfunction.

16. How is diastolic dysfunction recognized clinically?

Pure diastolic heart failure is identified when a patient with normal systolic function (by echocardiogram or radionuclide ventriculogram) experiences left heart failure (by symptoms, physical examination, and chest x-ray). Also look for the more specific findings of some of the disease states causing diastolic dysfunction, such as Kussmaul's sign seen in restrictive cardiomyopathy or the characteristic decrease in murmur intensity during Valsalva maneuver in hypertrophic obstructive cardiomyopathy. Recent advances in echocardiography have assisted in making the diagnosis of diastolic heart failure, but which parameter is the most useful for diagnosing and flowing diastolic dysfunction is still a subject of debate. In general, however, abnormal relaxation of the left ventricle is readily diagnosed by pulsed Doppler.

17. How do I classify heart failure?

The standard classification scheme for heart failure was produced by the New York Heart Association:

Class	Patient Description
I	Asymptomatic
II	Mild CHF symptoms with vigorous activity
III	Moderate to severe symptoms with routine activity
IV	Decompensated patients with symptoms at rest. Usually confined to a bed or chair.

18. What drugs are used in patients with heart failure?

In patients with **systolic dysfunction**, first consider treatment with angiotensin-converting enzyme (ACE) inhibitors, since these agents decrease mortality. It is importantto use the maximum tolerated dose. For patients who cannot tolerate ACE inhibitors, try angiotensin receptor blockers (ARBs). If neither ACE inhibitors nor ARBs are tolerated, treat patients with a combination of hydralazine and nitrates.

In most cases, the above-mentioned drugs are used in combination with a diuretic. In patients with symptomatic systolic dysfunction, digoxin may be added. Digoxin has been shown to improve the symptoms of, and decrease admissions due to, heart failure—but it does not decrease mortality. A landmark trial recently published shows a marked mortality benefit in heart failure patients treated with spironolactone.

In patients with **diastolic dysfunction**, treatment is aimed at the underlying cause, such as valve replacement in aortic stenosis. In hypertensive or obstructive disease states, first consider beta-blockers or verapamil. Some data supports the use of ACE inhibitors in patients with diastolic dysfunction because of their effect on ventricular remodeling.

19. Which patients with CHF should be admitted to the hospital for treatment?

Patients with known CHF who have unacceptable symptoms despite use of adequate doses of ACE inhibitors, diuretics, and digitalis should be considered for admission. Additionally, patients who previously did not carry the diagnosis of heart failure and who present with signs and symptoms of new-onset heart failure should be admitted for initial work-up and initiation of therapy.

20. If a patient's symptoms of heart failure persist despite appropriate use of these medications, what can be done?

Patients who are severely decompensated may benefit from "tailored therapy," in which drug dosing is adjusted based on data obtained from a pulmonary artery catheter. In conjunction with the use of Swan-Ganz catheters, short-term infusions of dobutamine, milrinone, or nitroprusside for 48–72 hours has benefit that may last up to a month. When drug treatment fails, heart transplantation is a treatment option in selected patients. Left ventricular assist devices or intra-aortic balloon pumps may be temporary bridges to transplantation in critically ill patients.

21. Are beta-blockers useful in the treatment of heart failure?

Yes. Because the negative inotropic properties of beta-blockers are so well known, it seems odd to suggest that they might be useful in the treatment of heart failure. Yet over the past 20 years a number of small-scale studies have done exactly that.

Both laboratory and clinical studies have shown that advancing heart failure is accompanied by increasing levels of activation of the sympathetic nervous system. Although this activation starts as a consequence of the physiologic abnormalities in heart failure, it leads to excessive peripheral vasoconstriction that increases afterload and to down-regulation of cardiac beta-receptors. These latter two actions contribute to a downward spiral of declining contractility. Some have speculated that this spiraling might be interrupted by blockading the peripheral effects of catecholamines with beta-blockers.

This question was presented under the heading "Controversy" in the first edition of this book. At that time there were few good studies addressing the issue, and no beneficial mortality data. However, there are now several trials showing mortality reduction with the use of beta-blockers in patients with NYHA Class I–III heart failure. The initiation of beta-blockers in patients with heart failure can be very complex, and should only be undertaken by clinicians experienced in their use.

CONTROVERSY

22. Does anticoagulant therapy improve morbidity or mortality in heart failure patients?

This is a well debated topic across the world, yet the existing data is scant. The impetus for the debate lies in the theoretical risk of stroke from ventricular thrombi in patients with severely depressed systolic function.

For: A few small trials suggest a benefit to anticoagulating patients with severe systolic dysfunction; however, these results have not been reproduced in randomized, controlled fashion. There is currently a trial underway randomizing patients with depressed systolic function to aspirin, warfarin, or clopidogrel. This is the first large-scale trial of its kind and should help to answer this question. Currently, most specialized heart failure centers use anticoagulants in patients with severely depressed systolic function.

Against: Currently there are no definitive randomized, controlled, blinded studies evaluating the efficacy of long-term anticoagulation in patients with severely depressed systolic function. Therefore, treatment is based on theoretical grounds, and carries increased risk of bleeding complications.

BIBLIOGRAPHY

1. Abrams J: Essentials of Cardiac Physical Diagnosis. Philadelphia, Lea & Febiger, 1987.
2. Digitalis Investigation Group: The effect of digoxin on mortality and morbidity in patients with heart failure. N Engl J Med 336:525–533, 1997.
3. Grossman W: Defining diastolic dysfunction. Circulation 101:2020–2021, 2000.
4. Leier CV, Huss P, Lewis RP, Unverferth DV: Drug-induced conditioning in congestive heart failure. Circulation 65:1382–1387, 1982.
5. Packer M, Bristow M, et al: The effect of carvedilol on morbidity and mortality in patients with chronic heart failure. N Engl J Med 334:1349–1355, 1996.
6. Philbin EF, Rocco TA Jr: Use of angiotensin-converting enzyme inhibitors in heart failure with preserved left ventricular systolic function. Am Heart J 134:188–195, 1997.
7. Pitt B, Zannad P, et al: The effect of spironolactone on morbidity and mortality in patients with severe heart failure. N Engl J Med 341:709–717, 1999.
8. SOLVD Investigators: Effect of enalapril on survival in patients with reduced left ventricular ejection fractions and congestive heart failure. N Engl J Med 325:293–302, 1991.
9. SOLVD Investigators: Effect of enalapril on mortality and the development of heart failure in asymptomatic patients with reduced left ventricular ejection fractions. N Engl J Med 327:685–691, 1992.

23. ENDOCARDITIS

Arnold Einhorn, M.D., Olivia V. Adair, M.D., and Douglas Paul Voorhees, R.R.T.

1. Discuss the incidence and mortality rate of infective endocarditis (IE).

Although the mortality rate of IE has declined from almost 100% to 5–15% with the use of antibiotics, the incidence probably has increased. The reason for this increase is multifactorial: an aging population, increased number of patients with prosthetic valves, adults surviving with congenital heart disease (CHD), improved detection, recurrence in survivors of endocarditis, virulence of pathogens, poor compliance or inadequate prophylaxis, and intravenous drug use. The majority of cases involve patients with prosthetic cardiac valves, users of illicit intravenous drugs, and patients with mitral valve prolapse or other nonrheumatic abnormalities. Underlying anatomy, clinical situation, and infecting organism serve as the basis for prognosis and management.

2. What are the predisposing risk factors for endocarditis of native valves in adults?

Native valve endocarditis in nonintravenous drug users has an identifiable predisposing cardiac lesion in 60–80% of patients, including mitral valve prolapse, degenerative lesions of the aortic and mitral valves, CHD, and rheumatic heart disease. Rheumatic heart disease was the most common underlying lesion in the past (37–76%) but now accounts for approximately 30% of lesions in adults with endocarditis. Other important risk factors are advanced age, male gender, and diabetes mellitus.

3. Which congenital heart diseases are associated with IE?

CHD accounts for the underlying cardiac lesion in 10–20% of adults with IE. The most common lesions are patent ductus arteriosus, ventricular septal defect, bicuspid aortic valve, coarctation of the aorta, and pulmonic stenosis. With improvement in echocardiographic technology, isolated IE of the pulmonic valve has been increasingly recognized, especially in patients with atrial and ventricular septal defects, patent ductus arteriosus, and tetralogy of Fallot. Additional risk factors for IE are bucuspid aortic valve, especially in men older than 60 years; hypertrophic obstructive cardiomyopathy, which accounts for 5% of adults who develop endocarditis; and Marfan syndrome associated with aortic insufficiency.

4. List the organisms that are associated with IE of native valves in patients who are not intravenous drug users.

In these patients, the majority of cases of IE are due to:
- Streptococci (50–70%) (alpha-hemolytic and *S. viridans* account for the majority)
- Staphylococci (25%) (especially *S. aureus*)
- Enterococci (10%)

Native valve infections due to *Staphylococcus epidermidis*, enteric bacilli, or fungi are uncommon.

5. Intravenous drug users are at high risk for IE. Describe the course of IE in this subgroup of patients.

Bacteremias in intravenous drug users are common, and the organisms most frequently originate on the skin. *S. aureus* is the most common organism in IE (50–60%), whereas various species of streptococci and enterococci account for approximately 20% of cases; gram-negative bacilli, especially Pseudomonas and Serratia spp., for 10–15%; and fungi, usually culture-negative, for approximately 5% of cases.

Infection still shows a slightly higher preference for the **tricuspid valve** (44%), followed by the mitral (43%), aortic (40%), and pulmonic (3%) valves; infection also may involve both right-

and left-sided valves (16%) or both left-sided valves (13%). The majority of patients with IE of the tricuspid valve (70–100%) have pneumonia or multiple septic emboli, and the majority of intravenous drug users with *S. aureus* (70–80%) have isolated IE of the tricuspid valve (see figure below).

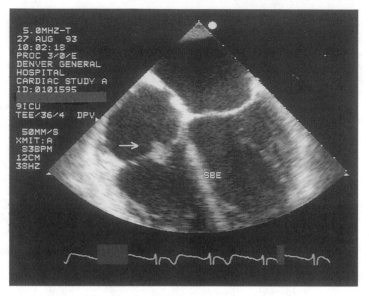

Endocarditis of the tricuspid valve with large mobile vegetation.

6. What are the most common organisms found in prosthetic valve endocarditis (PVE)?

PVE is divided into early (within 60 days of valve insertion) and late disease. **Early PVE** reflects perioperative contamination, either directly or through catheters (especially central lines). Staphylococcal infection accounts for 45–50% of cases, with *S. epidermidis* the most commonly isolated agent in early PVE (25–30%), followed by *S. aureus* (20–25%), gram-negative aerobic organisms (20%), and fungi (10–20%). **Late PVE** reflects seeding of the valve by transient bacteremia, especially from dental, genitourinary, or gastrointestinal manipulation; thus the organisms resemble those in native valve IE, with *S. viridans* being the most commonly isolated (25–30%), followed by *S. epidermidis* and *S. aureus* (25% and 10%, respectively).

7. Which prosthetic valve is more likely to acquire IE?

The rate of PVE is approximately the same for mechanical and tissue valves, but the aortic valve is 2–5 times more likely to be involved than the mitral valve.

8. What is the most common cause of culture-negative endocarditis?

The most common cause is inadequate therapy of prior endocarditis; culture-negative IE accounts for 5% of total cases.

9. What are the HACEK gram-negative organisms?

Haemophilus aphrophilus
Actinobacillus actinomycetemcomitans
Cardiobacterium hominis
Eikenella corrodens
Kingella kingae

10. Why is echocardiography important in the management of IE?

Echocardiography, especially **transesophageal echocardiography** (TEE) for patients with prosthetic valves, is important for both diagnosis and management decisions. A positive finding of vegetation constitutes a major criterion for diagnosis, second only to blood cultures. Echocardiography also provides important information about other valvular abnormalities, abscesses (see figure below), leaflet perforation, pericarditis, and ventricular function; serial studies are important in medically unresponsive patients to change management or to consider surgery.

Outcome is markedly affected by complications. Sensitivity for detecting vegetation is 50–70% by transthoracic echocardiography and > 95% with TEE. A negative study has some negative prognostic indicators, but does not exclude IE. Because of the numerous complications of PVE, patients with suspected IE should have TEE; the high mortality rate (up to 50% in late PVE and 40–80% in early PVE) is best countered with aggressive management.

Aortic valve endocarditis with a ring abscess on TEE

11. What are the definite indications for surgery in IE?

- Acute valvular dysfunction (i.e., severe mitral regurgitation or aortic insufficiency)
- Myocardial invasion
- Antibiotic-resistant organism and persistent sepsis
- Continuing (intractable) congestive heart failure
- Nonfatal emboli

12. If a clinical diagnosis of IE of a native valve is certain, which empirical therapy should be used while blood cultures are being incubated, barring regional-specific modifications?

Vancomycin and gentamicin should be used in suspected drug users, as *S. aureus* is resistant to beta-lactam antibiotics. If the clinical picture is acute endocarditis with methicillin-susceptible staphylococci, nafcillin or oxacillin plus gentamicin may be used.

13. In 1997, the American Heart Association changed its recommendations for antibiotic use and risk classification in IE prevention. What were the changes?

The recommendations from AHA and the American College of Cardiology will most likely continue to evolve. Therefore, a copy of the most recent recommendations should be kept available for reference (tel. 800/AHA-USA1). The major change is in post-procedure antibiotics, which are no longer advised for oral, dental, respiratory tract, and esophageal procedures (excluding sclerotherapy of esophageal varices and esophageal stricture dilatation). A single dose of amoxicillin (2 g) is suggested, 1 hour prior to the procedure. Also, while erythromycin was previously recommended for penicillin-allergic patients, azithromycin and clarithromycin have replaced it.

14. What is the empiric therapy for prosthetic valve endocarditis?
Ampicillin, vancomycin, and gentamicin.

15. Name four peripheral stigmata of IE.
Janeway lesions
Roth's spots
Splinter hemorrhages
Osler's nodes

16. What is Osler's or Austrian triad?
Osler's or Austrian triad consists of endocarditis, pneumonia, and meningitis. The most common organism is *Streptococcus pneumoniae*, which is especially prevalent in alcoholic (40%), elderly, and diabetic patients. The course is fulminant, with rapid valve destruction and abscess formation. The aortic valve is most often involved (see figure below), followed by the tricuspid valve. Infection is usually responsive to penicillin, but resistant strains that require vancomycin are becoming more common.

Aortic valve endocarditis.

17. Is anticoagulation helpful in the management of IE?
Although the vegetation is basically a thrombotic lesion and may embolize, no evidence suggests that anticoagulation is helpful in reducing embolization or preventing growth of vegetation. In fact, negative results, including increased rates of fatal intracerebral hemorrhage from mycotic aneurysms, cerebral embolus, and infarction, have been associated with use of heparin. However, recent data show that use of warfarin with antibiotic therapy is safe in patients with prosthetic

valve IE. The suggested protocol is to avoid heparin entirely unless there is a major indication (e.g., massive pulmonary embolism) and to use warfarin anticoagulation as necessary at the low range (international normalized ratio 2.5–3.5).

18. What are the common complications of IE?

- Heart failure: more common in IE of the aortic valve (75%) than in mitral valve (50%) or tricuspid valve disease (14%); poor prognostic sign (death rate with vs. without heart failure, 85% vs. 37%).
- Embolization: clinically seen in up to 35% of patients; pathologic evidence in up to 65%.
- Neurologic manifestations: 40–50% of patients.
- Mycotic aneurysm: 3–15% of patients; highest incidence in the proximal aorta.
- Renal failure: approximately 5%; dialysis can maintain the patient until bacterial antigens are cleared.

19. What is the prognosis of IE?

The prognosis depends on organism, type of valve, location, patient age, and complications. **Adverse prognostic indicators** are heart failure, renal failure, culture-negative disease, gram-negative or fungal infection, prosthetic valve, and abscess. **Favorable factors** are young age, early diagnosis and treatment, penicillin-sensitive streptococcal infection, and young intravenous drug users with *S. aureus* infection of the tricuspid valve (90% cure rate). Cure is 90% for native valve streptococcal infection, approximately 75–90% for enterococcal infection, and 30–60% for infection with *S. aureus*. Multiple valve involvement also has a higher mortality rate, as does aortic vs. mitral and left-sided vs. right-sided disease. Left-sided IE due to *S. aureus* carries a mortality rate of 25–40%. PVE has a worse prognosis: early PVE has a mortality rate of 41–80%, and late PVE of 20–50%.

IE involving both aortic and mitral valve.

20. What does the electrocardiogram (EKG) show in patients with IE? How often should the EKG be repeated?

An EKG should be done at admission for patients in whom IE is suspected and repeated according to response to treatment, initial findings, and echocardiographic data. Findings include possible silent MI or ischemia secondary to vegetation embolism involving a coronary artery. A prolonged P-R interval also may suggest extension into the conduction system, focal myocarditis, or abscess close to the conduction system. Other disturbances in conduction also may involve major complications, need for surgery, and worse prognosis.

21. Diagnosis and treatment of IE often are based on the belief that most cases are associated with dental work and that adherence to AHA guidelines is preventative. Is this belief founded on clinical trials?

Actually, there are several unfounded myths about IE. Only a fraction of the cases are associated with surgical or dental procedures, < 20%. About 4000–15,000 cases occur yearly, and 75% of patients have underlying cardiac lesions. The efficacy of prophylaxis is unknown; no prospective, randomized studies have been performed. Retrospective studies of high-risk patients with prosthetic valves suggest a 91–100% success rate with prophylaxis. A small study of 48 patients with IE following dental work found no significant benefits in treatment pre and post procedure, unless there was significant bleeding.

22. Does a past medical history of cardiac interventions or procedures mean prophylactic antibiotics are required?

No. A previous history of coronary artery bypass graft; percutaneous transluminal coronary angioplasty; stent, pacemaker, or defibrillator placement; as well as 6 months beyond repair of a ventricular or atrial septal defect, patent foramen ovale, or patent ductus arteriosus (without residual shunt) are all now considered negligible risk. Patients who have undergone these procedures are at no greater risk than the general population.

23. Do the minimal bactericidal concentrations (MBCs) help in treatment decisions?

Yes. Antimicrobial therapy should be established only after quantitative sensitivity tests of antibiotics—including MBC evaluation. In fact, especially in the case of a large (> 10 mm) vegetation, an MBC > 2 µg/ml may prompt early surgical consideration, because medical management is less likely to be successful. This is true even with established combination antibiotics.

24. Are there compelling factors to suggest that surgical intervention should be seriously considered?

Yes. The occurrence of the following complications prompts consideration of surgery:
• Large vegetations (> 10 mm) attached to the mitral valve are linked to a high incidence of thromboembolic complications. This usually is compelling for surgery, especially if, as in Question 23, the MBC of the optimally established combination of antibiotics (estimated by quantitative sensitivity tests of antibiotics) is high (> 2 µg/ml).
• Cerebral embolic events or MI thought to be due to an embolism
• Myocardial failure due to active valve incompetence
• Acute renal failure
• Mitral kissing vegetations
• Primary aortic valve IE
• Sepsis persisting > 48 hours despite adequate antimicrobial therapy

Note that there is controversy over the ability to predict embolic events. Therefore, evaluate the patient's condition and all of the above features when designing each individual's treatment plan.

25. What clinical features should I look for in IE?

Fever is the most common symptom and sign in patients with IE (80–90%). It is usually low grade, rarely > 39.4° C in subacute IE, but higher in acute IE. **Chills** are common (40–75%), but rigors are less often seen.

Heart murmurs are heard in 80–85% of patients with native valve endocarditis, except in tricuspid valve IE. Also, it's reported that with *S. aureus* the murmur is heard in only 30–45% on initial exam, but reaches the 80–85% range ultimately.

Splenomegaly is turning up less often recently, in 15–50% of patients.

Peripheral manifestations are reported in 25–75% of patients, but are less common and seem to be absent if there is only tricuspid valve IE.

Petechiae are common (10–40%). **Janeway lesions, Osler's nodes,** and **splinter hemorrhages** are seen in approximately 5–10% of patients.

26. Prophylaxis is still recommended for which high-risk categories?

- Prosethetic cardiac valves, including bioprosthetic and homograft
- Previous bacterial endocarditis
- Complex, cyanotic, congenital heart disease, i.e., single ventricle, transposition of great arteries, tetralogy of Fallot
- Surgically constructed systemic or pulmonary shunts or conduits

The regimen is now a single dose of antibiotic 1 hour pre-procedure: amoxicillin 2 g or, if penicillin-allergic, azithromycin or clarithromycin.

27. Which procedures are still moderate risk and require prophylaxis?

Most other cardiac malformations, acquired valvular dysfunction (e.g., rheumatic heart disease), hypertrophic cardiomyopathy, and mitral valve prolapse with either thickened leaflets or regurgitation.

BIBLIOGRAPHY

1. Birmingham GD, Rahko PS, Ballantyne F III: Improved detection of infective endocarditis with transesophageal echocardiography. Am Heart J 123:774–781, 1992.
2. Brydie AD, Clark AL: The changing face of endocarditis: Report of a series of cases. Hosp Med 60(5):378–380, 1999.
3. Castillo JC, Anguita MP, et al: Long-term outcome of infective endocarditis in patients who are not drug addicts: A 10-year study. Heart 83(5):525–530, 2000.
4. Chang FY: *Staphylococcus aureus* bacteremia and endocarditis. J Microbiol Immunol Infect 33(2):63–68, 2000.
5. Dajani AS, et al: Prevention of bacterial endocarditis by the American Heart Association. Circulation 96:358, 1997 and JAMA 277:1794, 1997.
6. De Castro S, Adorisito R, et al: Predicting embolic events in patients with infective endocarditis. Cardiology Review 17(3):29–34, 2000.
7. Durack DT: Infective and noninfective endocarditis. In Hurst JW (ed): The Heart, vol. 2, 8th ed. 1994, pp 1681–1704.
8. Frontera JA, Gradon JD: Right-side endocarditis in injection drug users: Review of proposed mechanisms of pathogenesis. Clin Infect Dis 30(2):374–378, 2000.
9. Horstkotte D: Endocarditis: Epidemiology, diagnosis, and treatment. Z Kardiol 89(suppl 4):2–11, 2000.
10. Korzeniowski OM, Kay D: Infective endocarditis. In Braunwald E (ed): Heart Disease: A Textbook of Cardiovascular Medicine, 5th ed. Philadelphia, W.B. Saunders, 1997.
11. Netzer RO, Zollinger E, Seiler C, Cerny A: Infective endocarditis: Clinical spectrum, presentation, and outcome. An analysis of 212 cases 1980–1995. Heart 84(1):25–30, 2000.

24. AORTIC DISSECTION AND DISEASES OF THE AORTA

Edward A. Gill, M.D.

1. What is aortic dissection?

Aortic dissection occurs when a separation develops within the media of the aorta, essentially causing the wall of the aorta to split into the true (original lumen) and false lumen.

2. What causes aortic dissection?

It is believed to be caused by a tear in the intimal layer of the aorta that results in the exposure of a typically diseased medial layer. Blood under pressure (common in patients who are hypertensive) then moves into the medial layer and begins traveling within the medial layer.

3. What is the direction of aortic dissection (antegrade or retrograde)?

Classically, the dissections proceeds antegrade down the aorta (from proximal to distal), but can also progress proximally or retrograde.

4. What are risk factors for developing aortic dissection?

The classic risk factor is hypertension. Patients are often elderly, in their sixth or seventh decade. Aortic dissection also develops in patients who have inherited connective tissue disorders, since connective tissue diseases affect the aorta frequently. Examples are Marfan syndrome and Ehlers-Danlos syndrome. Another common risk factor for dissection is a bicuspid aortic valve. Bicuspid valve has been found in 7–14% of all aortic dissections. The risk of aortic dissection appears to be unrelated to the degree of bicuspid aortic valve stenosis.

5. What is the relationship between pregnancy and aortic dissection?

The mechanism is unexplained, but often purported to be related to hormonal changes; about half of all aortic dissections in women under 40 years of age occur during pregnancy. The timing is typically in the third trimester, and occasionally in the early post-partum period.

6. Why is aortic dissection such an important diagnosis to make?

Aortic dissection, particularly of the ascending aorta, has a high mortality rate. Early studies suggested that the rate was 1% per hour when left untreated. The causes of death in this setting are rupture of the aorta and/or cardiac tamponade.

7. Describe the characteristic quality of the chest pain in patients with aortic dissection.

The chest pain has been described as "tearing," but perhaps a more constant finding is that the pain is most severe at onset. This is very different from classic angina, which comes on slowly and builds up in intensity.

8. List some important physical findings that can aid in the diagnosis of aortic dissection.

The presence of aortic regurgitation in the setting of chest pain should make you suspicious of aortic dissection, as the aortic valve is often part of the dissection syndrome either directly or secondarily related to aortic dilation. Another important physical finding is the absence of pulses or pulse deficits. They only occur in 50% of proximal dissection and 20% of distal aortic dissection.

9. What diagnostic modalities exist for aortic dissection?

The commonly employed diagnostic techniques include MRI, CT, transesophageal echo (TEE), and aortography.

10. Which of these methods has the highest sensitivity?
The sensitivity of both MRI and TEE were similar in series by Erbel and Nienaber, both nearing 99%.

11. Which of the methods has the highest specificity for the diagnosis?
MRI has a specificity of 98%.

12. So if the sensitivity and specificity of MRI is the best, why consider other tests?
MRI cannot be performed on all patients. Specific exclusions include patients with pacemakers, a situation that is not uncommonly encountered in cardiac patients; patients with intracranial clips; and patients with claustrophobia. In addition, the presence of coronary stents is a relative contraindication to MRI. Further, MRI is not always available 24 hours a day. CT is more likely to be available.

The sensitivity of CT has improved with the new spiral CT machines. Although the sensitivity of CT in Nienaber's series was only 83%, the sensitivity in recent series has been in the high 90s percentile.

Finally, TEE is much more portable than either MRI or CT, and therefore can be performed at the bedside of unstable patients.

13. Describe the treatment of aortic dissection.
The treatment of aortic dissection can be simplified just by stating that proximal dissections (Stanford type A involving the ascending aorta) are treated with emergency surgery. Distal dissections (Stanford type B involving the descending aorta distal to the left subclavian artery) are treated with blood pressure control and long-term medical treatment, unless vital organs such as the bowel or kidneys are involved. Note that initial treatment of type A dissections prior to surgery also requires aggressive blood pressure management.

14. What blood pressure medicines should be used in treating aortic dissections?
Absolute blood pressure must be controlled, but also the rate of rise of blood pressure with each cardiac cycle must be minimized. It is for this reason that beta-blockers are advocated for treatment of aortic dissection since they decrease dP/dT. Remember that part of blood pressure control is the **management of pain.** For the acute reduction of arterial pressure, the vasodilator sodium nitroprusside is very effective. The initial dose is 20 ug/min and can be titrated as high as 300 ug/min, depending on blood pressure response.

15. What are the downsides to using sodium nitroprusside?
Sodium nitroprusside or "nipride" can actually increase dP/dT, which is dangerous as this could lead to further propagation of the dissection. Therefore beta blockade should be given prior to the institution of nipride. Also, except when used at low doses (< 2 ug/kg/min), sodium nitroprusside infusion can result in important quantities of cyanide ion, which can be toxic. Thiocyanide levels can be followed. Sodium nitroprusside should not be used except by experts who are very familiar with its side effects and how to prevent them.

16. What are other choices for blood pressure control?
For the above reasons regarding nipride, labetolol is often a good substitute as it has both alpha- and beta-blocking actions. This drug can be started at a 2 mg/min infusion and titrated up to 5–20 mg/min.

17. What is the most common site for an atherosclerotic aneurysm involving the aorta?
The abdominal aorta (abdominal aortic aneurysm [AAA]). This is an important teaching point because aneurysm of the thoracic aorta is usually a different disease process than aneurysm of the abdominal aorta. The former is often due to underlying connective tissue illness, hypertension, bicuspid aortic valve, etc. The latter is usually due to atherosclerosis. However, atherosclerotic

aneurysms occasionally arise in the thoracic aorta and lead to penetrating ulcers that are life-threatening if they rupture.

18. When should abdominal aneurysms be repaired?

All patients with AAA > 6 cm should have surgical repair if they are surgical candidates. Aneurysms that are smaller, but symptomatic, should also be repaired. Note that nonsurgical modalities involving the placement of intra-aortic stents by interventional radiology and/or vascular surgery are evolving and improving. This therapy is likely to replace surgery for AAA in the near future for many, if not most, cases.

BIBLIOGRAPHY

1. Cooke JP, Kazmier FJ, Orszulak TA: The penetrating aortic ulcer: Pathologic manifestations, diagnosis, and management. Mayo Clinic Proc 63:718–725, 1988.
2. Crawford ES: The diagnosis and management of aortic dissection. JAMA 264:2537–2541, 1990.
3. Erbel R, Daniel W, Visser C, et al: Echocardiography in diagnosis of aortic dissection. Lancet 1:457, 1989.
4. Huang KK, Aberle DR, Lufkin R, et al: Advances in medical imaging. Ann Intern Med 112:203–220, 1990.
5. Karalis DG, Chadnrasekaran K, Victor MF, et al: Recognition and embolic potential of intraaortic atherosclerotic debris. J Am Coll Cardiol 17:73–78, 1991.
6. Marsalese DL, Moodie DS, Vacante M, et al: Marfan's syndrome: Natural history and long-term follow-up of cardiovascular involvement. J Am Coll Cardiol 14:422, 1989.
7. Nevitt MP, Ballard DJ, Hallet JW Jr: Prognosis of abdominal aortic aneurysms: A population-based study. N Engl J Med 321:1009–1014, 1989.
8. Nienaber CA, von Kodolitach Y, Nicolas V, et al: Definitive diagnosis of thoracic aortic dissection. The emerging role of noninvasive imaging modalities. N Engl J Med 328:1, 1993.
9. Pyeritz RE: Genetic and cardiovascular disease. In Braunwald E (ed): Heart Disease, 5th ed. Philadelphia, W.B. Saunders, 1997.
10. Sommer T, Fehske W, Holzknecht N, et al: Aortic dissection: A comparative study of diagnosis with spiral CT, multiplanar transesophageal echocardiography, and MR imaging [see comments]. Radiology 199(2):347–352, 1996.

25. PERICARDIAL DISEASE

Mark A. Perea, M.D., and Paul D. Sherry, M.D.

1. What are the normal functions of the pericardium?

The pericardium consists of two layers: the inner visceral layer, which is attached to the epicardium, and the outer parietal layer. The two layers are separated by approximately 15–50 ml of fluid. Normal functions of the pericardium include stabilizing the heart in anatomic position, reducing friction between the heart and adjacent structures, restricting the heart from overfilling, and providing a barrier against the spread of infections and neoplastic processes to the heart. The pericardium is clinically important because of its involvement in a number of disease states.

2. What are the most common causes of acute pericarditis?

In the outpatient setting, pericarditis is usually idiopathic. It is thought that viral infection probably causes many of the cases categorized as idiopathic. The coxsackie A and B viruses are highly cardiotropic and are two of the most common viruses that lead to pericarditis and myocarditis. Other viruses associated with pericarditis include mumps, varicella-zoster, influenza, Epstein-Barr, and human immunodeficiency virus (HIV).

In the inpatient setting some of the more common etiologies of pericarditis can be recalled with the mnemonic TUMOR.

T = **T**rauma

U = **U**remia

M = **M**yocardial infarction (acute and post); **M**edications (e.g., hydralazine and procainamide)

O = **O**ther infections (bacterial, fungal, tuberculous)

R = **R**heumatoid arthritis and other autoimmune disorders; **R**adiation

"Tumor" also serves as a useful reminder that metastatic cancer is a frequent cause of pericarditis and pericardial effusion in hospitalized patients.

3. What are the clinical manifestations in acute pericarditis?

The cardinal clinical features of acute pericarditis are chest pain, friction rub, and electrocardiogram (ECG) changes. Chest pain, which is almost always present, is characterized as pleuritic and postural and is relieved by sitting upright and leaning forward. The pain varies in location but is often substernal with radiation to the neck. The pericardial friction rub is the pathognomonic auscultatory finding. It characteristically has three components, but the ventricular systolic rub is the loudest component and the one that is usually present. The friction rub may vary in loudness and may be influenced by position. Thus, repeated cardiac auscultation with various positions is important.

Fever, leukocytosis, a mild elevated erythrocyte sedimentation rate, and pericardial effusion are often found in acute pericarditis.

4. What are the typical findings of acute pericarditis on ECG?

Conventionally, acute pericarditis causes ST segment elevation in most ECG leads, particularly the ones reflecting the epicardium (because the inflammation involves the epicardial surface of the heart), which are leads I, II, aVL, aVF, and V_3–V_6. Lead aVR usually shows ST depression. Unlike the ST elevation of acute myocardial infarction, which may concave downward like a cat's back, the ST elevation of pericarditis is concave upward. Depression of the PR segment occurs in the earlier stages of pericarditis and usually involves the limb and precordial leads. Another important distinguishing feature of pericarditis is that the T-wave inversion occurs *after* the ST segment returns to baseline. In myocardial infarction, there is often some degree of T-wave inversion accompanying the ST elevation.

An ECG from a patient with purulent pericarditis shows some of the classic features.

5. What is the treatment of acute pericarditis?

Addressing the underlying cause is the most appropriate treatment. However, treatment is generally symptomatic. Aspirin or other nonsteroidal anti-inflammatory agents (NSAIDs) such as indomethacin, usually suppress the symptoms within 24–48 hours. Corticosteroids may be beneficial in those who do not respond to NSAIDs. Narcotic agents such as meperidine and morphine may be given for pain. Anxiety responds well to diazepam or other anxiolytics.

6. Define pulsus paradoxus.

In normal physiologic conditions, blood pressure can decrease up to 10 mmHg during inspiration. In disorders that restrict normal right ventricular compliance, such as cardiac tamponade, the drop of systolic blood pressure on inspiration is greater than normal. This is due to an elevated right ventricular pressure, which causes bulging of the interventricular septum into the left ventricle. Thus, stroke volume is decreased with inspiration, which is then reflected as a drop in blood pressure.

7. How is pulsus paradoxus measured?

With the patient breathing normally, the blood pressure cuff is inflated and then deflated very slowly until Korotkoff sounds are heart intermittently (the sound during expiration). Then, the cuff is further deflated slowly until all beats are heard (the sound during inspiration). If the difference between the two pressures is abnormally elevated, it is defined as pulsus paradoxus. If severe, this condition can be detected by weakness or absence of the arterial pulse during inspiration. However, a sphygmomanometer is usually required.

8. What are the two classical ECG changes of pericardial effusion?

Diffuse low voltages and **electrical alternans** may be seen with pericardial effusions. Changes in the QRS are due to not only the amount of fluid but also the electrical conductivity of the fluid. In canine studies, saline introduced into the pericardial space produced a greater voltage reduction than blood.

Electrical alternans is a repetitive alternating change in the P, QRS, and T-wave amplitudes that occasionally occurs with cardiac tamponade. Most commonly, the QRS alone shows the alternating amplitude. The swinging motion of the heart in a relatively large volume of pericardial fluid is thought to produce electrical alternans. Sometimes electrical alternans is noticeable in only one lead and could therefore be missed on a bedside cardiac monitor. It should be noted that electrical alternans may occur in other conditions, such as paroxysmal supraventricular tachycardia, hypertension, and acute episodes of ischemia.

9. When does cardiac tamponade occur?
Cardiac tamponade occurs when the accumulation of fluid in the pericardial space increases pericardial pressure and thus decreases cardiac output. As the intrapericardial pressure rises, there is a progressive elevation and, usually, equalization of intracardiac chamber pressures. Ventricular diastolic filling becomes progressively limited, leading to a reduction in stroke volume. Compensatory adrenergic activation leads to tachycardia and increased myocardial contractility. If tamponade is unrelieved, the compensatory mechanisms are unable to keep the systemic arterial pressure from falling and hemodynamic collapse occurs.

10. What are the physical findings in cardiac tamponade?

Jugular venous distention	Pulsus paradoxus
Tachypnea	Diminished heart sounds
Tachycardia	Pericardial friction rub

11. Can the diagnosis of cardiac tamponade be excluded by chest x-ray?
Enlargement of the cardiac silhouette in adults usually is not manifest until at least 250 ml of fluid is present. Therefore, a normal chest x-ray does not reliably exclude the possibility of cardiac tamponade. Echocardiography is the most effective way of diagnosing cardiac tamponade because it is sensitive, specific, and noninvasive and can be performed rapidly.

12. What is the role of echocardiography in the diagnosis of pericarditis and cardiac tamponade?
The echocardiogram is the most sensitive test for the detection of pericardial effusion. As little as 15 ml of fluid can be detected by two-dimensional echocardiography. Pericardial fluid appears as an echo-free space between the walls of the heart and pericardium (see Figure). In tamponade, the cardiac chambers may appear underfilled and contracted. Collapse of the right atrium and right ventricle during diastole is virtually diagnostic of cardiac tamponade. Right atrial collapse tends to occur earlier and may be detected at a time when no clinical signs of tamponade exist, making it less specific for diagnosing tamponade than right ventricular collapse. The echocardiogram can also be used to guide placement of the needle used in pericardiocentesis.

Two-dimensional echocardiogram from a patient with pericardial effusion (LV = left ventricle, RV = right ventricle).

13. What is Dressler's syndrome?

This syndrome develops in a small number of patients a few days to several weeks and, in rare instances, months after an acute myocardial infarction. This post–myocardial infarction syndrome is characterized by low-grade fever, pericarditis with a friction rub, pleurisy, and pericardial effusion. Patients usually respond well to high doses of aspirin.

14. Describe constrictive pericarditis. Name some of its causes.

Constrictive pericarditis occurs when inflammation leads to thickened, fibrotic, adherent pericardium that restricts diastolic filling of the cardiac chambers.

The most common cause of constrictive pericarditis is idiopathic. However, other causes include radiation therapy, cardiac surgery, and neoplasm. Some uncommon causes are tuberculosis and histoplasmosis.

15. Describe the physical findings of constrictive pericarditis.

The jugular venous pattern yields the most significant finding in this condition so the neck should be the starting point of the examination.

Jugular veins. The jugular veins are distended with prominent x and y descents. There is usually an increase in the height of the jugular venous pulsation with inspiration (Kussmaul's sign).

Lungs. The lung fields are usually clear. Sometimes, a pleural effusion may be present and can be a clue to pericardial constriction in patients being evaluated for isolated pleural effusion of unknown etiology.

Heart. The apical impulse is usually soft and diffuse. S_1 and S_2 may be decreased in intensity. A diastolic pericardial knock may be heard along the left sternal border. The pericardial knock is a loud sound occurring early in diastole (0.09–0.12 seconds after A_2) and is sometimes accentuated with inspiration. Pericardial knocks may be confused with an S_3 but may be distinguished by a higher acoustic frequency and earlier occurrence than an S_3.

Abdomen. There may be distention from ascites. The liver is enlarged and pulsatile. In chronic cases, the spleen may also be enlarged.

Extremities. Peripheral edema is present.

BIBLIOGRAPHY

1. Ameli S, Shah P: Cardiac tamponade, pathophysiology, diagnosis, and management. Cardiol Clin 9:455–476, 1991.
2. Barach P: Pulsus paradoxus. Hosp Physician 36:49–50, 2000.
3. Chou T: Electrocardiography in Clinical Practice. Philadelphia. W.B. Saunders, 1991.
4. Diamond T: The ST segment axis: A distinguishing feature between acute pericarditis and acute myocardial infarction. Heart Lung 14:629–631, 1985.
5. Fauci AS, et al (eds): Harrison's Principles of Internal Medicine, 14th ed. New York, McGraw-Hill, 1998.
6. Lorell BH, Braunwald E: Pericardial disease. In Braunwald E (ed): Heart Disease: A Textbook of Cardiovascular Medicine, 5th ed. Philadelphia, W.B. Saunders, 1997.
7. Mehta A, Mehta M, Jain AC: Constrictive pericarditis. Clin Cardiol 22:334–344, 1999.
8. Soler-Soler J, Permanyer-Miralda G, Sagrista-Sauleda J: A systematic diagnostic approach to primary acute pericardial disease: The Barcelona experience. Cardiol Clin 8:609–620, 1990.

26. HYPERTENSION

Catalin Loghin, M.D.

1. Define hypertension. How widespread is it in the United States?

The Joint National Committee on Detection, Evaluation, and Treatment of High Blood Pressure, in its sixth report (JNC VI), defined hypertension as an average of two or more diastolic readings > 90 mmHg on at least two consecutive visits, or an average of multiple systolic readings > 140 mmHg. Systolic hypertension is diagnosed if systolic blood pressure (BP) is > 140 mmHg with a diastolic BP < 90 mmHg, in contrast to borderline hypertension: systolic BP 140–149 and diastolic BP < 90 mmHg. Mild, moderate, and severe hypertension subgroups have been defined as well. Based on these definitions, up to 24% of the adult population in the U.S. suffers from hypertension.

2. What is the significance of systolic and diastolic BP readings?

BP measurements should be done after at least 5 minutes of rest, with at least two averaged readings, in both arms and in seated as well as in standing positions. While a cuff device accurately measures systolic BP, diastolic readings are consistently higher than intra-arterial pressures by 10–15 mmHg, in particular in elderly or atherosclerotic patients. Traditionally, diastolic BP has been held responsible for the cardiovascular complications of hypertension, rather than systolic BP. Currently, more importance is given to the systolic BP, and the combination of a high systolic and normal diastolic pressure (resulting in a widened pulse pressure) seems to be the best predictor of cardiovascular risk.

Until recently, there was a concern about a J-curve effect in reducing systolic BP (over-reduction leading to increase in cardiovascular risk). As a subject of current controversy, excessive reduction of diastolic BP is regarded as a possible therapeutic caveat as it may precipitate coronary events by decreasing myocardial perfusion.

3. Is 24-hour blood pressure monitoring in an ambulatory setting beneficial?

The "white coat effect" is a well-established entity and is the cause of higher BP readings in the physician's office as compared to ambulatory measurement. The goal for treatment is to decrease BP below 140/90 mmHg, based on readings in the doctor's office. However, the World Health Organization (WHO) limit is 125/85 mmHg for ambulatory readings. An emerging therapeutic principle is to lower the BP as much as tolerated by the patient, keeping in mind that the optimal BP for cardiovascular risk reduction is 120/80 mmHg. The more severe the complications of hypertension, the more dramatic a decline in BP values is necessary.

Current (JNC VI and WHO/International Society of Hypertension) **indications for ambulatory BP monitoring** are: suspected white coat hypertension, episodic hypertension, autonomic dysfunction, apparent drug resistance, hypotensive symptoms with antihypertensive medications, office hypertension in subjects with low cardiovascular risk, and hypertension resistant to drug treatment. Note that there is no evidence that ambulatory BP monitoring improves cardiovascular risk stratification, although it is a precious tool in guiding therapy.

4. You have diagnosed a new case of hypertension. What is your next step?

Arterioles are the vessels to sustain the most damage from persistent elevation of BP. Therefore, the first step is to do a "damage assessment" by evaluating the target organs of hypertension, keeping in mind that their involvement is an expression of arteriolar damage with subsequent ischemia and ischemia-induced changes.

Kidney: signs of involvement range from minimal proteinuria or slight increase of serum creatinine to end-stage renal disease. Kidney size is evaluated by a variety of imaging methods and has prognostic significance. Hypertension is the second leading cause of renal failure in the U.S., in particular in African-Americans.

Brain: the eye fundus appearance is the "mirror" of the brain circulation. Findings range from minor atherosclerotic changes to papilledema and hemorrhages which are consistent with malignant hypertension. A careful neurologic examination may reveal signs of previously undiagnosed strokes, and history may reveal previous transient ischemic attacks.

Heart: the direct consequence is LV hypertrophy (LVH) with increased LV mass; this is easily documented by electrocardiogram, 2D and M-mode echocardiogram, or cardiac MRI. LVH is strongly associated with an increased risk of sudden death and MI, and constitutes the basis for decreased LV compliance and subsequent diastolic dysfunction. A thorough evaluation for the presence of coronary artery disease, guided by a skillful interview, is required. Holter monitoring may be necessary for evaluating LVH-associated arrhythmias. The last step in the natural history of the disease is LV dilatation and pump failure, with the classical signs of CHF.

5. What is secondary hypertension?

Up to 5% of all hypertension cases are "secondary," meaning that a cause can be identified. Some of these cases are curable if the source of hypertension can be removed, e.g., surgery for an adrenal tumor, stenting of a renal artery stenosis, correction of an aortic coarctation. Given the small incidence of secondary forms, routine screening for all possible etiologies is not recommended. A targeted approach is much more cost-effective, and clinical and laboratory clues are precious in "tailoring" the etiologic work-up.

6. Describe a targeted approach to secondary hypertension.

The following scenarios should trigger a search for possible causes of secondary hypertension:
- Onset at a young age (< 35 years).
- Unexplained muscular weakness, suggesting hypokalemia of primary hyperaldosteronism (in the absence of diuretic treatment). An exaggerated hypokalemia following regular doses of diuretics has the same significance.
- Paroxysmal crises of palpitations, sweating, and headaches suggest a pheochromocytoma.
- Abdominal/lumbar trauma may result in a perirenal hematoma with subsequent small unilateral kidney.
- A transient episode of periorbital swelling and dark-colored urine that went untreated may point to a chronic glomerulonephritis.
- Multiple episodes of cystitis or urinary infection left untreated or with incomplete treatment will lead to and suggest chronic pyelonephritis.
- Use of birth control pills by young women; laxative use by elderly people. (Note that the former may not report the pills unless specifically asked [drug-induced hypertension], and the latter generally do not consider their licorice-based, over-the-counter laxative to be "medication" [licorice has mineralocorticoid effects].)
- A history of chronic pain may be the clue for analgesic nephropathy.
- Renal calculi may be the sign of hyperparathyroidism or the cause of obstructive nephropathy.
- Reduced femoral pulses with high BP values only in the upper extremities suggests aortic coarctation (palpate the intercostal area space for exaggerated pulsations due to compensatory collateral circulation).
- Abdominal bruits (heard in systole and diastole without pressing with the stethoscope) are suggestive of renal artery stenosis. The cause may be either atherosclerosis in an elderly patient or fibromuscular dysplasia in a young woman. Renal artery stenosis is also suggested by an exaggerated drop in BP following initiation of treatment with ACE inhibitors or angiotensin-receptor blockers.
- Bilateral abdominal palpable masses are commonly due to policystic kidney. Typically, the history reveals the presence of hypertension with renal failure in other family members.
- Abdominal striae are the sign of Cushing disease along with the typical truncal obesity.

- Resistance to a multiple drug regimen (typically two or three drugs) can also point to a secondary cause of hypertension.
- Treating a pheochromocytoma with beta-blockers may result in a paradoxical increase in BP (unopposed alpha receptors stimulated by cathecolamines).

7. What is the recommended work-up for a hypertensive patient?

Any newly diagnosed patient with hypertension should have chest radiography, an electrocardiogram, measurement of vital capacity (directly related to cardiac diastolic function), urinalysis, and serum measurements of creatinine, sodium, and potassium. Other tests are based on clinical suspicion of a secondary form of hypertension.

8. Which tests are most commonly applied in secondary hypertension?

The most common causes of secondary hypertension are:

- Renal artery stenosis: Screening is done with the captopril test. The diagnosis requires either a noninvasive test, such as Doppler ultrasonography or magnetic resonance angiography, or a conventional iodine-based contrast selective angiography. Remember that the anatomical diagnosis of a renal artery stenosis, independent of its etiology, does not imply that the stenosis is the cause of hypertension. Causation can be confirmed by documenting the "functionality" of the lesion; this is accomplished by measuring renin activity in blood samples from the renal veins. A renin activity ratio > 1.5 between the two sides warrants intervention (stenting, balloon dilatation, surgical reconstruction) on the culprit lesion.
- Primary hyperaldosteronism: First step is to hold diuretics and give potassium supplements. Persistent hypokalemia requires measurement of plasma renin activity. If this is low, the aldosterone level is measured, and if the value is high and not suppressed by a saline load, then a localizing imaging procedure is performed (CT or MRI with specific adrenal protocol).
- Renal origin of hypertension: Requires imaging techniques to evaluate for kidney size, presence of hydronephrosis and obstructive nephropathy, calculi, polycystic kidney disease, or congenital malformations.
- Pheocromocytoma: see Question 9.

9. A 32-year-old man complains of intermittent episodes of headaches, palpitations, and profuse sweating. Over the last year, he has been treated three times in the emergency department for hypertensive crisis. He does not remember what his BP was, but he felt lightheaded when trying to stand, even before reaching the ED. In your office, he always has a BP below 120/70 mmHg. He has noticed low-grade fever at times and has lost a few pounds. After you examine him, he feels funny, so you measure his BP again. This time it is 165/110 mmHg, with a heart rate of 115 bpm. Laboratory studies only show a slightly elevated serum glucose and WBC of 18,000/μl with a normal differential. What is your diagnosis?

This is a typical presentation for a pheochromocytoma. The clues given by the patient's history are invaluable for diagnosis: many patients with pheochromocytoma have a normal baseline BP, with high BP values only on occasion. **Postural hypotension** is a classical feature. High serum catecholamine levels explain the sweating and palpitations as well as the low fever, elevation of serum glucose, and leukocytosis. Gentle palpation of the abdomen during physical examination may sometimes trigger a crisis. Because of the general and metabolic manifestations of the disease, it may mimic a large variety of conditions (e.g. vasculitis, diabetes), and a high level of suspicion is always necessary.

Some patients present with a high BP that is constant rather than paroxysmal. A "rule of 10" may be applied: 10% of all cases are familial, 10% are bilateral, 10% are due to a malignant adrenal tumor, 10% recur, 10% are extra-adrenal, 10% occur in children, 10% are associated with a MEN syndrome, and 10% present with a stroke as the inaugural symptom.

Diagnosis of a pheochromocytoma is rewarding, since this very sick patient who is prone to life-threatening complications can be virtually cured. The current recommendation for biochemical diagnosis of pheochromocytoma is urine testing for metanephrines and fractionated cate-cholamines. These tests only certify the presence of a cathecolamine-secreting tumor; therefore, the next step is to localize it (90% are in the adrenal medulla; the other 10% are scattered where chromaphin tissue is found). The preferred treatment is laparoscopic adrenalectomy.

10. What are the current strategies in hypertension treatment?

Hypertension treatment is a life-long process; therefore, obtaining **patient compliance** is fundamental in achieving good results. It is vitally important that patients have a good understanding of their condition—of their risk for severe target organ disease in the absence of warning signals (hypertension is known as the silent killer). Patient compliance is best achieved with combination therapy plus frequent visits to the physician's office and aggressive titration of medication.

Treatment is based on evaluation of disease severity and on thorough risk stratification. The presence of target organ disease and associated cardiovascular risk factors and/or CVD helps in choosing the right therapeutic option (guidelines detailed by JNC VI). **Lifestyle changes** are recommended in all patients: weight loss; regular exercise; reduced alcohol, fat, and salt intake; adequate supplements of calcium, potassium, magnesium, and fiber; and smoking cessation. A low-salt diet is fundamental for treatment of hypertension and cannot be replaced by an increased diuretic dosage.

Lifestyle modification for 6–12 months without **pharmacologic treatment** is appropriate if BP is 140–159/85–99 mmHg; in the absence of target organ disease, CVD, and diabetes; and if only one major cardiovascular risk factor is present. The presence of target organ disease, CVD, or diabetes, even in the absence of other risk factors, warrants drug therapy. As well, BP values of ≥ 160/≥ 100, even in the absence of target organ disease, CVD, and risk factors, require pharmacologic treatment.

11. How do I choose a drug therapy for a hypertensive patient?

The key is individualization of the therapeutic regimen, based on careful risk stratification (presence of target organ disease, cardiovascular pathology, and cardiovascular risk factors). The classical recommendation is to start with a diuretic or beta-blocker, or a combination of both drugs. These are the only antihypertensive drugs shown to reduce mortality rates in randomized, controlled trials. Moreover, they are less expensive and are associated with better compliance than some other options.

Elderly and African-American patients especially benefit from diuretics. A loop diuretic is preferred over a thiazide if serum creatinine is > 2 mg/dl. Potassium-sparing diuretics (e.g., spironolactone) are avoided in renal failure or in combination with ACE-inhibitors. Spironolactone is the drug of choice for medical treatment of hyperaldosteronism.

12. True or false: Diuretics are mandatory in the hypertensive patient with coronary artery disease (CAD).

False. Beta-blockers are mandatory in the presence of CAD, and are useful if mild or moderate CHF is present. Contraindications to beta-blockers must be carefully weighed against their tremendous therapeutic benefit. If CHF is present, dosage should be increased progressively and slowly. Withdrawal of beta-blockers in CAD patients must not be abrupt (increases mortality).

13. When are alpha-blockers appropriate?

Alpha-blockers are a good choice in treating pheocromocytoma, and they reduce HDL and total cholesterol. They are helpful in treating elderly men with benign prostate hyperplasia, but may induce significant postural hypotension. Central-acting alpha1-agonists (e.g., clonidine and methyldopa) typically are used. Abrupt withdrawal is the cause of a rebound phenomenon. A clonidine patch may be a better choice versus the short-acting form. Methyldopa is the drug of choice in pregnancy.

14. When are ACE inhibitors appropriate?

Initial drug choice may focus on ACE inhibitors if the patient has diabetes with proteinuria (compelling indication) or/and CHF is present. The benefit is slowing of the renal function deterioration and reduced mortality, respectively. ACE inhibitors are contraindicated in the second and third trimesters of pregnancy, and their dosage has to be reduced in the presence of renal failure. ACE inhibitors also prevent myocardial remodeling, heart failure, and death in post-infarct patients with decreased LV ejection fraction. IV preparations are useful for treating hypertensive emergencies. Angiotensin receptor blockers have similar antihypertensive efficacy and have an excellent tolerability.

15. Are there particular circumstances in which calcium antagonists or direct vasodilators are the ideal choice?

Calcium antagonists in their long-acting form are beneficial for older persons and CAD patients. Attention is given to the negative chronotropic effect of diltiazem, in particular when associated with beta-blockers or clonidine. Nifedipine in its short-acting form is no longer indicated in hypertensive crisis (increased mortality).

Direct vasodilators (e.g., hydralazine) are useful for treating hypertensive emergencies and are usually a late addition to the antihypertensive regimen. They may precipitate angina attacks in CAD patients.

BIBLIOGRAPHY

1. Carretero OA, et al: Essential hypertension. Part I: Definition and etiology. Circulation 101:329–335, 2000.
2. Carretero OA, et al: Essential hypertension. Part II: Definition and treatment. Circulation 101:329–335, 2000.
3. Graves JW: Management of difficult to control hypertension. Mayo Clin Proc 75:278–284, 2000.
4. Guidelines Subcommittee: World Health Organization-International Society of Hypertension guidelines for the management of hypertension. J Hypertens 17:151–183, 1999.
5. Hogan MJ: Hypertension. In Murphy JG, et al: Mayo Clinic Cardiology Review. Philadelphia, Lippincott Williams & Wilkins, 2000, pp 1067–1082.
6. Joint National Committee on Detection, Evaluation, and Treatment of High Blood Pressure: The Sixth Report of the Joint National Committee on Detection, Evaluation and Treatment of High Blood Pressure (JNC VI). Arch Intern Med 157:2413–2446, 1997.
7. Julius S: Trials of antihypertensive treatment—New agenda for the millennium. Am J Hypertens 13:11S–17S, 2000.
8. Kannel WB: Risk stratification in hypertension: New insights from the Framingham study. Am J Hypertens 13:3S–10S, 2000.
9. Messerli FH: Hypertension and sudden cardiac death. Am J Hypertens 12:181S–188S, 1999.
10. Smulyan H, et al: The diastolic blood pressure in systolic hypertension. Ann Intern Med 132:233–237, 2000.
11. Verdecchio P: Prognostic value of ambulatory blood pressure: Current evidence and clinical implications. Hypertension 35:844–851, 2000.
12. Weber MA: Interrupting the renin-angiotensin system: The role of angiotensin-converting enzyme inhibitors and angiotensin II receptor antagonists in the treatment of hypertension. Am J Hypertens 12:189S–194S, 1999.

27. SHOCK AND CARDIAC ARREST

Richard E. Wolfe, M.D.

1. Define shock.

Shock is the failure of the cardiovascular system to provide adequate blood flow to organs and tissues. It also has been defined as a reduction of cardiac output or a poor distribution of output to a point where potentially irreversible tissue damage occurs.

2. Give a pathophysiologic classification of shock.

Blood flow is determined by three entities: blood volume, vascular resistance, and pump function. Thus, there are three types of shock: hypovolemic, vasogenic or distributive, and cardiogenic. Examples of causes of **hypovolemic shock** are gastrointestinal bleeds, ruptured aortic aneurysm, and severe diabetic ketoacidosis. Examples of **vasogenic shock** include septic shock, anaphylactic shock, neurogenic shock, and shock from pharmacologic causes. There are many causes of **cardiogenic shock**, although acute myocardial infarction (MI) is the most common. Cardiogenic shock can be separated into *true cardiac causes*, such as MI, and *extracardiac causes* caused by obstruction to inflow (tension pneumothorax, cardiac tamponade) or outflow (pulmonary embolus).

3. Which clinical signs are helpful in classifying shock?

The patient's history usually makes the diagnosis, but patients may present with shock of undetermined etiology. The clinician must then rely on the clinical examination to classify the shock state. Feeling the extremities and examining the jugular veins provide vital clues:
- Warm skin is suggestive of a vasogenic cause; cool, clammy skin reflects enhanced reflex sympathoadrenal discharge leading to cutaneous vasoconstriction, suggesting hypovolemia or cardiogenic shock.
- Distended jugular veins, rales, or an S gallop suggest a cardiogenic cause rather than hypovolemia. Measured central venous pressure may aid in differentiating hypovolemia from cardiogenic shock.

Note that subclavian vein cannulation should be avoided if MI is suspected, as thrombolytic agents may be needed.

4. Do all patients in shock have an increased heart rate?

No. Although most patients in shock are tachycardic, this finding is far from consistent. Relative bradycardia is common in hypotensive trauma patients and patients with ruptured ectopic pregnancies. Patients with spinal shock lack sympathetic tone and lose the reflex tachycardia. Finally, many causes of cardiogenic shock present with bradycardia, including third-degree heart block, and beta-blocker and calcium antagonist poisonings.

5. What are the four determinants of central venous pressure?

The normal central venous pressure (CVP) is 5–12 cm HO. Intravascular volume, intrathoracic pressure, right ventricular function, and venous tone all affect the CVP. To reduce variability caused by intrathoracic pressure, CVP should be measured at the end of expiration.

6. List 10 causes of cardiogenic shock.

Acute myocardial infarction (the most common)	Arrhythmias
Acute myocarditis	Toxins, drugs
Chronic congestive cardiomyopathy	Hypothermia
Valvular heart disease	Hyperthermia
Myocardial contusion	Left atrial myxoma

7. What are the classic changes in systemic vascular resistance and cardiac output in septic shock?

In classic "warm" septic shock, the systemic vascular resistance is reduced and cardiac output is increased. The increase in cardiac output is a compensatory mechanism for the decrease in vascular resistance. It is not completely compensatory because of a circulating myocardial depressant factor released in sepsis. The identity of this factor has not yet been agreed upon.

8. How can septic shock appear like cardiogenic shock?

In hypodynamic or "cold" septic shock, seen more frequently in the elderly, there are two causes for reduced cardiac output. First, the myocardial depressant factor decreases the cardiac index. Second, in progressive sepsis, there are increases in pulmonary capillary resistance. These factors cause a significant decrease in cardiac output and present clinically like right-sided congestive heart failure. Cold septic shock has a very high mortality.

9. Describe the Killip classification of pump dysfunction in acute myocardial infarction.

The Killip classification is based on clinical criteria that correlate the degree of pump dysfunction with acute mortality in patients with MI.

Class I: no evidence of left ventricular failure and a 5% mortality

Class II: bibasilar rates, an S3 gallop, or heart failure by chest x-ray, and a 15–20% mortality

Class III: pulmonary edema and a 40% mortality

Class IV: cardiogenic shock, defined by (1) systolic blood pressure < 90 mmHg, (2) peripheral vasoconstriction, (3) oliguria, and (4) pulmonary vascular congestion; mortality 80%.

10. How significant is a loud holosystolic murmur in a patient with shock and an acute myocardial infarction?

Loud holosystolic murmurs with MI indicates either papillary muscle rupture or an acute ventricular septal defect (VSD). These may be indistinguishable, but acute VSD usually occurs with an anteroseptal MI and has an associated palpable thrill. Papillary rupture often does not have a thrill and is usually seen in inferior MI. These frequently cause shock on the basis of much reduced forward blood flow and can be differentiated by echocardiography or Swan-Ganz catheterization. Both require emergent cardiothoracic surgery for early repair. In some patients, the murmur may be soft or inaudible.

11. What are the signs and symptoms of massive pulmonary embolism?

Massive pulmonary embolism (PE) causes **shock** on the basis of reduced cross-sectional area of the pulmonary outflow tract. Shock occurs when the cross-sectional area is reduced by 50% or more. In an acute situation, the right ventricle can increase its systolic pressure only to a maximum of about 40 mmHg. This pressure is inadequate to overcome the increased resistance, blood flow is reduced, and shock develops.

Massive PE presents with dyspnea (78%), tachycardia (90%), syncope (76%), cyanosis (74%), chest pain (72%), systolic BP < 80 mmHg (87%), and cardiac arrest (85%).

12. What is the emergency treatment of cardiogenic shock?

Provide supplemental oxygen. Arrhythmias should be treated by protocols specified in the American Heart Association's textbook *Advanced Cardiac Life Support*. If the patient does not have PE, volume can be administered in aliquots of 200–300 ml of crystalloid. This is particularly true in inferior MI or if there is electrocardiographic evidence of right ventricular infarction.

Dopamine and dobutamine are the pressors of choice for improvement of hemodynamics. Dobutamine is likely to be a better choice, particularly if there is evidence of PE, since dobutamine, unlike dopamine, reduces left ventricular end-diastolic pressure. Dobutamine is also preferable in patients with a right ventricular infarct, although a combination of dopamine and dobutamine may be required. Dobutamine is always preferred over dopamine in the setting of myocardial ischemia/infarction because of reduced oxygen consumption. Emergency angioplasty may improve survival in patients with cardiogenic shock from MI.

13. What therapeutic measures may improve the condition of a patient with shock from a pulmonary embolism?

Massive PE should be treated similarly to cardiogenic shock from MI: oxygen (intubation if necessary), volume, and pressors. Thrombolytics have not been studied well enough in massive PE to show improved survival. However, the use of tissue plasminogen activator, streptokinase, and urokinase has been demonstrated to improve hemodynamics with reduced tricuspid regurgitation, reduced right ventricular dilatation, and improved cardiac output in patients with massive PE, and thus the use of thrombolytics should be considered. Emergency embolectomy should be considered.

14. What are the causes of traumatic cardiogenic shock?

Cardiac penetration with subsequent tamponade, myocardial contusion, tension pneumothorax, and air embolism from bronchial tears.

15. In which patients should I suspect pericardial tamponade?

Acute pericardial tamponade occurs in about 2% of penetrating chest trauma cases and is more common with stab wounds than gunshot wounds. Tamponade is rare after blunt trauma. Beck's classic triad of distended neck veins, decreased arterial pressure, and muffled heart sound occurs only in about a third of patients. A high central venous pressure with tachycardia and hypotension in penetrating trauma are reliable signs of tamponade. Examination and chest radiography will exclude tension pneumothorax.

16. Does cardiopulmonary resuscitation (CPR) resuscitate patients in cardiac arrest?

CPR rarely resuscitates patients from cardiac arrest without early institution of advanced life support interventions: defibrillation, airway management, and administration of appropriate drugs. All cardiac arrest victims should have a monitor placed as soon as possible, as immediate defibrillation is indicated in the presence of ventricular fibrillation.

17. How does the blood "flow" when CPR is being performed?

Two mechanisms have been proposed to explain blood flow with closed chest compressions: The **thoracic pump theory** suggests that the heart acts as the passive conduit, with systolic and mean arterial pressures and blood flow to the carotid artery augmented by increased thoracic pressure. Intrathoracic pressure is transmitted into the extrathoracic arteries to a greater extent than into the extrathoracic veins. This is reflected in an extrathoracic arteriovenous pressure gradient. The unequal transmission of intrathoracic pressure into the extrathoracic arteries and veins results from the presence of venous valves and unequal arterial and venous capacitance and collapsibility. Arteries resist collapse and therefore transmit the intrathoracic pressure into the extrathoracic arterial bed.

The **cardiac theory** suggests that the heart itself is compressed, creating a pressure gradient between intracardiac and extracardiac structures. However, there are not enough data at present to determine which mechanism predominates.

18. Describe the common reversible causes of cardiac arrest and their specific treatment.

Cardiac arrest may be successfully resuscitated if the underlying etiology is recognized and promptly treated.

Ventricular fibrillation and **ventricular tachycardia**. Perform immediate defibrillation, *before other procedures*, as the success rate decreases by 4% with every minute of delay.

Tension pneumothorax. Suspect this condition following positive-pressure ventilation in a cardiac arrest patient if breath sounds decrease on the affected side, subcutaneous air is present, or resistance to airflow with bagging occurs. The treatment is needle decompression at the fifth intercostal space, followed by thoracotomy.

Hyperkalemia. Heralded by wide QRS complexes and the absence of P waves, suspect hyperkalemia as the cause of arrest in patients with renal failure. Administer calcium chloride immediately, followed by sodium bicarbonate and an insulin-glucose drip.

Anaphylaxis. Consider anaphylaxis whenever cardiac arrest follows administration of parenteral medication. As asphyxia or shock is the underlying mechanism, immediately perform aggressive intervention with endotracheal intubation, fluids, and intravenous epinephrine.

19. When should intravenous calcium be used in the patient in cardiac arrest?

Overall, patients in cardiac arrest do not appear to benefit from the use of intravenous calcium. Indications are thus limited to three specific causes of cardiac arrest: hyperkalemia, hypocalcemia, and possibly calcium antagonist overdose. Calcium chloride should be administered at a dose of 24 mg/kg of a 10% solution intravenously every 10 minutes.

20. Can neurologic outcome be predicted following successful resuscitation of cardiac arrest?

Several reports have attempted to develop prognostic signs for cerebral recovery following CPR. The **duration of coma** is the most reliable prognostic sign. However, recovery of consciousness has occurred after 10 days of coma. Reactive pupils, oculocephalic reflexes, spontaneous respirations, and purposeful response to painful stimuli are associated with a higher percentage of neurologic recovery. Rarely, favorable outcomes do occur in patients with poor prognostic signs.

BIBLIOGRAPHY

1. Bresler MJ: Future role of thrombolytic therapy in emergency medicine. Ann Emerg Med 18:1331, 1989.
2. Dhainaut JF, et al: Right ventricular dysfunction in patients with septic shock. Intensive Care Med 14:488, 1988.
3. Donahue AM: Central venous pressure measurement. In Roberts JR, Hedges JR (eds): Clinical Procedures in Emergency Medicine. Philadelphia, W.B. Saunders, 1992, pp 332–338.
4. Ornato JP, Levine RL, Young DS, et al: The effect of applied chest compression force on systemic arterial pressure and end-tidal carbon dioxide concentration during CPR in human beings. Ann Emerg Med 18:732–737, 1989.
5. Schmidt RD, Wolfe R: Shock. In Rosen P, et al (eds): Emergency Medicine: Concepts and Clinical Practice, 3rd ed. St. Louis, Mosby, 1992, p 163.

28. MYOCARDITIS

Richard A. Stein, M.D., and Javier M. Gonzalez, M.D.

1. What mechanisms of injury to heart muscle cells play a role in myocarditis that is caused by infectious agents?
- Direct invasion of the myocardium
- Production of myocardial toxin
- Auto-antibodies
- Cellular immunity (activation of T-helper lymphocytes)
- Cytokine secretion (tumor necrosis factor alpha, interleukin)

The main cause of myocarditis in the United States is viral, and the mechanism of injury is thought to have an immunologic cause. Postulated mechanisms include viral-related creation of new cell surface antigens, antigen-antibody complex-related cell damage, and activation of T-helper lymphocytes with production of cytokines.

2. What are the major causes of myocarditis?
- Infectious agents
  - Viral
  - Rickettsial
  - Bacterial
  - Protozoan
  - Metazoal
- Allergic reactions
- Pharmacologic agents
- Systemic diseases such as vasculitis and connective tissue diseases
- Peripartum state (30 days before to 150 days after delivery)
- Toxic agents (alcohol, toxic metals such as cobalt)

3. Describe the patient complaints and clinical findings that frequently accompany myocarditis.

The symptoms vary with the etiology, but most commonly myocarditis is subclinical, especially when it accompanies a generalized infectious process. Patients may note fatigue, dyspnea, precordial discomfort, or palpitations. Frequently tachycardia is noted; the first heart sound may be muted, and an S_4 gallop is often described.

4. What electrocardiographic (ECG) changes are commonly seen in myocarditis?

ST-segment elevation or depression and T-wave inversions are the most frequently seen changes. Atrial arrhythmias are also common, and transient heart block (first, second, or third) may be noted.

5. How are patients with presumed viral myocarditis treated?

Treatment is supportive and responsive to the clinical presentation. Because atrioventricular (AV) conduction abnormalities are common in some forms of myocarditis, patients should be watched carefully for evidence of conduction disturbances. In addition, exercise has been shown in animal models to increase the cell damage in myocarditis, so rest is usually prescribed. When congestive heart failure is noted, the usual treatment is indicated (angiotensin-converting enzyme inhibitors, diuretics, and digoxin). Digoxin must be used carefully because of an increased incidence of digitalis toxic rhythms during active myocarditis. Beta-blockers and nonsteroidal anti-inflammatory drugs (NSAIDs) may increase mortality when used in early stages of myocarditis.

There is controversy over the use of corticosteroids and immunomodulators. They should not be used on every patient with the diagnosis of myocarditis; however, they must be considered in patients with rapidly progressive decompensation and those not improving with conventional therapy. Steroids should be used in myocarditis secondary to sarcoidosis, giant cell myocarditis, hypersensitivity myocarditis, eosinophilic myocarditis, possibly Lyme disease with AV block (see Question 8), and lupus myocarditis. Anticoagulation, pacemaker, or implantable cardioverter defibrillator (ICD) should be used as clinically indicated. Some patients with infectious myocarditis require antibiotic therapy.

6. **Which viral infections are associated with myocarditis?**
   - **Coxsackie B** virus is the most frequent cause of viral myocarditis. There is a presumed myocardial membrane affinity for these viral particles.
   - **Human immunodeficiency virus** (HIV) infection is associated with myocardial involvement in 20–25% of infected patients, but clinical disease is noted in only 10% of HIV-infected patients. Dilated cardiomyopathy manifesting as congestive heart failure is the usual presentation, although pericardial effusion is also observed with some frequency. Less commonly noted are marantic endocarditis, ventricular arrhythmia, and right ventricular dilatation or hypertrophy.
   - **Lassa fever** is caused by an arenavirus and is a major cause of death in West Africa. Involvement is usually subclinical with one half of the patients showing ST changes and low voltage on the ECG.
   - Myocarditis is frequently seen in fatal cases of **poliomyelitis**, especially during epidemics in the past.

7. **List the bacterial diseases often associated with myocarditis and their characteristic presentations.**
   Clostridium perfringens **infection**. These infections commonly involve the heart, with myocardial changes due to a toxin produced by the bacteria. The characteristic pathologic finding is gas bubbles in the myocardium. Abscess formation with resultant rupture into the pericardium and subsequent purulent pericarditis is seen.

   Diphtheria. Myocardial involvement is very common (up to 20% of cases) and is the most common cause of death from this organism. The bacteria-produced toxin, which interferes with protein synthesis, is the basis for the cardiac damage. On pathologic examination, the heart shows "streaks," and microscopic examination reveals fatty infiltration of the myocytes. Clinically, the myocarditis usually presents as cardiomegaly and severe congestive heart failure. Antitoxin should be administered as soon as the diagnosis is made, and antibiotic therapy then instituted. Conduction disturbances are common and may require a pacemaker. Some studies indicate that early treatment with carnitine ameliorates the course of the myocarditis.

   Meningococcal infection. Cardiac involvement is common in fatal infections. Congestive heart failure, pericardial effusion, tamponade, and involvement of the AV node with resultant heart block may occur.

   Mycoplasma pneumoniae. This infection commonly involves the heart, with subclinical findings such as ST and T wave changes on ECG. Pericarditis with an audible friction rub is noted on occasion.

   Psittacosis. Myocarditis is a common finding with this infection. Cardiac involvement treatment with tetracycline is indicated.

   Whipple's disease. Intestinal lipodystrophy is associated with rod-like organisms in the intestine and myocardium. The organism and mechanism of damage to the myocardium are not known. Cardiac involvement includes coronary artery lesions (panarteritis) and valvular fibrosis. Antibiotic therapy is reported to be effective in the treatment of the underlying disease.

   Spirochete infections. Leptospirosis (Weil's disease), Lyme carditis, syphilis, and, in Ethiopia, relapsing fever have myocardial involvement.

8. What are the cardiac findings in Lyme disease?

Lyme disease is caused by the tick-borne spirochete *Borrelia burgdorferi*. The initial infection is often marked by a rash, followed in weeks to months by involvement of other organ systems, including the heart, neurologic system, and joints. About 1 in 10 patients develops cardiac involvement, usually with severe AV node block, which is often associated with syncope because of concomitant depression of ventricular escape rhythms. Temporary pacing is indicated (the AV block usually resolves), as is antibiotic treatment with high-dose intravenous penicillin or oral tetracycline. (See Question 5.)

9. How long after the initial infection with *Trypanosoma cruzi* (Chagas' disease) do the cardiac manifestations occur?

The initial infection with *Trypanosoma* occurs when young adults are bit, usually around the eye, by a reduviid bug. A few individuals (about 1%) develop an acute myocarditis and pericarditis, which usually resolves over time. The major cardiac manifestation of Chagas' disease occurs about 20 years after the initial infection and is evident in 30% of the infected subjects. It involves cardiomegaly, congestive heart failure, arrhythmias, thromboembolism, right bundle branch block, syncope, and sudden death.

10. What are some unusual features of the cardiac involvement in Chagas' disease?

The pathologic appearance shows infiltration followed by fibrotic changes. There is a characteristic involvement of the right ventricle early in the process, which explains the early manifestations of right heart failure and tricuspid insufficiency. There is a predilection for involvement of the right bundle branch with subsequent right bundle branch block and an associated left anterior hemiblock. The fibrosis often extends into the apex of the left ventricle, resulting in a thin-walled, thrombus-filled ventricular aneurysm.

Laboratory and noninvasive testing yields some characteristic findings. The ECG shows characteristic right bundle branch block and left anterior hemiblock; ST and T-wave changes may be present. Ventricular arrhythmias are common, especially following exercise. Electrophysiologic testing often demonstrates inducible ventricular tachycardia. Echocardiography may reveal apical akinesis or a frank apical aneurysm, often with a ventricular thrombus. This pathophysiology explains in part the high incidence of sudden death and thromboembolic phenomena (seen in 50% of patients). However, mural thrombi have been reported in patients with myocarditis and normal wall motion, presumable secondary to the inflammatory process of the myocardial walls.

11. Describe the cardiac manifestations of a pheochromocytoma.

Patients may present with a reversible dilated cardiomyopathy. The cause is assumed to be the high level of circulating catecholamines resulting from the tumor, which may result in cell damage via a variety of pathways. The protective effect of aspirin suggests a role for platelet aggregation.

12. What tick bite–related infections are associated with myocarditis?

Borrelia burgdorferi (Lyme disease)
Rickettsia rickettsii (Rocky Mountain spotted fever)
Ehrlichia
Babesia infections
Relapsing fever
Colorado tick fever
Q fever

13. Describe the clinical course of cytomegalovirus myocarditis.

It is self-limited in the general population but frequently becomes severe if the infection starts after heart transplant. Early infection post-transplant correlates with allograft coronary artery disease—the major cause of death after the first year of heart transplant.

14. Which microorganisms are most frequently related to myocarditis in patients with HIV infection?

The most common pathogens are *Toxoplasma gondii*, *Mycobacterium tuberculosis*, and *Cryptococcus neoformans*. Reports of other microorganisms also implicate *M. avium-intracellulare* complex, *Aspergillus fumigatus*, *Candida albicans*, *Histoplasma capsulatum*, *Coccidioides immitis*, cytomegalovirus, herpes simplex, and HIV itself. Besides infectious agents, antiretroviral medications have been directly correlated to causing myocarditis (zidovudine).

15. Name the available diagnostic strategies and how they help in the diagnosis of myocarditis.

TEST	PURPOSE
Enteroviral IgG	Fourfold rise over a 4–6-week period documents acute infection
Echocardiography/cardiac catheterization	Helps to exclude treatable causes of heart failure
Creatine phosphokinase and troponins	Positive test suggests acute myocarditis
Antimyosin or gallium 67 scintigraphy	Negative test excludes active myocarditis
Endomyocardial biopsy	Standard diagnostic test for myocarditis

16. Describe common findings that point to specific etiologies of myocarditis.

PHYSICAL FINDING	PROBABLE ETIOLOGY
Post-transplant myocarditis	Cytomegalovirus
Illegal drug use	Cocaine
Enlarged lymph nodes	Sarcoidosis
Pruritic maculopapular rash with eosinophilia in blood	Hypersensitivity myocarditis
Rapid deterioration and ventricular arrhythmias in a young patient	Giant cell myocarditis
Erythema marginatum, polyarthralgias, chorea, subcutaneous nodules	Rheumatic fever
Endemic exposure (South or Central America) with right bundle branch block on the ECG	Chagas' disease

BIBLIOGRAPHY

1. Maguire JH, Hoff R, Sherlock I, et al: Cardiac morbidity and mortality due to Chagas' disease: Prospective electrocardiographic study of a Brazilian community. Circulation 75:1140–1145, 1987.
2. Mason JW, O'Connell JB, Gerskowitz A, et al: A clinical trial of immunosuppressive therapy for myocarditis. The Myocarditis Treatment Trial Investigators. N Engl J Med 333:269–275, 1995.
3. McAlister HF, Klementowicz PT, Andrews C, et al: Lyme carditis: An important cause of reversible heart block. Ann Intern Med 110:339–345, 1989.
4. Morris SA, Tanowitz HB, Wittner M, Bilezikian JP: Pathophysiological insights into the cardiomyopathy of Chagas' disease. Circulation 82:1900–1909, 1990.
5. National Heart, Lung, and Blood Institute and Office of Rare Diseases (National Institutes of Health) workshop recommendations and review: Peripartum cardiomyopathy. JAMA 238:1183–1188, 2000.
6. O'Connell JB: Diagnosis and medical treatment of inflammatory cardiomyopathies. In Topol EJ (ed): Textbook of Cardiovascular Medicine. Philadelphia, Lippincott-Raven, 1998, pp 2309–2326.
7. Rerkpattanapipat P, Wongpraparut N, Jacobs LE, Kotler MN: Cardiac manifestations of acquired immunodeficiency syndrome. Arch Intern Med 160:602–608, 2000.
8. Roberts WC, Berard CW: Gas gangrene of the heart in clostridial septicemia. Am Heart J 74:482–488, 1967.
9. Weinstein L, Shelokov A: Cardiovascular manifestations in acute poliomyelitis. N Engl J Med 244: 281–285, 1951.

29. DILATED CARDIOMYOPATHY

Catalin Loghin, M.D.

1. Define dilated cardiomyopathy.

Dilated cardiomyopathy is the most common form of all cardiomyopathies. It is defined by dilated chambers with depressed left ventricular (LV) systolic function and the presence of a variable degree of diastolic dysfunction. The presence of congestive heart failure (CHF) does not equal the definition or the diagnosis of dilated cardiomyopathy, as isolated diastolic dysfunction may exist, in the presence of normal LV systolic function. Dilated cardiomyopathy is the final evolutionary stage of many cardiac processes. Therefore, although it constitutes a diagnosis in itself, attempting an etiological diagnosis is always necessary as sometimes the original process leading to cardiac dilatation can be reversed.

2. Why is dilated cardiomyopathy an important form of cardiac disease?

In the U.S., there are 2 million cases of CHF with decreased LV ejection fraction, which is the typical clinical presentation for dilated cardiomyopathy. The prevalence of CHF is 1–2% in adult U.S. patients, and most of them meet the criteria of dilated cardiomyopathy. The incidence reaches 7.5/100,000 in the general population, and the typical patient is a 50-year-old African-American male. Approximately 400,000 new cases of CHF are diagnosed each year in the U.S. These patients have a global mortality of 50% at 5 years despite all the advances made by medical science, and 19% of them require a hospital admission within 1 year of their initial diagnosis. The mortality statistics have changed little over the last 40 years. From a prognostic standpoint, advanced CHF should be considered similar to very aggressive malignancies.

3. How broad is the etiologic spectrum of dilated cardiomyopathy?

Different etiologies have variable incidence, based on how extensive the efforts are in identifying the cause. Over 75 causes are described. If endomyocardial biopsy is added to the etiologic work-up of dilated cardiomyopathy, 51% of cases are still labeled as idiopathic. The second most important cause is myocarditis (9.2%), followed by coronary artery disease (7.7%), peripartum cardiomyopathy (4.5%), and hypertension (4.2%). Amyloidosis, HIV, and chronic alcohol abuse are each responsible for 2–3% of cases. Drugs account for less than 3% of cases, and interferon is a recent addition to the list.

4. What is the benefit of endomyocardial biopsy in the etiologic diagnosis of dilated cardiomyopathy?

The incidence of specific histological diagnosis brought by endomyocardial biopsy is only 16%, and myocarditis is the most common finding. Typical indications include monitoring of cardiac allograft rejection, monitoring of doxorubicin cardiotoxicity, diagnosis and follow-up of myocarditis, differentiation between restrictive cardiomyopathy and constrictive pericarditis, suspected infiltrative cardiomyopathy, recent onset of dilated cardiomyopathy with clinical suspicion of a reversible cause, and treatment-refractory patients. Endomyocardial biopsy has a role in diagnosis and guiding treatment, but does not influence long-term mortality.

5. What are the characteristics of peripartum cardiomyopathy?

The onset must occur during the last month of pregnancy or within 5 months of delivery. There must be no other cause for heart failure diagnosed prior or during this time interval. Peripartum cardiomyopathy is most common in twin pregnancies, multiparous and hypertensive women over 30 years old, and toxemic pregnancies (when tocolytic agents are used in excess).

A "50% rule" may be used: up to 50% of cases meet the Dallas pathological criteria for myocarditis, if endomyocardial biopsy is performed, and in general they do not respond to immunosuppressive treatment. Anticoagulant therapy is currently recommended, in view of the increased tendency for embolic events (50%). General mortality reaches up to 50%. If LV systolic function does not recover, subsequent pregnancies are considered extremely high risk.

6. Name the most common drugs known to induce a dilated cardiomyopathy.

The classic culprit is doxorubicin, followed by cocaine. Much less common are interferon, leukotrienes, lithium, and steroids. Doxorubicin-induced dilated cardiomyopathy is typically dose-dependent (in particular if the cumulative dose is > 500 mg/m^2, is related to myocardial oxidative stress induced by increased free radical formation, and responds poorly to treatment. Radiation therapy and other chemotherapeutic agents aggravate doxorubicin-induced cardiomyopathy. Interferon-induced dilated cardiomyopathy has specific histologic changes.

7. Which are the most common precipitating/aggravating factors for dilated cardiomyopathies and chronic heart failure in general?

In clinical practice, obtain a detailed history and perform a complete physical examination to discover a precipitating event in a patient presenting with CHF exacerbation. The importance of a good history cannot be overemphasized. Many of these precipitating factors are reversible; hence the importance of identifying them in a timely and accurate fashion.

- A **lack of compliance** with medical therapy and/or diet is common. Low-salt diet is often not well understood by patients and not emphasized enough by physicians.
- An **acute arrhythmia**, most commonly a rapid ventricular response of atrial fibrillation, must be ruled out.
- Fever and in general any infection, strenuous exercise, a coronary event (ranging from a common anginal attack with transitory depression of the LV pump to a massive transmural myocardial infarction) are all contributing factors.
- Some of the well-documented, beneficial therapies, such as ACE-inhibitors and beta-blockers, are either underused or are used improperly (e.g., rapid escalation of beta-blocker dosage or usage of a subtherapeutic dosage).
- Negative inotropic drugs, such as diltiazem or substances with direct toxic effect on the myocardium (e.g., ethanol), must always be sought.

8. Describe the role of echocardiography in the work-up of a dilated cardiomyopathy.

A complete echocardiographic study includes:

2-D and M-mode: provides information on the heart morphology; for example, chamber dimensions, wall thickness (typically diminished in dilated cardiomyopathy), and presence or absence of intracavitary thrombus. It may raise the suspicion of an infiltrative etiology (e.g., amyloidosis). Pericardial effusions are easily identified, but echocardiography is not a first choice for defining constrictive pericarditis. LV and RV systolic functions are assessed quickly and accurately. The presence of regional wall motion abnormalities usually suggests coronary artery disease but may also be caused by myocarditis with "patchy" involvement.

Doppler (pulsed, continuous and color): gives flow information in general and is particularly helpful in mitral regurgitation (detection and severity evaluation) and diastolic dysfunction (with possible quantification in degrees of severity). Patients displaying a restrictive pattern of the LV filling have a worse prognosis, with increased morbidity and mortality.

Dobutamine stress echocardiography: may reveal areas with myocardial viability versus scarred myocardium, and can be useful in decisions regarding myocardial revascularization in selected ischemic patients.

Of note, the recent advances in cardiac MRI are likely to make this technique the imaging modality of choice. The accuracy and wealth of information offered by MRI virtually make it a "one-stop shop" for evaluating the morphology and function of the failing heart. Limiting factors are the cost and the availability.

9. **List the recognized prognostic factors in dilated cardiomyopathy.**
   - Older patients with poor functional capacity tend to have a worse prognosis, in particular if ischemia is at the origin of their dilated cardiomyopathy.
   - Echocardiographic parameters: LV ejection fraction < 35%, a restrictive pattern of diastolic LV filling, thin walls, and severely dilated cardiac chambers have an adverse influence on prognosis.
   - A cardiac index of < 3.0 L/m^2 BSA and an LV end-diastolic pressure of > 20 mmHg are ominous signs.
   - A lack of heart rate variability on Holter monitoring may predict an adverse outcome.
   - The presence of cardiomegaly on chest x-ray, with an increased cardiothoracic ratio > 0.55 is not only a predictor of survival but also a useful way of following these patients.
   - Electrocardiogram can detect the presence of intraventricular conduction delays; ventricular arrhythmias (e.g., premature ventricular beats) and nonsustained ventricular tachycardia are controversial prognostic factors.
   - The presence of sinus tachycardia and a low systolic blood pressure appears to be associated to a worse prognosis.
   - Biochemical abnormalities—hyponatremia and increased serum levels of catecholamines, TNF, atrial natriuretic factor, ADH, and creatinine—are also related to a worse prognosis.

10. **What is the most common death mechanism in dilated cardiomyopathy?**
   The lack of heart rate variability on Holter monitoring is related to the often-encountered sudden death of these patients.

11. **Describe the current options for medical therapy of dilated cardiomyopathies.**
   - **ACE inhibitors** are indicated in all patients with LVEF < 40%, and they have been shown to reduce mortality. Alternatively, vasodilators like nitrates and hydralazine are used.
   - **Angiotensin II antagonists** are useful in combination with ACE inhibitors, and they also decrease mortality. However, they are not superior to ACE inhibitors, based on the results of the ELITE II Trial.
   - **Diuretics** are useful for volume overload symptoms.
   - **Spironolactone**, traditionally used for right-sided heart failure with ascites, can reduce mortality by 30% when administered in patients with LVEF < 35%.
   - **Beta-blockers** are now an established therapy for CHF. Carvedilol (FDA approved for CHF treatment), metoprolol, bisoprolol, and bucindolol are used. Guidelines exist for initiating the therapy and the key is slow increase of dosage with careful monitoring of the hemodynamic status. Beta-blockers can reduce mortality and morbidity in CHF and they are indicated mainly in mild and moderate pump failure.
   - **Digoxin** is safe and results in fewer hospital admissions when used in the appropriate dosage.
   - **Amiodarone** is still the subject of controversy regarding its ability to decrease mortality by suppressing ventricular arrhythmias, by exerting a slight beta-blocking effect along with mild dilatation of the coronary arteries. In myocarditis, immunosuppression typically is not indicated.
   - **Novel compounds**, such as endopeptidase inhibitors (increase ANP activity), endothelin receptor antagonists (vasodilator effect), and renin antagonists, might be added in the future to the therapeutic armamentarium.

12. **Is there a role for anticoagulation in dilated cardiomyopathy?**
   The incidence of embolic events in dilated cardiomyopathy is about 2% per year. Anticoagulation is a subject of great controversy, and warfarin is typically used. Classic indications include the documentation of an LV thrombus, documented arterial embolic events, the presence of atrial fibrillation, and peripartum cardiomyopathy. The presence of a large area of akinesis of the left ventricle may warrant long-term anticoagulation. In general, standard care is to anticoagulate patients with LVEF < 30%.

13. What does the term "dobutamine holiday" mean?

Patients with severely depressed LV ejection fraction may benefit from short-term administration of continuous or intermittent IV dobutamine (other positive inotropic drugs with beta-agonist activity have been used). Up to 21% of U.S. patients with New York Heart Association class III-IV CHF receive a "dobutamine holiday." However, more evidence is accumulating against the use of IV dobutamine since it may increase mortality. Its use should be reserved for end-stage heart failure, in patients unresponsive to conventional therapy, and when improving the quality of life is the only therapeutic goal.

14. How are pacemakers used in treating patients with dilated cardiomyopathy?

Pacing is indicated to control heart rate (with or without preliminary AV node ablation/modification) and to fine-tune atrioventricular synchrony and atrioventricular delay. Pacing with adequate parameters may have a significant impact on cardiac output and may increase exercise capacity, but there is no study to prove that pacing decreases mortality. The classic indication for pacing with AV node ablation is refractory atrial fibrillation with rapid ventricular response (the presence of atrial fibrillation may decrease cardiac output by up to 30%, in particular in patients with reduced LV compliance [e.g., "stiff heart"]).

There is growing evidence that biventricular pacing is more beneficial than right ventricular pacing. Since the incidence of ventricular arrhythmia (and arrhythmic sudden death) in these patients is high, a fair number of them become candidates for implant of a automatic implantable cardioverter defibrillator with biventricular pacing capabilities in conjunction with the use of amiodarone.

Several trials are underway to further evaluate pacing/defibrillation in heart failure, including Sudden Cardiac Death in Heart Failure Trial (SCD-HeFT) and Companion. At the time of this writing, 2112 patients have been enrolled in SCD-HeFT, with a goal of 2500. Recruiting should be complete by May 2001.

15. What is the role of left ventricular assist devices (LVADs) in treating patients with dilated cardiomyopathy?

LVADs are typically used to temporarily support the failing left ventricle until a heart transplant becomes possible. There is now evidence that recovery of the depressed LV systolic function after LVAD implantation is possible (5–30% of cases), leading to the options of either using these devices as permanent support or explanting them after a certain time without the need for subsequent heart transplant.

ACKNOWLEDGEMENT

The author wishes to thank Dr. Eddy Barasch for his valuable suggestions.

BIBLIOGRAPHY

1. Chuang ML, et al: Importance of imaging method over imaging modality in noninvasive determination of left ventricular volumes and ejection fraction: assessment by two- and three-dimensional echocardiography and magnetic resonance imaging. J Am Coll Cardiol 35:477–484, 2000.
2. Eichhorn EJ, Bristow M: Practical guidelines for initiation of beta-adrenergic blockade in patients with chronic heart failure. Am J Cardiol 79:794–798, 1997.
3. Felker GM, et al: The spectrum of dilated cardiomyopathy. The Johns Hopkins experience with 1278 patients. Medicine 78:270–283, 1999.
4. Investigators, The RESOLVD: Effects of Metoprolol CR in patients with ischemic and dilated cardiomyopathy: The randomized evaluation of strategies for left ventricular dysfunction pilot study. Circulation, 101:378–384, 2000.
5. Manolio TA, et al: Prevalence and etiology of idiopathic dilated cardiomyopathy (summary of a National Heart, Lung and Blood Institutes Workshop). Am J Cardiol 69:1458, 1992.
6. O'Connor CM, et al: Managing the patient with advanced heart failure: Current and novel pharmacologic approaches in advanced heart failure. Am Heart J 135:S249–263, 1998.
7. Peters RW, et al: Pacing for patients with congestive heart failure and dilated cardiomyopathy. Card Clinic 18: 55–66, 2000.

8. Pitt B, et al: The effect of spironolactone on morbidity and mortality in patients with severe heart failure. N Engl J Med 341:709–717, 1999.
9. Tajik AJ, et al: Dilated cardiomyopathy. In Murphy JG, et al: Mayo Clinic Cardiology Review. Philadelphia, Lippincott Williams & Wilkins, 2000, pp 445–454.
10. Wu AH, et al: Sudden death in dilated cardiomyopathy. Clin Cardiol 22:267–272, 1999.

30. HYPERTROPHIC CARDIOMYOPATHY

Ashraf ElSakr, M.D., Luther T. Clark, M.D., and Catalin Loghin, M.D.

1. What is hypertrophic cardiomyopathy?

Hypertrophic cardiomyopathy (HCM) is a primary disorder of the heart muscle characterized by inappropriate myocardial hypertrophy of a nondilated left ventricle (LV) and not secondary to a cardiovascular or systemic disease (i.e., hypertension or aortic stenosis). It most often
involves the interventricular septum (**asymmetric septal hypertrophy**) and may be associated
with dynamic LV outflow tract obstruction (**hypertrophic obstructive cardiomyopathy**).
Another term that has been used to describe HCM is **idiopathic subaortic stenosis**.

2. Is HCM genetic or acquired?

HCM is a genetically heterogeneous familial disorder, and more than half of patients inherit
it as an autosomal dominant trait. Patients with sporadic spontaneous mutations (up to 40% in the
elderly population and significantly less in the younger population) have a 50% chance of trans-
mitting the disease to each of their offspring. Therefore, screening of family members of these
patients is mandatory (echocardiography is the technique of choice). Multiple genotypes are described, the most common affecting the beta myosin heavy chain, with significantly different
phenotypic expression determining age of onset, symptoms, and survival.

3. What are the most common variants of HCM?

The pattern and extent of LV hypertrophy in patients with HCM vary greatly, and different patterns may occur in the same family pedigree. **Asymmetric septal hypertrophy**, the most common
variant, accounts for 90% of patients. The septal hypertrophy may affect the basal one-third of the
septum (subaortic area) only, the basal two-thirds (down to papillary muscles), or the entire septum
from base to apex. The other two common variants are **apical** (involving the apical one-third of the
ventricle) and **midventricle hypertrophy** (maximal thickening at the level of the papillary muscles).

4. Is the histology of HCM unique?

The histologic picture of HCM is characterized by myocardial hypertrophy and myocardial
fiber disarray. The muscle bundles and myofibrillar architecture are disorganized, and cell-to-cell
arrangements are abnormal, but these findings also may occur in other acquired and congenital
cardiac conditions. The disarray of HCM is unique only in its ubiquity and frequency, with virtually all patients having some degree of disarray and most having at least 5% of the myocardium
affected. In non-HCM patients, disarray usually involves only about 1% of the myocardium.

5. What are the most common symptoms in patients with HCM?

Most patients with HCM are asymptomatic and are identified during screening of relatives
with known disease. In patients who are symptomatic, the most common symptoms are:

Dyspnea
- Present in up to 90% of symptomatic patients
- Secondary to LV diastolic dysfunction, impaired ventricular filling, and elevation of left
  atrial and pulmonary venous pressures

Angina pectoris
- Occurs in up to 75% of symptomatic patients
- Secondary to imbalance between oxygen supply and demand, with greatly increased myocardial mass, impaired vasodilatory coronary reserve (due to thickened and narrowed
  small intramural coronary arteries), and subendocardial ischemia (due to increased oxygen
  demand in the presence of an outflow gradient and increased filling pressure)

Syncope and presyncope
- Due to inadequate cardiac output with exertion or to cardiac arrhythmias
- Identifies patients at increased risk for sudden death (especially in children and young adults, the first clinical presentation may be sudden death)

6. Describe the classic murmur of obstructive HCM and bedside maneuvers that help distinguish it from other common etiologies.

The classic murmur of obstructive HCM is a **crescendo-decrescendo systolic murmur**, typically harsh, that usually begins well after the first heart sound (since ejection is not impeded early in systole). Five bedside maneuvers can help differentiate this murmur from others.

Effect of Bedside Maneuvers on Systolic Murmurs

	VALSALVA	HANDGRIP	SQUATTING	AMYL NITRITE	LEG RAISING
Obstructive HCM	↑	↓	↓	↑	↓
Aortic stenosis	↓	↓	↑↓	↑	↑
Ventricular septal defect	↓	↑	No change	↓	↑
Mitral regurgitation	↓ (slight)	↑	No change	↓	↑

7. How does the carotid pulse in obstructive HCM differ from that in valvular aortic stenosis?

In patients with HCM, the carotid pulse has an initial brisk rise, followed by a decline, then a second rise ("spike and dome" pattern). In aortic stenosis, the carotid upstroke is slowed and the amplitude low (*pulsus parvus et tardus*).

8. Which noninvasive laboratory evaluations are helpful in evaluating patients with suspected HCM?

Useful noninvasive laboratory tests include electrocardiography (EKG), chest x-ray, and echocardiography. The **EKG** may be normal but is usually abnormal in symptomatic patients, showing nonspecific ST and T-wave changes, LV hypertrophy, deep broad Q waves in the inferolateral leads, left axis deviation, and left atrial enlargement. Arrhythmias (supraventricular and ventricular) may be present on ambulatory monitoring.

The **chest x-ray** may be normal but usually shows mild to moderate increase in the cardiac silhouette.

Echocardiography is the cornerstone of the diagnosis of HCM. Ventricular hypertrophy is the cardinal feature seen on the echocardiogram. The septum is usually > 15 mm thick with a septal-to-posterior wall ratio of > 1.3–1.5. Other features include narrowing of the LV outflow tract formed by the interventricular septum anteriorly and the anterior mitral valve leaflet posteriorly (accentuated further with the Valsalva maneuver or amyl nitrite), a small LV cavity, and partial systolic closure or fluttering of the aortic valve. Color flow Doppler imaging may reveal mitral regurgitation.

9. What is systolic anterior motion (SAM)? What causes it?

SAM refers to abnormal movement of the anterior (and occasionally posterior) mitral valve leaflet during mid-systole. The role of SAM in producing the outflow gradient is controversial, although the degree of SAM and size of the outflow gradient are related. Three explanations have been offered for SAM:

1. A Venturi effect that draws the mitral valve toward the septum because of the early high-velocity jet of ejected blood and the decreased pressure at the outflow tract

2. Pulling of the mitral valve against the septum by the contraction of the papillary muscles, which are abnormally located and orientated

3. Pushing of the mitral valve against the septum, perhaps by the posterior wall because of its abnormal position in the LV outflow tract (see figures on next page).

Apical four-chamber view showing SAM (*arrow*) of the anterior mitral leaflet during midsystole. (RV = right ventricle, LV = left ventricle, RA = right atrium, LA = left atrium.)

This figure shows two M-mode echocardiographic views in a patient with HCM. *Left*, The M-mode of the aortic root and left atrium. There is late systolic notching (arrow) of the aortic valve leaflets due to partial closure and reopening of the aortic valve. *Right*, SAM of the mitral valve during midsystole (arrow).

10. Which patients with HCM are at greatest risk for sudden death?

Sudden death in patients with HCM is presumed (but not proven) to be due to a ventricular arrhythmia. Sudden death may occur in patients who are asymptomatic or whose clinical course has been otherwise stable. Markers of increased risk include:

• Age < 30 years at diagnosis
• Family history of HCM and sudden death
• History of syncope (in children)
• Nonsustained ventricular tachycardia on ambulatory EKG monitoring (in adults)
• Genetic mutation in the troponin T gene. Results in mild phenotypic changes to the heart in
  terms of only mild thickening, but a significant risk of sudden death.
• Bradyarrhythmias
• Aborted sudden death

Symptoms, degree of functional limitation, and severity of the outflow tract gradient do *not* correlate with risk of death. In young, competitive athletes who die suddenly, unsuspected HCM is the most common diagnosis at autopsy.

11. Which clinical manifestations of HCM are amenable to medical or surgical therapy?

The goals of management in patients with HCM are to improve symptoms, prevent complications, and reduce the risk of sudden death. The three manifestations of HCM that are amenable to specific medical or surgical therapy are: (1) ventricular outflow obstruction, (2) impaired ventricular relaxation during diastole, and (3) atrial and ventricular arrhythmias.

12. What are the effects of different drugs on the LV outflow tract gradient in HCM?

Decreasing contractility significantly affects the LV outflow tract gradient. Beta-adrenergic blockers may relieve symptoms by their negative inotropic effect as well as by decreasing the heart rate—resulting in longer diastolic filling time of the left ventricle. Disopyramide decreases contractility, but also has a pro-arrhythmic effect (induces torsade de pointes). Verapamil can either decrease the LV outflow tract gradient, or increase it due to its vasodilatory effect. Diltiazem may improve the diastolic filling of the left ventricle.

Decreasing preload (hypovolemia, diuretics, nitrates) enhances the dynamic obstruction and gradient by increasing the LV outflow tract obstruction. Chest pain in HCM is *not* to be treated with nitroglycerin, and dehydration must be avoided. Use diuretics with caution only when heart failure develops and in association with beta-blockers.

Decreasing afterload (nitrates, vasodilators) also leads to increased LV outflow tract gradient and obstruction. Dihydropyridines are contraindicated due to their pronounced vasodilatory effect and induction of tachycardia.

Note that in asymptomatic patients, there is no evidence that pharmacologic treatment prolongs survival.

13. What alternatives other than pharmacologic treatment can be offered to HCM patients?

Dual chamber pacing was initially thought to relieve symptoms in 90% of patients. Further blind randomized trials showed that up to 42% had improved symptoms when the pacer was inactivated, thereby raising the issue of the placebo effect of pacing. Pacing is offered to patients who are refractory to pharmacologic treatment or are not candidates for surgery, but evidence that pacing prolongs survival is lacking.

Myomectomy (resection of a segment of the basal septum), possibly accompanied by mitral valve replacement, is the radical solution with the best long-term results in terms of symptomatology and survival.

Transcoronary ablation of septal hypertrophy (TASH) is performed by alcohol injection into the first major septal branch of the left anterior descending coronary artery, leading to a limited myocardial infarction with reduced septal thickness. Initial follow-up results of TASH are encouraging, but further studies are needed.

14. What is the natural history of HCM?

The clinical course of patients with HCM is variable. Many patients remain asymptomatic or only mildly symptomatic for years. In those with resting obstruction, approximately two-thirds progress to New York Heart Association class III-IV over a 4-year period. The degree of ventricular hypertrophy usually remains stable over time, but may increase. In about 10% of patients, HCM progresses to LV dilatation and a dilated cardiomyopathy. The onset of atrial fibrillation usually results in worsening of symptoms. Mortality tends to be higher in those with outflow obstruction, who also tend to have the most extensive hypertrophy and the highest incidence of atrial and ventricular arrhythmias. The annual mortality of patients with HCM is about 3% in adults and 6% in children.

BIBLIOGRAPHY

1. De Luca M, Tak T: Hypertrophic cardiomyopathy. Tools for identifying risk and alleviating symptoms. Postgrad Med 107(7):127–139, 2000.
2. Erwin JP III, Nishimura RA, Lloyd MA, Tajik AJ: Dual chamber pacing for patients with hypertrophic obstructive cardiomyopathy: A clinical perspective in 2000. Mayo Clin Proc 75(2):173–180, 2000.
3. Fatkin D, Seidman JG, Seidman CE: Hypertrophic cardiomyopathy. In Willerson JT, Cohn JN (eds): Cardiovascular Medicine, 2nd ed. Philadelphia, Churchill Livingstone, 2000, pp 1055–1074.
4. Frank S, Braunwald E: Idiopathic hypertrophic subaortic stenosis: Clinical analysis of 126 patients with emphasis on the natural history. Circulation 37:759–788, 1968.
5. Maron BJ, Fananapazir L: Sudden cardiac death in hypertrophic cardiomyopathy. Circulation 85(Suppl I):I-57–I-63, 1992.
6. Romeo F, Pelliccia F, Cristofan R, et al: Hypertrophic cardiomyopathy: Is a left ventricular outflow tract gradient a major prognostic determinant? Eur Heart J 11:233–240, 1990.
7. Sasson Z, Rakowski H, Wigle ED, et al: Echocardiographic and Doppler studies in hypertrophic cardiomyopathy. Cardiol Clin 8:217–232, 1990.
8. Seiler C, Hess OM, Schoenbeck M, et al: Long-term follow-up of medical versus surgical therapy for hypertrophic cardiomyopathy: A retrospective study. J Am Coll Cardiol 17:634–642, 1991.
9. Solomon SD, Jarcho JA, McKenna W, et al: Familial hypertrophic cardiomyopathy is a genetically heterogenous disease. J Clin Invest 86:993–999, 1990.
10. Takagi E, Yamakado T, Nakano T: Prognosis of completely asymptomatic adult patients with hypertrophic cardiomyopathy. J Am Coll Cardiol 33(1):206–211, 1999.
11. Wynne J, Braunwald E: Hypertrophic cardiomyopathy. In Braunwald E (ed): Heart Disease: A Textbook of Cardiovascular Medicine, 5th ed. Philadelphia, W. B. Saunders, 1997.
12. Zieman J, Fortuin N: Hypertrophic and restrictive cardiomyopathies in the elderly. Cardiol Clin 17(1):159–172, 1999.

31. SYNCOPE AND DIZZINESS

Olivia V. Adair, M.D., and Catalin Loghin, M.D.

1. What is syncope? How common is it?

Syncope is a transient loss of consciousness, usually for seconds to minutes, with loss of postural tone. It resolves with spontaneous recovery. Syncope may also be associated with near-syncope or presyncope, which is described as dizziness and/or almost blacking out. Syncope is not associated with stupor or coma. The condition is seen in 30–50% of the adult population and accounts for approximately 1–2% of hospital admissions and 3% of emergency department visits per year.

2. How common is dizziness?

Dizziness is one of the most common complaints in ambulatory care and accounts for nearly 8 million outpatient visits/year in the U.S.; after fatigue, it is the most common complaint in general medical clinics. Dizziness is a heterogeneous symptom, including sensations of vertigo, presyncope, disequilibrium, and light-headedness.

3. What prognosis is associated with syncope or dizziness?

The prognosis depends on the underlying cause. Cardiac syncope carries the worse prognosis. Therefore, syncope usually initiates a thorough diagnostic evaluation to rule out a cardiac etiology. Dizziness, on the other hand, is often self-limiting and only rarely relates to life-threatening events, even in elderly patients.

4. What causes dizziness?

Based on a recent meta-analysis of 12 studies, the most common causes of dizziness are:
- Peripheral vestibular vertigo (4–44%), labyrinthitis (3–23%), Meniere's disease (0–10%); benign positional vertigo is the most common specific peripheral vestibular diagnosis.
- Central vestibular cerebrovascular (0–20%), tumor (0–6%).
- Psychiatric disorders (2–26%) and hyperventilation (0–24%), usually in younger patients
- Multicausal (13%)

Dizziness accounts for 1% of office visits, and a patient may use the term to describe vertigo (the illusion of motion accompanied by nausea, vomiting, pallor, and perspiration), presyncope (perception of an oncoming fainting episode accompanied by pallor, diaphoresis, nausea), dysequilibrium (losing balance without the illusion of movement), or lightheadness.

5. Describe the work-up for dizziness.

Dizziness is often self-limiting, but when it does persist, a directed history and physical examination can establish a presumptive diagnosis in most patients. The best supplemental tests are vestibular function and psychiatric evaluation. If a brain lesion is suspected, auditory evoked potentials and brain imaging by MRI yield the best results.

6. What are the major causes of syncope?

Three major categories each account for approximately one-third of the cases of syncope: noncardiac, cardiac, and unknown causes. Syncope is a symptom, not a disease; therefore, the etiology is diverse and includes numerous disorders.

Some causes of **cardiac syncope** are tachyarrhythmias or bradyarrhythmias (or a combination of both, as in the sick sinus syndrome), atrioventricular conduction defects, pacemaker failure or pacemaker-induced tachycardia, acute MI, massive pulmonary embolism, aortic stenosis (fixed obstruction in valvular lesions and dynamic obstruction in hypertrophic cardiomyopathy), and cardiac tamponade.

Lately, a more important role is attributed to **vasovagal syncope** (neurocardiogenic syncope); this syndrome is considered to be one part of a large group of autonomic disorders associated with defective blood pressure control and orthostatic intolerance. The group also includes carotid sinus syndrome, Shy-Drager syndrome, diabetic neuropathy, multisystem atrophy, tabes dorsalis, familial dysautonomia, and amyloidosis.

The 1-year mortality rates are: cardiac syncope 30%, noncardiac syncope 12%, syncope with an undetermined etiology 6%. The latter two, though lower, still represent a higher mortality than in a general, healthy population. The symptom of syncope should be considered serious, and a cause should be identified.

7. What is the most important evaluation step or test in identifying the cause of syncope?

A careful **history and physical examination** form the cornerstone of a proper diagnosis of syncope. One study showed that the history and physical exam were sufficient in establishing the diagnosis in 85% of patients. Also, if the answer is not found in the history and physical exam, it may never be found. The surrounding circumstances are important to establish, e.g., loss of consciousness, chest pain, palpitations, running after a bus, or watching TV. Also, other medical problems and medications should be evaluated for a possible effect. Physical examinations should include postural maneuvers, attention to murmurs, carotid pulse, carotid sinus massage (unless contraindicated), careful neurologic examination, as well as rectal examination (to rule out gastrointestinal bleeding).

Routine laboratory studies, a chest x-ray, and an **electrocardiogram** (ECG) are recommended. If heart disease is suspected, an echo-Doppler study should be included in the initial work-up. Unfortunately, only about one-half of patients will have a correct diagnosis after the routine clinical evaluation.

8. How helpful is 24-hour Holter monitoring for the diagnosis of syncope?

Not as helpful as *48-hour* monitoring. In a large study of patients with syncope unexplained by history or physical examination, 86 patients (mean age, 61 years) underwent three serial 24-hour Holter evaluations. The first Holter showed at least one major abnormality in 14 patients (16%); the second showed a major abnormality in 9 (12%) of the remaining 72 patients; only 3 patients (5%) had major abnormalities on the third Holter. The factors associated with major abnormalities on Holter were age > 65 years, male gender, history of heart disease, and initial non-sinus rhythm (highest relative risk, 3.5). Therefore, in the 26 patients identified with major abnormalities, 23 of them were identified with 48-hour Holter evaluation. Extending the monitoring duration from 24 to 48 hours almost doubled the diagnostic benefit.

Perhaps even better are event recorders, activated by the patient at the onset of symptoms. Recently, an implantable version became available. Note that symptoms must correlate with the Holter monitoring findings to establish a causal relationship. If they don't correlate, the ECG findings probably don't play a role in the syncope.

9. Does syncope ever occur as the initial presentation of an acute myocardial infarction?

Yes. Five percent to 10% of patients with acute myocardial infarction have syncope as their initial presentation. This most commonly occurs in association with Q-wave inferior wall infarction and may be fatal. The mechanism is most likely activation of the Bezold-Jarisch reflex, predominantly a vasovagal reaction.

10. Should I perform a different evaluation of syncope in the elderly patient?

Yes. The incidence of syncope is increased in the elderly (6–7% annually and 30% recurrence rate), as cerebral blood flow decreases with aging. Also, syncope in the elderly may be the first manifestation of various serious illnesses and thus of graver prognosis. One study reported that patients over 70 years old who experienced syncope had a mortality in 1 year of 16–27% versus a mortality in a young population of 1–8%. The physical injury that may result from a syncopal episode may be especially devastating in elderly persons.

11. How common is carotid sinus syncope?

Hypersensitivity to carotid sinus stimulation has been shown in recent studies to be more common than previously thought. Carotid sinus stimulation may cause a vasodepressor reaction, a predominant vasovagal reaction, or both. Drugs known to aggravate carotid sinus syncope are digitalis, beta blockers, and calcium channel blockers. The hypersensitivity may be secondary to an abnormality of the carotid sinus mechanism or to underlying conduction system disease.

Diagnosis can be made with carotid massage in a head-up tilt position with blood pressure and ECG monitoring. Never perform carotid massage if a carotid bruit is present. In patients taking digoxin, carotid massage may induce fatal arrhythmias. A positive response is reproduction of symptoms in the presence of an induced ventricular electrical pause > 5 seconds; a decrease in the ventricular rate by > 50%; or symptomatic hypotension.

12. What is the therapy for carotid sinus syncope?

Therapy includes patient education and evaluation of their medications, with possible carotid sinus denervation and pacemaker implantation if symptoms are refractory or associated with significant bradycardias. Dual-chamber pacing is required since single-chamber pacing commonly produces pacemaker syndrome. Pacer therapy reduces the incidence of syncope even without a direct affect on vasodepressor response.

13. When should arrhythmic syncope be suspected?

Arrhythmia is more likely if the patient has underlying heart disease, symptoms of palpitations, abrupt syncope with injury, and syncope not associated with posture changes. Arrhythmic syncope is usually the result of a heart rate either too fast or slow occurring in a patient with limited cardiac reserve (secondary to valvular or myocardial disease). These patients are also more likely to have conduction abnormalities, predisposing them to low cardiac output with an arrhythmia.

14. A 28-year-old man presents to the emergency department complaining of an episode of exercise-related syncope. His physical examination reveals a right ventricular gallop. A 12-lead EKG shows anterior right precordial T-wave inversion, with a QRS duration of 130 msec. Subsequently, a Holter monitor documents multiple episodes of nonsustained ventricular tachycardia, with left bundle branch block configuration. An echocardiogram reveals a dilated right ventricle with depressed ejection fraction and a normal left ventricle. How is the diagnosis established? What is the diagnosis?

MRI establishes the diagnosis of arrhythmogenic right ventricular dysplasia (ARVD), by providing tissue characterization information.

Image courtesy of S. Flamm, M.D.

"Black-blood" spin-echo MRI of the outflow tract of the right ventricle demonstrates fatty infiltration of the myocardium (*white arrows*) in this patient with ARVD. The fat-infiltrated myocardium is bright on this spin-echo sequence, while normal myocardium is gray, as seen throughout the left ventricle.

15. What is the best approach for work-up of a suspected arrhythmic syncope?

The work-up of syncope can be costly and timely. Therefore, it should usually start with the less expensive and least invasive studies, unless special circumstances dictate otherwise (see table). Obviously, if a specific exertional etiology is suspected from the history and physical examination, it should dictate the work-up strategy. It's an excellent idea to include echo-Doppler in the evaluation of almost all syncope patients, because of the importance of left ventricular function in the prognosis of these patients.

Laboratory Evaluation of Arrhythmic Syncope

TEST	PURPOSE
Electrocardiogram (ECG)	Defines conduction system disease, Wolff-Parkinson-White syndrome, myocardial infarction, left ventricular hypertrophy, atrial and ventricular ectopy, and occasionally arrhythmia.
Signal-averaged ECG	Screens for ventricular tachycardia after myocardial infarction.
Ambulatory monitoring	Documents arrhythmia and relates to symptoms; aids in defining therapeutic response.
Echocardiography	Evaluates for valve disease, myocardial disease, left ventricular function.
Patient-activated monitoring devices	Documents paroxysmal arrhythmias in low-risk subsets.
Exertional exercise test	Reproduces exertional arrhythmia; evaluates role of ischemia.
Invasive electrophysiologic study	Defines conduction system disease, elicits supraventricular and ventricular tachycardia, and measures hemodynamic effect of arrhythmias and response to pharmacologic and pacing interventions.
Head-up tilt	Elicits vasodepressor or hemodynamic response to arrhythmia.

Modified from Weissler AM, Boudoulas HB, Lewis RP, et al: Syncope: Pathophysiology, recognition, and treatment. In Hurst JW (ed): The Heart, 7th ed. New York, McGraw-Hill, 1990, p 581.

16. How helpful is signal-averaged ECG in evaluating recurrent syncope?

Signal-averaged ECG is especially helpful in identifying patients with ventricular tachycardia with late potentials. The presence of a late potential predicts ventricular tachycardia as the etiology of syncope with a sensitivity of 73% and specificity of 89%. The combination of heart disease (in particular, dilated cardiomyopathy and post MI) and late potentials is highly predictive of the eventual clinical diagnosis of ventricular tachycardia. Also, combining results of other noninvasive test, such as Holter monitoring and echocardiogram, greatly increases the usefulness of signal-averaged ECG. The absence of a late potential provides a strong negative predictor of ventricular tachycardia and is therefore a useful screening test in patients with syncope.

17. When should electrophysiology studies (EPS) be considered for arrhythmia detection?

Patients who are best served by EPS are those strongly suspected of having arrhythmic syncope as indicated by the noninvasive test and underlying heart disease. In these patients, EPS reveals a mechanism in 71% of patients who undergo the procedure. Also, patients with a negative study have a very low short-term mortality, but may have recurrent nonarrhythmic syncope. The most common arrhythmia detected is ventricular tachycardia, and the most powerful predictor of a positive EPS is an ejection fraction of < 40%. The therapeutic strategies formulated by the diagnostic tests are very effective in preventing syncope in most patients (96%) during an 18-month follow-up.

A **head-up tilt table test** often accompanies EPS and more than doubles the chance of revealing the cause of the syncope. Specificity of the tilt test is close to 90%. Sensitivity can be enhanced by a low-dose infusion of isoproterenol.

18. Can I expect to find the cause of syncope in most patients? What should I do if no cause is identified?

With the more common use of EPS and tilt-table testing, fewer patients are given the diagnosis of syncope of unknown cause. However, about 20% of patients have no etiology established after extensive work-ups. These may include patients with multiple causes, especially older patients. Close follow-up is important because about one-third will have recurrence. Also, counseling on avoidance of potentially dangerous activities and predisposing factors is essential.

19. What is the pharmacologic treatment of neurocardiogenic syncope?

Treatment is indicated only if the episodes are frequent, lead to significant changes in lifestyle, prevent employment, or pose a major risk of injury to the patient or others. Simple reassurance and nonpharmacologic measures (e.g., support hose, increase salt and fluid intake) are often enough to prevent recurrence.

Agents currently used are **beta-blockers**, **disopyramide**, **vasoconstrictors** (midodrine, etilephrine), **serotonin reuptake inhibitors** (sertraline, fluoxetine), and **volume-retention drugs** (fludrocortisone). Beta-blockers are indicated in patients with a positive tilt test to block the effects of epinephrine (which facilitates vasodilatation, increases the sensitivity of trigger sites for afferent neural reflexes, and enhances responsiveness to the efferent parasympathetic response "accentuated antagonism").

Disopyramide is a controversial choice and should probably be reserved for young, active patients with no underlying heart disease. Such patients generally prefer this drug over a beta-blocker, because the latter decreases their exercise tolerance.

Midodrine is an alpha-1 agonist that achieves good results in orthostatic hypotension and neurally mediated syncope, but long-term therapy may be hampered by the occurrence of tachyphylaxis.

Note that the only *well-proven* therapies are beta-blockers and SSRIs.

BIBLIOGRAPHY

1. Bass EB, Curtiss EI, Arena VC, et al: The duration of Holter monitoring in patients with syncope. Arch Intern Med 150:1073–1078, 1990.
2. Benditt DG, Fabian W, Sakaguchi S: Syncope. In Willerson JT, Cohn JN (eds): Cardiovascular Medicine, 2nd ed. New York, Churchill Livingstone, 2000, pp 1055–1074.
3. Benditt DG, Fahy GJ, et al: Pharmacotherapy of neurally mediated syncope. Circulation 100(11):1242–1248, 1999.
4. Derebery MJ: The diagnosis and treatment of dizziness. Med Clin North Am 83(1):163–167, 1999.
5. Grubb BP: Pathophysiology and differential diagnosis of neurocardiogenic syncope. Am J Cardiol 41(4):247–254, 1999.
6. Kroenke K, Lucas CA, Rosenberg ML, et al: Causes of persistent dizziness: A prospective study of 100 patients in ambulatory care. Ann Intern Med 117:898–904, 1992.
7. Kroenke K, Hoffman R, Einstadter D: How common are various causes of dizziness? A critical review. South Med J 93(2):160–167, 2000.
8. Manolis AS, Linzer M, Salem D, Estes NA 3d: Syncope: Current diagnostic evaluation and management. Ann Intern Med 112:850–863, 1990.
9. Sra JS, Anderson AJ, Sheikh SH, et al: Unexplained syncope evaluated by electrophysiologic studies and head-up tilt testing. Ann Intern Med 114:1013–1019, 1991.
10. Wehrmacher WH: Syncope among the aging population. Am J Geriatr Cardiol 2:50–57, 1993.

32. TRAUMATIC HEART DISEASE

Fernando Boccalandro, M.D.

1. What is the most common cause of cardiac injury?
Motor vehicle accidents.

2. List the physical mechanisms of injury in cardiac trauma.
- Penetrating trauma (e.g., ribs, foreign bodies, sternum)
- Non-penetrating trauma
  Massive chest compression or crush injury
  Deceleration, traction, or torsion of the heart or vascular structures
  Sudden rise in blood pressure due to acute abdominal compression
  Myocardial contusion

3. What is myocardial contusion?
Myocardial contusion is a common, reversible injury and is the consequence of a non-penetrating trauma to the myocardium. It is detected by elevations of specific cardiac enzymes with no evidence of coronary occlusion and by reversible wall motion abnormalities detected by echocardiography. It can manifest in the ECG by ST/T changes or by more complex arrhythmias. Myocardial contusion is pathologically characterized by areas of myocardial necrosis and hemorrhagic infiltrate that can be recognized on autopsy.

4. Which cardiac structures are most commonly involved in a cardiac trauma?
- Right ventricle contusion
- Aortic valve tear
- Left ventricle or left atrium rupture
- Innominate artery avulsion
- Aortic isthmus rupture
- Left subclavian artery traumatic occlusion
- Tricuspid valve tear

5. What bedside findings should be carefully sought in a patient with suspected cardiac trauma?
Obvious clinical signs in this group of patients are not common, but a complete evaluation to detect possible life-threatening complications can be made in a few minutes:

1. Carefully observe **vital signs** to assess the hemodynamic status. Pseudo-coarctation or decreased blood pressure in the left arm may occur in patients with a rupture of the aortic isthmus.

2. Inspect conjunctiva, palms, skin color, and oral mucosa for **pallor** suggestive of important blood loss. Cervical and supraclavicular hematomas are common in carotid rupture. Subcutaneous emphysema and tracheal deviation suggestive of pneumothorax may also be detected on **palpation**.

3. Check the patient's **jugular venous pulse**; a high jugular venous pressure with inspiratory raise (i.e., Kussmaul sign) is suggestive of cardiac tamponade or tension pneumothorax. A prominent systolic V wave suggests tricuspid insufficiency, which is most likely acute. Note that these patients may be extremely hypovolemic and the jugular venous distention may be difficult to interpret even in the presence of cardiac tamponade.

4. A **non-palpable apex** and/or **distant heart sounds** are suspicious for pericardial effusion in a non-obese patient. Check carefully for **pericardial rubs, heart murmurs, and thrills**, which can suggest pericarditis, regurgitant valves, ventricular septal defect, or arterio-venous fistulas. Palpate all pulses in all extremities, including in the subclavian location.

5. Always confirm **bilateral breath sounds** and perform **percussion** and **tactile fremitus** to exclude pneumothorax or hemothorax, if clinically suspected. Always perform **pulsus paradoxus** if cardiac tamponade is considered, since its presence heralds an impending cardiac tamponade.

6. Can an acute myocardial infarction (MI) complicate a cardiac trauma?

Yes, chest trauma can injure a coronary artery, leading to MI based on coronary spasm, thrombosis, or dissection of the arterial wall. Patients with established severe coronary artery disease have perfect pathophysiologic conditions for an acute myocardial event during significant trauma due to limited coronary flow reserve, excess of circulating catecholamines, and hypovolemia if there is significant blood loss. Always consider the possibility that when a patient has an acute MI and trauma, the MI could be the primary cause of the traumatic event due to cardiac syncope. Chest trauma can elevate cardiac-specific enzymes without significant coronary stenosis; therefore, carefully interpret these indicators in this setting.

7. What is the preferred treatment for an acute MI in the event of chest trauma?

The treatment of choice is emergent coronary angiography. Thrombolytics and anticoagulants are contraindicated. Also withhold nitrates, ACE inhibitors, and beta-blockers until the patient is hemodynamically stable. Aspirin may be considered in patients with no evidence of severe bleeding. Aortic balloon pumps are contraindicated in patients with acute MI, cardiogenic shock with acute traumatic aortic regurgitation, or any suspected aortic lesions.

8. List the causes of shock in patients with heart trauma.

The first cause to address is **hypovolemic shock** due to acute blood loss, usually from an abdominal source. If the shock persists despite fluid resuscitation or the degree of hemodynamic compromise is not in proportion to the degree of blood loss, consider cardiogenic causes.

Two other important causes are **cardiac tamponade** and **ventricular akinesia**. Rupture of any intrapericardial vessel or cardiac structure (e.g., coronary arteries, proximal aorta, great veins, ventricle) produces a rapid state of shock because of cardiac tamponade, unless there is a concomitant pericardial tear.

Cardiac akinesia or **severe hypokinesia** with temporary myocardial stunning could be a consequence of cardiac trauma and could lead to cardiogenic shock or acute heart failure.

Pericardial tamponade requires immediate treatment with a surgical subxyphoid approach as the preferred option, or with a percutaneous approach. Cardiac akinesia requires volume resuscitation to increase the cardiac pre-load and inotropic support until contractile recovery is achieved.

9. What work-up should be considered in a patient with suspected heart trauma?

Laboratories: hemoglobin, hematocrit, chemistries, cardiac enzymes, blood typing, and coagulation panel are routine.

Chest x-ray: to evaluate the cardiac silhouette, mediastinum, and lung fields.

Electrocardiogram: not a sensitive or specific tool, but may reveal nonspecific ST/T changes, conduction abnormalities, sinus tachycardia, premature atrial contractions, ventricular premature beats, or more complex arrythmias suggestive of myocardial contusion. Low voltage is suggestive of pericardial effusion, while electrical alternans is very suspicious for impending cardiac tamponade.

If the patient is stable, no further work-up may be needed.

If more complex heart lesions are suspected, including any pericardial involvement, an **echocardiogram with Doppler imaging** is the test of choice. This test is fast, inexpensive, and readily available to provide a vast amount of information regarding the pericardial space, wall motion, valvular damage, myocardial rupture, fistulas, and proximal aorta. Pay special attention to the right ventricle, due to its anterior location, and to the possible presence of ventricular thrombus.

Transthoracic echo may have important limitations in patients with complicated trauma (e.g., unstable chest, ventilated patients, chest tube drainages) because of limited windows. New echo contrast agents and transesophageal echo could play an important role in this group of patients. Transesophageal echo may not be possible in those with an unstable neck or facial trauma. In suspected aortic involvement, a contrast CT is the test of choice.

10. What are the mechanisms of injury of the thoracic great vessels?

Deceleration and traction are the most common mechanisms of injury of the thoracic arteries. Sudden horizontal **deceleration** creates marked shearing stress at the aortic isthmus (i.e., the junction between the mobile aortic arch and the fixed descending aorta), while vertical deceleration displaces the heart caudally and pulls the ascending aorta and the innominate artery. Rapid extension of the neck or **traction** on the shoulder can also overstretch the arch vessels and produce tears of the intima, disruption of the media, or complete rupture of the vessel wall, leading to bleeding, dissection, thrombosis, or pseudoaneurysm formation. Aortic rupture leads to immediate hypovolemic shock and death in the vast majority of cases (90%).

11. Describe the management of thoracic arterial lesions.

Usually, all arterial lesions require surgical repair, except benign ones like wall hematomas and limited dissections. An effort should be made to control the blood pressure with beta-blockers in all arterial lesions if the patient is hemodynamically stable. Venous lesions due to low pressure usually do not lead to a rapid hemodynamic compromise unless the implicated vessel drains to the pericardium, possibly leading to cardiac tamponade.

12. What are the potential late complications of heart trauma?

• Fistulas between different structures
• Constrictive pericarditis as a late consequence of hemopericardium
• Embolization from mural thrombus
• Ventricular aneurysm formation
• Valvular insufficiency
• Post-pericardiotomy syndrome

13. What is commotio cordis?

Sudden death following a blunt chest trauma is a rare phenomenon known as commotio cordis. It is theorized that commotio cordis is caused by ventricular fibrillation secondary to an impact-induced energy transmission via the chest wall to the myocardium during its vulnerable repolarization period. This can cause lethal arrythmias resulting in sudden death.

14. Describe the cardiac complications of electrical or lightning injuries.

Patients in whom an electric current has a vertical pathway are at high risk for cardiac injury. Arrhythmias are frequently seen. Damage to the myocardium is uncommon and occurs mainly because of heat injury or coronary spasm, causing myocardial ischemia. DC current and high-tension AC current are more likely to cause ventricular asystole, whereas low-tension AC produces ventricular fibrillation. The most common ECG abnormalities are sinus tachycardia and nonspecific ST-T wave changes.

The effect of lightning on the heart has been called "cosmic cardioversion" and results in ventricular standstill and, in some reports, ventricular fibrillation. Standstill usually returns to sinus rhythm, but often with a persistent respiratory arrest that causes deterioration of the rhythm. If initial ECG changes are not seen, it is unlikely that significant arrhythmias will occur later.

BIBLIOGRAPHY

1. Biffl WL, Moore FA, Moore EE, et al: Cardiac enzymes are irrelevant in the patient with suspected myocardial contusion. Am J Surg 168:523–528, 1994.
2. Chapelle JP: Cardiac troponin I and troponin T: Recent players in the field of myocardial markers. Clin Chem Lab Med 37(1):11–20, 1999.

3. Eddy AC, Rusch VW, Marchioro T, et al: Treatment of traumatic rupture of the thoracic aorta: A 15-year experience. Arch Surg 125:1351–1356, 1990.
4. Feliciano DV, Rozycki GS: Advances in the diagnosis and treatment of thoracic trauma. Surg Clin North Am 79(6):1417–1429, 1999.
5. Fish RM: Electric injury, part I: treatment priorities, subtle diagnostic factors, and burns. J Emerg Med 17(6):977–983, 1999.
6. Fulda G, Brathwaite CEM, Rodriguez A, et al: Blunt traumatic rupture of the heart and pericardium: a ten-year experience (1979-1989). J Trauma 31:167–173, 1991.
7. Galan G, Penalver JC, Paris F, et al: Blunt chest injuries in 1696 patients. Eur J Cardiothorac Surg 6:284–287, 1992.
8. Jain S, Bandi V: Electrical and lightning injuries. Crit Care Clin 15(2):319–331, 1999.
9. LeBlang SD, Dolich MO: Imaging of penetrating thoracic trauma. J Thorac Imaging 15(2):128–135, 2000.
10. May AK, Patterson MA, Rue LW 3rd, et al: Combined blunt cardiac and pericardial rupture: review of the literature and report of a new diagnostic algorithm. Am Surg 65(6):568–574, 1999.
11. Pretre R, Chilcott M: Blunt trauma to the heart and great vessels. N Engl J Med 336(9):626–632, 1997.
12. Pretre R, LaHarpe R, Cheretakis K, et al: Blunt injury to the ascending aorta: Three patterns of presentation. Surgery 119:603–610, 1996.
13. Shorr RM, Crittenden M, Indeck M, et al: Blunt thoracic trauma: analysis of 515 patients. Ann Surg 206:200–205, 1987.
14. Smith DC, Bansal RC: Transesophageal echocardiography in the diagnosis of traumatic rupture of the aorta. N Engl J Med 333:457–458, 1995.
15. Wang J, Tsai Y, Chen S, et al: Dangerous impact—commotio cordis. Cardiology 93(1–2):124–126, 2000.

33. CARDIAC TUMORS

Karen Cooper, M.D.

1. A 45-year-old woman with a history of metastatic breast cancer develops shortness of breath, cardiomegaly, and elevated neck veins. What findings are consistent with pericardial involvement by tumor?

Generally, signs of pericardial tamponade include equalization of pressures in the pericardial space, right atrium, pulmonary artery wedge, right ventricle, and pulmonary artery during diastole. In tamponade, there is a prominent x descent with a small y descent on the jugular venous pressure contour. The echocardiogram characteristically shows right ventricle free-wall diastolic collapse.

2. What is the most common type of primary cardiac tumor?

Benign myxoma. Most frequently, these arise in the left atrium, where auscultation may reveal a "tumor plop" in diastole as the tumor hits the ventricular wall. Myxomas usually are sporadic but can be familial with autosomal-dominant inheritance. Features of familial syndromes include pigmented nevi, nodular disease of the adrenal cortex, mammary fibroadenomas, and testicular or pituitary tumors.

3. Are recurrent myxomas the result of seeding or multifocal disease?

After complete resection of atrial myxomas, 85% of the recurrences appear at or close to the original site. Regeneration usually occurs between 3 months and several years afterward, with an average of 3.9 years. Review of the literature implies these recurrences are not due to inadequate resections or seeding, but rather to multifocal disease. The postmortem examination of one patient revealed no fewer than six separate myxomas in the left atrium even though the patient had had two resections while alive.

4. What primary malignant cardiac tumor is seen most frequently in adults?

Sarcoma occurring most frequently in the right atrium. The most common morphologic subtypes include angiosarcoma, rhabdomyosarcoma, mesothelioma, and fibrosarcoma. In general, these tumors are fatal, and the interval between diagnosis and death is very short. These sarcomas infiltrate the heart extensively so that resection is not possible, and they tend to extend locally into the pericardium, lung, and other surrounding structures. Eighty percent of these tumors have distant metastases at the time of discovery. Symptoms can range from nonspecific, such as anemia and weight loss, to frank congestive heart failure. On occasion, the first sign can be from a symptomatic metastasis.

5. Name the most common benign cardiac tumor seen in children.

Rhabdomyoma. These tumors arise from the ventricular surfaces and affect the right and left sides equally. They vary in size and cause symptoms either by obstructing intracardiac blood flow or by interfering with normal cardiac conduction. A high percentage (30%) of these tumors are associated with tuberous sclerosis, which ultimately determines their prognosis. They are congenital. Resection has been performed successfully.

6. What mode of imaging the heart best detects primary cardiac tumors?

It could be argued that most cardiac tumors are initially diagnosed by echocardiography. At this point in time, magnetic resonance imaging (MRI) of the chest is superior to computed tomography (CT) scan. Whether positron emission tomography (PET) scans will be more useful in the future remains to be seen. If you suspect a rare pheochromocytoma in the heart, the indium-111 octreotide uptake scintillation scan is the most useful.

7. Which tumor has the greatest propensity for cardiac metastases?

Malignant melanoma, with 50–65% of patients have cardiac metastases.

8. What four tumors are commonly associated with most cardiac metastases?

1. Leukemia
2. Bronchogenic carcinoma
3. Carcinoma of the breast
4. Lymphoma (Hodgkin's and non-Hodgkin's)

The tumors spread to the heart by direct extension from surrounding intrathoracic structures or by hematogenous or lymphatic spread. Direct extension is seen most often with bronchogenic carcinoma that has extended through the pericardium into the left atrium. Malignant pericardial effusions from noncardiac neoplasms can lead to the implantation of viable cells on the epicardial surface.

9. How are cardiac metastases detected?

Most myocardial metastases are symptomatic. Although the metastases can interfere with conduction, valve function, or intracardiac blood flow, most commonly they are relatively small and do not affect global cardiac function. As the tumors become larger, symptoms can occur. Atrial arrhythmias, fibrillation or flutter, occur most often, and these findings in a patient with known carcinoma should arouse suspicion of cardiac metastasis. Diagnosis can be made by two-dimensional echocardiography or cytologic examination of pericardial fluid.

10. What class of cancer drugs is most often associated with electrocardiographic (ECG) abnormalities and arrhythmias?

Anthracycline antibiotics. ECG changes can occur over a wide range of doses and develop as a cumulative effect. The most frequent abnormalities are nonspecific ST-T wave changes, decreased QRS voltage, sinus tachycardia, supraventricular tachyarrhythmias, premature ventricular and atrial contractions, T-wave abnormalities, and QT-interval prolongation. The changes occur during or within a few days of drug administration but are reversible within a few hours after discontinuation of treatment. Most ECG abnormalities commonly encountered with doxorubicin or daunorubicin therapy are benign, and usually it is not necessary to stop therapy, although sudden death and life-threatening ventricular tachyarrhythmias have been reported.

11. Describe the pericarditis seen after treatment of Hodgkin's disease.

Radiation-induced pericarditis occurs following radiotherapy, and its effects are related to the dose of radiation administered. The acute pericarditis usually occurs within 12 months of the initiation of radiation therapy but may manifest years later. The clinical course may be mild, but in 50% of patients, a mild to severe tamponade may develop, requiring pericardiocentesis or a pericardial window. Chronic pericarditis is generally benign, with many patients having an asymptomatic enlarged pericardial silhouette on chest x-ray. An effusion may develop 2–5 years after treatment and clears spontaneously. A constrictive pericarditis may occur with an acute pericarditis or chronic effusion, appearing 6–30 months after radiation therapy. Other clinical radiation-induced heart diseases include myocardial fibrosis, accelerated coronary heart disease, and valvular dysfunction.

12. Name four potential sources of cerebrovascular or cardiac ischemia/infarction.

1. Emboli from a cardiac source
2. In-situ thrombosis of a major cerebral vessel
3. Atheroemboli from a central vessel
4. Primary cardiac tumor. Papillary fibroelastoma is the third most common cardiac tumor. Eighty percent are found on valvular endocardium. These tumors are more common in elderly patients with long-standing heart disease. Transient ischemic attack or stroke are the most common presenting symptoms. These tumors are diagnosed best with echocardiography and are generally successfully excised.

13. Which cancer drugs have been associated with myocardial ischemia and infarction?

Although rare findings, drug-induced ischemia and infarction are most commonly associated with **5-fluorouracil**, **doxorubicin**, and the **vinca alkaloids** (vinblastine and vincristine). Rarely do patients who experience 5-fluorouracil-induced myocardial infarction have preexisting coronary artery disease. Chest pain occurs after 3–4 days of consecutive administration. With daunorubicin and doxorubicin, few cases of myocardial ischemia and infarction have been reported, with episodes occurring within hours of drug administration. The vinca alkaloids have been associated with coronary artery–related toxicities that include accelerated atherosclerosis, coronary vasospasm, angina, and myocardial infarction. Prophylactic treatment with nitrates and calcium channel blockers may be useful in abolishing pain and allowing continuation of treatment when necessary.

14. What is the most important factor in the development of cardiomyopathy secondary to anthracycline chemotherapy?

Total dose of drug received. The overall incidence of clinical doxorubicin cardiomyopathy is low, at 1–2%, but is dose-dependent. It is rare at doses < 450 mg/m^2 body surface area, but increases along a continuum with an average incidence of 7% at 550 mg/m^2, 15% at 600 mg/m^2, and 30–40% at 700 mg/m^2. Congestive heart failure occurs generally 30–60 days after the last dose but can occur during treatment or years later.

15. How should a patient's cardiac status be followed during treatment with anthracycline drugs?

Recommended guidelines for monitoring patients are based on the patient's cardiac function as measured by the left ventricular ejection fraction (LVEF):

Normal baseline LVEF ($\geq$ 50%)

• A second LVEF should be determined after administration of 250–300 mg/ml of anthracycline.

• In patients with risk factors (heart disease, radiation, abnormal echocardiogram, cyclophosphamide), LVEF should be measured again at 400 mg/ml; in those with no risk factors, at 450 mg/ml.

• Sequential studies should then be performed prior to each dose.

• Treatment should be discontinued if the LVEF shows an absolute decrease of 10% or more or a decline to 50% or less.

Abnormal baseline LVEF (< 50% but > 30%)

• Sequential studies should be performed prior to each dose.

• Treatment should be discontinued if the LVEF shows an absolute decrease of 10% or more and/or a final LVEF of 30% or less.

16. What is the most accurate method for detecting anthracycline-induced cardiac damage?

The most accurate method is endomyocardial biopsy. The main disadvantages of the biopsy are its invasive nature, limited availability, and expense.

17. How is anthracycline-induced cardiomyopathy treated?

Treatment of congestive heart failure or cardiomyopathy secondary to anthracyclines is with digoxin, diuretics, vasodilators, and/or ACE inhibitors (e.g., captopril). Cardiac dysfunction can improve with standard therapy in some cases, as evidenced by improved long-term assessment.

BIBLIOGRAPHY

1. Haq MM, Legha SS, Choksi J, et al: Doxorubicin-induced heart failure in adults. Cancer 56:1361–1365, 1985.
2. Howard RA, Aldea GS, Shapira OM, et al: Papillary fibroelastoma: Increasing recognition of a surgical disease. Ann Thorac Surg 68:1881–1885, 1999.
3. Labianca R, Beretta G, Clerici M, et al: Cardiac toxicity of 5FU: A study on 1083 patients. Tumori 68:505–510, 1982.

4. Lin JC, Palafox BA, Jackson HA, et al: Cardiac pheochromocytoma: Resection after diagnosis by one one one-indium octreotide scan. Ann Thorac Surg 67:555–558, 1999.
5. McAllister HA: Primary tumors and cysts of the heart and pericardium. Curr Probl Cardiol 4(May):1–51, 1979.
6. Piehler JM, Lie JT, Giuliani ER: Tumors of the heart. In Brandenbury RO, et al (eds): Cardiology: Fundamental and Practices. Chicago, Year Book, 1987, pp 1671–1689.
7. Prichard RW: Tumors of the heart: Review of the subject and report of one hundred and fifty cases. Arch Pathol 51:98–128, 1951.
8. Ritchie JL, Singer JW, Thorning D, et al: Anthracycline cardiotoxicity: Clinical and pathologic outcomes assessed by radionuclide ejection fraction. Cancer 46:1109–1116, 1980.
9. Schwartz RG, McKenzie WB, Alexander J, et al: Congestive heart failure and left ventricular dysfunction-complicated doxorubicin therapy: Seven years' experience using radionuclide angiocardiopathy. Am J Med 82:1109–1118, 1987.
10. Shinefeld A, Katsumata T, Westaby S: Recurrent cardiac myxoma: Seeding or multifocal disease? Ann Thorac Surg 66:285–288, 1998.
11. Stewart JR, Fajardo LF: Radiation-induced heart diseases: Clinical and experimental aspects. Radiol Clin North Am 9:511–531, 1971.
12. Tori FM, Lum BL: Cardiac toxicity. In DeVita VT Jr, Hellman S, Rosenberg SA (eds): Cancer: Principles and Practice of Oncology, 3rd ed. Philadelphia, J.B. Lippincott, 1989, pp 2153–2161.
13. Van Hoff DD, Layard MW, Basa P, et al: Risk factors for doxorubicin-induced congestive heart failure. Ann Intern Med 91:710–717, 1979.

34. ADULT CONGENITAL HEART DISEASE

Ira M. Dauber, M.D.

1. What are the most common congenital heart diseases in adults?

The spectrum of congenital heart disease in adults is considerably different from that in infants and children. **Bicuspid aortic valve** and **atrial septal defect** are the most common congenital heart lesions found in adults. **Coarctation of the aorta** and **pulmonary stenosis** occur considerably less frequently. In children, ventricular septal defects are the most common malformations, but most children who survive to adulthood without surgical correction will have spontaneous closure of the defect. Adults are much less likely than children to have complex congenital lesions: the lesions are either corrected in childhood or cause death before adulthood. Adults with corrected congenital heart disease are increasingly more common.

2. What is the most common congenital lesion to escape detection until adulthood? Does early detection matter?

Atrial septal defect is the most common undetected congenital heart defect. Often, it is an isolated finding allowing survival to adulthood with few or no signs or symptoms. Detection is important because the left-to-right shunting of blood through the atrial septal defect causes pulmonary blood flow overload, which can eventually result in irreversible pulmonary hypertension and right ventricular overload (Eisenmenger's syndrome). This can be prevented by early detection and closure of the atrial septal defect.

3. Can cyanotic congenital heart disease occur in adults?

Yes! In adults, as in children, cyanotic heart disease is caused by right-to-left shunting of blood. In adults, shunting is most often due to increased pulmonary vascular resistance, but obstructive lesions causing reduced pulmonary blood flow (which are more common in children) are also seen. Atrial and ventricular septal defects and patent ductus arteriosus involve acyanotic left-to-right shunting. Increased pulmonary blood flow from these lesions can increase pulmonary vascular resistance with subsequent right-to-left shunting of cyanotic blood (Eisenmenger's complex). Some patients with obstruction to pulmonary blood flow and an associated right-to-left-shunt survive to adulthood. The most common anomaly with pulmonary obstruction is **tetralogy of Fallot**.

4. Do bicuspid aortic valves cause symptoms?

Bicuspid aortic valves can be functionally normal at birth and therefore go undetected. Even though a murmur is audible, some bicuspid valves remain functional. Most bicuspid valves eventually develop **aortic stenosis, aortic regurgitation**, or both. Progressive fibrocalcific thickening of a bicuspid valve is a common cause of aortic stenosis accounting for nearly one-half of adult cases requiring valve surgery. Bicuspid valves are the most common cause of isolated valvular aortic regurgitation. The development of both aortic stenosis and aortic regurgitation is usually gradual. Sudden aortic regurgitation can result from infective endocarditis because bicuspid valves are at increased risk for endocarditis.

5. Describe the signs and symptoms of atrial septal defects.

Many atrial septal defects are detected only at autopsy because the physical signs may be subtle and symptoms absent. Life expectancy is shortened, but there is usually a long asymptomatic phase and most patients do not develop symptoms until after age 40. Increased left-to-right shunting associated with age-related reduced left ventricular compliance can lead to **dyspnea on exertion** and **fatigue**. New onset **atrial arrhythmias**, especially atrial fibrillation, occur and may precipitate congestive heart failure. Patients with **pulmonary hypertension** from long-standing left-to-right shunting may also have symptoms of effort-related cyanosis, hemoptysis, and chest pain.

6. **What are the classic features of atrial septal defects?**
   - Widened and fixed splitting of the second heart sound (due to increased pulmonic blood flow)
   - Pulmonic systolic heart murmur (due to increased flow across the pulmonic valve)
   - Electrocardiographic (EKG) findings of right axis deviation with evidence of right-sided forces (especially in lead V_1) and incomplete right bundle branch block. These are the classic findings of a secundum ASD, the most common type of ASD, accounting for 70%.
   - Left axis deviation and cleft mitral valve, which are associated with primum ASD—a defect in the distal interatrial septum near the atrioventricular valves.

Pulmonary hypertension secondary to the atrial septal defect can cause cyanosis, clubbing, accentuated pulmonary component of S_2, and right-sided regurgitant murmurs. Because there is an association between ostium secundum atrial septal defect and mitral valve prolapse, findings of a mitral valve click or murmur of mitral regurgitation may occur. An ectopic atrial rhythm may be present in patients with sinus venosus atrial septal defect.

7. **Is echocardiography useful for the assessment of atrial septal defects?**
   Echocardiography can suggest the presence of an atrial septal defect by identifying an attenuated or absent atrial septum, associated atrial or right ventricular enlargement, or pulmonary hypertension from right-to-left shunting. Transesophageal echocardiography may provide better visualization of the atrial septum than standard transthoracic echo studies. Doppler studies may localize a high-velocity flow pattern across the atrial septum. Contrast echocardiography may be diagnostic of an atrial septal defect, especially with right-to-left shunting. Injections of saline microbubbles into a peripheral vein can demonstrate transit of the contrast from right to the left at the atrial level. In patients with left-to-right shunting, a negative image of contrast-free blood may be seen in the right atrium due to washout from contrast-free left atrial blood.

8. **Should atrial septal defects be surgically repaired?**
   Symptomatic atrial septal defects should be closed whether symptoms are due to left-to-right or to right-to-left shunting. In asymptomatic patients, recommendations for closure of the defect are intended to prevent the development of pulmonary hypertension, which can develop from persistently increased pulmonary blood flow from left-to-right shunting. Closure is recommended for patients with pulmonary to systemic blood flow ratios of 1.5:1.0 or greater. In patients younger than 45 years, surgical risk is < 1%. Closure is commonly done by open surgical repair, but catheter-based closure techniques are rapidly evolving, although still largely under experimental protocol. It is anticipated that catheter-based closure will become widely available in the next 2 years. Further, it is expected that the technique will widen the indications for closure of atrial septal defects.

9. **Which congenital heart lesions are at increased risk of endocarditis?**
   - Bicuspid aortic valve
   - Aortic coarctation
   - Ventricular septal defect
   - Tetralogy of Fallot
   - Pulmonic stenosis (moderate or severe)
   - Mitral or tricuspid regurgitation (severe—even if normal valve anatomy)
   - Patent ductus arteriosus

Patients with surgically corrected congenital heart disease involving placement of a prosthetic valve or prosthetic conduit are at even higher risk. Antibiotic prophylaxis is recommended for these patients. Unfortunately, < 20% of endocarditis cases of congenital heart lesions are associated with identifiable events or medical procedures.

10. How important are congenital anomalies of the coronary arteries?

Congenital coronary artery anomalies have been described with increased frequency because of the increased use of coronary angiography, but most are asymptomatic. **Myocardial bridging** due to an intramuscular course of a portion of the coronary artery (usually the left anterior descending) is the most common anomaly. In some patients sufficient systolic compression of the artery occurs to produce symptoms of ischemic heart disease (angina, myocardial infarction, sudden death). Ectopic aortic origin of either the right or left coronary artery is asymptomatic unless its course is altered to pass between the aorta and the right ventricular outflow tract, which can cause proximal obstruction of the artery and resultant ischemic symptoms. Anomalous origins from the pulmonary artery and congenital coronary arteriovenous fistulas usually become symptomatic during infancy and childhood.

11. Are arrhythmias a problem in congenital heart disease?

Approximately 25% of patients with congenital heart disease have arrhythmias, especially patients who have undergone corrective intracardiac surgery. More than 50% of patients with corrected transposition, 30% with tetralogy of Fallot, 25% with Fontan repair, and 10% with ventricular or atrial septal defect have postoperative arrhythmias. Supraventricular arrhythmias are most common, but sudden death due to ventricular arrhythmias is believed to occur in 5–10% of these patients. Complete heart block is particularly a risk for patients who have had correction of tetralogy of Fallot, and undoubtedly a cause of sudden death.

12. Ventricular arrhythmias are most common after repair of tetralogy of Fallot. What are the risk factors for sudden death in these patients?

- Older age at the time of repair
- Prolonged postoperative recovery
- Right ventricular end-systolic pressure > 60 mmHg
- Right ventricular end-diastolic pressure > 10 mmHg
- Depressed right ventricular systolic function
- Significant tricuspid or pulmonic regurgitation

Fifteen percent of postoperative patients have inducible ventricular tachycardia during electrophysiologic testing.

13. What is a coarctation of the aorta?

Coarctation of the aorta is a congenital narrowing of the descending thoracic or abdominal aorta. It usually occurs just distal to the origin of the left subclavian artery. Coarctation occurs 5 times more often in men than in women. There is a significant association with bicuspid aortic valve and Turner's syndrome (gonadal dysgenesis).

14. Does aortic coarctation have any classic findings?

The physical exam clue to coarctation is **differential pulses** in the arms (strong) versus the legs (weak and delayed). There is often a systolic murmur from the coarctation best heard in the posterior left thorax. Chest x-ray may show notching of the ribs due to enlargement of the intercostal arteries. Coarctation is one of the causes of surgically correctable hypertension in the adult. Later symptoms include heart failure and endocarditis.

15. Describe the features of Eisenmenger's syndrome. How is it different from Eisenmenger's complex?

Eisenmenger's syndrome is a broad term applied to any anomaly in which the pathophysiologic process (e.g., increased pulmonary blood flow) leads to obliterative pulmonary vascular disease with resultant pulmonary hypertension whether or not there is an associated right-to-left shunt and cyanosis. **Eisenmenger's complex** refers to congenital heart disease involving shunts with pulmonary hypertension severe enough to cause reversal of a left-to-right shunt with resultant right-to-left shunting through the defect. Eisenmenger originally described patients with ventricular septal defects. Pulmonary hypertension due to Eisenmenger-type pathophysiology is usually irreversible, but it may improve after corrective surgery if the associated pulmonary vascular anatomic changes are not too severe.

16. Who were Blalock and Taussig?

Dr. Helen B. Taussig and Dr. Alfred Blalock collaborated in establishing the Blalock-Taussig procedure in 1945. This subclavian-to-pulmonary artery anastomosis created a systemic-to-pulmonic shunt. This procedure established the first surgical treatment for "blue babies" suffering from pulmonic stenosis or pulmonic atresia, a previously fatal condition.

17. Name the four features of tetralogy of Fallot.
   1. Ventricular septal defect
   2. Obstruction to right ventricular outflow
   3. Overriding of the aorta
   4. Right ventricular hypertrophy

Tetralogy of Fallot accounts for approximately 10% of all congenital heart lesions (including pediatric) and is the most common cause of cyanotic disease presenting after 1 year of age. The degree of obstruction to pulmonary blood flow is the major factor in the clinical presentation.

18. Is mitral valve prolapse a congenital heart disease?

Although some cases of mitral valve prolapse are associated with congenital heart diseases, mitral valve prolapse itself is not due to congenital malformation of the valve. Mitral valve prolapse results from a variety of pathogenetic mechanisms affecting the mitral valve apparatus of which myxomatous degeneration is the most frequent cause.

19. How are patients with adult congenital heart disease who need noncardiac surgery managed?

They are managed similarly to other adult patients with cardiac disease undergoing noncardiac surgery. Preoperative cardiac risk assessment and intraoperative management are based on the patient's underlying clinical status and cardiac disease process as well as the type of surgery planned and its associated hemodynamic stress. Sufficient data are not available to make specific recommendations for patients with congenital heart disease. However, the presence of cyanotic heart disease, pulmonary hypertension, secondary erythrocytosis, or intracardiac shunts likely further increase operative risk.

CONTROVERSIES

20. Can patients with congenital heart disease participate in athletics?

In general, yes. Some general guidelines are available, but specific recommendations are based on the judgment of the patient's individual physician. The risks of athletic activity vary with the type of disease, functional cardiac status of the patient, and type of activities. Echocardiography and exercise testing are helpful in assessment of the athlete's cardiac status. The intensity and duration of exercise, risk of body collision or trauma, conditioning required, and the risk of injury (to both the athlete and spectators) if the athlete developed syncope are also factors in assessing risk.

Congenital aortic stenosis of mild degree (resting gradient < 20 mmHg) does not require restriction of activities if EKG and exercise stress test are normal and both left ventricular function and Holter monitor evaluations are benign. Patients with moderate or severe aortic stenosis should be advised to avoid strenuous activities or athletics until after surgical (or catheter-based) correction. They are at increased risk not only of angina and syncope but of sudden death as well. Similarly, patients with mild **pulmonic stenosis** (gradient < 25 mmHg) can participate in unrestricted athletic activity but not if there is moderate or severe obstruction unless the stenosis has been corrected. Patients with **tetralogy of Fallot** can have increased right-to-left shunting with exercise causing breathlessness, cyanosis, and risk of exercise-induced arrhythmias. They require careful assessment prior to participation in athletics. **Anomalous origin of the left coronary artery**, which courses between the aorta and right ventricular outflow tract, is associated with obstruction of the artery. Ischemic symptoms such as angina, myocardial infarction, or sudden death may develop with exertion. These patients should be advised against vigorous activity unless the defect is surgically corrected. Fortunately, if no myocardial injury has developed, surgery can be curative and allow normal athletic activity. The presence of pulmonary vascular disease, especially **pulmonary hypertension**, is associated with exercise-induced syncope, which carries a risk of sudden death. Athletic activities requiring strenuous or sudden exercise should be avoided. The risks of **atrial septal defect** are not due to the defect itself but relate to its functional consequences. Exercise limitation and risks of athletic activity depend on the degree of shunting, any associated impairment of ventricular function, and the presence of pulmonary hypertension. Patients who require anticoagulant therapy for either native or corrected malformations need to consider the risks of trauma-induced bleeding in their athletic activities.

21. Is congenital heart disease a contraindication to pregnancy?

The most common congenital malformations in women surviving to childbearing age are atrial septal defect (secundum), patent ductus arteriosus, pulmonary valvular stenosis, aortic coarctation, aortic valve disease, and tetralogy of Fallot. Few congenital heart lesions interfere with the initiation of pregnancy. Maternal mortality is related to functional class and varies from 0.4% for New York Heart Association functional class I and II to 6.8% for classes III and IV. Fetal mortality varies from essentially 0% in class I to 30% for class IV.

The effects of pregnancy on common congenital defects also relates to clinical status. Asymptomatic atrial septal defects, bicuspid aortic valves, and aortic coarctation require special attention to risks of embolism and endocarditis but have little effect on mortality. In contrast, elevations of pulmonary vascular resistance significantly increase the risks of pregnancy, and Eisenmenger's complex is associated with cumulative maternal death rates of 30–70% during pregnancy and the early postpartum period. Risks of problems during pregnancy are lower in patients with surgically corrected disease but are still determined by the degree of cardiac and vascular reserve and the residual defects after surgery. The major risks to the fetus stem from functional class of the mother, presence of maternal cyanosis, and the use of anticoagulants to manage the mother's heart disease (especially warfarin for prosthetic heart valves).

BIBLIOGRAPHY

1. Dajani AS, Taubert KA, Wilson W, et al: Prevention of bacterial endocarditis: Recommendations by the American Heart Association. Circulation 96:358–366, 1997.
2. Eagle KA, Brundage BH, Chaitman BR, et al: Guidelines for perioperative management for noncardiac surgery: Report of the American College of Cardiology/American Heart Association Task Force on Practice Guidelines. J Am Coll Cardiol 27:910–948, 1996.
3. Foster E, Webb G, Human D, et al: The adult with tetralogy of Fallot. Am Coll Cardiol Curr J Rev March/April:62–66, 1998.
4. Graham TP, Bricker JT, James FW, Strong WB: Twenty-sixth Bethesda Conference: Recommendations for determining eligibility for competition in athletes with cardiovascular abnormalities. J Am Coll Cardiol 24:867–873, 1994.
5. Liberthson RR: Congenital Heart Disease: Diagnosis and Management in Children and Adults. Boston, Little, Brown, 1989.
6. Maron BJ, Thompson PD, Puffer JC, et al: Cardiovascular preparticipation screening of competitive athletes. Circulation 94:850–856, 1996.
7. Perloff JK, Child JS: Congenital Heart Disease in Adults. Philadelphia, W.B. Saunders, 1991.
8. Perloff JK: Congenital heart disease in the adult. In Braunwald E (ed): Heart Disease, 5th ed. Philadelphia, W.B. Saunders, 1997, pp 963–987.
9. Pitkin RM, Perloff JK, Koos BJ, Beall MH: Pregnancy and congenital heart disease. Ann Intern Med 112:445–454, 1990.
10. Zuppiroli A, Rinaldi M, Kramer-Fox R, et al: Natural history of mitral valve prolapse. Am J Cardiol 75:1028–1032, 1995.

35. HEART DISEASE IN WOMEN

Olivia V. Adair, M.D.

1. Is ischemic heart disease a problem in women?

Yes. Ischemic heart disease causes 250,000 deaths/year in women in the U.S. This represents 23% of all deaths in women, making ischemic heart disease the leading cause of death in women over age 50.

2. What are the risk factors for coronary artery disease (CAD) in women?

The effects of risk factors are not well studied, but age, smoking, hypertension, lipoprotein profile, obesity, diabetes, and family history do predict CAD in women. Also, oral contraceptives and menopause increase the risk, while postmenopausal hormonal replacement decreases the risk.

3. Does the natural history of atherosclerotic CAD differ in females and males?

Yes. The Framingham Study has shown that 23% of all female mortality and 52% of all cardiovascular female deaths are due to atherosclerotic CAD, whereas figures for males are 34% and 64%, respectively. Sudden cardiac death is less common in women, and women manifest symptoms approximately 10 years later than men.

4. Do women and men present with the same symptoms when they have CAD?

Common Presenting Manifestations of CAD

	MALES	FEMALES
Angina	33%	50%
Myocardial infarction	33%	33%
Sudden death	33%	17%

5. What tests have been used for diagnosing CAD in women?

The **exercise treadmill test** alone is of limited value in the diagnosis of CAD in women, having a sensitivity and specificity of 70%; however, the addition of thallium increases the specificity to 90%. **Radionuclide ventriculography** with exercise has also been disappointing in diagnosing CAD in females. The diagnostic accuracy for the presence of CAD is increased with stress testing in women if two or more cardiac risk factors are present; mitral valve prolapse is excluded; the ST segments normalize after > 6 minutes into recovery; target heart rate is achieved; or exercise duration is < 5 minutes on a full Bruce protocol.

6. Why is thallium perfusing imaging less sensitive in diagnosing CAD in women?

Though studies predominantly in men show exercise thallium perfusion imaging to improve the sensitivity of the stress test for CAD diagnosis, in women with single-vessel and multi-vessel disease the sensitivity is lower. This may be influenced by women's inability to attain target heart rate, low exercise levels, or imaging artifact from breast attenuation.

7. Is there another test to diagnose CAD in women before going to angiography?

Exercise echocardiography (ECG) has excellent accuracy, independent of chest pain being typical or atypical. Also, exercise ECG can detect noncoronary causes of chest pain, such as mitral valve prolapse, pericardial effusion, pulmonary hypertension, hypertrophic cardiomyopathy, and valvular disease.

Coronary angiography should be used when noninvasive risk stratification and testing suggest a high probability of significant CAD. Women who—despite medical therapy—are symptomatic during low-level exercise in their daily routine or who have had frequent noninvasive testing for multiple bouts of chest pain (even with minimal risk factors) should be considered for coronary angiography.

8. Is there a difference in the extent of CAD in females compared to males?

Yes. As a subset study in the Coronary Artery Surgery Study, Chaitman et al. showed less extensive left main and triple-vessel CAD in women as compared to men in coronary angiography studies. Women also retained angiographic systolic function to a greater extent, suggesting a resistance to developing chronic left ventricular dysfunction and heart failure.

9. Do women fare as well as men post heart transplantation?

Although this issue has not been studied well, the Italian Multicenter Study Group followed 65 women and 238 men with documented idiopathic cardiomyopathy. Though the women presented with a more advanced phase of the disease—i.e., more dilated left ventricles, thicker left ventricular walls, shorter exercise duration, and worse symptoms—the 18-month follow-up transplant-free survival was not significantly different by gender, and there was no difference in prognosis. Therefore, although women presented with more symptomatic disease after transplant, they did equally well as men.

10. Should women be treated differently than men for CAD?

There is little information available comparing the efficacy of medical management for CAD by gender. In two studies, the protective effects of beta-blockers and aspirin as secondary prevention of CAD were shown not to extend to women, whereas one study showed a regimen of 1–6 aspirin/week decreased the risk of the first myocardial infarction (MI) in women. Recent studies show success of percutaneous transluminal coronary angioplasty is no longer adversely influenced by female gender. Coronary artery bypass surgery in women is associated with an increased operative mortality, perhaps related to smaller vessels, and vein graft (including the internal mammary artery) patency is less at 5 years (87–97% survival in women vs. 90–94% in men). These differences post-bypass, however, disappear at 10-year follow-up studies.

11. Diabetes is an important risk factor for CAD. Are there gender differences in risk when diabetes and CAD coexist?

In a study of 585 men and 389 women with CAD assessed by angiography, diabetic women had greater than two times the relative risk of death over a 4 to 6-year follow-up for all causes of death as well as cardiac death; whereas in nondiabetic patients, death was significantly lower in women. Therefore, diabetes confers a substantially higher risk of mortality in women when it coexists with CAD than in men, and the favorable cardiac risk profile premenopausal women have compared to men is lost in the presence of diabetes. Hypertriglyceridemia may also be of greater risk for women than men.

12. How does estrogen replacement affect the risk of atherosclerosis and myocardial infarction in postmenopausal women?

Estrogen reduces the risk of atherosclerosis and MI in postmenopausal women. There is a reduction of up to 50% in MI and stroke and a reduction in the incidence of hypertension.

13. Do cardiac rehabilitation programs show similar results for women and men?

A recent study showed older women were less likely to enter cardiac rehabilitation than older men, due primarily to the stronger recommendations to men by their physicians. Although before entrance to programs, women were less fit than men (peak oxygen consumption 18% lower in women), both groups improved aerobic capacity similarly in response to a 12-week aerobic conditioning program.

14. List some other gender-specific characteristics of MI in CAD.

Non–Q-wave MI, supraventricular arrhythmias, and infarct expansion are all more common in women, whereas pericarditis and ventricular arrhythmias are more common in men.

15. Are there new guidelines suggesting better treatment of hyperlipidemia in women?

Yes. Women were not receiving aggressive preventive therapy; therefore, joint guidelines were published by the American Heart Association and the American College of Cardiology (AHA/ACC). The first cardiovascular event in women is often fatal, and risk factor modification must be aggressive.

The recent Heart and Estrogen/Progestin Replacement study (HERS) found that hormone replacement alone is not adequate for women with CAD and hyperlipidemia. The use of **statins** is recommended. Such usage is also important in primary therapy with initial presentation of MI or sudden death in women with CAD.

Weight management, including physical activity, appropriate diet, and vitamin supplements, also needs to be part of risk management. High-density lipoprotein (HDL) and triglyceride (TG) levels are powerful predictors of events in women. AHA/ACC recommends HDL-C > 45 mg/dl and < TG 150 mg/dl. These levels are best accomplished with statins if a brief effort of lifestyle management is not *totally* successful in addressing low-density lipoprotein, TG, and HDL.

The recent Women's Health Initiative (WHI) study actually showed a slight increase in MI and stroke blood clots in the hormone replacement therapy group, possibly related to the prothrombotic effect and new recommendations for initial lower-dose replacement.

16. Discuss the gender differences recently uncovered that encourage aggressive risk factor management in women.

We are finally able to look at studies that include adequate populations of women, to address the female-identified reversal of CVD decline—which is most likely due to underdiagnosis and undertreatment. A recent study demonstrated that in a group of 1000 women, 203 will die of CVD and only 33 of breast cancer by the age of 85. Another showed that women < 50 years old are twice as likely to die during hospitalizations after MI than men of the same age. In fact, the younger the age, the higher the risk of death among women relative to men. This age-related difference does level off after age 74. Women have more complications than men hospitalized for angina and MI, and have a higher 30-day mortality.

Diabetes removes any advantage women have against CVD: women's risk increases 3 to 7 times vs. men's risk increase of 2 to 3 times. It also appears that HDL-C is not as sensitive in women at similar risk for CVD as men. TG levels are more predictive in women than men to identify CVD.

17. What is the new controversy regarding hormone replacement therapy (HRT)?

New data suggests that in primary CVD prevention there is still no clear answer regarding HRT. The WHI study showed a slight increase in MI, stroke, and deep venous thrombosis, but the event rate was 4%—*not* statistically significant. In fact, this rate could have occurred by chance. Also, these are preliminary results and did not stop the study.

The secondary prevention studies HERS and Estrogen Replacement and Atherosclerosis suggest lower doses for the first year of HRT, as this is the high-risk period. After 4–5 years, the maximum benefit/risk ratio starts increasing.

BIBLIOGRAPHY

1. American Heart Association/American College of Cardiology: Guide to preventive cardiology for women. Circulation 99:2480–2484, 1999.
2. Becker RC, Alpert JS: Cardiovascular disease in women. Cardiology 77(suppl 2):1–39, 1990.
3. De Maria R, Gavazzi A, Recalcati F, et al: Comparison of clinical findings in idiopathic dilated cardiomyopathy in women versus men: The Italian Multicenter Cardiomyopathy Study Group (SPIC). Am J Cardiol 72:580–585, 1993.

4. Liao Y, Cooper RS, Ghali JK, et al: Sex differences in the impact of coexistence of diabetes on survival in patients with coronary heart disease. Diabetic Care 16:708–713, 1993.
5. Rehnquist N, Hartford M, Schenck-Gustafsson K, et al: Coronary artery disease in women. J Myocard Ischemia 5:29–35, 1993.
6. Salvage MP, et al: Clinical and angiographic determinants of primary coronary angioplasty success. J Am Coll Cardiol 17:22–28, 1991.
7. Shlipak MG, Simon JA, et al: Estrogen and progestin, lipoprotein (a), and the risk of recurrent coronary heart disease events after menopause. JAMA 283:1845–1852, 2000.
8. Superko HR, Hecht HS, et al: Small LDL, IDL, and HDL: Should cardiologists use these measures? [abstract] American College of Cardiology 49th Annual Scientific Session, March 2000.
9. Vaccarino V, Parsons L, et al: Sex-based differences in early mortality after myocardial infarction. New Engl J Med 341:217–225, 1999.
10. Wren BG: The effect of estrogen on the female cardiovascular system. Med J Aust 157:204–208, 1992.

36. HEART DISEASE IN THE ELDERLY

Evelyn Hutt, M.D.

1. What cardiovascular changes are part of normal aging?

This question is a difficult one to answer because coronary artery disease is so prevalent among the elderly, affecting 50% of Americans aged 65–74 years and 60% of those > 75 years. There are virtually no studies that address this question in the oldest old, those over 80. Studies that were careful to screen out underlying atherosclerotic disease indicate the following:

The heart ages well.
- Normal morphology changes little except for a mild increase in left ventricular wall thickness.
- Contractile function is well preserved.
- Decrease in early diastolic filling results from diminished myocardial compliance, increased isovolumic relaxation time, and sclerosis of the mitral valve.

Resting heart rate does not change.
- Maximum heart rate declines (about 1 beat/year due to diminished beta-adrenergic responsiveness).
- Cardiac output in both rest and exercise is preserved.
- End-diastolic volume and stroke volume increase.

Arteries and veins do not fare so well.
- Arterial media thickens and becomes less elastic.
- Vascular resistance increases.
- Autonomic nervous system becomes less efficient.
- Blood pressure falls significantly on standing (baroreceptor reflex attenuated).

2. What is diastolic dysfunction?

Diastolic dysfunction is increased resistance to filling of one or both cardiac ventricles and is particularly prevalent in older patients, especially in association with hypertension and senile amyloidosis and in women and blacks. The cellular mechanism is thought to be a decline in the cells' ability to sequester calcium after contraction, mediated by cyclic adenosine monophosphate (AMP). A decrease in cyclic AMP may be related to the decreased beta-adrenergic responsiveness of normal aging.

Diastolic dysfunction should be suspected when a patient presents with dyspnea and fatigue without the classic x-ray findings of congestive heart failure or obvious pulmonary disease. The diagnosis is important because it is treated differently than systolic failure, responding best to agents that increase the diastolic filling time, such as beta blockers and calcium channel blockers.

3. Are myocardial infarctions more difficult to recognize clinically in older people?

Yes. The older a patient is, the more likely he or she is to present with dyspnea, syncope, delirium, or stroke and the less likely to have chest pain. This change again may be related to diminished adrenergic responsiveness. Given the prevalence of atherosclerotic disease in older men *and* women, the clinician should consider infarction high in the differential diagnosis of any acutely ill older patient.

4. Do people over 70 benefit from bypass grafting and angioplasty as much as young people do?

Limited data suggest that, in well-selected patients, a low operative mortality and good symptom relief can be achieved for patients 75 and older by **coronary artery bypass grafting**. Preoperative factors that predict mortality include emergency operation, cachexia, New York

Heart Association functional class IV disease, and previous myocardial infarction. The major perioperative risk factor for death is prolonged pump and cross-clamp time. Postoperative problems include atrial fibrillation, delirium, depression, anorexia, and delays in starting ambulation.

Several case series have looked at success rates and complications from **percutaneous transluminal angioplasty** in elders. Clinical and arteriographic success rates are similar for middle-aged, young-old (60–69 years), middle-old (70–79 years), and old-old (> 80 years), but complication rates are higher for old-old patients (who had more extensive atherosclerotic disease and a higher prevalence of preoperative heart failure). Mortality from both procedures is decreasing in patients over age 65 despite a concomitant increase in comorbidity.

5. Is age over 75 a strong contraindication to thrombolytic therapy in acute myocardial infarction?

This is a controversial question. On one hand, the risk of major hemorrhagic complications during thrombolysis clearly rises with age. However, the mortality associated with myocardial infarction also rises with age. Subgroup analyses of larger trials (ISIS-2 in particular) show a reduction in mortality from 37% to 20% in patients over 80 who were given thrombolytic therapy.

The decision to use thrombolysis in the elderly must be individualized. Vigorous patients with classic signs, symptoms, and a large area of involved myocardium who present early in the course of their event should not be denied thrombolytic therapy solely because of their age.

6. What is the most common valvular heart disease in older people?

Aortic stenosis. Autopsy studies show that it occurs in 4–6% of people over 65. In the absence of symptoms, it is very difficult to distinguish true stenosis from the much more common murmur of aortic sclerosis, which occurs in about one-third of patients over 65. Concern over this murmur should prompt echocardiography with Doppler flow studies. Several case series indicate that the aortic valve can be replaced with acceptable mortality rates in otherwise vigorous octogenarians.

7. How does orthostatic hypotension affect the elderly?

Orthostatic hypotension, a drop in blood pressure of ≥ 20 mmHg as a person moves from lying to standing, is caused by decreased beta-adrenergic responsiveness and is a common cause of syncope. It may be worse in the morning on first arising and after meals, and especially affects patients with systolic hypertension, whose treatment may exacerbate it. Blood pressure should be checked with the patient lying down for a minute, immediately upon standing, and after 1 and 5 minutes of standing.

8. How should orthostatic hypotension be managed in the elderly?

In patients without hypertension, control of symptoms can be achieved without medication. Patients should arise more slowly, increase salt and caffeine intake, and elevate the head of the bed at night (lessens diurnal fluid shifts). More refractory cases that cause the patient to fall can be treated with a very low dose of mineralocorticoid, watching carefully for signs of volume overload.

Patients with hypertension and orthostatic hypotension need careful selection of antihypertensive drugs to minimize symptoms. Avoid diuretics and vasodilators.

9. At what age can you stop checking cholesterol?

It is known that approximately 10 years' treatment of elevated cholesterol levels is required to effect a change in risk for myocardial infarction. Given the average life expectancy of 80 years for men and 85 for women, it is probably reasonable to stop screening the general population at about age 70. This does *not* pertain to cholesterol management in patients with symptomatic atherosclerotic heart disease, in whom lowering cholesterol achieves much more rapid benefits.

10. Does estrogen replacement therapy affect the incidence of heart disease in older women?

The answer to this question is not known. Both epidemiologic and biochemical evidence suggests that it should decrease risk for myocardial infarction. Epidemiologically, the incidence of atherosclerotic disease rises dramatically after menopause and is the leading cause of death in older women. Biochemically, estrogen raises high-density lipoprotein (HDL) and lowers low-density lipoprotein (LDL) cholesterol, which should improve cardiac risk. A recent, large, randomized, double-blind, placebo-controlled trial of estrogen and progesterone in women with known coronary artery disease, however, revealed no effect of hormone replacement therapy on further cardiac events or mortality at 4 years.

11. What are appropriate goals and treatment regimens for controlling cholesterol in the elderly?

In attempting cholesterol lowering, a reasonable goal is to get the LDL cholesterol below 100 + the patient's age. As in younger people, the first step is an adequate trial of diet, exercise, and, for women, estrogen replacement. Because constipation is common in the elderly, psyllium can be added early and is generally well tolerated *if* the patient drinks sufficient water.

Choosing a medical regimen involves balancing side effects and cost. The bile acid–binding residues and niacin are generally poorly tolerated. Gemfibrozil is less expensive than the HMG-CoA reductase inhibitors, is the only cholesterol-lowering agent that raises HDL, and is generally effective and well-tolerated. The HMG-CoA reductase inhibitors have the advantages of once-daily dosing and greatest efficacy.

12. What common side effects of cardiac medications are the elderly most vulnerable to?

Side effects of cardiac medications that present a real danger to the elderly can be divided into four broad categories:

    1. Mental status changes

        Antihypertensives

        Antianginals

        Antiarrhythmics

        Drugs with anticholinergic effects (e.g., atropine)

        Centrally acting alpha agonists (e.g., clonidine)

        Lipophyllic beta blockers (e.g., propranolol)

    2. Orthostatic hypotension

        Antihypertensives

        Antianginals (e.g., isosorbide, nitroglycerin)

    3. Cardiac conduction delays

        Drugs with anticholinergic effects

        Antiarrhythmics

        Calcium channel blockers (e.g., verapamil)

        Beta blockers

    4. Gastrointestinal problems

        Nausea and anorexia

          Digoxin (even below toxic levels)

          Angiotensin-converting enzyme inhibitors

          Peripherally acting calcium channel blockers (e.g., nifedipine)

        Constipation

          Centrally acting calcium channel blockers (e.g., verapamil)

          Drugs with anticholinergic effects

13. How common is atrial fibrillation in the elderly?

Atrial fibrillation affects 5–10% of ambulatory elderly. The incidence among hospitalized elderly is probably twice that. Unlike in younger people, atrial fibrillation is a harbinger of underlying cardiac disease in the elderly. The rate of stroke is 10 times higher in older than younger patients with atrial fibrillation.

14. Is anticoagulation therapy more risky in an elderly patient with atrial fibrillation than in younger patients?

Solid evidence demonstrates that the risk of bleeding from appropriately dosed and monitored warfarin does not rise with age alone. Instead, increased risk of bleeding is associated with frailty, a tendency to fall, history of peptic ulcer disease, and underlying malignancy.

15. Who is too old for a pacemaker?

No one. Sinus and atrioventricular nodal dysfunctions are more common in the elderly and are a common cause of syncope and falls. Both quality and length of life can be improved by appropriate use of pacemakers.

16. What role should beta-adrenergic blockade play in the management of congestive heart failure in the elderly?

There is a growing body of evidence that beta-blockade improves mortality in all patients with heart failure, but no trials have addressed this issue directly in the elderly. There is better evidence that beta-blockade after a myocardial infarction benefits the elderly and those with heart failure and is underutilized in this circumstance. As with the initiation of any therapy in the elderly, it is advisable to "start low and go slow," watching carefully for signs of cardiac decompensation or orthostatic hypotension.

BIBLIOGRAPHY

1. Aranki SF, Rizzo RJ, Couper GS, et al: Aortic valve replacement in the elderly. Circulation 88:17–23, 1993.
2. Bayer AJ, Chadha JS, Farag RR, Pathy MSJ: Changing presentation of myocardial infarction with increasing old age. J Am Geriatr Soc 34:263–266, 1986.
3. Ezekowitz MD, Bridgers SL, James KE, et al: Warfarin in the prevention of stroke associated with non-rheumatic atrial fibrillation. N Engl J Med 327:1406–1412, 1992.
4. Forman DE, Berman AD, McCabe CH, et al: PTCA in the elderly: The 'young old' versus the 'old-old.' J Am Geriatr Soc 40:19–22, 1992.
5. Gottlieb SS, McCarter RJ, Vogel RA: Effect of beta-blockade on mortality among high-risk and low-risk patients after myocardial infarction. N Engl J Med 339:551–553, 1998.
6. Grossman W: Diastolic dysfunction in congestive heart failure. N Engl J Med 325:1557–1564, 1991.
7. Heidenreich PA, Lee TT, Massie BM: Effect of beta-blockade on mortality in patients with heart failure: A meta-analysis of randomized clinical trials. J Am Coll Cardiol 30:27–34, 1997.
8. Hulley S, Grady D, Bush T, et al: Randomized trial of estrogen plus progestin for secondary prevention of coronary heart disease in postmenopausal women. JAMA 280:605–613, 1998.
9. Krumholz HM, Pasternak RC, Weinstein MC, et al: Cost effectiveness of thrombolytic therapy with streptokinase in elderly patients with suspected acute myocardial infarction. N Engl J Med 327:7–13, 1992.
10. Muller DWM, Topol EJ: Selection of patients with acute myocardial infarction for thrombolytic therapy. Ann Intern Med 113:949–960, 1990.
11. Peterson ED, Jollis JG, Bebchuk JD, et al: Changes in mortality after myocardial revascularization in the elderly. Ann Intern Med 121:919–927, 1994.
12. Pritchett ELC: Management of atrial fibrillation. N Engl J Med 326:1264–1271, 1992.
13. Topol EJ, Traill TA, Fortiun NJ: Hypertensive hypertrophic cardiomyopathy of the elderly. N Engl J Med 312:277–283, 1985.

37. HEART TRANSPLANTATION

Sumant Lamba, M.D., William T. Abraham, M.D., Brian D. Lowes, M.D.,
and JoAnn Lindenfeld, M.D.

1. How common is heart failure?

It is estimated that at least 500,000 new cases of heart failure are diagnosed annually in the United States. Despite advances in medical therapy, heart failure is the principal cause of 40,000 deaths and a contributing cause of another 250,000 deaths each year. In the U.S., more than $38 billion is spent annually for the direct care of persons with heart failure. The donor shortage, which limits heart transplants in the U.S. to about 2500 procedures per year, underscores the alarming discrepancy between the number of patients with heart failure who might benefit from transplantation (approximately 40,000) and those fortunate enough to receive a suitable donor organ.

2. Who should be considered for heart transplantation?

Adult patients are considered to be candidates for transplantation when there is progressive deterioration of ventricular function or clinical functional status despite optimal medical therapy, including use of ACE inhibitors, beta-blockers, diuretics, digoxin, and aldosterone antagonists. Patients with malignant arrhythmias or refractory myocardial ischemia, those who are unresponsive to conventional treatment, and those with the need for ongoing intravenous inotropic support also benefit from transplantation. Objectively, patients with a maximum myocardial oxygen consumption < 14 ml/kg/min and a left ventricular ejection fraction < 20% benefit the most from transplantation.

3. Are there patients who cannot be considered for a heart transplant?

Yes. Contraindications to transplantation include coexisting systemic illness that limits a patient's survival:

- Severe irreversible pulmonary, renal, or liver disease
- Irreversible pulmonary hypertension (pulmonary vascular resistance > 6 Wood units)
- Acute infection
- History of recent malignancy
- Insulin-dependent diabetes mellitus with end-organ damage
- Acute pulmonary embolism
- Severe peripheral vascular disease
- Psychosocial disability

4. What quality of life can patients reasonably expect post transplantation?

Approximately 30–50% of patients return to work after transplantation, and 80–85% consider themselves to be physically active. One-year survival post transplantation is about 85–90%, and the 5-year survival is about 75%.

The function of a transplanted heart is not completely normal. It remains largely, but not entirely, denervated throughout the life of the recipient. The cardiac response to exercise or stress is less than normal, but adequate for almost all activities. The resting heart rate is higher due to the absence of vagal tone. Other factors, which contribute to decreased cardiac function, are altered neurohormonal activity, organ preservation injury, and differences in the donor and recipient body size. Thus, while transplant recipients have a better functional capacity than pretransplantation, they typically are impaired compared to normal controls.

5. Which medicines are commonly used for immunosuppression in heart transplant patients?

Currently, most transplant centers use triple combination therapy with **cyclosporine**, **azathioprine** (or the newer agent mycophenolate), and **prednisone** as standard immunosuppressive therapy. Cyclosporine is generally titrated to specific plasma levels depending on the renal function and manifestations of toxicity. Azathioprine is usually adjusted to maintain a white cell count of 4000-6000/ml. Immediately after transplantation, patients receive methylprednisolone and then are switched to prednisone at a dose of approximately 1 mg/kg/day, which is gradually weaned to a maintenance dose of 0.1 mg/kg/day over the next 6 months. Some centers have discontinued steroids in about half of patients; others maintain patients on a low dose of prednisone indefinitely.

Two newer immunosuppressive agents are increasingly used in preventing rejection in heart transplant patients. **Mycophenolate mofetil** acts by inhibiting de novo pathways of purine (guanine) synthesis. It is substituted for azathioprine and reduces the incidence of early acute rejection after heart transplantation without affecting the lymphocyte subpopulation when compared to azathioprine. **Tacrolimus**, a macrolide antibiotic, is a novel immunosuppressive drug that is more potent than cyclosporine. It prevents helper cell amplification by blocking interleukin-2 synthesis and is used as a rescue agent when the use of cyclosporine is undesirable or inefficient.

6. What are the side effects of the commonly used immunosuppressive medicines?

Cyclosporine: nephrotoxicity, believed to be secondary to renal arterial vasoconstriction and from a direct vasoconstrictor effect; hypertension, in up to 90% of patients; also hyperkalemia, hyperuricemia, cholelithiasis, hirsutism, gingival hyperplasia, facial flushing, sexual dysfunction, and essential tremors. Many of cyclosporine's side effects can be avoided by close monitoring of trough levels and adjusting the dose as needed to maintain safe levels.

Azathioprine: dose-related bone marrow suppression, generally responsive to decreased dosage; drug-induced cholestasis or hepatitis.

Steroids (at high doses): numerous side effects include osteoporosis, avascular necrosis of the femoral head, hyperlipidemia, glucose intolerance.

Tacrolimus: nephrotoxicity; hypertension; thrombocytopenia.

Mycophenolate: thrombocytopenia; leukopenia; gastrointestinal distress.

7. Name common infections in heart transplant patients. When do they usually occur?

Infection remains a major cause of death in the transplant population. The overall incidence of infections is 41–71% in various series. In a multicenter analysis of 814 consecutive patients undergoing heart transplanation, approximately half suffered acute infection within 6 months.

Within the first month post transplant, nosocomial bacterial infections with staphylococci or gram-negative organisms tend to predominate. Other early bacterial infections involve Legionella, *Pseudomonas aeruginosa*, Proteus, Klebsiella, and *Escherichia coli*.

Herpes simplex mucocutaneous infections tend to occur within the first few months after transplant.

Late post-transplant infections are more diverse and include a variety of opportunistic organisms: viruses (cytomegalovirus [CMV], herpes), *Pneumocystis carinii* (PCP), and fungi (Candida and Aspergillus).

Regular prophylactic therapy of trimethoprim-sulfamethoxazole three times a week on a long-term basis is now recommended routinely by most transplant programs to prevent PCP and toxoplasma infection.

8. Which is the most common infection? What is the most frequent *site* of infection in transplant patients?

CMV remains the most common single infection. The lung tends to be the most frequent site of infection in heart transplant patients.

9. What malignancies are common in heart transplant patients? What predisposes patients to them?

Cancer is an unfortunate consequence of chronic immunosuppression. In general, transplant recipients have a three-fold increase in the incidence of various cancers when compared with age-matched controls. Perhaps the most important neoplasms are the **lymphoproliferative**

tumors that occur early after transplantation, more frequently in younger recipients. Most of these tumors are thought to be the result of Epstein-Barr viral infection and consist of B-cell proliferation because of T-cell suppression or depletion. Patients with this disease often respond to decreased levels of immunosuppression and possibly antiviral therapy. Use of OKT3 and other antilymphocyte antibodies also may increase the risk of lymphoproliferative disorders.

Skin and lip cancers are the most common post-transplant neoplasms. Squamous cell tumors are more frequent than basal cell tumors by a ratio of 2:1. Other common tumors are are non-Hodgkin's lymphoma, Kaposi's sarcoma, and uterine, cervical, vulvar, and perineal tumors.

10. What is the leading cause of death in heart transplantation after the first year?

Coronary artery disease (CAD; graft atherosclerosis). Graft atherosclerosis can develop within months of transplantation, but usually appears gradually, so that 5 years after transplantation 30–50% of patients have angiographic evidence of CAD.

The cause of graft atherosclerosis is controversial and is probably multifactorial. It is believed to be secondary to immune-mediated endothelial injury.

11. How is CAD detected in heart transplant patients? How is it treated?

Detection of graft atherosclerosis is a difficult clinical problem since cardiac transplant patients usually do not have angina, due to cardiac denervation. In addition, noninvasive tests such as exercise testing and radionuclide scans are less reliable in the cardiac transplant patient. Thus, yearly coronary angiography is still routinely employed in these patients. Patients with severe disease usually present with sudden death or congestive heart failure secondary to MI. Due to diffuse involvement of the coronary arteries rather than focal disease, some centers routinely employ intravascular ultrasound to diagnose graft atherosclerosis.

The diffuse nature of CAD in heart transplant patients makes them poor candidates for revascularization by angioplasty or surgery, and leaves retransplantation as the only definitive therapy for this life-threatening process.

12. What predisposes heart transplant patients to CAD?

Several studies have attempted to identify risk factors for graft atherosclerosis. Humoral rejection, circulating HLA antibodies, HLA mismatch at the DR locus, hyperlipidemia, and CMV infection all have been variably associated with its development. Newer risk factors such as hyperhomocystenemia and elevated lipoprotein (a) seem to play an important part. Medical attempts to prevent or slow this process, such as exercise, lipid-lowering therapy, and blood pressure control, have not met with success. The addition of diltiazem to the post-transplant regimen has retarded progression of allograft coronary disease, and its cyclosporine-sparing effect has also reduced costs.

13. Which noninvasive tests are useful for the diagnosis of CAD in heart transplant patients?

Unfortunately, routine exercise testing, nuclear myocardial blood flow scans with thallium and sestamibi, and dobutamine stress echocardiography all lack the sensitivity to be useful tests in screening for graft atherosclerosis. This is likely due to the diffuse nature of disease. **Surveillance angiography** is the gold standard for screening graft atherosclerosis, and noninvasive tests are used predominantly to assess functional capacity and discern the physiologic significance of coronary stenosis.

14. What are some of the signs and symptoms of rejection?

The clinical diagnosis of rejection is often difficult. Frequently, patients have rejection on biopsy without symptoms. Less often, patients may have nonspecific complaints of fatigue or malaise as the presenting symptom. If left untreated, patients progress to symptoms of overt heart failure such as dyspnea on exertion, orthopnea, and paroxysmal nocturnal dyspnea. Signs on physical examination include jugular venous distension, tricuspid regurgitation, and a third heart sound. Atrial arrhythmias often herald the onset of acute rejection. Fevers without a source and hypotension also may be presentations of cardiac allograft rejection.

15. How is the diagnosis of rejection made?

Endomyocardial biopsy remains the gold standard for the diagnosis of rejection. The International Society of Heart and Lung Transplantation developed a scale for grading the severity of cellular rejection that is now widely used and is based on amount of lymphocytic infiltration and degree of myocyte necrosis (see table).

International Society of Heart and Lung Transplantation Scale for Cardiac Rejection

GRADE	PATHOLOGIC FINDINGS ON BIOPSY
0	No rejection
1	1A—Focal (perivascular or interstitial) infiltrate without necrosis 1B—Diffuse but sparse infiltrate without necrosis
2	One focus only, with aggressive infiltration or focal myocyte damage
3	3A—Multifocal infiltrates or myocyte damage 3B—Diffuse inflammatory process with necrosis
4	Diffuse aggressive infiltrate with necrosis, edema, vasculitis, or hemorrhage

16. Are noninvasive tests such as cardiac echocardiography useful in the diagnosis of rejection?

In general, cardiac imaging studies lack the sensitivity and specificity to be useful in diagnosing rejection. By the time left ventricular dysfunction supervenes, the level of rejection is fairly advanced and more difficult to treat. Echocardiography is useful to assess systolic and diastolic dysfunction. Other echocardiographic findings such as increased wall thickness or edema may provide important clues about humoral rejection that are not routinely detected by standard biopsy staining techniques. Echocardiography can also provide evidence of wall motion abnormalities, suggesting ischemic disease, and can assist in the evaluation of valvular dysfunction, which may explain worsening cardiac function.

17. What are the different kinds of rejection?

Rejection currently accounts for a minority of deaths in transplanted patients (less than 15–20%). There are three broad classifications of rejection: hyperacute, cellular, and humoral.

Hyperacute rejection usually occurs immediately after transplantation as severe graft dysfunction and has an extremely poor prognosis. It results when the recipient has preformed antibodies from prior transfusion, pregnancy, or ABO incompatibility. Prompt retransplantation is required. Screening recipients for anti-HLA antibodies prior to transplantation can prevent most instances of hyperacute rejection. Patients who have had broad-spectrum anti-HLA antibodies are required to undergo crossmatching prior to transplantation.

Cellular rejection is the most common form of rejection. T-lymphocytes mediate this process, which involves perivascular and myocytic lymphocytic infiltrates. This form of rejection is diagnosed by H&E staining of biopsy specimens and usually responds to increased levels of immunosuppression. Cellular rejection occurs most frequently and most aggressively in the first few months following transplantation. It is uncommon after the first 6 months unless the recipient has a concurrent infection or has had a recent reduction in immunosuppression or frequent episodes of rejection.

Humoral (vascular) rejection is much less common than cellular rejection, although it may occur in up to 20% of patients receiving antilymphocyte preparations. It carries a much worse prognosis. Patients with this type of rejection characteristically have deposition of immunoglobin and complement in a vascular pattern by immunofluorescent staining. They also have generalized endothelial cell swelling by light microscopy. Vascular rejection is seen more commonly in patients with sensitization to OKT3.

18. How is rejection treated?

Treatment of rejection depends on the type and severity of the pathologic grade as well as clinical symptoms and presence of hemodynamic changes (see table at Question 15). Patients with grade 1 rejection without hemodynamic changes often are not treated, but are followed closely for progression. Rejection often resolves spontaneously, avoiding the risks of additional immunosuppression. Grade 2 rejection is treated with oral steroids. Grades 3 and 4 rejection are usually treated with high doses of intravenous or oral steroids for 3 days, followed by a steroid taper. Steroid-resistant episodes are treated with OKT3, a mouse monoclonal antibody to the CD 3 molecule, which is part of a multimolecular complex found on mature lymphocytes. Initial doses of OKT3 may cause hypotension, bronchospasm, fever, or diarrhea mediated by lymphokines. These side effects can be minimized by pretreatment with steroids and antihistamines.

19. Who may be considered as a potential donor candidate?

Due to shortage of donor organs and the poor prognosis of patients awaiting cardiac transplantation, the initial screening of donors should be very liberal. The initial step involves the recognition and declaration of brain death in the donor. After consent has been obtained, the donor is screened for suitability by the designated organ recovery system. The relative contraindications could potentially complicate a transplantation, but this must be weighed against the recipient's clinical situation and short-term survival.

Contraindications to Organ Donation

ABSOLUTE CONTRAINDICATIONS	RELATIVE CONTRAINDICATIONS
HIV-positive status	Sepsis
Death due to CO poisoning	Prolonged inotropic support or CPR
Structural heart disease	Prolonged hypotension
Previous myocardial infarction	Noncritical coronary artery disease
Intractable ventricular arrhythmias	Hepatitis B or C positivity
Severe occlusive coronary artery disease	History of metastatic cancer
	Evidence of cardiac contusion
	History of intravenous drug abuse

BIBLIOGRAPHY

1. Baldwin J, Anderson JL, Boucek M, et al: Donor Guidelines. J Am Coll Cardiol 22:15–20, 1993.
2. Baumgartner WA, Reitz BA, Achuff SA: Heart and Heart-Lung Transplantation. Philadelphia, W.B. Saunders Company, 1990.
3. Boyd D, Mego N, Khan B, et al: Doppler echocardiography in cardiac transplant patients: allograft rejection and its relationship to diastolic function. J Am Soc Echocardiography 10:526–531, 1997.
4. Brann WM, Bennett LE, Keck BM, Hosenpud JD: Morbidity, functional status, and immunosuppressive therapy after heart transplantation: an analysis of the joint International Society for Heart and Lung Transplantation/United Network for Organ Sharing Thoracic Registry. J Heart Lung Transplant 17:374–382, 1998.
5. Constanzo MR, Augustine S, Bourge R, Bristow M: Selection and treatment of candidates for heart transplantation. Circulation 92:3593–3612, 1995.
6. Gao SZ, Hunt SA, Schroeder JS, et al: Early development of accelerated graft coronary artery disease: risk factors and course. J Am Coll Cardiol 28:673–679, 1996.
7. Gill EA, Borrego C, Bray BE, et al: Left ventricular mass increases during vascular rejection: Comparison with cellular rejection. J Am Coll Cardiol 15:922–926, 1995.
8. Hammond EH, Taylor DO, Yowell RL, et al: The repetitive histologic pattern of vascular cardiac allograft rejection. Transplantation 62:205–210, 1996.
9. Hosenpud JD, Bennett LE, Keck BM, et al: The Registry of the International Society for Heart and Lung Transplantation: Sixteenth Official Report–1999. J Heart Lung Transplant 18:611–626, 1999.
10. Mudge G, Goldstein S, Addonizio LJ, et al: Recipient guidelines/prioritization. J Am Coll Cardiol 22:21–30, 1993.
11. United Network for Organ Sharing: 1997 Report of Center-Specific Graft and Patient Survival Rates. Rockville, Maryland, Department of Health and Human Services, 1997.
12. Weis M, von Scheidt W: Cardiac allograft vasculopathy: a review. Circulation 96:2069–2077, 1997.
13. Young JB: Cardiac Transplantation: Three Decades of Experience Define Our Challenge. Transplant Proc 30:1885–1888, 1998.

38. PERIPHERAL VASCULAR OCCLUSIVE DISEASE

Eric S. Weinstein, M.D., and David Tanaka, M.D.

1. What is peripheral vascular occlusive disease (PVOD)?

This term refers to a subset of atherosclerotic disease, the other subset being aneurysmal disease. PVOD is characterized by stenoses or occlusions affecting arteries throughout the body, except in the heart. It is commonly referred to as "hardening of the arteries."

2. Describe the types of symptoms that are produced by PVOD.

The symptoms produced by PVOD are determined by the vascular bed that is being supplied by the affected arteries. For example, PVOD affecting the carotid arteries may produce strokes or transient ischemic attacks. PVOD affecting the visceral circulation may produce symptoms of chronic intestinal ischemia, such as post-prandial pain and weight loss. Renal arterial involvement may produce hypertension or renal insufficiency. Lower extremity arterial involvement may produce symptoms such as claudication, ischemic rest pain, or tissue loss.

3. What is claudication?

The term claudication is derived from the Latin word *claudical*, which means "to limp." Claudication is intermittent pain experienced in a muscle group (usually immediately below the area of stenosis or occlusion), and it results from inadequate perfusion during exercise. It is very reproducible and is relieved by rest. The symptom may be characterized by patients as pain, cramping, numbness, or muscle fatigue.

4. Are there other causes for claudication besides PVOD?

Yes. Similar symptoms of lower extremity pain with exercise can be produced by compression or irritation of spinal nerve roots, which can be seen in cauda equina syndrome or degenerative lumbosacral spine/disk disease. This is called **neurogenic claudication**. It sometimes can be differentiated from vasculogenic claudication in the history by the patient noting that he/she has to sit down to relieve the symptoms (which takes the stretch off the affected nerve), and in the physical examination by the presence of normal pulses at rest and after exercise.

5. What causes claudication symptoms in young patients?

Atherosclerosis tends to be a disease primarily affecting older patients; however, it can manifest itself in younger patients who have familial hyperlipidemic syndromes. Buerger's disease (thromboangitis obliterans), or hypercoagulable disorders. In addition, several anatomic conditions can present as claudication in young patients. **Popliteal entrapment syndrome** is an anatomic abnormality in which the popliteal artery gets compressed either by an abnormal muscle band or because it has taken an abnormal (medial) course behind the knee and is compressed by a normal gastrocnemius muscle. **Popliteal adventitial cystic disease** is also in the differential diagnosis of claudication in young patients; it produces a popliteal stenosis that gives a classic "scimitar sign" on angiography. **Exercise-induced compartment syndrome** may produce similar symptoms of leg pain with exercise that are relieved by rest.

6. What is limb-threatening ischemia?

Whereas claudication is produced by decreased perfusion to the muscles with exercise, limb-threatening ischemia refers to inadequate tissue perfusion *at rest*. It is characteristically manifested as rest pain or tissue loss. Rest pain refers to the specific symptom of a burning or aching pain, usually experienced in the toes or heel, that occurs at night when the foot is elevated and is relieved by dependent positioning. Patients often tell the examiner that they have to sleep in a chair because of the pain. Tissue loss may be seen in limb-threatening ischemia as either a non-healing ulcer (present for more than 4 weeks) or gangrene. Arterial insufficiency ulcers usually are distal to the malleolus and are painful (as opposed to venous ulceration, which tends to be above the malleoli and generally is not painful unless infected).

7. **Do patients with claudication invariably progress to limb-threatening ischemia?**
   No. In 80% of these patients, symptoms stabilize or improve with smoking cessation and an exercise program. Approximately 10% go on to require revascularization due to progressive ischemia, and 10% require subsequent amputation.

8. **Are the risk factors for coronary artery disease (CAD) and PVD the same?**
   Yes and no. The general risk factors are the same, but there are some differences:
   • **Smoking** is more pervasive in patients with PVD (80%). Smoking status influences limb prognosis, patency of vessels after surgery or angioplasty, and mortality.
   • **Diabetes** increases the risk of progression of disease. Diabetics also have a higher incidence of vascular disease distal to the popliteal artery.
   • **Hyperlipidemia** is a risk factor for PVD, but the risk profile is different than for CAD. Low levels of high-density lipoprotein cholesterol and elevated triglycerides are independent risk factors for PVD, but elevated low-density lipoprotein cholesterol is not.
   • **Hypertension** is a risk factor for PVD, but there is no evidence that treatment of hypertension influences the prognosis of PVD. Most patients with claudication can be treated for hypertension without worsening their claudication, although in some patients with severe disease symptoms might worsen. In general, beta blockers can be safely used to treat hypertension or angina in the presence of claudication.

9. **Which noninvasive vascular studies are useful in PVD?**
   • **Ankle:brachial index** (ABI) is the ankle systolic pressure as determined by Doppler divided by the brachial systolic pressure. An abnormal index is < 0.90. The sensitivity is approximately 90% for diagnosis of PVD.
   • **Plethysmography** measures changes in volume of toes, fingers, or parts of limbs that occur with each pulse beat as blood flows into or out of the extremity. This method may be used to determine toe pressures and pulse volume recordings, which are helpful when ankle pressures are falsely elevated because of calcified lower extremity vessels. A toe:brachial index of < 0.6 is abnormal, and values of < 0.15 are seen in patients with rest pain (toe pressures of < 20 mmHg).
   • **Ultrasound: Doppler velocity, duplex, and color-flow Doppler** are methods of evaluating artery stenosis and blood flow. These methods can localize and quantify the degree of stenosis. They are dependent on operator skill and are not as sensitive as the ABI for screening purposes.
   • **Transcutaneous oxygen tension measurements** are useful in assessing tissue viability for wound healing. Measurements > 55 mmHg are considered normal, and < 20 mmHg are associated with nonhealing ulcers.
   • **Exercise testing** measures treadmill walking time and pre-exercise and post-exercise ABIs. In those without significant PVD, the ABI is unchanged after exercise. In patients with PVD, the ABI falls after exercise. This test is more sensitive for detecting disease than a resting ABI alone.

10. **What is the general approach to outpatient management of PVD?**
    First, treat other conditions that might adversely affect tissue oxygen delivery, such as congestive heart failure, anemia, and hypoxia. Modify risk factors. Smoking cessation improves the morbidity and mortality of patients with PVD. Despite the lack of firm evidence, it is prudent to

treat hypertension, control hyperglycemia, and lower cholesterol. In severe cases, especially in diabetics, meticulous local care of skin, feet, and nails is necessary if infection and limb loss are to be prevented. Have your patient take off their shoes and socks during the examination.

11. Can claudication be improved?

Exercise has been shown to improve pain-free walking time. The magnitude of the improvement has been up to 190%, with an average of approximately 134%. Encourage patients to walk to the point of claudication; rest until pain-free; and then resume walking.

Pentoxifylline initially was the only medication for claudication. It is believed to improve erythrocyte deformability, platelet reactivity, and blood viscosity. Recently, cilostazol was shown to be significantly better than pentoxifylline or placebo for increasing walking distances. Cilostazol has antiaggregation effects on platelets, beneficial effects on serum lipids, and vasodilator effects.

12. What about anticoagulation, aspirin, and vasodilators?

None of these medications has been proved to reduce claudication or prevent progression of atherosclerosis in PVD patients. Aspirin should be prescribed routinely because it reduces the incidence of myocardial infarctions and strokes in patients with PVD.

13. When is surgery or angioplasty indicated?

- Limb-threatening ischemia
  Rest pain
  Nonhealing ulceration
  Gangrene
- Life-style limiting claudication

14. Is angioplasty preferable over surgery?

The answer to this question is complex. In certain situations angioplasty may be recommended because it is less invasive and does not necessarily preclude future surgery. Once it is determined that an intervention is necessary to treat PVD, a patient's risk factors for surgery must be weighed against both the initial success rate for the procedure as well as long-term patency rates associated with angioplasty.

15. Which lesions are appropriate for angioplasty?

Angioplasty is most effective for localized disease, especially of the common iliac arteries. Extensive disease (lesion < 10 cm in length) or disease at multiple sites is often best treated surgically. These decisions are best made in consultation with a vascular surgeon and interventional radiologist.

16. How do I evaluate operative risk in a patient scheduled for vascular surgery?

The major concern for PVD patients is evaluating risk of a perioperative cardiac complication. This is the most common cause of mortality with vascular surgery because approximately one-half of such patients have significant CAD. Many of these patients do not have angina and cannot exercise because of their PVD.

The proper preoperative evaluation of the patient for vascular surgery has been extensively studied, but remains controversial. One approach is based on the clinical evaluation and begins with the assessment of the patient for the following risk factors: age > 70, diabetes, previous myocardial infarction, angina, or history of ventricular ectopy.

If the patient has **no risk factors** and can walk approximately two blocks, then he or she is at low risk and can proceed to surgery.

If the patient has **three or more risk factors**, then he or she is at high risk for surgery. Consideration should be given to performing a lower-risk procedure, such as axillofemoral bypass or angioplasty, or foregoing surgery altogether. Coronary angiography may be an option, but risks inherent in this procedure plus vascular surgery risks must be considered. Invasive monitoring with Swan-Ganz and arterial catheters, perioperative use of beta blockers and nitrates, and careful monitoring for ST depression perioperatively (up to 48 hours postoperatively) may decrease the risk of cardiac complications.

If the patient has **one or two risk factors** or is unable to walk two blocks, then he or she is an intermediate risk. Dipyridamole-thallium imaging should be done. If the study is negative, the patient is at low risk and can proceed to surgery. If the study is positive, then the patient is at high risk and is approached as above.

BIBLIOGRAPHY

1. Consensus Document: Chronic Critical Leg Ischemia. Eur J Vasc Surg 6(supplA):1–32, 1992.
2. Criqui MH, Fronek A, Kjauber MR, et al: The sensitivity, specificity and predictive value of traditional clinical evaluation of peripheral arterial diseases: Results from noninvasive testing in a defined population. Circulation 71:516–522, 1985.
3. DeWeese JA, Leather R, Porter J: Practice guidelines: Lower extremity revascularization. J Vasc Surg 18:280–294, 1993.
4. Eagle KA, Coley CM, Newell JB, et al: Combining clinical and thallium data optimizes preoperative assessment of cardiac risk before major vascular surgery. Ann Intern Med 110:859–866, 1989.
5. Hertzer NR, et al: Coronary artery disease in peripheral vascular patients. Ann Surg 199:223–233, 1984.
6. Hiatt WR, Regensteiner JG: The value of exercise programs and risk factors modifications in claudicators. Semin Vas Surg 4:88–194, 1991.
7. Mannick JA: Evaluation of chronic lower extremity ischemia. N Engl J Med 309:841–843, 1983.
8. Turnipseed W, Metmer DE, Girdley F: Chronic compartment syndrome: An unusual cause for claudication. Ann Surg 210:557–563, 1989.
9. Wilt TJ: Current strategies in the diagnosis and management of lower extremity peripheral vascular disease. J Gen Intern Med 7:97–101, 1992.
10. Dawson DL, Cutler BS, Hiatt WR, et al: A comparison of Cilostazol and Pentoxifylline for treating intermittent claudication. Am J Med 109:523–530, 2000.

39. PULMONARY EMBOLISM

Michael E. Hanley, M.D.

1. What three primary factors promote thromboembolic disease?

Development of venous thrombosis is promoted by (1) venous blood stasis, (2) injury to the intimal layer of the venous vasculature, and (3) abnormalities in coagulation and/or fibrinolysis.

2. List the risk factors for thromboembolic disease.

Previous history of thromboembolic disease
Obesity
Pregnancy
Prolonged immobilization
Lower-extremity or pelvic trauma or surgery
Surgery with greater than 30 minutes of general anesthesia
Congestive heart failure
Nephrotic syndrome
Cancer
Estrogen-containing compounds
Advanced age

3. What is the natural history of venous thrombosis?

Resolution of fresh thrombi occurs by fibrinolysis and organization. **Fibrinolysis** results in actual clot dissolution. **Organization** re-establishes venous blood flow by re-endothelializing and incorporating into the venous wall residual clot not dissolved by fibrinolysis. In the absence of new clot formation, the two processes generally are complete in 7–10 days.

4. Can patients with deep venous thrombosis be accurately diagnosed clinically?

No. The clinical diagnosis of deep venous thrombosis is neither sensitive nor specific. Less than 50% of patients with confirmed deep venous thrombosis present with classic symptoms of pain, erythema, and edema. Similarly, radiologic tests confirm the diagnosis in only 50% of patients who present with a high clinical suspicion of deep venous thrombosis.

5. How is the diagnosis of lower extremity deep venous thrombosis confirmed?

The test of choice depends on the likely location of the deep venous thrombosis. Contrast venography remains the gold standard, but is associated with a higher incidence of adverse effects, primarily phlebitis. Radiolabeled fibrinogen scanning is highly sensitive for deep venous thromboses in the calf and lower thigh, but loses sensitivity above mid-thigh, because accumulated radiofibrinogen in the large pelvic blood pool interferes with scanning. In contrast, impedance plethysmography is sensitive above but not below the knee. Similarly, Doppler/ultrasound has a sensitivity and specificity of 90–95% for proximal clots located cephalad of the popliteal vein. Its accuracy for vein thromboses in the calf is not well defined.

6. When should prophylaxis of deep venous thromboses be considered?

Two factors must be weighed in deciding to initiate prophylaxis of deep venous thrombosis: the degree of risk for thrombosis (see Questions 1 and 2) and the risk of prophylaxis. The risk factors for deep venous thrombosis are cumulative. The primary risk of pharmacologic prophylaxis is hemorrhage, which is generally uncommon if no coagulation defects or lesions with bleeding potential exist.

7. What prophylactic measures are available?

Approaches to prophylaxis of deep venous thrombosis (DVT) include antithrombotic drugs and pneumatic-compressive devices. **Heparin, low-molecular-weight (LMW) heparin**, and **warfarin** are effective in preventing DVT. Subcutaneous heparin offers a low risk of bleeding and rapid onset of prophylaxis, but is ineffective in patients undergoing prostate or hip surgery. Low-dose warfarin (with prolongation of the prothrombin time to 1.2–1.3 times normal) also has a low risk of bleeding and is effective in patients with trauma, burns, and hip surgery. However, it takes several days to develop a full antithrombotic effect. Antiplatelet drugs such as aspirin and dipyridamole are not effective in prophylaxis.

Intermittent pneumatic-compressive devices effect prophylaxis by maintaining venous flow in the lower extremities and are especially efficacious in patients who cannot receive anticoagulant medications. Modalities available include compressive devices applied to the feet alone, covering the calves, or extending to the thighs. No version has been shown to provide superior prophylaxis.

8. Should all deep venous thromboses be treated with anticoagulation?

No. DVTs are treated primarily to prevent fatal pulmonary embolism (PE). Because the risk of fatal embolism is low for DVTs limited to calf veins, many authorities do not recommend anticoagulant therapy in this setting. Lack of extension into the popliteal system must be confirmed and followed (for 14 days) by impedance plethysmography. If this or other reliable tests for popliteal extension are not available, DVTs in the calf should be treated.

9. Can deep venous thrombosis be safely treated in an outpatient setting?

Yes. LMW heparin compounds have revolutionized the management of *simple* DVT. With regard to safety and efficacy, these agents are at least equivalent to unfractionated heparin. Their comparatively excessive cost, however, has limited their use in the management of hospitalized DVT patients. LMW heparin can be delivered in a single or twice-daily dose and doesn't require daily monitoring of the activate partial thromboplastin time to assure therapeutic effect. These advantages have led to the development of outpatient treatment protocols for *selected patients*. The costs saved by avoiding prolonged hospitalization and daily lab tests are enormous.

10. Where do most pulmonary emboli originate?

Thromboses in the deep veins of the lower extremities account for 90–95% of pulmonary emboli. Less common sites of origin include thromboses in the right ventricle; in upper-extremity, prostatic, uterine, and renal veins; and, rarely, in superficial veins.

11. Are pulmonary embolism and pulmonary infarction synonymous terms?

No. The pulmonary parenchyma is supplied by both the pulmonary and bronchial (systemic) circulations. Pulmonary infarction results when embolized lung parenchyma is inadequately perfused by the bronchial circulation. Infarction complicates only 10% of pulmonary emboli. The two conditions are treated in the same fashion.

12. What are the most common findings on chest x-ray and electrocardiogram (EKG) in patients with pulmonary emboli?

Most patients with PE have a normal chest x-ray. When it is abnormal, the findings are non-specific and include an elevated hemidiaphragm, focal or multifocal infiltrates, pleural effusion, plate-like atelectasis, enlarged pulmonary arteries, focal oligemia (Westermark's sign), and right ventricular enlargement.

Most patients with PE present with sinus tachycardia only evident on EKG. Other EKG findings include arrythmias (premature atrial and ventricular beats, first-degree atrioventricular block, supraventricular arrhythmia); right ventricular strain (right axis deviation, right ventricular hypertrophy); p-pulmonale; right bundle-branch block; $S_1S_2S_3$ and $S_1Q_3T_3$ pattern; and depression, elevation, or inversion of S-T and T waves. ST-T changes, when present, often are most marked in the right precordial leads.

13. **What is the differential diagnosis of the patient suspected of having pulmonary emboli?**
Infectious pneumonitis
Viral pleuritis
Atelectasis
Cardiovascular collapse secondary to sepsis or hemorrhage
Pulmonary edema
Bronchial asthma
Hyperventilation syndrome
Ischemic chest pain
Pericarditis

14. **How is the diagnosis of pulmonary embolism confirmed?**
Laboratory confirmation is required, because clinical diagnosis is quite unreliable. Helpful diagnostic tests include tests for lower-extremity DVT (see Question 5), ventilation/perfusion (V/P) lung scans, and pulmonary angiography. **Pulmonary angiography** remains the gold standard. Although angiography is safe when performed by experienced angiographers, morbidity and mortality are increased in patients with pulmonary hypertension, cor pulmonale, or acute right ventricular strain. V/P lung scanning is safer and less invasive than angiography, but also less specific. Specificity is improved when only segmental or larger perfusion defects are considered significant. When V/P lung scans are nondiagnostic, some authorities advocate evaluation for evidence of lower-extremity DVTs before proceeding to angiography. Although definitive proof of DVT does not prove PE, it renders the issue inconsequential, because anticoagulation is generally indicated for both conditions.

15. **What is the role of D-dimers in diagnosing pulmonary embolism?**
The quantitative D-dimers assay can be helpful in excluding the diagnosis of pulmonary thromboembolic disease. The assay measures cross-linked fibrin degradation products and—when positive—indicates activation of the coagulation cascade and fibrinolysis. Elevated levels of D-dimers are nonspecific, but a level < 500 ug/L has a sensitivity of 98–100% in excluding the diagnosis of thromboembolic disease.

Some authors have suggested incorporating this assay into diagnostic algorithms for pulmonary emboli. However, this approach has not been adequately validated to justify widespread application at this time.

16. **What is the role of spiral (helical) computed tomography of the chest in diagnosing pulmonary embolism?**
Spiral CT angiograms are gaining popularity in the diagnosis of pulmonary emboli. The sensitivity and specificity generally exceed 90%, especially if clot is present in large central vessels. However, the sensitivity and specificity are highly dependent on the experience of the radiologist interpreting the study and the amount of time devoted to interpretation.

A negative result doesn't abrogate the need for a formal pulmonary angiogram (*especially* in the setting of moderate to high clinical suspicion), as it only excludes clot in larger vessels. For this reason, the primary role of spiral CT in the diagnosis of PE is similar to that of V/P scans: it is a **screening test** that can confirm the diagnosis. In institutions well versed in its use, it may be the test of choice.

Note that spiral CT is likely superior to V/P scans in patients with significant underlying lung disease; there is a high incidence of nondiagnostic V/P scans in these patients.

17. **Describe the treatment of pulmonary embolism.**
Treatment of PE includes cardiopulmonary supportive measures (fluids and vasopressors for hemodynamic support, oxygen) and specific measures for thromboembolism, such as anticoagulant therapy, placement of an intracaval filter, or thrombolytic therapy. **Anticoagulant therapy** remains the treatment of choice for most patients. The primary debate regards length of therapy.

The goal of therapy is to prevent new clot formation and/or thrombus growth while existing clots become organized or resolve. Because organization and resolution require 7–10 days, all patients must receive anticoagulant therapy for this period. Although most authorities recommend anticoagulant therapy for 3 months for DVT and 6 months for proved PE, some advocate therapy beyond 7–10 days only if there is a high risk for recurrence (continued thromboembolic risk factors [see Questions 1 and 2] and/or persistent venous obstruction, as assessed by impedance plethysmography).

Oral warfarin, subcutaneous heparin, or subcutaneous LMW heparin compounds are effective if chronic anticoagulant therapy is indicated.

18. What are the indications for intracaval filters?

Absolute indications for interruption of the inferior vena cava through insertion of a filter include **failure of, and/or a contraindication to, anticoagulant therapy**. In addition, some experts advocate placement of an intracaval filter for massive PE, because failure of anticoagulation in this setting frequently has a fatal outcome.

19. When is thrombolytic therapy indicated for pulmonary embolism?

Although thrombolytic therapy for PE in general is associated with more rapid clot dissolution than anticoagulant therapy (heparin) alone, no well-controlled studies have demonstrated a difference in morbidity or mortality between the two therapeutic modalities. Thrombolytic therapy is therefore indicated only for **massive PE characterized by refractory hypotension and/or refractory hypoxemia**. In the setting of right ventricle failure based on echocardiographic criteria, thrombolytics may be considered.

CONTROVERSIES

20. Is surgery indicated in massive pulmonary embolism?

Massive PE is a life-threatening occurrence with significant morbidity and mortality. Surgical embolectomy (via thoracotomy, suction catheter, or balloon catheter) is a potentially life-saving procedure. Attempts at medical therapy may waste precious time, and if unsuccessful almost certainly result in a fatal outcome.

On the other hand, many patients with massive PE die within the first hour of presentation— before surgical services can be mobilized. Medical therapy is highly effective if instituted quickly; results of surgical embolectomy are not impressive.

Therefore, surgical embolectomy should be reserved for rare cases when the diagnosis is irrefutable, medical therapy has failed or is contraindicated, and surgical intervention can be performed immediately.

21. Are intracaval filters contraindicated in patients with thromboembolic disease?

A recent study questions the safety of inferior vena cava filters in patients receiving prophylaxis for PE. Patients with proximal DVT were randomly assigned to at least 3 months of anticoagulant therapy with or without filter placement. Although there were fewer short-term (by day 12) PE in the group with filters, there was no difference in 2-year mortality between the two groups. Long-term follow-up revealed that once anticoagulant therapy was discontinued, the patients with filters had a significantly higher incidence of symptomatic DVT.

However, in this study the indications for filter placement were not those listed in Question 18. Indeed, patients in whom anticoagulant therapy was contraindicated or had previously failed were excluded from the study. Furthermore, DVTs that complicated the filter group may have resulted from venous stasis due to filter obstruction by trapped emboli, which suggested that the filters were acting efficaciously. Finally, although the authors did not offer statistical analysis, the incidence of fatal PE at 2 years was lower in the filter group than the non-filter group (one versus five).

The conclusions of this study are controversial, but at minimum they suggest that physicians should:

Be cautious in recommending filter placement

Re-examine the validity of traditionally accepted contraindications to anticoagulant therapy

Continue life-long anticoagulant therapy in patients with filters, if possible (including restarting therapy after resolution of the process that contraindicated it).

BIBLIOGRAPHY

1. Clagett GP, Anderson FA, Heit J, et al: Prevention of venous thromboembolism. Chest 108:312S–334S, 1995.
2. Cross JL, Kemp PM, Walsh CG, et al: A randomized trial of spiral CT and ventilation perfusion scintigraphy for the diagnosis of pulmonary embolism. Clin Radiol 53:177–182, 1998.
3. Decousus H, Leizorovicz A, Parent F, et al: A clinical trial of vena caval filters in the prevention of pulmonary embolism in patients with proximal deep-vein thrombosis. New Engl J Med 338:409–415, 1998.
4. Heijboer H, Buller HR, Lensing AWA, et al: A comparison of real-time compression ultrasonography with impedance plethysmography for the diagnosis of deep-vein thrombosis in symptomatic outpatients. New Engl J Med 329:1365–1369, 1993.
5. Hyers TM: Venous thromboembolism. Am J Respir Crit Care Med 159:1–14, 1999.
6. Levine M, Gent M, Hirsh J: A comparison of low-molecular-weight heparin administered primarily at home with unfractionated heparin administered in the hospital for proximal deep-vein thrombosis. N Engl J Med 334:677–681, 1996.
7. Perrier A, Desmarais S, Goehring C, et al: D-dimer testing for suspected pulmonary embolism in outpatients. Am J Respir Crit Care Med 156:492–496, 1997.
8. PIOPED Investigators: Value of the ventilation/perfusion scan in acute pulmonary embolism: Results of the prospective investigation of pulmonary embolism diagnosis (PIOPED). JAMA 263:2753–2795, 1990.
9. Rathbun SW, Raskob GE, Whitsett TL: Sensitivity and specificity of helical computed tomography in the diagnosis of pulmonary embolism: A systematic review. Ann Intern Med 132:227–232, 2000.
10. Ryu JH, Swensen SJ, Olson EJ, Pellikka PA: Diagnosis of pulmonary embolism with use of computed tomographic angiography. Mayo Clin Proc 76:59–65, 2001.
11. Stein PD, Terrin ML, Hales CA, et al: Clinical, laboratory, roentgenographic, and electrocardiographic findings in patients with acute pulmonary embolism and no pre-existing cardiac or pulmonary disease. Chest 100:598–603, 1991.
12. Wells PS, Ginsberg JS, Anderson DR, et al: Use of a clinical model for safe management of patients with suspected pulmonary embolism. Ann Intern Med 129:997–1005, 1998.
13. Yusen RD, Haraden BM, Gage BF, et al: Criteria for outpatient management of proximal lower extremity deep venous thrombosis. Chest 115:972–979, 1999.

40. PULMONARY HYPERTENSION

Karen A. Fagan, M.D., and David B. Badesch, M.D.

1. What are the typical presenting symptoms in patients with pulmonary hypertension?

Dyspnea on exertion is most common. Because this symptom is nonspecific, patients are often thought to have some other respiratory or cardiac disorder. Other symptoms include chest pain, presyncope or syncope, edema, and ascites.

2. What are the usual physical findings in patients with pulmonary hypertension?

By the time most patients present, pulmonary hypertension is already severe. Findings on physical examination might include:

Loud pulmonic valve closure sound (P_2)
Right ventricular heave
Murmur of tricuspid regurgitation (a systolic murmur over the left lower sternal border)
Murmur of pulmonic insufficiency (a diastolic murmur over the left sternal border)
Jugular venous distention (indicating elevated central venous pressures)
Peripheral edema
Hepatomegaly
Hepatojugular reflux
Ascites
Cyanosis
Clubbing

3. How is pulmonary hypertension classified?

Etiology: primary vs. secondary. Primary pulmonary hypertension is not associated with any of the known causes of pulmonary hypertension. Secondary pulmonary hypertension is due to an underlying disease.

Location: precapillary vs. post-capillary. Precapillary pulmonary hypertension is caused by increased resistance to flow in the pulmonary arteries and arterioles. Post-pulmonary hypertension is caused by back pressure from the left heart and/or increased resistance to flow in the pulmonary veins.

Duration: acute vs. chronic. Acute pulmonary hypertension is caused by such things as thromboembolism or adult respiratory distress syndrome. Most other forms of pulmonary hypertension are chronic.

Histopathology: plexiform vs. thrombotic. The plexiform lesion is characterized by focal medial disruption and aneurysmal dilatation, with formation of a complex proliferative tuft of intimal cells and channels. Thrombotic histopathology is characterized by intravascular thrombus.

4. Is pulmonary hypertension a genetic disease?

About 6% of patients with PPH have a close relative also with primary pulmonary hypertension. Recently, mutations in the gene encoding the bone morphogenetic receptor 2 (BMPR2) were found in families with familial pulmonary hypertension. How mutations in this gene are responsible for pulmonary hypertension is unknown.

5. What should the clinical evaluation for possible pulmonary hypertension include?

As always, the evaluation begins with a thorough history and physical examination. Possible causes of secondary pulmonary hypertension should be addressed in the history. In addition, travel to or residence in an area endemic for schistosomiasis should be considered. All patients should receive a basic initial screening evaluation, consisting of chest x-ray, electrocardiogram, and echocardiogram.

Patients with no clues to the etiology on history or physical examination are given a broad "detailed" evaluation; patients with a suspected secondary cause receive a "focused" evaluation to verify that etiology, followed by the broad evaluation if necessary. In addition to these tests, arterial blood gases and pulmonary angiography may be indicated. If undertaken, pulmonary angiography should be performed by someone experienced in working with pulmonary hypertension patients.

6. List some causes of secondary pulmonary hypertension.
Recurrent pulmonary emboli
Chronic exposure to high altitude
Chronic lung diseases, especially COPD and pulmonary fibrosis
Sleep apnea
Obesity with hypoventilation
Sickle cell disease
Schistosomiasis
Left heart failure
Mitral valve disease, especially stenosis
Pulmonary veno-occlusive disease
Collagen vascular disease

7. Which connective tissue diseases most commonly cause pulmonary hypertension?
Scleroderma (especially CREST syndrome)
Mixed connective tissue disease
Systemic lupus erythematosus
Rheumatoid arthritis
Dermatomyositis

8. Which occurs more frequently: primary or secondary pulmonary hypertension?
Primary (unexplained) pulmonary hypertension is a rare disorder. Secondary pulmonary hypertension is seen considerably more often in practice.

9. What population group is most frequently affected by primary pulmonary hypertension (PPH)?
Although PPH occurs in both sexes and virtually all age groups, it has a tendency to affect young females. The female-to-male predominance is 1.7:1, and the mean age is 36 years.

10. Is surgical therapy now an option for patients with pulmonary hypertension secondary to chronic recurrent thromboembolism?
Appropriate prevention of recurrent thromboembolism continues to be extremely important. In addition to this prevention, it is now possible to remove organized thrombus surgically from the proximal pulmonary arteries of patients with pulmonary hypertension secondary to chronic recurrent thromboembolism. Operative mortality was 8.7% in a study from the most experienced center. Life-long anticoagulation is essential in all of these patients.

11. What is the average survival for the patient with PPH?
According to the National Institutes of Health Registry on Primary Pulmonary Hypertension, the median survival is approximately 2.8 years from the date of diagnosis. It should be noted, however, that there is large interindividual variability. Although some patients progress quickly to death over a period of months, others live for years with little change in symptoms or hemodynamics. Improved life expectancy has been reported with the use of vasodilators (both oral and intravenous).

12. What is now considered "conventional therapy" for patients with PPH?
Conventional therapy includes **supplemental oxygen** as needed to maintain an oxygen saturation of at least 91%, **diuretics** if the patient has clinically significant edema or ascites,

vasodilators (oral or intravenous), **anticoagulation** in the absence of contraindications, and occasionally *digitalis*.

13. How are vasodilators used in the treatment of PPH?

Until recently, only orally active vasodilators (usually calcium channel blockers) were available for use in patients with primary pulmonary hypertension. About 25% of patients with PPH have a favorable response to calcium channel blockers, leading to a better prognosis. However, despite an initial improvement, these patients may later deteriorate, requiring additional treatment and close follow-up.

Currently, intravenously administered vasodilators are used successfully in the treatment of PPH. Despite the complexity of administering the drug, continuous infusion of prostacyclin has led to improvement in both functional status and survival.

14. How do I determine which vasodilator is best for patients with pulmonary hypertension?

Since only about 25% of patients with PPH respond favorably to oral vasodilators, it is important to attempt to predict who these individuals might be since the alternative is the use of complicated intravenous therapy. To determine the likelihood of responding to oral vasodilators, the acute response to vasodilators is determined with invasive hemodynamic monitoring in the cardiac catheterization laboratory or in the intensive care unit. In this setting, patients are given short-acting pulmonary vasodilators, and hemodynamic measurements are taken to determine if there is any significant improvement. A wide variety of vasodilators are used in clinical practice, including nitric oxide, prostacyclin, and adenosine. If patients have a favorable response to acutely administered vasodilators, this predicts a response to calcium channel blockers. If patients do not have a favorable response to acutely administered vasodilators, then consider treatment with intravenous prostacyclin.

15. What is considered a favorable response to acutely administered vasodilators?

A decrease in mean pulmonary artery pressure by 10 mmHg, an increase in cardiac output by 25%, and a decrease in pulmonary vascular resistance by 25% are all indicative of a favorable response to acutely administered vasodilators.

16. What are the complications of vasodilator therapy?

None of the vasodilators are selective for the pulmonary circulation (except possibly inhaled nitric oxide), so a common complication is systemic hypotension. Other commonly reported side effects of treatment, especially with prostacyclin, include flushing, headaches, nausea, diarrhea, and jaw pain. Because intravenous administration of prostacyclin requires central venous access, line infections and catheter associated thrombosis are unfortunately common. Careful care of the catheter and anticoagulation help lessen these risks, but there is still the chance for significant and life-threatening complications.

17. How do you treat secondary forms of pulmonary hypertension?

Treat the underlying disease, if possible. Thus, for pulmonary hypertension associated with lung disease, maintaining adequate oxygen saturation is key. For patients with sleep apnea syndrome, effective treatment with CPAP is necessary. If congenital heart disease is the cause of pulmonary hypertension, definitive repair may be undertaken. Vasodilators have been used with variable success for treatment of secondary pulmonary hypertension, but great care must be taken when considering this treatment, as clinical worsening has been reported occasionally in patients with underlying lung disease.

18. How do I treat the pulmonary hypertension associated with CREST syndrome?

Pulmonary hypertension is a common, life-threatening complication of the CREST syndrome and accounts for the significant morbidity and mortality of this disease. Orally available vasodilators have been notoriously ineffective in the treatment of pulmonary hypertension associated with CREST. Recently, infused prostacyclin has been shown to improve the functional status of patients with CREST and pulmonary hypertension and is being used in this clinical setting more commonly.

19. Is transplantation possible in patients with PPH?

Yes. Lung transplantation is an additional option especially for patients that do not respond to aggressive treatment. A combined heart and lung transplant is no longer believed to be required, as the right ventricle appears to recover function after lung transplantation. Occasionally, heart-lung transplantation is required in patients with uncorrectable congenital heart defects with Eisenmenger's syndrome.

BIBLIOGRAPHY

1. Badesch DB, Tapson VF, McGoon MD, et al: Continuous intravenous epoprostenol for pulmonary hypertension due to the scleroderma spectrum of disease. A randomized, controlled trial. Ann Intern Med 132(6):425–434, 2000.
2. Barst RJ, Rubin LJ, Long WA, et al: A comparison of continuous intravenous epoprostenol (prostacyclin) with conventional therapy for primary pulmonary hypertension. New Engl J Med 334:296–301, 1996.
3. D'Alonzo GE, Barst RJ, Ayres SM, et al: Survival in patients with primary pulmonary hypertension: Results from a national prospective registry. Ann Intern Med 115:343–349, 1991.
4. International PPH Consortium—Lane KB, Machado RD, et al: Heterozygous germline mutations in BMPR2, encoding a TGF-b receptor cause familial primary pulmonary hypertension. Published electronically, Nature Genetics July 28, 2000.
5. Jamieson SW, Auger WR, Fidulo PF, et al: Experience and results with 150 pulmonary thromboendarterectomy operations over a 29 month period. J Thoracic Cardiovasc Surg 106:116–127, 1993.
6. Rich S, Kaufman E, Levy PS: The effect of high doses of calcium-channel blockers on survival in primary pulmonary hypertension. N Engl J Med 327:76–81, 1992.

41. PULMONARY DISEASE AND THE HEART

David A. Kaminsky, M.D., and Olivia V. Adair, M.D.*

1. How can diseases of the left heart affect the lungs?

The heart and lungs are intimately linked by the pulmonary vasculature; thus, it is not surprising that the pulmonary vasculature is most commonly affected by left-heart disease. Any process that raises left ventricular (LV) end-diastolic pressure or left atrial pressure results in elevated pulmonary venous pressure (PVP). Such processes include diseases that *reduce LV contractility*, such as ischemic heart disease, mitral regurgitation, or cardiomyopathy, as well as processes that *decrease LV compliance*, such as ischemic heart disease, aortic stenosis, and hypertension. Mitral stenosis results in elevated left atrial pressures. In all of these circumstances, PVP is increased and leads to elevations of pulmonary capillary and pulmonary arterial pressures.

2. What are the mechanical effects of the heart on the lungs?

The heart and lungs both occupy an enclosed space within the thoracic cavity. Any process that results in changes in the size or position of the heart may alter pulmonary function. Cardiomegaly may produce pulmonary symptoms such as cough, dyspnea, and wheezing by compressing mediastinal structures such as the trachea or bronchi. A dilated main pulmonary artery or enlarged left atrium may cause gas trapping and hyperinflation by occluding bronchi. Massive cardiomegaly or pericardial effusion may cause left lower lobe atelectasis.

3. Describe the pulmonary vascular consequences of elevations in PVP.

Pulmonary capillary pressures are elevated in the setting of increased PVP. Normal Starling forces in the alveolar interstitium yield a net filtration force of 4 mmHg outward from the pulmonary capillaries to the interstitium. However, net fluid accumulation does not occur due to the absorptive capacity of the pulmonary lymphatics, which may increase fluid transport 5- to 10-fold in response to increased fluid formation. Eventually, the lymphatics reach their limit, and net fluid formation in the form of interstitial edema occurs, usually at capillary pressures > 20 mmHg. Alveolar flooding, or pulmonary edema, may be seen with elevations in pressure > 25 mmHg.

These pressure limits apply to acute pulmonary edema. Situations in which PVP is chronically elevated, such as mitral stenosis, may require much higher pressures before alveolar edema occurs.

4. What are the two primary diagnoses to consider when Kerly B lines are seen on chest x-ray?

Left-heart disease (congestive heart failure [CHF] or mitral stenosis) and lymphangitic carcinomatosis. Radiographically, pulmonary congestion, with redistribution of flow to the upper zones of the lung, is typically seen with pulmonary capillary pressures of 18–20 mmHg. As pressure increases further, interstitial edema occurs with the appearance of perihilar haze, peribronchial cuffing, and Kerly B lines. So-called periacinar rosettes, or radiolucent grapelike clusters surrounded by radiodense fluid, may appear as fluid encroaches upon the alveolar space. At 25–30 mmHg pressure, frank pulmonary edema occurs, with fluffy alveolar infiltrates typically in a perihilar distribution. Fairly accurate assessments of true pulmonary capillary pressures, as measured by Swan-Ganz catheter readings, can be made by looking closely at the chest radiograph.

* The authors acknowledge Thomas A. Neff, M.D., whose text from the first edition is incorporated in this chapter.

5. Describe the pulmonary function abnormalities associated with elevations in PVP due to cardiac disease.

Patients with elevated PVP, such as seen in chronic CHF, may show a combined restrictive and obstructive ventilatory defect on pulmonary function testing. Restriction occurs as a result of loss of lung volume due to increased blood and fluid within the interstitial and alveolar spaces; compliance is reduced.

Airflow limitation is evident as a fall in **forced expiratory volume** in the first second (FEV1) and **forced vital capacity** (FVC). Since both FEV1 and FVC fall, the ratio of FEV1/FVC may be normal. A very low ratio usually implies the concurrence of additional airways disease, such as chronic obstructive pulmonary disease (COPD). Increased airway resistance due to elevations of PVP occurs predominantly in the lung periphery.

Diffusing capacity for carbon monoxide (DLCO) may be *increased* early on due to increased pulmonary blood volume, but with worsening interstitial edema and ultimate injury to the pulmonary vessels, DLCO normalizes and is then reduced.

6. What is cardiac asthma?

Patients with elevations in PVP, such as in CHF or mitral stenosis, have airflow limitation due to increased airways resistance. On physical examination, this may be manifested as wheezing. Although blood vessel engorgement and edema are thought to be responsible for this process, smooth muscle constriction may also be involved. Bronchial hyperresponsiveness to methacholine and acetylcholine has been demonstrated in cardiac asthma.

Obviously, it is important to distinguish wheezing due to heart failure from wheezing due to intrinsic airway disease, as the treatment is substantially different. A careful history and physical examination, followed by a therapeutic trial of diuretics or bronchodilators, will answer the question.

7. Besides wheezing, patients with CHF often have coarse crackles. What other pulmonary diseases can cause crackles?

• Bronchiectasis
• Chronic obstructive pulmonary disease (COPD, especially chronic bronchitis)
• Pneumonia
• Interstitial lung disease

As with cardiac asthma, a careful history is the best initial approach to diagnosis. Sophisticated analysis of crackles in different disease states has shown that cardiac crackles are typically more coarse and prolonged than the fine, late-inspiratory, short-duration crackles of interstitial lung disease. COPD crackles also tend to be of short duration, but are early in inspiration and are relatively infrequent and scant. Differentiating crackles of CHF from those of pneumonia and bronchiectasis is more difficult.

8. What respiratory care modality can be used to treat cardiogenic pulmonary edema and CHF?

Continuous positive airway pressure (CPAP). CPAP is applied via a tight-fitting mask over the mouth and nose or nose alone. It is usually used to treat respiratory insufficiency due to obstructive sleep apnea or severe COPD. However, CPAP has also been shown to be effective in improving symptoms of acute pulmonary edema and may buy time if you are trying to avoid intubation while waiting for pharmacologic therapy to take effect.

9. What are the long-term consequences of elevations in PVP?

Pulmonary hypertension. The typical pathologic change associated with left-heart-related pulmonary hypertension is medial thickening due to vascular smooth muscle hypertrophy and/or hyperplasia. Pulmonary parenchymal abnormalities may also be seen, especially in advanced mitral stenosis. These include alveolar wall thickening, fibrosis, hemosiderosis, and even parenchymal calcification.

10. Can other classes of cardiac disease alter the pulmonary vasculature?

Congenital heart disease with left-to-right shunting affects the pulmonary vasculature by causing large increases in pulmonary blood volume and flow. These diseases include atrial septal defect, ventricular septal defect, patent ductus arteriosus, and anomalous pulmonary venous return. The increased flow seen with these lesions may ultimately cause pulmonary hypertension. Patients may develop pulmonary vascular resistance that is high enough to equalize shunt flow, or reverse it right-to-left (Eisenmenger's syndrome).

11. What are the pleural manifestations of cardiac disease?

Normally, a thin layer of fluid exists between the visceral and parietal pleura. Net filtration is favored by Starling forces into the pleural space from the parietal pleura, but the visceral pleura absorbs the fluid to prevent its accumulation. However, increased hydrostatic pressure as in heart failure results in a transudative pleural effusion. The parietal pleura is supplied by the systemic circulation, so any increase in systemic venous pressure, as occurs in right-heart failure, promotes increased fluid formation. The visceral pleural is supplied by the pulmonary circulation, so any increase in pulmonary pressure, as in left heart failure, impedes fluid resorption.

Effusions from heart failure are usually bilateral, but when unilateral, they occur more frequently on the right side.

12. How can heart disease cause an *exudative* pleural effusion?

Following many forms of cardiac injury, including myocardial infarction (MI), surgery, or trauma, a syndrome of pericarditis, pleuritis, and rarely pneumonitis may develop over the ensuing 1–12 weeks. This process is called **Dressler's syndrome** and may be seen in 1–3% of patients following MI and up to 30% of cardiac surgery patients. Symptoms include pericardial and pleuritic chest pain, and signs of fever, pericardial or pleural friction rub, and elevated white blood cell count and sedimentation rate are typically seen. Pleural effusions occur in 60–80% of cases, and 50% have an enlarged cardiac silhouette due to pericardial effusion. The pleural effusion is exudative with high protein (usually > 3 g/100 ml), pH (> 7.40), lactate dehydrogenase, and red blood cell count.

The etiology of Dressler's syndrome is unknown but is thought to be due to an antibody-mediated response to myocardial antigens exposed upon injury. Treatment is supportive with nonsteroidals or corticosteroids.

13. A patient presents with fevers, hemoptysis, and multiple pulmonary infiltrates with central radiolucencies on chest x-ray. What is the diagnosis?

Right-sided endocarditis with septic pulmonary emboli. Cardiac disease may lead to pulmonary embolism in the setting of right-sided endocarditis affecting the tricuspid valve. Rarely, septic emboli may arise from indwelling catheters in the superior vena cava. Right-sided endocarditis accounts for 5–10% of all cases of endocarditis and is most often seen in intravenous drug abusers. The most common infecting organism is *Staphylococcus aureus*, although Streptococcus, gram-negative, and Candida species also may be involved.

The radiographic appearance is very characteristic and includes multiple, patchy, ill-defined densities scattered throughout the lung fields, especially in the periphery. They may appear to change in number and size on serial x-rays, reflecting the ongoing shower of emboli to the lungs. Cavitation is seen in 25% of patients.

14. What are the pulmonary effects of various cardiovascular drugs?

Angiotensin-converting enzyme inhibitors cause cough in approximately 15% of all patients, but twice as frequently in women than men. The mechanism is not known. **Beta-blockers** precipitate bronchospasm in patients with asthma and occasionally in those with bronchitis. The drugs **procainamide** and **hydralazine** may cause a lupus-like syndrome in susceptible individuals. With procainamide, the reaction is much more common and involves a positive antineutrophil antibody test in 50–80% of patients, with 30–40% developing pulmonary infiltrates and 40–50%

having pleuropericardial disease. The latter manifestations are rare with hydralazine. **Amiodarone** causes pulmonary toxicity, with 5–15% of treated patients developing a severe pneumonitis, which is fatal in 5–10%. This side effect is dose-dependent, usually occurring only in patients who have been treated with > 400 mg/day for > 4 months.

15. What are the main pulmonary complications of cardiac surgery?

Atelectasis, pneumonia, and exacerbation of COPD. Atelectasis and pneumonia are usually due to the inability of the patient to cough adequately or deep breathe following surgery, often because of the pain of the thoractomy and the heavy use of analgesics and sedatives. These complications are less common following median sternotomy than after lateral thoracotomy. Left lower lobe atelectasis may also be due to concomitant phrenic nerve dysfunction, which may result from mechanical injury or from the cooling associated with cardioplegia. Phrenic nerve function usually recovers within the first 30 days to 1 year but may take as long as 2 years. Bronchospasm may be worsened. Pleural effusions are also common. Some special pulmonary concerns in cardiac transplant surgery, in addition to those above, include postoperative elevations in pulmonary vascular resistance and the numerous infectious complications associated with immunosuppression.

16. Differentiate dyspnea due to cardiac disease from that due to pulmonary disease.

This is a common clinical problem, as many patients have concomitant cardiac and pulmonary disease, often in association with cigarette smoking. Clues of underlying disease are critical in distinguishing these two etiologies. Thus, a history of angina, hypertension, or previous MI, together with signs of heart failure on examination, make cardiac disease more likely; whereas a history of bronchitis and heavy smoking, *diminished* breath sounds on examination, and a normal cardiac silhouette with hyperinflated lungs on chest x-ray suggest primary pulmonary disease. In many cases, however, further testing including pulmonary function, arterial blood gases, and a cardiac function assessment with echocardiography or radioisotope scanning are necessary. Exercise testing with measurement of expired gases can be helpful in difficult cases.

17. Can the pattern of dyspnea help distinguish between cardiac and pulmonary causes?

Yes and no. **Paroxysmal nocturnal dyspnea** (PND) is thought to be specific for heart failure, but patients with COPD may also complain of PND due to the development of increased secretions upon lying down. Asthmatics may also have PND due to nocturnal worsening of bronchospasm. **Orthopnea** is likewise not specific for CHF because COPD patients sometimes complain of orthopnea due to partial loss of diaphragmatic and accessory muscle function when supine. **Sleep apnea** is often associated with hypertension or left-heart failure, but secondary pulmonary hypertension may result from years of hypoxia. **Cheyne-Stokes respirations**, or periodic breathing, is characteristic of LV dysfunction and rarely associated with pulmonary disease per se. A recent study of patients with CHF and Cheyne-Stokes respirations found that such patients were more likely to have awake hypocapnia due to hyperventilation. Such patients may complain of PND during periods of hyperpnea.

18. Which occult cause of hypoxia is commonly overlooked?

Obstructive sleep apnea (OSA). Chronic hypoxia is an important cause of pulmonary hypertension and can lead to pulmonary vasoconstriction.

19. What are the cardiovascular consequences of obstructive sleep apnea?

In addition to causing pulmonary hypertension and cor pulmonale, OSA is associated with systemic hypertension. Grote and colleagues recently showed that the relative risk for systemic hypertension increases with the severity of the sleep-related breathing disorder, especially in patients younger than 50 years. Postulated mechanisms include elevated sympathetic activity in sleep-related breathing disorders and the possibility of a genetic trait shared among obestiy, hypertension, and sleep apnea.

20. Can pulmonary function predict cardiovascular morbidity and mortality?

Yes. Recent studies have shown an inverse relationship between pulmonary function, as measured by FEV1 or FVC, and the incidence of coronary artery disease and CHF, independent of cigarette smoking. One explanation for these findings is that decreased pulmonary function is a marker of centripetal obesity and decreased physical activity, which are themselves related to increased insulin resistance, lower high-density lipoproteins, and higher triglycerides. Hyperinsulinemia is associated with increased sympathetic nervous activity and therefore may result in increased risk of hypertension and MI.

21. Is age a contributing risk factor for increased arrhythmias at high altitude?

A 75-year-old man climbing 5100 meters (m) on Mt. Kilimanjaro was observed via Holter monitor. The findings were compared to those 10 years earlier when the same individual climbed 5895 m. Arterial oxygen saturation by finger oximeter and sea-level testing to rule out any evidence of cardiac tamponade also were recorded. At age 75, oxygen saturation dropped to 70% at 4710–5100 m, heart rate increased, and LV arrhythmias were more frequent and complex. Ventricular tachycardia was noted, including runs of 14 beats at 250 bpm.

These findings suggest that aging may increase the sympathetic response or perhaps the sensitivity to hypoxia. This increased sympathetic stimulation may play an important role in high-altitude arrhythmias, meaning that pulmonary hypertension can no longer be considered the only likely cause.

22. What is the strategy for diagnosis and treatment of pulmonary embolism (PE)?

Advances in diagnosis of PE are seen in new-generation spiral CT scanning and MRI. The choice of imaging is based on the quality of the test center.

Treatment includes third-generation fibrolytics and safer anticoagulants, such as low-molecular-weight heparin. Indications for fibrinolysis include hypotension or right ventricular (RV) dysfunction and/or severe symptoms. The International Cooperative Pulmonary Embolism Registry reported that RV dysfunction doubled the risk of death at 3 months.

23. Is hypotension the sign I should look for to start fibrinolysis for PE?

No. Goldhaber and colleagues found that 40% of their study patients had baseline RV dysfunction on echocardiogram, but were normotensive. RV function showed striking improvement with tPa and heparin (89%) versus heparin alone (44%). Additionally, morbidity and mortality were much higher in the heparin-only group (28% versus 6%).

Other patients who may benefit from fibrinolysis are those with massive deep vein thrombosis; the treatment can help prevent reoccurrence.

Fibrinolysis for PE

	PREVIOUS NOTIONS	CURRENT THEORY
Diagnosis of PE	Mandatory pulmonary angiogram	High-probability lung scan or suggestive echocardiogram (if hypotensive, or angiogram) or chest CT scan
Indications for fibrinolysis	Systemic arterial hypotension	Hypotension or normotension with accompanying moderate or severe right ventricular hypokinesis
Time window	≤ 5 days	14 days or less
Fibrinolytic agents	SK or UK*	tPA, rPA, SK, or UK*
Dosing regimens	24 h for SK; 12–24 h for UK*	100 mg/2 h tPA; 10 U + 10 U rPA (double bolus separated by 30 minutes)
Route of administration	Pulmonary artery catheter	Peripheral vein

(Table continued on next page.)

Fibrinolysis for PE (Continued)

	PREVIOUS NOTIONS	CURRENT THEORY
Coagulation tests	DIC screens every 4–6 h during infusion	PTT at conclusion of fibrinolysis to help dose heparin
Location	Intensive care unit	Intermediate care (step-down) unit

* UK is no longer available in the United States
SK = streptokinase; UK = urokinase; tPA = alteplase; rPA = reteplase; DIC = disseminated intravascular coagulation; PTT = partial thromboplastin time
Adapted from Goldhaber SZ: Thrombolytic therapy. Adv Intern Med 44:311–325, 1999.

24. A patient is admitted for PE. The next day, an echocardiogram shows RV dysfunction. Should any treatment be added to her IV heparin?

Yes, fibrinolysis should be started. Daniels et al. found that fibrinolysis was beneficial for up to 14 days in patients with symptoms.

25. PE is rather common. Do I really need to worry about poor outcome?

Yes! PE remains the third most common cause of cardiovascular death, with 50,000 deaths in the U.S. annually. The mortality rate is > 15%. Wider use of fibrinolysis is expected to decrease not only this rate, but also recurrent PE. Moreover, striking improvement in RV function, prevention of resultant pulmonary hypertension (by preventing release of serotonin and other neurohumoral factors), and treatment of the source of thrombus in DVT may be expected.

BIBLIOGRAPHY

1. Alexander JK: Cardiac arrhythmia at high altitude: The progressive effect of aging. Tex Heart Inst J 26:258–263, 1999.
2. Badgett RG, Tanaka DJ, Hunt DK, et al: Can moderate chronic obstructive pulmonary disease be diagnosed by historical and physical findings alone? Am J Med 94:188–196, 1993.
3. Baratz DM, Westbrook PR, Shah PK, Mohsenifar Z: Effect of nasal continuous positive airway pressure on cardiac output and oxygen delivery in patients with congestive heart failure. Chest 102:1397–1401, 1992.
4. Brunnee T, Graf K, Kastens B, et al: Bronchial hyperreactivity in patients with moderate pulmonary circulation overload. Chest 103:1477–1481, 1993.
5. Daniels LB, Parker JA, et ai: Relation of duration of symptoms with response to thrombolytic therapy in pulmonary embolism. Am J Cardiol 80:184–188, 1997.
6. Ettinger NA, Trulock EP: Pulmonary considerations of organ transplantation: State of the art. Am Rev Respir Dis 144:433–451, 1991.
7. Goldhaber SZ: Thrombolytic therapy. Adv Intern Med 44:311–325, 1999.
8. Goldhaber SZ, Visani I, De Rosa M: Acute pulmonary embolism: Clinical outcomes in the International Cooperative Pulmonary Embolism Registry. Lancet 353:1386–1389, 1999.
9. Grote L, et al: Sleep-related breathing disorder is an independent risk factor for systemic hypertenstion. Am J Respir Crit Care Med 160:1875–1882, 1999.
10. Hanly P, Zuberi N, Gray R: Pathogenesis of Cheyne-Stokes respiration in patients with congestive heart failure. Chest 104:1079–1084, 1993.
11. Higgins M, Keller JB, Wagenknecht LE, et al: Pulmonary function and cardiovascular risk factor relationships in black and in white young men and women: The CARDIA Study. Chest 99:315–322, 1991.
12. Krowka MJ: Pulmonary hypertension: Diagnostics and therapeutics. Mayo Clin Proc 75:625–630, 2000.
13. McParland C, Krishnan B, Wang Y, Gallagher CG: Inspiratory muscle weakness and dyspnea in chronic heart failure. Am Rev Respir Dis 146:467–472, 1992.
14. Messner-Pellenc P, Ximenes C, Brasileiro CF, et al: Cardiopulmonary exercise testing: Determinants of dyspnea due to cardiac or pulmonary limitation. Chest 106:354–360, 1994.
15. Piirila P, Sovijarvi ARA, Kaisla T, et al: Crackles in patients with fibrosing alveolitis, bronchiectasis, COPD and heart failure. Chest 99:1076–1083, 1991.
16. Rosenow EC III, Myers JL, Swenson SJ, Pisani RJ: Drug-induced pulmonary disease: An update. Chest 102:239–250, 1992.

42. PREOPERATIVE EVALUATION FOR CARDIAC RISK

David Van Pelt, M.D., and Jeffrey Pickard, M.D.

1. What is perioperative cardiac morbidity?

It is defined as the onset of myocardial infarction (MI), unstable angina, congestive heart failure (CHF), serious dysrhythmias, or cardiac death during the intraoperative or in-hospital postoperative periods. It affects more than 1 million of the 30 million patients who undergo noncardiac surgery annually in the United States. Myocardial ischemia and infarction in the first postoperative week are the most serious risk factors for cardiovascular morbidity and mortality.

2. Which noncardiac procedures carry the highest cardiac risk?

The American College of Cardiology/American Heart Association (ACC/AHA) Task Force breaks down procedures into high-, intermediate-, and low-risk categories (see table). High-risk procedures (> 5% cardiac risk) are emergent major operations (particularly in the elderly), surgical procedures involving the aorta and other major vascular or peripheral vascular vessels, and prolonged surgical procedures associated with large fluid shifts and/or blood loss.

Risk Categories for Noncardiac Surgical Procedures*

High Risk (> 5%)
• Emergent major operations, particularly in the elderly
• Aortic and other major vascular
• Peripheral vascular
• Anticipated prolonged surgical procedures associated with large fluid shifts and/or blood loss
Intermediate Risk (< 5%)
• Carotid endarterectomy
• Head and neck
• Intraperitoneal and intrathoracic
• Orthopedic
• Prostate
Low Risk (< 1%)[†]
• Endoscopic procedures
• Superficial procedure
• Cataract
• Breast

* Combined incidence of cardiac death and nonfatal myocardial infarction.
[†] Do not generally require further preoperative cardiac testing.
Adapted from ACC/AHA Task Force Report: Guidelines for Perioperative Cardiovascular Evaluation for Noncardiac Surgery. Circulation 93(6):1278–1317, 1996.

3. Why is the risk of cardiac complications higher in vascular surgery than in other types of surgery?

Many vascular surgery patients have asymptomatic myocardial ischemia; because they are made sedentary by claudication, they are not active enough to induce angina and thus their coronary artery disease (CAD) is undiagnosed. In one study from the Cleveland Clinic, a series of 1000 patients underwent catheterization prior to vascular surgery. Only 8% had normal coronary arteries: 13% had triple or left main disease; 19% had two-vessel disease, and 27% had single-vessel disease. Increased cardiac risk is also due to advanced age of the patient population and adverse hemodynamic changes associated with aorta cross-clamping and traction on the mesentery.

4. What is the rate of perioperative reinfarction?

Risk of reinfarction is highest the first 3 months after an MI. The risk is lowest after 6 months.

A 1974 Mayo Clinic study showed that patients with a history of prior MI had a 27% risk of reinfarction if surgery was performed in the first 3 months post-MI, 11% if 3–6 months post-MI, and 4–5% if surgery was more than 6 months post-MI. A more recent study shows improved outcome. Rao et al. in 1983 found that overall reinfarction occurred in only 1.9% of patients with a prior MI. In patients less than 3 months post-MI the risk was 5.7% and at 4–6 months the risk was 2.3%. Use of better hemodynamic monitoring and more careful management of problems with electrolytes, anemia, and oxygenation are explanations for the improved patient outcome. The patients in this study had lengthy stays in the intensive care unit.

5. What are the clinical predictors of perioperative cardiac morbidity?

Several authors have established scoring systems to calculate a cardiac risk index. These include the Dripps-American Society of Anesthesiologists classification (1963), Goldman's cardiac risk index (1977), and Detsky's modified risk index (1986). Such indexes provide useful information to identify high-risk patients (see tables).

The Dripps-American Society of Anesthesiologists Classification of Physical Status[*]

1: A normal healthy patient
2: A patient with a mild systemic disease
3: A patient with a severe systemic disease that limits activity but is not incapacitating
4: A patient with an incapacitating systemic disease that is a constant threat to life
5: A moribund patient not expected to survive 24 h with or without operation

---

[*] In the event of emergency operation, precede the number with an E.
Adapted from the American Society of Anesthesiologists: New classification of physical status. Anesthesiology 24:111, 1963.

The Goldman Multifactorial Cardiac Risk Index

CRITERIA	MULTIVARIATE DISCRIMINANT-FUNCTION COEFFICIENT	POINTS
• History		
Age > 70 years	0.191	5
MI in previous 6 months	0.384	10
• Physical examination		
S_3 gallop or JVD	0.451	11
Important VAS	0.119	3
• Electrocardiogram		
Rhythm other than sinus or PACs on last preoperative ECG	0.283	7
> 5 PVCs/min documented at any time before operation	0.278	7
• General status		
Po_2 < 60 or Pco_2 > 50 mmHg, K < 3.0 or HCO_3^- < 20 meq/L, BUN > 50 or Cr > 3.0 mg/dL, abnormal SGOT, signs of chronic liver disease or patient bedridden from noncardiac causes	0.132	3
• Operation		
Intraperitoneal, intrathoracic, or aortic operation	0.123	3
Emergency operation	0.167	4
Total		53

MI = myocardial infarction, JVD = jugular-vein distention, VAS = valvular aortic stenosis, PAC = premature atrial contractions, ECG = electrocardiogram, PVC = premature ventricular contractions, Po_2 = partial pressure of oxygen, Pco_2 = partial pressure of carbon dioxide, K = potassium, HCO_3 = bicarbonate, BUN = blood urea nitrogen, Cr = creatinine, SGOT = serum glutamic oxaloacetic transaminase.
Adapted from Goldman L, Caldera DL, Nussbaum SR, et al: Multifactorial index of cardiac risk in noncardiac surgical procedures. N Engl J Med 297:845–850, 1977.

The Modified Multifactorial Cardiac Risk Index

VARIABLES	POINTS
CAD	
MI within 6 months	10
MI more than 6 months previously	5
Canadian Cardiovascular Society angina	
Class 3	10
Class 4	20
Unstable angina within 3 months	10
Alveolar pulmonary edema	
Within 1 week	10
Ever	5
Valvular disease	
Suspected critical aortic stenosis	20
Arrhythmias	
Sinus plus atrial premature beats or rhythm	5
other than sinus on last preoperative ECG	
More than 5 ventricular premature beats at any	5
time before surgery	
Poor general medical status*	5
Age over 70 years	5
Emergency operation	10

* Oxygen pressure < 60 mmHg; carbon dioxide pressure > 50 mmHg; serum potassium < 3.0 meq/L (< 3.0 mmol/L); serum bicarbonate < 20 meq/L (< 20 mmol/L); serum urea nitrogen > 50 mg/dL (> 18 mmol/L); serum creatinine > 3 mg/dL (> 260 mmol/L); aspartate aminotransferase, abnormal; signs of chronic liver disease; and/or bedridden because of noncardiac causes.

Adapted from Detsky AS, Abrams HB, Forbath N, et al: Cardiac assessment for patients undergoing noncardiac surgery. Arch Intern Med 146:2131–2134, 1986.

The more recent ACC/AHA Task Force guidelines put forth a simpler criteria by grouping predictors into major, intermediate, and minor categories.

Clinical Predictors of Increased Perioperative Cardiovascular Risk (MI, CHF, Death)

Major

Unstable coronary syndromes
  • Recent MI* with evidence of important ischemic risk by clinical symptoms or noninvasive study
  • Unstable or severe† angina (Canadian Class III or IV)

Decompensated CHF

Significant arrhythmias
  • High-grade atrioventricular block
  • Symptomatic ventricular arrhythmias in the presence of underlying heart disease
  • Supraventricular arrhythmias with uncontrolled ventricular rate

Severe valvular disease

Intermediate

Mild angina pectoris (Canadian Class I or II)

Prior myocardial infarction by history or pathological Q waves

Compensated or prior congestive heart failure

Diabetes mellitus

(*Table continued on next page.*)

Clinical Predictors of Increased Perioperative Cardiovascular Risk (MI, CHF, Death) (cont.)

Minor

Advanced age

Abnormal EKG (left ventricular hypertrophy, left bundle branch block, ST-T abnormalities)

Rhythm other than sinus (e.g., atrial fibrillation)

Low functional capacity (e.g., inability to climb one flight of stairs with a bag of groceries)

History of stroke

Uncontrolled systemic hypertension

EKG = electrocardiogram.

* The American College of Cardiology National Database Library defines recent MI as > 7 days but ≤ 1 month (30 days).

† May include "stable" angina in patients who are unusually sedentary.

Adapted from ACC/AHA Task Force Report: Guidelines for Perioperative Cardiovascular Evaluation for Noncardiac Surgery. Circulation 93(6):1278–1317, 1996.

6. Describe the limitations of using a cardiac risk index.

To use a risk index accurately, the clinician must define perioperative MI using the same method as the authors who developed the index. Also, these indexes only predict cardiac morbidity, not overall patient morbidity. A more significant problem, however, is their limited sensitivity for identifying significant CAD in patients with low cardiac risk.

7. Which patients should undergo preoperative cardiac testing?

The ACC/AHA Task Force has proposed an algorithm for cardiac assessment. A series of questions is used as a guide for the evaluation (see figure, next page):

Step 1. What is the urgency of noncardiac surgery?

Step 2. Has the patient undergone coronary revascularization in the past 5 years?

Step 3. Has the patient had a coronary evaluation in the past 2 years?

Step 4. Does the patient have an unstable coronary syndrome or a major clinical predictor of risk?

Step 5. Does the patient have intermediate clinical predictors of risk?

Step 6. Patients without major but with intermediate predictors of clinical risk and moderate or excellent functional capacity can generally undergo intermediate-risk surgery with little likelihood of perioperative death or MI. Conversely, further noninvasive testing is often considered for patients with poor functional capacity or moderate functional capacity but higher-risk surgery and especially for patients with two or more intermediate predictors.

Step 7. Noncardiac surgery is generally safe for patients with neither major nor intermediate predictors of clinical risk and moderate or excellent functional capacity (4 METs or greater). Further testing may be considered on an individual basis for patients without clinical markers but poor functional capacity who are facing higher-risk operations, particularly those with several minor clinical predictors of risk who are to undergo vascular surgery.

Step 8. The results of noninvasive testing can be used to determine further preoperative management.

8. When should a prior cardiac work-up be repeated?

After 2 years; or in the event of increasing frequency or severity of cardiac symptoms; or if new clinical findings (changes) are noted on EKG.

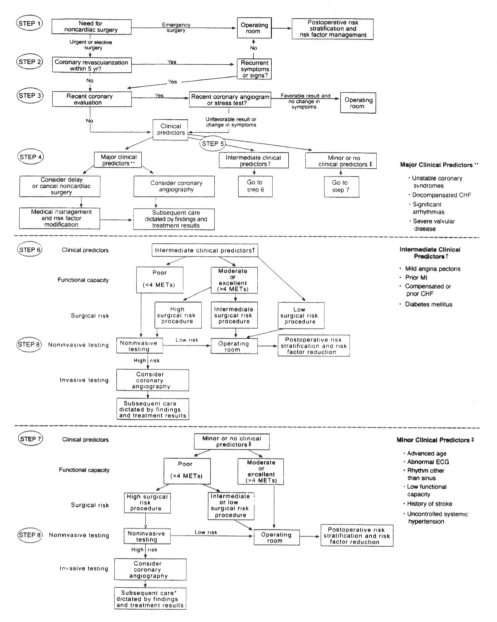

ACC/AHA algorithm for cardiac assessment. (From ACC/AHA Task Force Report: Guidelines for Perioperative Cardiovascular Evaluation for Noncardiac Surgery. Circulation 93(6):1278–1317, 1996 ; with permission.)

9. What is the value of the history in assessing functional status?

Patients without major clinical predictors who can accomplish tasks requiring more than 4 METs can undergo intermediate- or low-risk procedures without further testing (see table, next page).

10. Who needs a preoperative EKG?

A preoperative EKG is indicated in all patients over age 40 and in younger patients with cardiovascular risk factors. Special indications include emergency operations, conditions that affect cardiac function, medications that can alter the EKG, risk for major electrolyte disorders, and neurosurgery, intrathoracic surgery, or aortic surgery.

The preoperative EKG is useful for postoperative comparison in the event of complications. Undiagnosed MI is found on up to 4% of EKGs. Other important findings include ventricular hypertrophy, conduction abnormalities, and nonspecific ST-T changes.

Estimated Energy Requirements for Various Activities

| 1 MET | Can you take care of yourself? Eat, dress, or use the toilet? Walk indoors around the house? Walk a block or two on level ground at 2–3 mph or 3.2–4.8 km/h? Do light work around the house like dusting or washing dishes? | 4 METs | Climb a flight of stairs or walk up a hill? Walk on level ground at 4 mph or 6.4 km/h? Run a short distance? Do heavy work around the house like scrubbing floors or lifting or moving heavy furniture? Participate in moderate recreational activities like golf, bowling, dancing, doubles tennis, or throwing a baseball or football? |
| 4 METs | | > 10 METs | Participate in strenuous sports like swimming, singles tennis, football, basketball, or skiing? |

MET = metabolic equivalent.
Adapted from ACC/AHA Task Force Report: Guidelines for Perioperative Cardiovascular Evaluation for Noncardiac Surgery. Circulation 93(6):1278–1317, 1996.

11. Which preoperative tests are preferred in assessing cardiac risk?

The optimal test depends on individual patient characteristics. A meta-analysis comparing dipyridamole thallium scanning, dobutamine stress echocardiography, radionuclide ventriculography, and ambulatory EKG to assess cardiac risk in vascular surgery showed that they all had a similar predictive value.

In ambulatory patients the test of choice is exercise EKG testing. It can provide information about both functional capacity and risk for MI. Those with abnormalities on resting EKG (e.g., left bundle branch block or left ventricular hypertrophy [LVH] with strain pattern) should undergo additional imaging such as exercise echocardiogram or a myocardial perfusion study.

Patients unable to exercise are often tested by dipyridamole thallium imaging or dobutamine echocardiography. Dipyridamole should be avoided in patients with significant bronchospasm, those requiring theophylline, and patients with critical carotid stenosis. Dobutamine should be avoided in patients with arrhythmias, severe hypertension, or hypotension.

12. How is vasodilator myocardial imaging done?

The technique involves administration of a vasodilator (usually dipyridamole) and a contrast agent (**thallium-201**), followed by myocardial perfusion scanning. Intravenous **dipyridamole** dilates normal coronary arteries by enhancing their sensitivity to adenosine, a potent coronary artery dilator. Stenotic or occluded vessels remain unaffected. After dipyridamole is infused, thallium-201 is injected, and myocardial scanning is done immediately and 4 hours later. Patients with adequate myocardial perfusion have normal scans. Patients with defects on the initial scan and no defects after 4 hours have ischemic myocardium. Perfusion defects that do not change after 4 hours usually indicate old infarction.

Adenosine-thallium scanning appears to be equally accurate in predicting perioperative risk. It may have an advantage over dipyridamole-thallium scanning because adenosine is rapidly metabolized and so side effects are transient. However, adenosine causes a higher incidence of chest pain.

13. When is preoperative coronary revascularization indicated?

Coronary artery bypass grafting (CABG) should only be performed when a patient's symptoms or coronary anatomy would benefit from revascularization. This includes patients with left main disease, three-vessel CAD with LV dysfunction, two-vessel disease involving severe proximal LAD obstruction, and patients with intractable angina despite maximal medical management.

The operative mortality of patients with significant CAD undergoing noncardiac surgery is 2.4%. This is comparable to the 2.3% combined risk of coronary revascularization followed by noncardiac surgery. Therefore, prophylactic CABG is *not* routinely indicated prior to noncardiac surgery.

14. How long is coronary revascularization protective from perioperative MI or death?
Follow-up data from the Coronary Artery Surgery Study shows that revascularization is protective for at least 6 years.

15. What is the value of perioperative cardiovascular medication?
Atenolol use beginning preoperatively and continued up to 7 days postoperatively has been shown to reduce the incidence of cardiovascular complications for as long as 2 years following surgery. **Nitroglycerin** and **calcium channel blockers** have also been studied, but the trials are smaller and not as convincing. Intraoperative nitroglycerin is indicated for high-risk patients previously on nitroglycerin who have evidence of myocardial ischemia and are not hypotensive.

16. How is a patient with a prosthetic valve managed perioperatively?
If cardiac function is relatively normal, there are two major risks to which patients with prosthetic valves are exposed: infective endocarditis and thromboembolism.
Individuals with a prosthetic cardiac valve (including bioprosthetic and homograft) are in a high-risk category for development of bacterial endocarditis. (For information on procedures for which endocarditis prophylaxis is recommended and prophylactic regimens, see tables.)

Nondental Procedures

ENDOCARDITIS PROPHYLAXIS RECOMMENDED	ENDOCARDITIS PROPHYLAXIS NOT RECOMMENDED
• Respiratory tract	• Respiratory tract
Tonsillectomy and/or adenoidectomy	Endotracheal intubation
Surgical operations that involve respiratory	Bronchoscopy with a flexible bronchoscope,
mucosa	with or without biopsy[†]
Bronchoscopy with a rigid bronchoscope	Tympanostomy tube insertion
• Gastrointestinal tract[*]	• Gastrointestinal tract
Sclerotherapy for esophageal varices	Transesophageal echocardiography[†]
Esophageal stricture dilation	Endoscopy with or with gastrointestinal biopsy[†]
Endoscopic retrograde cholangiography with	• Genitourinary tract
biliary obstruction	Vaginal hysterectomy[†]
Biliary tract surgery	Vaginal delivery[†]
Surgical operations that involve intestinal	Cesarean section
mucosa	In uninfected tissue:
• Genitourinary tract	Urethral catheterization
Prostatic surgery	Uterine dilatation and curettage
Cystoscopy	Therapeutic abortion
Urethral dilation	Sterilization procedures
	Insertion or removal of intrauterine devices
	• Other
	Cardiac catheterization, including balloon
	angioplasty
	Implanted cardiac pacemakers, implanted
	defibrillators, and coronary stents
	Incision or biopsy of surgically scrubbed skin
	Circumcision

[*] Prophylaxis is recommended for high-risk patients; optional for medium-risk patients.
[†] Prophylaxis is optional for high-risk patients.
Adapted from Dajani AS, Taubert KA, Wilson W, et al: Prevention of bacterial endocarditis: Recommendations by the American Heart Association. JAMA 277(2):1794–1801, 1997.

Prophylactic Regimens for Dental, Oral, Respiratory Tract, or Esophageal Procedures

	DRUG	REGIMEN*
Standard general prophylaxis	Amoxicillin	Adults: 2.0 g; children: 50 mg/kg orally 1 h before procedure
Unable to take oral medications	Ampicillin	Adults: 2.0 g intramuscularly (IM) or intravenously (IV); children: 50 mg/kg IM or IV within 30 min before procedure
Allergic to penicillin	Clindamycin *or*	Adults: 600 mg; children: 20 mg/kg orally 1 h before procedure
	Cephalexin† or cefadroxil† *or*	Adults: 2.0 g; children: 50 mg/kg orally 1 h before procedure
	Azithromycin or clarithromycin	Adults: 500 mg; children: 15 mg/kg orally 1 h before procedure
Allergic to penicillin and unable to take oral medications	Clindamycin *or*	Adults: 600 mg; children: 20 mg/kg IV within 30 min before procedure
	Cefazolin†	Adults: 1.0 g; children: 25 mg/kg IM or IV within 30 min before procedure

* Total children's dose should not exceed adult dose.
† Cephalosporins should not be used in individuals with immediate-type hypersensitivity reaction (urticaria, angioedema, or anaphylaxis) to penicillins.
Adapted from Dajani AS, Taubert KA, Wilson W, et al: Prevention of bacterial endocarditis: Recommendations by the American Heart Association. JAMA 277(2):1794–1801, 1997.

Prophylactic Regimens for Genitourinary Gastrointestinal (Excluding Esophageal) Procedures

	DRUGS*	REGIMEN†
High-risk patients	Ampicillin plus Gentamicin	Adults: ampicillin 2.0 g intramuscularly (IM) or intravenously (IV) plus gentamicin 1.5 mg/kg (not to exceed 120 mg) within 30 min of starting the procedure; 6 h later, ampicillin 1 g IM/IV or amoxicillin 1 g orally Children: ampicillin 50 mg/kg IM or IV (not to exceed 2.0 g) plus gentamicin 1.5 mg/kg within 30 min of starting the procedure; 6 h later, ampicillin 25 mg/kg IM/IV or amoxicillin 25 mg/kg orally
High risk patients allergic to ampicillin/amoxicillin	Vancomycin plus Gentamicin	Adults: vancomycin 1.0 g IV over 1–2 h plus gentamicin 1.5 mg/kg IV/IM (not to exceed 120 mg); complete injection/infusion within 30 min of starting the procedure Children: vancomycin 20 mg/kg IV over 1–2 h plus gentamicin 1.5 mg/kg IV/IM; complete injection/infusion within 30 min of starting the procedure
Moderate-risk patients	Amoxicillin or Ampicillin	Adults: amoxicillin 2.0 g orally 1 h before procedure, or ampicillin 2.0 g IM/IV within 30 min of starting the procedure Children: amoxicillin 50 mg/kg orally 1 h before procedure, or ampicillin 50 mg/kg IM/IV within 30 min of starting procedure

(Table continued on next page.)

Prophylactic Regimens for Genitourinary Gastrointestinal (Excluding Esophageal) Procedures (cont.)

	DRUGS*	REGIMEN†
Moderate-risk patients allergic to ampicillin/amoxicillin	Vancomycin	Adults: vancomycin 1.0 g IV over 1–2 h; complete infusion within 30 min of starting the procedure Children: vancomycin 20 mg/kg IV over 1–2 h; complete infusion within 30 min of starting the procedure

* Total children's dose should not exceed adult dose.
† No second dose of vancomycin or gentamicin is recommended.
Adapted from Dajani AS, Taubert KA, Wilson W, et al: Prevention of bacterial endocarditis: Recommendations by the American Heart Association. JAMA 277(2):1794–1801, 1997.

Patients on oral anticoagulation for a prosthetic heart valve or atrial fibrillation should have four doses held if INR is 2–3, or longer if INR is > 3. Generally an INR of 1.5 is acceptable for surgery. Vitamin K 1 mg subcutaneously is recommended for a preoperative INR of 1.8 or greater.

In patients with a history of recent arterial embolism, elective surgery should be avoided for the first month after the event. The risk of acute arterial embolism 1 month after an initial event is 15%. If surgery cannot be postponed, then IV heparin should be started when the INR is < 2. Anticoagulation is reversed using protamine sulfate immediately before surgery. IV heparin is also recommended for patients with a prosthetic valve that causes a high risk of thrombosis, such as a caged-ball valve.

17. What type of anesthesia is the safest?

It is a common misconception that spinal anesthesia is safer and better tolerated than general anesthesia. Both confer equal risks of postoperative fatal and nonfatal MI. Regional or local anesthesia may be less risky than the same procedure done under general or spinal anesthesia. The type of anesthesia is best determined by the anesthesiologist.

18. How does postoperative MI present?

The incidence of postoperative MI after noncardiac surgery in the general population is 0–0.7%, and 1.1% in patients with CAD. Most perioperative MIs occur in the first 4 days postoperatively and are often clinically silent. Studies have shown a tendency for non-Q-wave infarction to occur in the first 48 hours. Q-wave infarctions tend to occur later, in days 3 to 5, when the patient is in a hypercoaguable state. One study by Hollenberg et al. identified five major preoperative risk factors in men associated with postoperative ischemia: EKG evidence of LVH, history of hypertension, diabetes mellitus, definite CAD, and use of digoxin.

BIBLIOGRAPHY

1. American Society of Anesthesiologists: New classification of physical status. Anesthesiology 24:111, 1963.
2. Dajani AS, et al: Prevention of bacterial endocarditis: Recommendations by the American Heart Association. JAMA 277:1794–1801, 1997.
3. Detsky AS, Abrams HB, Forbath N, et al: Cardiac assessment for patients undergoing noncardiac surgery. Arch Intern Med 146:2131–2134, 1986.
4. Eagle KA, Charanjit SR, et al: Cardiac risk of noncardiac surgery: Influence of coronary disease and type of surgery in 3368 operations. Circulation 96:1882–1887, 1997.
4a. Foster ED, Davis KB, Carpenter JA, et al: Risk of noncardiac operation in patients with defined coronary disease: The Coronary Artery Surgery Study (CASS) registry experience. Ann Thorac Surg 41:42–50, 1986.
5. Goldman L, Caldera DL, Nussbaum SR, et al: Multifactorial index of cardiac risk in noncardiac surgical procedures. N Engl J Med 297:845–850, 1977.
6. Granieri R, MacPherson DS: Perioperative care of the vascular surgery patient: The perspective of the internist. J Gen Intern Med 7:102–113, 1992.

7. Kearon C, Hirsch J: Management of anticoagulation before and after elective surgery. N Engl J Med 336:1506–1511, 1997.
8. Mangano DT: Perioperative cardiac morbidity. Anesthesiology 72:153–184, 1990.
9. Mangano DT, Layug EL, et al: Effect of atenolol on mortality and cardiovascular morbidity after noncardiac surgery. N Engl J Med 335:1713–1720, 1996.
10. Massie BM, Mangano DT: Assessment of perioperative risk: Have we put the cart before the horse? J Am Coll Cardiol 21:1353–1356, 1993.
11. Massie BM, Mangano DT: Risk stratification for noncardiac surgery: How and why? Circulation 87:1752–1755, 1993.
12. Report of the American College of Cardiology/American Heart Association Task Force on Practical Guidelines (Committee on Perioperative Cardiovascular Evaluation for Noncardiac Surgery): Guidelines for perioperative cardiovascular evaluation for noncardiac surgery. J Am Coll Cardiol 27:910–948, 1996 and Circulation 93:1278–1317, 1996.
13. Schlant RC, Eagle KA: Perioperative evaluation and management of patients with known or suspected cardiovascular disease who undergo noncardiac surgery. In Alexander RW, Schlant RC, Fuster V (eds): Hurst's The Heart: Arteries and Veins, 9th ed. New York, McGraw-Hill, 1998, pp 2243–2255.

43. RHEUMATIC HEART DISEASE AND MITRAL STENOSIS

Rajesh Bhola, M.D., and Edward A. Gill, M.D.

1. What causes most cases of mitral stenosis?

Rheumatic heart disease.

2. What is rheumatic fever?

Rheumatic fever is an acute, systemic, inflammatory disease that occurs as a reaction to a recent streptococcal soft-tissue infection, most commonly pharyngitis.

3. How long does it take from the onset of rheumatic fever until mitral stenosis develops?

It can be as short as 2 years. Progression seems to be particularly rapid in developing countries, for reasons which are not entirely understood but could relate to the lack of appropriate penicillin treatment of rheumatic fever or nutritional factors.

4. What are the Jones criteria?

The Jones criteria are guidelines for making the diagnosis of an initial attack of rheumatic fever. There is a high likelihood that the disease is present if there is supporting evidence of antecedent group A streptococcal infection (positive throat culture, positive rapid streptococcal antigen test, elevated or rising streptococcal antibody titer), as well as either two major or one major plus two minor manifestations.

Major manifestations	*Minor manifestations*
Carditis	Arthralgia
Polyarthritis	Fever
Chorea	Elevated sedimentation rate
Erythema marginatum	Elevated C-reactive protein
Subcutaneous nodules	Prolonged PR interval

5. Besides mitral stenosis, how does rheumatic disease affect the heart?

Aortic regurgitation is the second most common lesion, followed by mitral regurgitation and aortic stenosis. The tricuspid valve is less commonly involved, either with stenosis or regurgitation. Involvement of the pulmonary valve is rare. Constrictive pericarditis is thought not to be a sequela to rheumatic fever.

6. What are the typical symptoms of mitral stenosis?

Dyspnea on exertion is the classic presenting symptom. However, mitral stenosis can present with an arrhythmia, such as atrial fibrillation, or a systemic embolic event, since left atrial thrombi are common in mitral stenosis.

7. What are less typical presentations?

Severe mitral stenosis can present as pulmonary edema or severe right-sided heart failure if pulmonary pressures become severely elevated. Approximately 15% of patients with mitral stenosis experience angina. Although this symptom may arise from right ventricular hypertension, concomitant atherosclerosis, or embolization of a left atrial thrombus to a coronary artery, in many cases the explanation for chest pain in mitral stenosis cannot be determined.

8. What are the physical findings in mitral stenosis?

Most notable are a loud S_1, an opening snap early in diastole, followed by a diastolic murmur that is mostly decrescendo. By phonocardiogram, the murmur actually has two brief crescendo periods, the first just after the opening snap and the second with atrial contraction. These periods of crescendo murmur correspond to the two periods of the greater transvalular gradient in diastole.

9. Why is the first heart sound (S_1) accentuated?

The explanation for this is uncertain. McCall and others have suggested that the mitral valve leaflets must be pliable for the S_1 to be accentuated. The accentuated S_1 then is caused in part by the rapidity of the upstroke of the left ventricular pressure at the time of mitral valve closure. In addition, the wide excursion or displacement of the mitral valve leaflets prior to closure is felt to play a role in the accentuated S_1. Marked calcification or thickening of the mitral valve reduces the amplitude of S_1. Finally, the presystolic accentuation of mitral blood flow caused by atrial contraction blends into S_1 and may contribute to the perceived accentuation.

10. What are the hemodynamic findings in mitral stenosis?

The most important finding is the presence of a pressure gradient across the mitral valve. That is, during diastole, the pressure in the left atrium is greater than the pressure in the left ventricle. This gradient is measured by recording the left ventricular diastolic pressure simultaneously with the pulmonary capillary wedge pressure (PAW). The PAW is used as a close approximation of the left atrial pressure. The mean gradient across the mitral valve can then be determined, and with the Gorlin formula, the valve area (in cm^2) can be calculated:

$$\text{Valve area} = \frac{\text{Cardiac output/(heart rate} \times \text{avg. diastolic period)}}{37.7 \times \sqrt{\text{mean gradient}}}$$

(Note: 37.7 is a constant empirically derived for the mitral valve.)

11. Describe the echocardiographic findings in mitral stenosis.

M-mode echocardiography. The most specific finding by M-mode echocardiography is the posterior mitral valve leaflet moving in an anterior direction with the anterior mitral valve leaflet in diastole. This demonstrates the tethering of the valve leaflets caused by fusion of the commissures (Fig. 1). Other, less specific findings include increased echoes from the mitral valve due to thickening or calcification and decreased E-F slope due to low flow across the mitral valve (Fig. 1). Decreased E-F slope is a frequent finding in severe heart failure and could be confused with mitral stenosis in this setting.

Two-dimensional echocardiography. The findings of mitral stenosis include diastolic bowing ("hockey stick" formation) of the anterior mitral leaflet (Figs. 2 and 3); thickening and increased echogenicity of the mitral valve leaflets, annulus, and subvalvular apparatus (Fig. 4); and narrowed orifice of the valve as measured by short axis. The actual valve area can be measured by two-dimensional echocardiography in the short-axis view (Fig. 5). It also allows estimates of chamber size and pulmonary artery pressure, and an indication of presence or absence of associated valvular abnormalities.

Doppler echocardiography. Findings in mitral stenosis include an elevated velocity across the mitral valve (> 1.3 m/sec or 130 cm/sec), indicating an abnormally high transvalvular gradient, and prolonged pressure half-time.

12. How is the pressure half-time calculated from Doppler echocardiography?

The pressure half-time is the time required for the peak transvalvular pressure gradient to be reduced by one-half and is quantitatively related to the degree of mitral stenosis. The pressure gradient is measured by calculating the velocity of flow across the mitral valve and converting the velocity to pressure, using the modified Bernoulli equation: $P = 4V^2$, where P = pressure and V = velocity of flow. Figure 6 shows a typical velocity envelope across the mitral valve. The maximum velocity is 207 cm/sec. A normal pressure half-time is about 70 msec. In severe mitral stenosis, the pressure half-time is > 200 msec. The mitral valve area can be calculated using the formula MVA = 220/pressure half-time. For example in a patient with severe mitral stenosis, the pressure half-time might be 250 ms and the MVA = 220/250, or 0.7 cm^2.

FIGURE 1.   M-mode echocardiogram obtained from the parasternal long-axis view at the level of the mitral valve. *A*, The posterior and anterior mitral valve leaflets (PMVL, AMVL) can be seen tracking together. The posterior leaflet moves anterior (toward the top of the figure) during diastole. Ordinarily, the posterior leaflet should move posterior when it opens. Note that the E-F slope is markedly reduced compared to that seen in *B*, an example of a normal mitral valve. This is a semiquantitative measure to show that the mitral valve does not open briskly during diastole.

13. How do regurgitant lesions affect the calculation of valve area?

The presence of severe aortic regurgitation will cause a slight underestimation of the severity of the mitral stenosis (overestimation of the valve area) determined by Doppler pressure half-time,

FIGURE 2. Parasternal long-axis view of the left atrium (LA), left ventricle (LV), and mitral valve. Note the diastolic bowing of the anterior mitral valve leaflet (*arrow*).

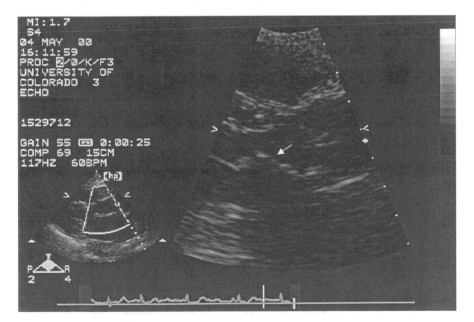

FIGURE 3. Enlarged view of the mitral valve (same patient as in Figure 3), with arrow again depicting the bowing ("hockey stick" appearance) of the anterior mitral valve leaflet.

because the gradient between the left atrium and left ventricle decreases faster due to the aortic regurgitation (hence a shorter pressure half-time). On the other hand, the valve area as determined by cardiac catheterization will tend to overestimate the severity of the mitral stenosis

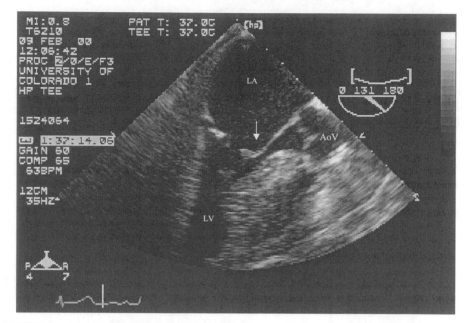

FIGURE 4. Transesophageal view of a patient with mitral stenosis. Note that both the mitral valve leaflets are thickened and again there is bowing of the anterior leaflet (*arrow*). LA = left atrium, LV = left ventricle, AoV = aortic valve.

FIGURE 5. Short axis view of the left ventricle at the level of the mitral valve. The orifice of the mitral valve can be measured by planimetry.

(underestimate the valve area), because the cardiac output is in the numerator of the Gorlin equation. The cardiac output used in the formula often is the forward cardiac output measured by the Fick equation and therefore does not take into account the regurgitant volume, underestimating

FIGURE 6. Continuous-wave Doppler measurement of mean and peak velocity (207 cm/sec and 119 cm/sec, respectively), mean and peak pressure gradients (17.1 mmHg and 6.6 mmHg, respectively), and pressure half-time (P$\frac{1}{2}$ time) of 153 msec resulting in a valve area (220/P$\frac{1}{2}$ time) of 1.43 cm^2.

the flow across the valve. Also the mean gradient across the valve will be overestimated when there is significant regurgitation because flow across the valve will increase. Since the mean gradient is in the denominator of the Gorlin equation, the valve area will be underestimated and, again, the severity of the valvular stenosis will be overestimated. Mitral regurgitation does not affect the pressure half-time significantly, but it does affect the Gorlin area, as with aortic regurgitation.

14. What is a normal mitral valve area? When is the mitral valve orifice small enough to warrant surgical or other intervention?
A normal mitral valve orifice is 4–6 cm^2, and intervention is usually considered warranted when the orifice is ≤ 1.0 cm^2. However, some patients with valve areas of 1.0–1.5 cm^2 may have pulmonary hypertension or exertional dyspnea, warranting intervention.

15. What treatment options are available?
  • Surgical (open) commissurotomy where the fused commissures are surgically split
  • Balloon mitral valvotomy (i.e., done with percutaneous balloon technique) (Figs. 7, 8, and 9)
  • Surgical replacement of the valve with either metallic prosthetic valve or bioprosthetic valve
Percutaneous mitral valvotomy (PMV) is a preferred method in most cases of mitral stenosis. PMV is advantageous because of the lower cost, elimination of thoracotomy and cardiopulmonary bypass during surgery, and comparable immediate and long-term results to surgical commissurotomy. PMV has a clear advantage in cases where surgical risk is high.
Patients with severe subvalvular thickening or fusion, heavy calcification, and poor mitral valve mobility (i.e., a high valve score) are best treated with surgical valve replacement.

16. List the complications of PMV.
  • PMV resulted in severe mitral regurgitation in 4–6% of cases in one large series of patients.
  • Left-to-right interatrial shunt is detectable by Doppler echocardiography in 10% of patients, but this is rarely clinically significant and typically resolves in the months after the procedure.

FIGURE 7.   Transesophageal view of the left atrial appendage (LAA) showing spontaneous echo contrast ("smoke") in the appendage but no discrete thrombus. Transesophageal echocardiography to rule out left atrial/left atrial appendage thrombus is mandatory prior to percutaneous mitral valvotomy.

FIGURE 8.   Short-axis view of the left ventricle at the mitral valve level showing the stenotic mitral valve pre–balloon valvotomy (*left*) and post–balloon valvotomy (*right*). Arrows depict the fused commissures.

- Clinical restenosis of the mitral valve may occur but is quite uncommon, particularly if the postprocedure valve area is > 1.8 cm^2.
- Cerebral embolic events also may occur but are exceedingly rare. Preprocedure transesophageal echocardiography (TEE) identifies those with left atrial thrombosis who should not have the procedure until the thrombus is resolved, typically by 3 months of anticoagulation.

17. When is PMV contraindicated?
- Left atrial thrombus. Most patients (at the authors' institution) undergo routine TEE prior to surgical or percutaneous commissurotomy (see Figure 7).
- Moderate-to-severe mitral regurgitation (> 2+ angiographically)
- Need for other cardiac surgery, such as severe aortic stenosis, severe tricuspid regurgitation, and severe coronary artery disease (left main stenosis or equivalent)

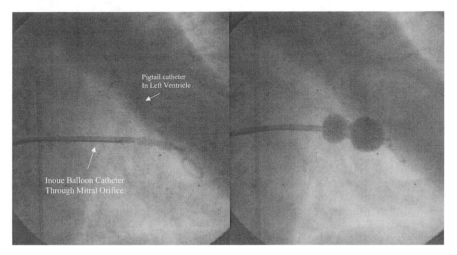

FIGURE 9.   Radiograph of the single Inoue balloon prior to (*left*) and during (*right*) inflation. Note the "dog-bone" appearance of the balloon as it is blown up with the stenotic mitral valve surrounding it.

18. What are the predictors of late clinical outcomes after PMV?

PMV has become an established nonsurgical treatment for mitral stenosis. Therefore, it is important to be able to detect factors that may identify patients who are likely to benefit from this procedure. Benefit (i.e., success of the procedure) can be stratified by early (1–5 years) or late event free survival (no mitral valve repair, no death).

Outcome Predictors of PMV

BEFORE THE PROCEDURE*	AFTER THE PROCEDURE
Age	Valve area
Atrial fibrillation	Mean valve gradient
New York Heart Association functional classification	Mitral regurgitation
Echo score (based on degree of valve deformity)	
Prior surgical or percutaneous commissurotomy	

* Note that none of these predictors is strong, particularly of early results. The echo score only weakly correlates with 5-year event-free survival.

19. What are the indications to perform PMV?

- Symptomatic patient
- Wilkens echo score of 8 or less with no left atrial thrombus
- Hemodynamically severe stenosis
- Elderly patients with other medical risk factors
- Associated ischemic heart diseases
- Pregnancy with symptomatic mitral stenosis
- Asymptomatic patients who have (1) at least moderate mitral stenosis, (2) suitable valve morphology for PMV who are about to undergo major physiologic stress (pregnancy, major noncardiac surgery), or (3) physiologic evidence of important mitral stenosis (e.g., pulmonary hypertension)

20. What echocardiographic parameters are used to predict the success of mitral valvuloplasty?

The mitral valve is more amenable to valvuloplasty if the valve is pliable and the valve and subvalvular apparatus are not severely calcified or thickened. An echocardiographic grading system has been developed by Weyman et al. based on valve mobility, thickening or calcification, and subvalvular thickening. Each of these four variables is assigned a score from 1 to 4 (4 being most severe), with a maximum score of 16. In general, a score of 8 or less suggests that the valve would respond well to valvuloplasty. The presence of more-than-mild mitral regurgitation precludes valvuloplasty, because in most cases this procedure will increase the degree of mitral regurgitation.

21. What is the role of an exercise evaluation in a patient with mitral stenosis?

One of the most common clinical applications of simultaneous exercise and hemodynamic measurements is in the patient with mitral stenosis and borderline resting measurements. Exercising such a patient to the level of a symptomatic state with simultaneous Doppler measurement of mitral valve gradient and pulmonary artery pressure (or similar measurements made in the catheterization laboratory) may better elucidate the physiologic severity of the mitral valvular disease. With regard to Doppler measurements of pulmonary artery pressures and mitral gradients with exercise, performing exercise with a bicycle ergometer is useful in order to obtain measurements at true peak exercise (as opposed to post-treadmill walking).

22. What is the emerging role of three-dimensional echocardiography in the diagnosis and management of mitral stenosis?

- Improved visualization and evaluation of degree and length of commissural fusion
- Evaluation of mitral valve in situ using surgeon's view of mitral valve from the left atrium
- ? Equivalent or better predictor of outcomes from PMV—still to be resolved
- ? Quantitation of mitral regurgitation by regurgitant volume

 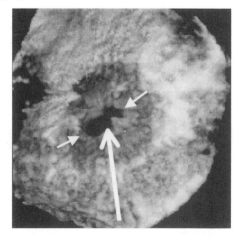

FIGURE 10. Three dimensional echocardiography showing the stenotic mitral valve viewed from the left atrial side. The large arrow points to the valve orifice; small arrows point to the fused commissures.

FIGURE 11. Three-dimensional echocardiography showing the stenotic mitral valve viewed from the left ventricular side. Large arrow points to valve orifice, and small arrows point to the fused commissures.

23. What are the other causes of mitral stenosis besides rheumatic heart disease?

Congenital mitral stenosis is the second most common cause of mitral stenosis and is far less frequent than rheumatic fever. Rarely, mitral stenosis can be a complication of malignant carcinoid, systemic lupus erythematosus, rheumatoid arthritis, and the mucopolysaccharidoses of the Hunter-Hurler phenotype. Two obscure causes of mitral stenosis are eosinophilic fibroelastosis and the drug methysergide (a vasodilator used for headaches), which is now rarely, if ever, used. Degenerative mitral annular calcification also can cause stenosis.

24. What myocardial tumor can mimic mitral stenosis?

Atrial myxoma, specifically left atrial myxoma, can present with similar findings on physical examination, including a diastolic rumble and a loud S_1. An opening snap is characteristically absent. The presence of systemic symptoms, such as fever, arthralgia, malaise, cachexia, rash, and Raynaud's phenomenon, can be clues to the presence of myxoma.

25. What is the NAME syndrome?

This syndrome is the association of:

N = Nevi
A = Atrial myxoma
M = Myxoid neurofibromas
E = Ephelides (freckles)

The syndrome is inherited with an autosomal dominant pattern. Seven percent of all atrial myxomata are inherited.

26. What is Ortner's syndrome?

Hoarseness caused by a dilated left atrium compressing the left recurrent laryngeal nerve.

27. What is Lutembacher's syndrome?

It is the combination of mitral stenosis and atrial septal defect. The significance of this lesion is the presence of a left-to-right shunt that is increased by worsening severity of mitral stenosis. In addition, the mitral valve gradient and pressure half-time will be inaccurate because of rapid deterioration of the pressure gradient due to left atrial–to–right atrial shunting.

ACKNOWLEDGMENT

The author thanks Doug Voorhees and Sue Rainguet for preparation of the echocardiography figures, and Dr. John Carroll for his help reviewing the manuscript.

BIBLIOGRAPHY

1. Ben Farhat M, Ayari M, Maatouk F, et al: Percutaneous balloon versus surgical closed and open mitral commissurotomy: Seven-year follow-up results of a randomized trial. Circulation 97:245–250, 1998.
2. Gorlin R, Gorlin G: Hydraulic formula for calculation of area of stenotic mitral valve, other cardiac valves and central circulatory shunts. Am Heart J 41:1, 1951.
3. Hernandez R, Banuelos C, Alfonso F, et al: Long-term clinical and echocardiographic follow-up after percutaneous mitral valvuloplasty with the Inoue balloon. Circulation 99:1580–1586, 1999.
4. Iung B, Garbarz E, Michaud P, et al: Late result of percutaneous mitral commissurotomy in a series of 1024 patients: Analysis of late clinical deterioration: Frequency, anatomic findings, and predictive factors. Circulation 99:3272–3278, 1999.
5. Narula J, Chandrasekhar Y, Rahimtoola S: Diagnosis of active rheumatic carditis: The echoes of change. Circulation 100:1576–1581, 1999.
6. Reyes VP, Raju BS, Wynne J, et al: Percutaneous balloon valvuloplasty compared with open surgical commissurotomy for mitral stenosis. N Engl J Med 331:961–966, 1994.

V. Valvular Heart Disease

44. AORTIC STENOSIS AND REGURGITATION

Edward P. Havranek, M.D., and Olivia V. Adair, M.D.

1. What is the classic triad of symptoms in significant aortic stenosis?
Dyspnea, syncope, and angina.

2. What are the usual physical findings in aortic stenosis?
The hallmark of aortic stenosis is a **crescendo-decrescendo systolic murmur**. This murmur is heard best at the upper right or left sternal border, radiates to the carotids, and is harsh. The murmur of significant aortic stenosis typically is at least III/VI in intensity; in severe stenosis with left ventricular (LV) systolic failure, the murmur may be less intense.

The **carotid pulses** offer important clues in the diagnosis of aortic stenosis. As the valvular disease progresses, the carotid upstroke becomes slowed, the contour sustained, and the amplitude small. In elderly patients, however, relatively inelastic arteries may make the pulse seem normal even in severe disease.

Palpation of the precordium may demonstrate the findings of left ventricular hypertrophy (LVH)—a sustained, forceful apical impulse and a palpable atrial filling wave.

The **second heart sound** (actually the aortic component of S2) is diminished in intensity. In aortic stenosis caused by a congenitally bicuspid valve, an ejection sound may be heard.

In advanced disease, when systolic dysfunction occurs, the findings of **congestive heart failure** are present: a displaced apical impulse, rales, jugular venous distension, hepatomegaly, and the like.

3. Which noninvasive tests are useful in evaluating suspected significant aortic stenosis?
The single most useful test is **Doppler echocardiography**, which allows measurement of the velocity of blood flow through the stenotic valve: the more severe the stenosis, the higher the velocity. A simple formula relates the velocity to the estimated pressure gradient across the valve:

$$\Delta P = 4V^2$$

where ΔP is the pressure gradient (in mmHg), and V is the maximum outflow tract velocity (in m/s). When ventricular function is normal, a pressure gradient of > 50–60 mmHg is likely to be associated with hemodynamically significant stenosis. The remainder of the echocardiogram should demonstrate a calcified, poorly mobile aortic valve and LVH.

Examine an **electrocardiogram**. The presence of LVH and left atrial enlargement suggests significant stenosis. The **chest radiograph** may show evidence of a calcified aortic valve, cardiomegaly, and congestive heart failure.

4. List the causes of aortic stenosis.
In patients over age 70 years, the most common cause is senile calcific degeneration. In younger patients, the most common cause is calcific degeneration of a congenitally bicuspid valve. Rheumatic heart disease is diminishing in importance as a cause for aortic stenosis. In children and young adults, congenital stenosis is most common. Methysergide, a vasodilator medication used for migraines, is a rare cause of aortic stenosis.

5. Of what value is cardiac catheterization?

The main value of catheterization is to define the degree of stenosis accurately. This is done by estimating the valve orifice area through use of an equation that relates area to cardiac output, pressure gradient across the valve, and duration of systole, all of which are measured during catheterization. The procedure is also useful for defining LV function and for assessing coronary artery disease in patients over age 40. Significant coronary stenoses should be bypassed at the time of valve replacement.

6. Describe the natural history of aortic stenosis.

In patients with mild to moderate stenosis (valve area > 1 cm^2), the prognosis is excellent. The mean time between diagnosis and surgery is well over a decade. In patients with severe stenosis, the outlook is not as good. In one study of patients who refused surgery, survival rates depended on symptoms. Mean survival was 45 months for those with angina, 27 months for those with syncope, and only 11 months for those after the onset of left-heart failure. Patients with severe stenosis seldom die suddenly prior to the onset of symptoms.

7. The poor clinical prognosis of aortic stenosis is established, but what is the clinical importance of a milder degree of aortic valve disease?

A 5-year study of patients with aortic valve sclerosis—thickening and calcification of the aortic valve without significant obstruction of flow—indicated an increased risk of cardiac events (MI, congestive heart failure). Death from cardiovascular causes was found to be 50% higher in patients with aortic valve sclerosis than in those with normal aortic valves. Aortic valve sclerosis is a common finding in the elderly: approximately 21–26% in those older than 65 years. However, aortic *stenosis* affects only 2–9% of this same population. Therefore, it would seem that aortic valve sclerosis is not entirely a benign finding, but may represent a spectrum of aortic valve disease associated with increased clinical problems.

Aortic valve sclerosis is not entirely benign and may represent a spectrum of AV disease.

8. When should aortic valve surgery be considered?

Most agree that aortic valve replacement should be performed only when stenosis causes symptoms. Some believe that valve replacement should be performed in asymptomatic patients when the valve reaches a critical degree of narrowing, usually defined as a valve area < 0.8 cm^2 as determined at catheterization. Firm evidence that this latter approach improves outcome is lacking, however.

9. When is balloon valvuloplasty a useful procedure?

This procedure has not replaced surgical valve replacement because of high rates of restenosis and complications. It may be useful in patients with severe symptoms whose lifespans are limited by other diseases and malignancy. It may also "buy time" in patients with severe heart failure or intercurrent illness, such as pneumonia, allowing surgical risk to improve. The procedure may be more useful in children or young adults with congenital stenosis.

10. Can chronic aortic regurgitation cause heart failure?

Yes. Although aortic regurgitation is generally better tolerated than stenosis, it may lead to irreversible LV dysfunction. This may occur *prior to the development of symptoms*. Thus, patients with severe aortic insufficiency must be followed carefully.

11. What symptom is found with aortic regurgitation?

Dyspnea.

12. What are the major physical findings in aortic regurgitation?

They vary with the severity of disease. The murmur is diastolic, decrescendo, and heard along the left sternal border. It is frequently missed because it is very similar to normal breath sounds. Listening during held expiration improves chances of correctly identifying the murmur.

A **third heart sound** is common. An **Austin-Flint murmur** may be present. This murmur sounds exactly like that of mitral stenosis. Its pathogenesis is incompletely understood, but results from interaction between the regurgitant jet and mitral valve inflow. Significant aortic regurgitation is usually accompanied by a **wide pulse pressure**. This pulse pressure is typically at least 60 mmHg, and the diastolic pressure is typically < 70 mmHg.

13. What are the peripheral pulse findings?

The wide pulse pressure can produce many abnormalities in the peripheral pulses:
• Bifid carotid pulse
• Visible carotid pulsations (Corrigan's pulse)
• Head bobbing (de Musset's sign)
• Bobbing of the uvula (Müller's sign)
• Femoral artery bruit induced by light pressure over the artery (Duroziez's murmur)
• Pistol shot sound over the femoral artery (Traube's sound)
• Visible pulsations in the nail beds (Quincke's pulses).

14. Is the ejection fraction a reliable index to follow aortic regurgitation?

No, evaluation of LV function with regurgitation is problematic, as ejection indices (including the ejection fraction) are dependent on preload and afterload. Thus, they are not reliable to evaluate contractility when loading conditions are altered. Attempts have been made to develop corrected indices by using other LV parameters such as mitral and aortic stroke volume (calculated cross-sectional area × timed velocity integral). The advantages of this type of evaluation are that it is noninvasive and able to predict the immediate postoperative clinical course.

15. How are the noninvasive tests useful?

In severe regurgitation, the **electrocardiogram** generally shows LVH, and the **chest radiograph** shows cardiomegaly. **Doppler echocardiography** can confirm the diagnosis and grade the severity of the regurgitation. Because irreversible LV dysfunction can occur prior to the onset of symptoms, noninvasive tests provide clues to early decompensation, such as a progressive increase in LV end-systolic diameter and decrease in measures of contractility. Thus, serial echocardiography is useful in following patients with severe regurgitation. Some cardiologists find **serial radionuclide ventriculography** to be useful for the same purpose.

16. Can color-flow Doppler imaging assess the severity of aortic regurgitation?

A prospective study evaluated color-flow Doppler imaging of the vena contracta, the smallest area of regurgitant flow. There was good correlation with simultaneous quantitative measures, and it appeared to be a simple and reliable technique. An especially impressive aspect is no loss of accuracy with eccentric jet.

17. What are the causes of aortic regurgitation?

Causes of Aortic Regurgitation

Long-standing hypertension (most common)

Inflammatory disease of the valve and aortic root (rheumatic fever, rheumatoid arthritis, ankylosing spondylitis, tertiary syphilis)

Connective tissue disorders (Marfan's syndrome, Ehlers-Danlos syndrome)

Congenital disease (congenitally malformed aortic valve, prolapse from long-standing ventricular septal defect)

Aortic insufficiency

Torn cusp (blunt chest trauma, dissecting aortic aneuryms, infective endocarditis)

---

18. What are the causes of *acute* aortic regurgitation?

Unlike chronic aortic regurgitation, acute regurgitation is generally poorly tolerated. Because the ventricle does not have sufficient time to dilate, the volume of blood flowing back into the ventricle produces a dramatic rise in end-diastolic pressure, which in turn produces signs and symptoms of heart failure. Acute aortic regurgitation generally requires early surgical treatment.

BIBLIOGRAPHY

1. Abd-El-Aziz TA, Frerer AE, et al: Study of the value of corrected ejection fraction in the evaluation of left ventricular function in patients with mitral or aortic regurgitation. Angiology 51(7):55–64, 2000.
2. Otto CM, Lind DK, Kitzman D, et al: Association of aortic valve sclerosis with cardiovascular mortality and morbidity in the elderly. New Engl J Med 341:142–147, 1999.
3. Tribouilloy CM, Enriquez-Sarano M, et al: Assessment of severity of aortic regurgitation using the width of the vena contracta: A clinical color Doppler imaging study. Circulation 102(5):558–564, 2000.

45. MITRAL VALVE PROLAPSE AND MITRAL REGURGITATION

Howard D. Weinberger, M.D., FACC

1. Describe mitral valve prolapse and the mitral valve prolapse syndrome.

Mitral valve prolapse refers to protrusion or prolapse of a portion of the mitral valve into the left atrium during systole, when the mitral valve should be closed. The mitral valve prolapse syndrome, also called the systolic click-murmur syndrome and Barlow's syndrome (among other terms), is a clinical syndrome that includes mitral valve prolapse and may include mitral regurgitation and/or a myxomatous or thickened mitral valve. Clinical manifestations of the mitral valve prolapse syndrome can be quite variable.

2. How common is mitral valve prolapse? Who is most likely to be affected?

Mitral valve prolapse is one of the most common cardiac valvular abnormalities. Most sources report an incidence of 3–5%, with a 2:1 female predominance. A recent study of 3491 subjects in the Framingham Heart Study offspring study by Freed revealed an incidence of 2.4% using strict criteria for the diagnosis of mitral valve prolapse. There was no difference in the frequency of mitral valve prolapse between men and women in this study.

3. What findings on physical examination suggest mitral valve prolapse?

A mid-systolic click, usually best heard over the apex, is the classic auscultatory finding for prolapse of the mitral valve. A systolic murmur follows the click if mitral regurgitation is present.

4. Describe maneuvers that can enhance the systolic click and murmur of mitral valve prolapse on physical examination.

Maneuvers that decrease left ventricular filling or volume tend to move the click closer to the first heart sound (occurs earlier in systole) and increase the intensity of the mitral regurgitation murmur. Likewise, maneuvers that increase left ventricular filling or volume tend to move the click closer to the second heart sound (occurs later in systole) and decrease the intensity of the mitral regurgitation murmur.

A relatively simple maneuver is to listen to the patient's heart while the patient goes from a standing to a squatting position, and then back to a standing position. Squatting increases left ventricular filling or volume, delaying the click and decreasing the intensity of the mitral regurgitation murmur. As the patient returns to a standing position, left ventricular filling and volume decreases, leading to an earlier click and a louder mitral regurgitation murmur.

5. What are the echocardiographic findings of mitral valve prolapse?

The mitral valve leaflets may be myxomatous and thickened. During systole, one or both of the mitral leaflets prolapse superiorly into the left atrium. This can be seen on 2-dimensional and M-mode echocardiography. Doppler echocardiography (ECG) can identify mitral regurgitation if present.

6. What symptoms do patients with mitral valve prolapse experience?

Many patients with mitral valve prolapse are asymptomatic. Patients with "classic" mitral valve prolapse syndrome may demonstrate a variety of nonspecific symptoms, such as fatigue, palpitations, anxiety, chest pain, and/or symptoms of autonomic dysfunction. The chest pain is often atypical for myocardial ischemia, and tends to be stabbing, prolonged and not related to exertion.

7. Outline the management of patients with mitral valve prolapse.
- Asymptomatic patients without mitral regurgitation, arrhythmias, or ECG changes can be reassured about their favorable prognosis, and every 3–5 years a re-evaluation with an echocardiogram should be performed.
- Patients with mitral valve prolapse and mitral regurgitation should be followed every 6–12 months, and educated about the need for antibiotic prophylaxis to decrease the chance of developing infective endocarditis.
- Patients with palpitations or chest pain may benefit from treatment with beta-adrenergic receptor blockers.
- Patients with lightheadedness, dizziness, syncope, prolonged QT interval on ECG, or arrhythmias should undergo electrophysiologic evaluation.

8. List the common causes of mitral regurgitation.
Mitral regurgitation may be caused by problems with one or more of the following: the mitral valve leaflets, mitral annulus, chordae tendinae, papillary muscles, or left ventricular myocardium. Abnormalities of the mitral leaflets can result from rheumatic valve disease, systemic lupus erythematosis, infective endocarditis, or mitral valve prolapse. Myocardial ischemia or infarction may disrupt the papillary muscles leading to mitral regurgitation, as can rupture of chordae tendinae. Left ventricular enlargement may dilate the mitral annulus and lead to mitral regurgitation.

9. What are the common findings of mitral regurgitation on physical examination?
The murmur of mitral regurgitation is holosystolic (starting with the first heart sound and ending with the second heart sound), and is best heard over the apex. The murmur usually radiates towards or into the left axilla, and may be best appreciated with the patient examined in the left lateral decubitus position. The intensity of the murmur does not always correlate with the severity of the regurgitation.

CONTROVERSY

10. When should patients undergo surgery for mitral regurgitation?
Timing of surgery for mitral regurgitation is controversial. It is generally agreed that patients with severe, acute mitral regurgitation require urgent surgery. Timing of surgery for chronic mitral regurgitation is less well defined. Most feel that left ventricular enlargement or significant or progressive symptoms despite medical therapy indicate the need for surgery. Once left ventricular systolic dysfunction occurs, improvement with surgery may be reduced. When possible, mitral valve *repair*, as opposed to replacement, is an attractive option because it helps maintain more normal ventricular geometry as well as maintain the relationship of the native papillary muscles, chordae tendinae, and mitral annulus.

BIBLIOGRAPHY

1. Anwar A, Kohn SR, Dunn JF, et al: Altered beta adrenergic receptor function in subjects with symptomatic mitral valve prolapse. Am J Med Sci 302:89–97, 1991.
2. Bouknight DP, O'Rourke RA: Current management of mitral valve prolapse. Am Fam Physician 61(11): 3343–50, 3353–4, 2000.
3. Braunwald E: Valvular heart disease. In Braunwald E (ed): Heart Disease, 5th ed. Philadelphia, W.B. Saunders, 1997.
4. Devereux RB, Kramer-Fox R, Kligfield P: Mitral valve prolapse: Causes, clinical manifestations, and management. Ann Intern Med 111:305–317, 1989.
5. Farb A, Tang AL, Atkinson JB, et al: Comparison of cardiac findings in patients with mitral valve prolapse who die suddenly to those who have congestive heart failure from mitral valve regurgitation to those with fatal noncardiac conditions. Am J Cardiol 70:234–239, 1992.
6. Freed LA, Levy D, Levine RA, et al: Prevalence and clinical outcome of mitral valve prolapse. N Eng J Med 341:1–7, 1999.

7. Galloway AC, Colvin SB, Bauman G, et al: Long-term results of mitral valve reconstruction with Carpentier techniques in 148 patients with mitral insufficiency. Circulation 78(Suppl I):I-97–I-105, 1988.
8. Weyman AE (ed): Principles and Practice of Echocardiography, 2nd ed, Philadelphia, Lea & Febiger, 1994.
9. Wooley CF, Baker PB, Kolibash AJ, et al: The floppy, myxomatous mitral valve, mitral valve prolapse, and mitral regurgitation. Prog Cardiovasc Dis 33:397–433, 1991.

46. PROSTHETIC VALVES

Michael Staab, M.D., and Norman Krasnow, M.D.

1. When is a mechanical prosthesis preferred over a bioprosthetic valve?

Bioprosthetic valves in the aortic position may not require anticoagulation, whereas mechanical valves always require such therapy. **Bioprosthetic valves** are therefore preferred in patients for whom anticoagulation poses additional risks or problems: young, vigorous patients whose occupations or sports activities present risks of trauma, patients who have clotting disorders or bleeding problems (e.g., peptic ulcer disease), and patients who are unable to follow instructions or have appropriate monitoring of clotting factors. However, bioprosthetic valves have much higher long-term failure rates than mechanical valves, which must be taken into account when selecting a valve. Bioprosthetic failure rates may decrease with changes in preservation techniques. **Mechanical prostheses** may be preferred in young patients with expected considerable longevity, those for whom anticoagulation is not difficult to manage, those who may calcify tissue excessively (e.g., patients with renal failure), and those who may have already failed a bioprosthetic implant.

2. Which type of valve has the lower incidence of bacterial endocarditis? Which has the lower overall complication rate?

Bacterial endocarditis (or, more broadly, infective endocarditis to include fungal organisms) occurs in about 1% of valve replacement per year of implant. The incidence is approximately the same for bioprosthetic and mechanical valves. When infection occurs on a bioprosthetic valve, cure with antibiotics alone is feasible in many cases, especially when the infection is on the leaflet. When infection is present in mechanical prostheses, the valve ring is always involved, and therefore medical cure is extremely difficult (though not impossible). Surgical therapy is usually required, with valve replacement.

The complication rate is somewhat lower with bioprosthetic valves than mechanical valves, but when the reduced longevity of the bioprosthetic is considered, the overall patient survival and requirement for reoperation are about the same for both types.

3. When is replacement indicated for aortic regurgitation in a patient without symptoms?

When congestive heart failure occurs in association with aortic regurgitation, it is generally agreed that surgical valve replacement is the treatment of choice. In patients with definite severe aortic regurgitation but who have no symptoms and may be fully functional, one or more parameters of left ventricular (LV) function are measured, usually by echocardiography, and followed serially. An end-systolic diameter of 5.5 cm has been advocated by some as an upper limit beyond which surgery leads to worse functional results and survival. Similarly, a decrease in ejection fraction from normal to borderline (e.g., 45–50%) is also used. The absolute end-diastolic diameter of the LV is a less reliable parameter indicating surgery, though markedly enlarged hearts (e.g., diameter of 8 cm by echocardiography) are perhaps less likely to return entirely to normal even if surgery is performed; increasing end-diastolic diameters serve to alert the physician to the need for surgery in the near future.

4. Is Doppler echocardiography accurate in diagnosing prosthetic aortic stenosis?

When bioprosthetic leaflets thicken and calcify, they may become stenotic. Doppler echocardiography may accurately define the pressure gradient in these cases, just as in stenosis of native valves. However, mechanical prostheses have a variety of orifices, depending on the type of valve. In these cases, the spectral Doppler recording can be challenging to interpret, particularly leading to overestimate of the gradient because of the phenomenon of pressure recovery.

St. Jude Medical valves, for example, have a narrow central orifice between the two leaflets. The velocity of blood flow through this slit may be very high, leading to a false diagnosis of prosthetic stenosis. This misinterpretation can be avoided by using the mean gradient (or velocity) rather than the peak gradient (or velocity). In addition, evaluation of the ratio of LVOT velocity to velocity across the aortic valve

(LVOT velocity)/(Velocity across aortic valve)

is helpful (normal ratio for St. Jude valves 0.35–0.50).

When there is doubt about the severity of prosthetic obstruction, transesophageal echocardiography, cardiac fluoroscopy, or cardiac catheterization with hemodynamic recording of pressure is extremely helpful.

5. When is valve replacement indicated for aortic stenosis?

When congestive heart failure, angina pectoris, and syncope appear. Usually, the aortic valve area associated with such symptoms is about 0.7–1.0 cm^2 or less. Because aortic stenosis occurs most often in older patients, knowledge of the coronary artery anatomy and its contribution to the angina and congestive heart failure is required. Patients with significant aortic stenosis but without symptoms may be followed closely without surgery. Occasionally, severe LV hypertrophy may be present causing LV diastolic dysfunction with symptoms of pulmonary congestion but with well-maintained systolic function; in these cases, surgery is often warranted.

6. How are prosthetic mitral valves evaluated for stenosis?

When a patient with a prosthetic mitral valve begins to develop new or increased symptoms of pulmonary congestion, the possibility of prosthetic stenosis due to thrombus formation, fibrosis with leaflet restriction (for bioprosthetic valves), or valve dysfunction must be considered. The appearance of the leaflets, both bioprosthetic and mechanical, on the two-dimensional echocardiographic image is of considerable use, especially if the leaflets are well visualized and are seen to move well. Because such visualization is often not achieved, alternative approaches are necessary. Bioprosthetic valves may be evaluated reasonably well with spectral Doppler recordings. The peak inflow velocity and the pressure half-time of the deceleration phase of inflow may be used to compute a mitral valve area. These parameters are not accurate with mechanical prostheses, although abnormal values may be useful clues to dysfunction. In these cases, transesophageal echocardiography and hemodynamic study by cardiac catheterization may be needed.

7. When is valve replacement indicated for mitral regurgitation?

When mitral regurgitation is severe (or at least moderate), it may be associated with LV failure and symptoms of dyspnea on exertion, orthopnea, and edema. When LV function is well maintained despite the volume overload causing symptoms, surgical correction is indicated. Depending on the cause of the regurgitation—e.g., rheumatic valvular disease, prolapse, or ruptured chordae tendineae—the surgeon may elect to repair the valve without replacement. Such repair is being done increasingly, as it leads to better preservation of ventricular function. When repair is not possible, valve replacement offers a good alternative.

However, when LV function has already deteriorated due to the chronic volume overload and the ejection fraction is about 30% or less, surgical mortality and late results are less favorable. This is because implanting a competent valve where there was previously a low-resistance regurgitant "shunt" to the left atrium in effect imposes a significant afterload on the ventricle; if function is already poor, it may then decrease further.

Patients who are asymptomatic but have evidence of severe mitral regurgitation pose a difficult problem in the timing of surgery. By analogy with aortic regurgitation, some recommend surgery based on deterioration of echocardiographic parameters of LV size and/or function. An ejection fraction < 60% is already cause for concern. Also, evidence of deteriorating right ventricular function and development of pulmonary hypertension are used as guides. With mitral valves that have a high likelihood of repair (especially posterior leaflet prolapse), earlier surgical intervention improves outcome.

8. How is mitral regurgitation across a prosthetic valve diagnosed?

Valve dehiscence, thrombotic obstruction of leaflets, or endocarditis are among common causes for prosthetic valve dysfunction with regurgitation. Ordinarily, mitral regurgitation may be usefully evaluated by color-flow Doppler and semi-quantitative estimation based on various parameters of the visualized jet. However, prosthetic mitral valves, especially mechanical types, cause severe shadowing artifacts on the color-flow image, leading to significant underestimation of the degree of regurgitation. In these cases, imaging by the transesophageal route eliminates the shadowing artifact, especially in the mitral position, allowing more accurate visualization of the regurgitant jet. Thereafter, angiography is used to define somewhat more quantitatively the degree of regurgitation.

9. Are anticoagulants needed for bioprosthetic mitral valves?

Mechanical mitral prostheses require anticoagulation. Aortic mechanical prostheses generally require anticoagulation, although the risk of thrombosis is less than in mitral mechanical valves. Bioprosthetic valves may require anticoagulation for related indications such as atrial fibrillation or prior systemic embolism. Many surgeons will anticoagulate for 1 month while epithelialization of the valve sewing ring occurs.

10. How does an apparently normally functioning mitral prosthesis cause recurrent symptoms?

Implantation of a prosthesis in the mitral annulus sometimes causes the prosthesis to project into the outflow tract of the LV, causing obstruction to outflow. This was more common in the past, when prostheses were larger and bulkier. With modern low-profile valves of various types (e.g., Carpentier-Edwards, St. Jude Medical), the problem is less common but occasionally accounts for failure to improve—either acutely at the time of surgery or postoperatively. Careful Doppler echocardiography can document the presence of a gradient across the outflow tract despite a normal aortic valve and septal thickness. Valve prosthesis–patient mismatch occurs when a valve is too small for the patient's body size and can result in elevated gradients and ongoing symptoms.

11. What is a homograft/allograft?

A homograft, or allograft, is a valve removed from a cadaver or transplanted heart, most often used as an aortic valve replacement. The primary benefit is that anticoagulation is not required; it also has a role in the treatment of infective endocarditis. With changes in preservation techniques such as cryopreservation, there has been a resurgence in the use of these valves.

12. What is the Ross procedure?

The Ross procedure entails transplantation of the patient's own pulmonary valve into the aortic position with a homograft implanted in the pulmonary position. In experienced centers, this has become the procedure of choice for younger patients.

13. What characteristics make a stenotic mitral valve unsuitable for percutaneous valvuloplasty?

A mitral valve with calcified leaflets, especially in the commissures, does not do as well as pliable, noncalcified leaflets. More-than-mild mitral regurgitation is also a contraindication to valvuloplasty. Aortic valvuloplasty has fallen out of favor because the calcific leaflet characteristics of aortic stenosis tend to tear and result in regurgitation.

BIBLIOGRAPHY

1. American College of Cardiology/American Heart Association Committee on Management of Patients with Valvular Heart Disease: Guidelines for the management of patients with valvular heart disease. Circulation 98:1949–1984, 1998.
2. Baumgartner H, Khan S, DeRobertis M, et al: Discrepancies between Doppler and catheter gradients in aortic prosthetic valves in vitro: A manifestation of localized gradients and pressure recovery. Circulation 82:1467–1475, 1990.

3. Bloomfield P, Wheatley DJ, Prescott RJ, Miller HC: Twelve-year comparison of a Bjork-Shiley mechanical heart valve with porcine bioprostheses. N Engl J Med 324:573–579, 1991.
4. Bonow RO: Asymptomatic aortic regurgitation: Indications for operation. J Cardiol Surg 9(Suppl):170–173, 1994.
5. Enriquez-Sarano M, Schaff HV, Orszulak TA, et al: Valve repair improves the outcome of surgery for mitral regurgitation. Circulation 91:1022–1028, 1995.
6. Rahimtoola SH: The problem of valve prosthesis-patient mismatch. Circulation 58:20–24, 1978.
7. Staab ME, Nishimura RA, Dearani JA, Orszulak TA: Aortic valve homografts in adults: A clinical perspective. Mayo Clin Proc 73:231–238, 1998.

VI. Cardiovascular Pharmacology

47. ANTIARRHYTHMIC THERAPY

Olivia V. Adair, M.D., and Charles E. Fuenzalida, M.D.

1. What major clinical trials have influenced the management of arrhythmias?
Ongoing studies of beta blockers, amiodarone, and sotalol, both oral and intravenous, and their effect on arrhythmia in postinfarction patients (n = 20), have shown an average reduction of approximately 20% in mortality rates.

Evaluation of Pharmacologic Therapy for Arrhythmia

STUDY	PURPOSE/DESIGN	CLINICAL FINDINGS
CAMIAT (Canadian Amiodarone Myocardial Infarction Arrhythmia Trial)	To evaluate the efficacy of amiodarone in reducing arrhythmic death post-MI.	1. Amiodarone did not affect total cardiac mortality either by on-drug or intention-to-treat analysis (6.3% vs. 8.5%, p > 0.05 on drug, 7.3% vs. 9.6%, p = 0.1 intention to treat). 2. Amiodarone reduced SD or recurrent VF compared with placebo (3.3% vs. 6%, p < 0.05 on drug, and 4.9% vs. 6.9%, p < 0.5 intention to treat). 3. There was concordance between PVC suppression and reduced SD and recurrent VF 4. Early discontinuance of drug due to intolerance or side effects was common (42.3% for amiodarone group; 28.5% for placebo group). In this post-MI study, amiodarone did not improve overall mortality, but it did reduce SD or recurrent VF. Improvement was concordant with PVC suppression.
CHF STAT (Congestive Heart Failure—Survival Trial of Antiarrhythmic Therapy) 1995	To evaluate the efficacy of amiodarone in reducing mortality in patients with CHF and asymptomatic ventricular arrhythmias.	The amiodarone group had the same overall mortality as the placebo group (39% vs. 42%, p = NS). Actuarial survival at 2 years was the same in the 2 groups (69.4% vs. 70.8%). There was a trend in favor of amiodarone in patients with nonischemic heart disease (p = 0.07). Amiodarone suppressed PVCs and improved LVEF. This study showed a disparity between PVC suppression and improved mortality (as had CAST). In this mixed group of patients, amiodarone was found to have no effect on overall mortality or SD despite PVC suppression. There was a favorable trend seen in patients with nonischemic cardiomyopathy.

(Table continued on next page.)

Evaluation of Pharmacologic Therapy for Arrhythmia (cont.)

STUDY	PURPOSE/DESIGN	CLINICAL FINDINGS
EMIAT (European Myocardial Infarction Amiodarone Trial)	To assess the efficacy of prophylactic anti-arrhythmic therapy in post-MI patients with asymptomatic complex ventricular ectopy.	1. There was no difference in overall mortality between the 2 groups. 2. There was a reduction in arrhythmic death in the amiodarone group (p = 0.052 by intention-to-treat analysis, p < 0.01 by on-treatment analysis). 3. Drug discontinuance due to side effects or intolerance was high in the amiodarone group (45% by 2 y). In this study of patients with depressed LV function and ischemic heart disease, amiodarone did not decrease overall mortality but did reduce SD, particularly seen in the "on-treatment" analysis.
AVID (Antiarrhythmics Versus Implantable Defibrillators) 1997	To compare overall survival in patients with VT/VF initially treated with an ICD vs. those treated with empiric amiodarone or EP-guided sotalol.	1. 507 patients randomized to ICD group and 509 to drug therapy. 2. In ICD group: 93% nonthoracotomy ICD, 5% epicardial ICD, 2% no device implanted. 3. In drug therapy group: 356 impiric amiodarone, 153 random assignment—79 to amiodarone, 74 to sotalol—13 (2.6%) suppressed on sotalol. The remainder received amiodarone (58), other antiarrhythmic (1), or ICD (2). 4. Fewer deaths occurred in the ICD groups than in the drug therapy group. Death rates at 18 mo = 15.8 ± 3.2% for ICD vs. 24.0 ± 3.7% for drugs (p < 0.02). 5. RR reductions with ICD were 39 ± 20% at 1 y, 27 ± 21% at 2 y, and 31 ± 21% at 3 y. This study provides strong evidence that ICDs prolong life compared to drug therapy in patients who have survived near lethal arrhythmias. The absolute prolongation of life was modest—just over 3 mo. The estimated cost per y of life saved was $114917.[49]
CIDS (Canadian Implantable Defibrillator Study) 1998	To determine whether ICD was superior to amiodarone in patients surviving a cardiac arrest or VT.	1. A 3-y risk reduction of 19.6% was seen in the ICD group; p = NS 2. 22% of the control group crossed over to ICDs 3. 30% of ICD group received appropriate shocks by 5 y. The benefit of ICD was marginal, but the results may have been masked by high cross-over rates. The inclusion of the unmonitored syncope group may have introduced a lower risk group of patients.

(Table continued on next page.)

Evaluation of Pharmacologic Therapy for Arrhythmia (cont.)

STUDY	PURPOSE/DESIGN	CLINICAL FINDINGS
MADIT (Multi-center Automatic Defibrillator Implantation Trial) 1996	To determine whether ICD would reduce death as compared with conventional pharmacologic therapy in high-risk patients with CAD and potentially life-threatening ventricular arrhythmias.	1. ICD therapy demonstrated a 54% reduction in overall mortality as compared with the conventional therapy group. 2. More patients in the conventional therapy arm received amiodarone than in the ICD group (80% vs. 2%) 3. More patients in the ICD arm received a beta-blocker than in the conventional therapy arm (28% vs. 9%). 4. Overall mortality in patients noninducible at baseline EPS was 25%. 5. Overall mortality in patients rendered noninducible by I.V. procainamide was 30%.

CHF = congestive heart failure, EPS = electrophysiologic study, ICD = implantable cardioverter defibrillator, LVEF = left ventricle ejection fraction, PVC = premature ventricular contractions, SD = septal defect, VT = ventricular tachycardia

2. What information should be gathered to determine if an arrhythmia is the cause of a patient's symptoms?

The first essential element in evaluation of a possible arrhythmia is a good **history**. Of special interest are frequency, duration, mode of onset, and mode of cessation, along with associated symptoms and any history of medications.

Physical examination focuses on blood pressure, peripheral pulses, jugular venous pulsation, heart auscultation for measurement of gallops and variations of first heart sound, and evidence of cardiomegaly, congestive heart failure (CHF), or thyroid dysfunction.

Laboratory tests should include electrolytes, especially calcium and magnesium; antiarrhythmic level; thyroid function; chest radiography; EKG with a long rhythm strip; and event monitor recording (loop or wrist recorder) if patient has arrhythmia symptoms, or Holter monitoring for symptoms that are daily (an implantable recorder, which can remain for up to 1 year or until arrhythmia is recorded, can be used).

3. In view of the side effects shown in recent studies, what options remain for management of arrhythmias?

- No therapy
- Pharmacologic therapy
- Electrical therapy
    Direct current conversion
    Implantible cardioversion defibrillator
    Radiofrequency ablation
- Surgical therapy

4. How should treatment of a patient with an arrhythmia be determined?

Treatment must be individualized, with consideration of:

Electrocardiographic analysis of the arrhythmia, with evaluation of atrial and ventricular activation and atrioventricular conduction pattern; whether the arrhythmia is triggering additional arrhythmias; and whether the arrhythmias are sustained.

Assessment of the clinical setting, including categorization of arrhythmia as acute or chronic, and as transient, persistent, or recurrent. Anatomic and physiological substrate also should be evaluated.

Defining the goal or endpoint of therapy, which depends on the previous evaluations. Appropriate diagnostic tools in addition to history, physical examination, routine laboratory tests, and electrocardiogram include: (1) special leads to identify the P waves (esophageal lead, intra-atrial electrode, or Lewis leads), (2) Holter monitoring; (3) echocardiography; (4) exercise testing; (5) tilt table test; (6) signal-averaged electrocardiography, (7) electrophysiologic studies, and (8) heart variability analysis. Note that suppression of ventricular ectopy (e.g., in the Electrophysiologic Study Versus Electrocardiographic Monitoring [ESVEM] trial) requires a 100% reduction of non-sustained or sustained ventricular tachycardia; a 90% reduction of back-to-back premature ventricular contractions (PVCs); and an 80% reduction of PVCs over a span of 24 hours.

5. Discuss the categories of patients who do not require antiarrhythmic therapy.
Because of the risk of proarrhythmia or exacerbation of pre-existing arrhythmia by antiarrhythmic drugs, the trend to suppress ventricular ectopy has diminished. Although controversy still surrounds arrhythmic therapy, by general agreement it is not indicated in specific circumstances:
• Asymptomatic atrial ectopy and unsustained supraventricular tachycardia (SVT)
• Asymptomatic ventricular ectopy without runs of ventricular tachycardia (VT)
• Simple ventricular ectopy in acute myocardial infarction (MI), not associated with hemodynamic compromise
• Asymptomatic, unsustained VT with no structural heart disease or other risk indicators
• Asymptomatic Wolff-Parkinson-White (WPW) syndrome without known SVT
• Mildly symptomatic, simple atrial or ventricular ectopy

6. What is programmed electrical stimulation (PES)?
PES studies use percutaneous catheter electrodes placed in the atria and ventricle (usually right venous) to record intracardiac electrograms and to evaluate SVT, ventricular arrhythmias, including VT and ventricular fibrillation (VF), and bradycardia without clinical or Holter criteria for pacer implantation.

7. When should PES be used in the management of a suspected arrhythmia?
The **primary indications** for PES are:
1. Identification of the tachycardia and its mechanisms
2. Selection of appropriate therapy
3. Mapping of the substrate of the arrhythmia for ablation or (rarely) surgical intervention.
Complication rates are low: death 0.06%; perforation 0.2%; major hemorrhage 0.05%; atrial injury 0.1%; and major venous thrombosis, 0.2%. PES is especially accurate in evaluation of SVT with induction in 90–95% of patients with clinical atroventricular nodal reentrant tachycardia or WPW. Ablation is used after the mechanism is defined, with deliverance of radiofrequency current through the catheter positioned at the site of the pathway.

PES is used extensively in VT evaluation; sustained VT/VF is reproducible in 75% of survivors of sudden cardiac death and 95% of patients with sustained monomorphic VT. The efficacy of antiarrhythmic therapy also can be evaluated with PES; a 10% recurrence rate is expected over 2 years, compared with 50% recurrence with no therapy identified. Note that an implantable cardioverter defibrillator is recommended for the majority of patients with *sustained* VT, based on findings from the MADIT trial, the CHF STAT trial, and the AVID trial.

8. How do PES and Holter monitoring compare in evaluation of antiarrhythmic drug efficacy?
The ESVEM trial examined this question in patients with VT. Holter monitoring predicted efficacy in 77% of cases; PES, in only 45%. In addition, Holter monitoring required only about one-half the number of hospital days. Thus in this selected sample, PES offered no advantage over Holter monitoring in accurate evaluation of drug efficacy. The negative predictive value of PES is good (approximately 90%), but the positive predictive value is weak (25%). Therefore, Holter monitoring may offer an alternative to PES in evaluation of antiarrhythmic agents.

Note that, in general, malignant ventricular arrhythmias are now treated predominantly with ICDs.

9. Are antiarrhythmic drugs still classified according to their electrophysiologic effects?

Yes. The Vaughn Williams classification of antiarrhythmic agents is still used despite multiple attempts to develop a more clinically oriented system, based, for example, on channels, pumps, and receptors. The Vaughn Williams system serves as a useful means of communication:

Class 1—local membrane-stabilizing activity; blocks the fast sodium channel

Class 2—blocks the beta-adrenergic receptors

Class 3—prolongs duration of cardiac action potential and repolarization; blocks potassium channels

Class 4—blocks the slow calcium channel

This classification is based on the repolarization/depolarization curve of the action potential.

10. Should lidocaine be initiated in all patients with acute MI?

Although some data suggested that lidocaine decreases VF in patients admitted within 6 hours of onset of acute MI symptoms, the untreated group had no increased risk of death, and all patients were resuscitated. Likewise, two meta-analyses in over 9000 patients showed a reduction in primary VF, but no benefit in survival, perhaps because the toxic effects of lidocaine produce conduction abnormalities and increased asystole, which negate the benefit of decreased VF.

No evidence suggests that routine or prophylactic use of lidocaine in acute MI is beneficial. Use of lidocaine is recommended: (1) for frequent, multiform ventricular ectopy, especially R-on-T phenomenon, or short runs of nonsustained VT; (2) after an episode of VT or VF requiring electrical conversion or after cardiopulmonary resuscitation; and (3) for ventricular ectopy so frequent or so timed that it significantly impairs hemodynamics. Amelioration of left ventricular failure is essential in the treatment of arrhythmias in patients with acute MI. Aggressively treat ischemia, which also may contribute to ectopy. Always consider the possibility of drug-induced VT or hypokalemia.

Note that recent studies give strong support to the use of beta blockers in acute ischemic syndromes, especially in VT storm.

11. When is cardioversion indicated?

Attempt immediate cardioversion if an arrhythmia causes angina, hypotension, or heart failure. Use the lowest possible energy level to reduce complications. Major complications are infrequent, and success is seen in approximately 90% of recent-onset arrhythmias.

Atrial fibrillation, the most commonly cardioverted arrhythmia, requires at least 100 Joules (J) and has a higher rate of systemic emboli if the arrhythmia has a > 3-day duration. Atrial flutter is the easiest rhythm to convert to sinus; it requires low energy (approximately 50 J), but may be converted to atrial fibrillation if too little energy is used (5–10 J); re-entrant SVT due to atrioventricular nodal pathways can be converted with 25–100 J. VT can be converted with low energy, but in the presence of hemodynamic compromise, immediately deliver 200 J, followed by 360 J if the first attempt is not successful.

12. What are the contraindications to cardioversion?

Relative contraindications to cardioversion include: (**1**) digoxin toxicity (in emergencies, start cardioversion with low energy levels and progressively increase prophylactic lidocaine and energy delivery; (**2**) short repetitive runs of VT; (**3**) multifocal atrial tachycardia; (**4**) immediately before or after surgery in patients with stable atrial fibrillation; (**5**) SVT and hyperthyroidism; (**6**) SVT with complete heart block; and (**7**) inadequate anticoagulation in patients with chronic atrial fibrillation.

13. Amiodarone is frequently used in patients with a history of ventricular tachycardia. Why is it so popular? What are its side effects?

Amiodarone has class 3 activity, with prolongation of both refractoriness and duration of cardiac action potential as well as antiarrhythmic, beta-blocker, and vasodilator effects. Many authorities believe that amiodarone is the most effective single agent for many arrhythmias, including

SVT and VT. Its ability to prolong survival has been studied in various disease states, such as MI and CHF. Amiodarone is approved by the Food and Drug Administration for treatment of life-threatening ventricular arrhythmias when other drugs are ineffective or not tolerated.

Amiodarone is quite effective in many cases of SVT, atrial fibrillation conversion and rate control, atrioventricular nodal re-entry, and WPW. Long-term therapy is well tolerated hemodynamically in patients with CHF and severe cardiomyopathies. Two controlled trials showed an improvement in longevity among survivors of MI. Another study suggested that amiodarone therapy prolongs life in patients with CHF and arrhythmias, but a short-term study showed no benefit in patients with CHF and ventricular ectopy.

The major disadvantage of amiodarone is adverse reactions, which include the potentially lethal interstitial pneumonitis.

14. What are the indications for, and side effects of, sotalol?

Sotalol is a class 3 drug and beta blocker that prolongs the action potential and increases its refractoriness. It is effective for many supraventricular and ventricular arrhythmias, including sustained inducible VT. In the ESVEM study, sotalol was more effective than the other antiarrhythmic drugs evaluated (31% vs. 12%).

The major side effects are QT prolongation, which may result in torsade de pointes (2%); proarrhythmic events (4.5% at higher doses of 640 mg/day); and worsening heart failure (3%).

15. Procainamide and quinidine are class 1A agents that used to be popular. Are they still used as much as before?

No. As a result of the CAST study, class 1 agents have fallen into disfavor. Both procainamide and quinidine are effective against supraventricular or ventricular arrhythmias. **Procainamide** has a high rate of intolerable side effects; 40% of patients stop the drug in the first 6 months. As a class 1A agent, it prolongs QT and may produce torsade de pointes as well as lupus-like syndrome in 20% of patients; agranulocytosis is another possible side effect. **Quinidine** has been shown in two meta-analyses to increase mortality compared with untreated patients and with other agents, but it is still one of the most widely used antiarrhythmic agents. However, most physicians are cautious, and stratify risk to justify antiarrhythmic use as well as to individualize therapy.

16. What is the role of class 1C agents in antiarrhythmic therapy?

Type 1C agents are quite helpful in the setting of atrial fibrillation without structural heart disease. They are the treatment of choice. Overall efficacy at 1 year, however, is only 55–60%, maintaining patients in sinus rhythm. Furthermore, an exercise treadmill test performed 7–10 days following institution of type 1C antiarrhythmic agents is necessary to establish if the patient will have any proarrhythmia (QRS widening) or sustained VT at maximal heart rates.

17. How are implantable cardioverter defribrillators (ICD) used in the treatment of arrhythmias?

Monitoring systems have shown that the principal cause of sudden cardiac death in outpatients is VF, with > 80% of deaths due to progression of abrupt-onset VT to VF. The mortality rate of out-of-hospital cardiac arrest is high (> 75%), mainly because of delay in effective therapy. The ICD is able to deliver an initial electrical countershock within 10–20 seconds of arrhythmia onset, a delay in which the potential for reversed arrhythmia approaches 100%. Because of this immediate response, ICDs are the most effective method for aborting sudden death due to life-threatening ventricular arrhythmias.

The indications for ICDs continue to broaden and change with new technology and more experience. There are basically five categories of patient for which ICDs are indicated:

• Survivors of cardiac arrest with documented VF or VT
• Patients with drug-refractory, clinical, and inducible sustained VT

• Patients without documented sustained ventricular arrhythmias at high risk for future life-threatening arrhythmic events because of inducible arrhythmias at electrophysiologic study
• Patients with nonsustained VT and/or asymptomatic, but inducible, ventricular dysrhythmias that are nonsuppressed with procainamide (MADIT criteria)
• Patients with a family history of structural heart disease that renders a very high risk of sudden cardiac death (family history of recurrent sudden cardiac death, long QT interval, or hypertrophic cardiomyopathy with syncope).

18. A 34-year-old man is referred for recurrent palpitations. A Holter monitor documents paroxysmal atrial tachycardia, which degenerates into atrial fibrillation. An echocardiogram shows normal LV and RV performance and dimension, and there is no evidence of valvular heart disease. Upon further questioning, the patient admits that he drinks excessively. What is the most appropriate recommendation or therapy?

Numerous antiarrhythmic agents are available for the treatment of paroxysmal atrial fibrillation. An initial recommendation to absolutely abstain from alcohol, caffeine, and chocolate is paramount. Monitoring the patient's blood pressure may be necessary because many patients who abuse alcohol have associated hypertension/left ventricular hypertrophy (not evident in this case).

Initial antiarrhythmic therapy depends on the patient's compliance and age. The absence of structural heart disease in this patient suggests that flecainide or propafenone could be used. Flecainide is perhaps the best tolerated of the current first-line antiarrhythmic agents.

Flecainide 100 mg PO bid was instituted in this case. Verapamil also was prescribed, to keep the ventricular response and atrial tachycardia controlled by blocking the AV node. An exercise treadmill test performed 4–5 days later showed no evidence of QRS prolongation or exercise-induced VT.

19. The patient presented above did well for 5 years. He then experienced recurrent atrial fibrillation, despite abstaining from alcohol. His blood pressure was normal. What additional antiarrhythmic therapy or testing is necessary at this point?

Repeat echocardiography can reassess for structural heart disease, which may now be evident due to progression. Another exercise treadmill test can reveal reversible ischemia. Neither of these disorders were found in the present patient, and, although he is middle-aged, he has no symptoms to suggest coronary disease. Flecainide was incremented to 150 mg PO bid.

20. The patient's symptoms persisted, and flecainide was incremented to 200 mg PO bid. On this dosage, the patient complained of paresthesias. Which alternative antiarrhythmic agents should be considered?

If flecainide fails, then propafenone, sotalol, and dofetilide can be considered. Amiodarone would not be an ideal agent in a patient of this young age due to the potential for serious side effects (lung, thyroid, retinal, liver, neurologic).

21. Sotalol, disopyramide, and propafenone failed in this patient. Dofetilide was not available. What alternative therapy can be considered?

Nonpharmacologic therapy was elected by the patient. Electrophysiologic studies with mapping revealed that the atrial tachycardia was located in the right atrium at the superior vena cava junction. Successful **radiofrequency transcatheter ablation** was performed, and a cure was established on follow-up 9 months later.

22. Describe new, acute antiarrhythmic therapy for field initiation by paramedics.

Data from the ARREST study (Amiodarone in Out-of-Hospital Resuscitation of Refractory Sustained Ventricular Tachyarrhythmias) presented at the American Heart Association's 72nd session, November 1999, showed that patient survival to hospital admission improved by 29% with amiodarone administered. This study provides a major advance in cardiac arrest resuscitation. Patients were screened and treated by paramedics (504 patients, mostly male with heart disease and in their 60s): those failing three resuscitation efforts (cardioversion, intubation, epinephrine and an initial antiarrhythmic agent administered [e.g., lidocaine, magnesium]) were given amiodarone 300 mg IV. The most frequent side effects were hypotension and bradycardia.

Life-support guidelines are expected to change to include amiodarone *before* intubation, and use of vasopressin instead of epinephrine IV, so that the patient's condition does not continue to destabilize.

BIBLIOGRAPHY

1. Bansch D, Castrucci M, et al: Ventricular tachycardia above the initially programmed tachycardia detection intervals in patients with implantable cardioverter defibrillators: Incidence, prediction, and significance. J Am Coll Cardiol 36:557–565, 2000.
2. Cairns JA, et al: Randomized trial of outcome after myocardial infarction in patients with frequent or repetitive ventricular premature depolarization: CAMIAT. Lancet 349:675–682, 1997.
3. Echr DS, Liebson PR, Mitchell LB, et al: Mortality and morbidity in patients receiving encainide, flecainide, or placebo. The Cardiac Arrhythmia Suppression Trial. N Engl J Med 324:781–788, 1991.
4. Fonarow GC, Feliciano Z, et al: Improved survival in patients with nonischemic advanced heart failure and syncope with an implantable cardioverter debrillator. Am J Cardiol 85:981–985, 2000.
5. Jackman WM, Wang XZ, Friday KJ, et al: Catheter ablation of accessory atrioventricular pathways (Wolff-Parkinson-White syndrome) by radiofrequency current. N Engl J Med 324:1605–1611, 1991.
6. Jideus L, Blomstrom P, et al: Tachyarrhythmias and triggering factors for atrial fibrillation after coronary artery bypass operations. Ann Thorac Surg 69:1064–1069, 2000.
7. Julian DG, et al: Randomized trial of effect of amiodarone on mortality in patients with left ventricular dysfunction after recent myocardial infarction: EMIAT. Lancet 349:667–674, 1997.
7a. Kudenchuk PJ, Cobb LA, Copass MK, et al: Amiodarone for resuscitation after out-of-hospital cardiac arrest due to ventricular fibrillation: ARREST [see comments]. N Engl J Med 341(12):871–878, 1999.
8. Lau C, Camm AJ: Rate-responsive pacing: Technical and clinical aspects. In El-Sherif N, Samet P (eds): Cardiac Pacing and Electrophysiology. Philadelphia, W. B. Saunders. 1991, pp 534–544.
9. Malik M, Camm AJ, et al: Depressed heart rate variability identifies postinfarction patients who might benefit from prophylactic treatment with amiodarone: A substudy of EMIAT (The European Myocardial Infarct Amiodarone Trial). J Am Coll Cardiol 35:1263–1275, 2000.
10. Mass AJ, et al: Improved survival with an implanted defibrillator in patients with coronary disease at high risk for ventricular arrhythmias: MADIT. N Engl J Med 335:1933–1940, 1996.
11. Myerburg RJ, Kessler KM, Castellanos A: Recognition, clinical assessment, and management of arrhythmias and conduction disturbances. In Schlant RC, Alexander RW (eds): The Heart Arteries and Veins, 8th ed. New York, McGraw-Hill, 1994, pp 705–758.
12. Opie LH: In Drugs of the Heart, 3rd ed. Philadelphia, W.B. Saunders, 1991.
13. Richards DA, Byth K, Ross DL, Uther JB: What is the best predictor of spontaneous ventricular tachycardia and sudden death after myocardial infarction? Circulation 83:756–763, 1991.
14. Roy D, Talajic M, et al: Amiodarone to prevent recurrence of atrial fibrillation. N Engl J Med 342:913–920, 2000.
15. Sobel RM, Dhruva NN: Termination of acute wide QRS complex atrial fibrillation with ibutilide. Am J Emerg Med 18:462–464, 2000.
16. Woosley RL: Antiarrhythmic drugs. In Schlant RC, Alexander RW (eds): The Heart Arteries and Veins, 8th ed. New York, McGraw-Hill, 1994, pp 775–805.

48. BETA-ADRENERGIC RECEPTOR BLOCKERS

Olivia V. Adair, M.D., John T. Madonna, M.D., Mark E. Dorogy, M.D., and Richard C. Davis, M.D., Ph.D.

1. Name some of the beta-adrenergic receptor blockers (beta blockers) and their important pharmacologic properties.

Pharmacologic Properties of Commonly Used Beta Blockers

	AVERAGE DAILY DOSE (MG)	CARDIO-SELECTIVITY	LIPID SOLUBILITY	ISA*	MEMBRANE-STABILIZING ACTIVITY
Acebutolol	400–1200	Yes	Moderate	Yes	Yes
Atenolol	50–200	Yes	Weak	No	No
Esmolol	50–150†	Yes	Weak	No	No
Labetalol	400–800	No	Weak	Possible	No
Metoprolol	100–200	Yes	Moderate	No	No
Nadolol	40–80	No	Weak	No	No
Pindolol	5–30	No	Moderate	Yes	Yes
Propranolol	40–160	No	High	No	Yes
Sotalol	80–320	No	Weak	No	No

* Intrinsic sympathomimetic activity.
† Dose in µg/kg/min, parenteral.

2. What are the mechanisms of action of beta blockers?

Beta blockers are competitive antagonists of beta-adrenergic receptors. There are two receptor classes. **Beta-1 receptors**, located in the heart, lead to increases in heart rate, contractility, and atrioventricular conduction when stimulated. Blockade of beta-1 receptors attenuates these increases, particularly during exercise or stress, but also during rest if resting adrenergic tone is increased. Several beta blockers produce low-level receptor stimulation, offsetting the effects of receptors blockade in the resting state while maintaining antagonism during exercise or stress—this is referred to as **intrinsic sympathomimetic activity**.

Beta-2 receptors are more widespread than beta-1 receptors. Activation of these receptors results in such diverse actions as bronchodilation, peripheral vasodilation, and lipolysis. Many adverse effects of beta blockers, such as bronchospasm, are due to beta-2 receptor blockade. Agents that are beta-1 specific, or **cardioselective**, have been developed to minimize these adverse effects. This preferential blockade is not complete however, and some beta-2 receptor antagonism can be observed at standard pharmacologic doses.

3. What are the cardiovascular indications for beta-blocker therapy other than hypertension and angina pectoris?

Acute myocardial infarction (MI)	Hypertrophic cardiomyopathy
Postinfarction	Mitral valve prolapse
Supraventricular arrhythmias	Prolonged QT syndrome
Ventricular arrhythmias	Heart failure
Aortic dissection	Digitalis-induced ventricular arrhythmias

4. When is the use of beta blockers contraindicated?

Contraindications:
  Hypotension
  Asthma
  Chronic obstructive pulmonary disease
Relative contraindications:
  Bradydysrhythmias
  Atrioventricular conduction disturbances
  Congestive heart failure (LV systolic function)
  Raynaud's phenomenon

5. What are the signs and symptoms of beta-blocker toxicity? How is this best treated?

Beta-blocker toxicity, although rare, should be considered in any patient experiencing the sudden onset of bradycardia and hypotension. Generalized seizures can also occur, especially with use of agents that are both lipophilic and have membrane-stabilizing effects. Other reported symptoms include peripheral cyanosis and coma. A history of hypertension, coronary artery disease, or chronic beta-blocker therapy should heighten the suspicion for this diagnosis.

Glucagon is the most effective agent for treating the hemodynamic disturbances due to beta-blockers; epinephrine should be considered second-line therapy, and atropine and isoproterenol are frequently ineffective. Glucagon exerts both positive inotropic and chronotropic effects on the heart. The inotropic effects are not affected by beta blockade, but the increase in heart rate with glucagon may be blunted by beta blockade, and temporary transvenous pacing may be necessary. The initial dose of glucagon is 3 mg or 0.05 mg/kg given intravenously over 30 seconds followed by a continuous infusion at 5 mg/hr or 0.07 mg/kg/hr. The infusion is tapered slowly as the patient improves.

6. How is beta-blocker therapy used following MI?

Beta blockers decrease the risk of death in approximately 20% of patients following MI. This benefit is due almost entirely to a reduction in cardiovascular deaths, both sudden and non-sudden, and is independent of the timing of drug administration. Administration of beta-blocker therapy within hours after infarction provides the additional benefits of limiting infarct size and reducing the risks of nonfatal reinfarction and recurrent ischemia.

The advantages of long-term therapy may be diminished in low-risk subgroups, but data are lacking on which patients can forgo therapy. For example, a 45-year-old man presenting with his first MI who has been treated successfully with thrombolytics and has a normal ejection fraction, inferior location, and single-vessel coronary disease is at low risk and may not benefit from long-term beta-blockade. Characteristics of postinfarction survivors likely to receive maximum benefit from long-term administration include:
- Impaired LV function
- Persistent ischemia (angina, abnormal postinfarction stress test, significant coronary disease supplying viable myocardium)
- Complex ventricular ectopy
- Coexisting illness treatable with beta blockade (e.g., hypertension, supraventricular tachycardia, anxiety)

7. A 19-year-old woman is referred for recurrent fainting spells. A head-up tilt test elicits hypotension and bradycardia, and her symptoms are reproducible. Why might beta-blocker therapy be appropriate?

Neurocardiogenic syncope (common faint) is often a cause of temporary loss of consciousness in young people. Syncope follows profound vasodilatation, bradycardia, or a combination of these responses. It is postulated that in response to a diminished venous return to the heart, such as from prolonged standing, adrenergic tone is enhanced. This results in vigorous myocardial contraction, which stimulates intramyocardial mechanoreceptors (C fibers). Activation of these fibers may override the normal baroreceptor-mediated reflex and produce bradycardia and vasodilatation, which leads to hypotension and syncope.

It may seem paradoxical that beta blockers are effective in treating this disorder. Nevertheless, the negative inotropic effects of beta blockers can diminish C-fiber activation, allowing normal reflex physiology to prevail.

In this patient, a follow-up tilt test should be attempted after therapy, to reproduce her symptoms and ensure the effectiveness of therapy.

8. What types of ventricular arrhythmia are effectively treated with beta blockers?

Beta blockers are effective in preventing ventricular fibrillation during acute myocardial infarction and sudden cardiac death in the postinfarction period; treating digitalis-induced ventricular arrhythmias; suppressing torsade de pointes in the long QT syndrome; treating exercise-induced ventricular tachycardia; and suppressing premature ventricular contractions and complex ventricular ectopy. Some recent studies suggest they may be as effective as sole agents in selected patients with sustained ventricular tachycardia or primary ventricular fibrillation.

9. A middle-aged woman with long-standing hypertension is currently on an antihypertensive regimen of clonidine and propranolol. She complains of symptoms referable to the clonidine. What should you consider before you withdraw clonidine?

Rapid withdrawal of clonidine can provoke a hypertensive rebound thought secondary to increased catecholamine release. Concurrent beta blocker use may greatly enhance the hypertension as a result of unopposed alpha-adrenergic receptor stimulation. Consider a prolonged clonidine taper or withdrawal of the beta blocker prior to tapering.

10. A 39-year-old man with hypertension presents to the emergency department with resting chest pressure and a 4-mm ST-segment elevation in the inferior leads on EKG. Both the chest pressure and EKG changes are relieved by nitroglycerin. Cardiac catheterization demonstrates normal coronary arteries, and spasm of the right coronary artery is subsequently provoked with ergonovine. He currently takes nadolol and a diuretic for hypertension. How should you alter his medical regimen?

This presentation is typical of coronary vasospasm (Prinzmetal's angina). Use of a beta blocker in this disorder has been associated with increased frequency and severity of angina. Discontinuation of the beta blocker and initiation of a calcium channel blocker or nitrate are recommended. When coronary vasospasm occurs in the setting of obstructive coronary disease, beta-blocker administration may be desirable in combination with a calcium channel blocker.

11. A 43-year-old man, referred for management of severe hypertension, was found at the initial visit to have a blood pressure of 190/120 mmHg and tachycardia. He has been followed by a local psychiatrist for several years for episodic anxiety with recurrent spells of apprehension, diaphoresis, nausea, and headache. Antihypertension therapy with a beta blocker was begun. Several days later he returned with pulmonary edema, confusion, and a blood pressure of 260/140 mmHg. What is the most likely diagnosis? Could the accelerated hypertension be related to beta blocker therapy?

This is a classic presentation of pheochromocytoma. Precipitation of the hypertension crisis is directly related to initiating beta blockade. The resultant unopposed alpha-adrenergic stimulation may cause intense peripheral vasoconstriction. While beta blockers may be beneficial in treating this disorder, they should be withheld until alpha-blocker therapy is started. The diagnosis of pheochromocytoma, although not established definitively in this example, should be suspected and beta-blocker therapy avoided until the appropriate diagnostic tests are performed.

12. A 29-year-old woman with a history of mitral valve prolapse complains of palpitations and light-headedness. A rhythm strip taken during her symptoms is shown on the next page. Would beta blockers be effective in treating this disorder?

Yes. This case is an example of an atrioventricular (AV) nodal reentrant tachycardia. Beta blockers interrupt the reentrant circuit by prolonging AV nodal refractoriness and conduction and provide effective treatment and prevention of this arrhythmia. Beta blockers also are effective in treating other supraventricular arrhythmias, including sinoatrial reentrant tachycardia, AV reciprocating tachycardia, and atrial fibrillation and flutter.

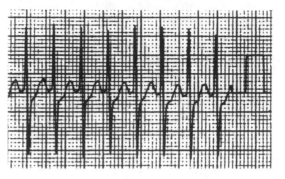

13. What is the proposed mechanism of action for beta blockers in the treatment of heart failure?

Increased adrenergic activity in patients with congestive heart failure can downregulate cardiac beta-adrenergic receptors and cause peripheral vasoconstriction. Beta blockers can attenuate these deleterious effects of chronic catecholamine stimulation. Clinically, this has translated into improvements in hemodynamics, symptoms, exercise tolerance, and left ventricular function. Beta blockers, however, have not been shown to decrease mortality in this setting.

14. In patients with left ventricular (LV) hypertrophy induced by hypertension, do beta blockers reduce LV mass? How do they compare with other agents?

Beta blockers have been shown to cause regression of LV mass in hypertensive patients with LV hypertrophy. In a meta-analysis, LV mass was reduced an average of 8%, as compared to 15% for angiotensin-converting enzyme (ACE) inhibitors, and 8.5% for calcium channel blockers. Diuretics decreased LV mass an average of 11.3%, but this was attributed to a reduction in LV volume and not reversal of wall hypertrophy as seen with the other drug classes.

15. A hypertensive patient presents with an acute aortic dissection. What would proper emergency management include?

While immediate lowering of blood pressure is essential acute therapy for aortic dissection, initial use of nitroprusside may increase the force and velocity (dP/dT) of ventricular contraction, which may increase aortic shear forces and accelerate the propagation of the dissection. By reducing dP/dT, beta blockers decrease aortic shear forces and allow safer introduction of nitroprusside. Labetalol, with its combined beta- and alpha-adrenergic blockade, can be administered intravenously and is a single-agent alternative to the more traditional therapy.

16. What is an "electrical storm" (ES)?

A phenomenon of rapid and recurrent clusters of ventricular fibrillation (VF) that requires multiple cardioversions to maintain a stable rhythm. ES is an independent risk factor for sudden death, especially over the 3 months following the episode.

17. What condition is associated with or causes electrical storm?

Usually the patient has had a recent myocardial infarction, within 3 months. Also, cardiomyopathy with depressed systolic function is seen in these patients. The prognosis is quite poor if only treated at presentation with present guidelines.

18. What treatment plan improves the long- and short-term outcome of electrical storm?

In a recent study, after the patients in ES received the usual ACLS core protocol, they also received beta blocker IV (esmolol or propranolol) or left stellate ganglionic blockade for sympathetic blockade. In the **short term** (1 wk), 24 of the 49 patients died. The mortality rate was 82% in the patients treated with ACLS protocol only, and 72% in the patients who received sympathetic blockade. In the **long term** (1 yr)), 20 of 27 blockade patients lived, but only 2 of the 22 patients not treated with sympathetic blockade lived.

New data shows even greater benefit with amiodarone and beta blocker combined.

19. How do beta blockers compare to implanted cardiac defibrillators (ICDs) for survivors of cardiac arrest?

In the recent CASH study, a comparison of amiodarone, metoprolol, and ICDs showed reduced mortality in cardiac arrest survivors in the ICD patient group. There was no difference in the reduction of mortality between metoprolol and amiodarone. Also, the benefit of ICD therapy was more effective in the first 5 years of follow-up. This may indicate the need for addition of medical therapy to ICD use, e.g., amiodarone and/or metoprolol.

20. Should beta-blockers be withdrawn from patients with dilated cardiomyopathy (DCM)?

No. Morimoto, et al. looked at the influence of tapering and then stopping metoprolol in patients with DCM. The patients had been receiving metoprolol for ≥ 30 months. Four died suddenly out of 13, and an additional 3 had severe deterioration and worsening of heart failure.

21. In the acute management of atrial fibrillation or flutter, what treatment options are now suggested?

Calcium channel blockers IV and **beta blockers** IV are still being used frequently with good results. However, the time to conversion may be many hours or not at all, rate control is usually successful. Also 1–2 g of IV magnesium infusion should be given. **Ibutilide** IV is effective in conversion of atrial fibrillation (80%) and flutter (78%) and more than 90% conversion within 1 hour. Ibutilide is a class III antiarrhythmic drug, given in long infusion IV over 10 minutes; you can repeat a second time after a 10-minute wait between doses.

The pharmacodynamics involve a prolongation of the myocardial action potential and effective refractory. This is rapidly achieved by a dual ionic mechanism involving activation of a slow inward sodium current and blockade of a delayed rectifier potassium current.

Incidence and magnitude of CK-MB elevation in prior β-blocker therapy versus no β-blocker therapy groups. (From Sharma SK, Kini A, Marmur JD, Fuster V: Cardioprotective effect of prior β-blocker therapy in reducing creatine kinase-MB elevation after coronary intervention. Circulation 102:166–172, 2000, with permission.)

Intermediate-term mortality in relation to prior β-blocker therapy and CK-MB elevation. *A*, Mortality in relation to prior β-blocker therapy at the time of intervention. *B*, Mortality in relation to CK-MB levels. *C*, Mortality in relation to prior β-blocker therapy and CK-MB levels. (From Sharma SK, Kini A, Marmur JD, Fuster V: Cardioprotective effect of prior β-blocker therapy in reducing creatine kinase-MB elevation after coronary intervention. Circulation 102:166–172, 2000, with permission.)

22. If a patient presents with threat of infarct (angina), but undergoes intervention that opens the artery, are there any benefit(s) post myocardial infarction?

Though studies had shown increased survival and decreased reinfarction in patients with infarction, the benefit and protective value of intervention had not been examined. Sharma et al. looked at this question using pre-procedure beta-blocker therapy. The group receiving pre-therapy had significantly lower incidence of CK-MB elevation (2.2%) vs. nontreated (13.2%). The former group also had lower heart rates and blood pressure and less occurrence of chest pain.

In the intermediate outcome follow-up (15 months), the pre-intervention beta-blocker group had lower mortality rates, 0.78% vs. 1.96%. These benefits are seen as well in patients with small CPK-MB rise and an open artery.

Note: The opinions and assertions contained herein are the private views of the authors and are not to be construed as official or reflecting the views of the Department of the Army or Department of Defense.

BIBLIOGRAPHY

1. Bocker D, Breithardt G: Evaluating AVID, CASH, CIDS, CABG-patch, and MADIT: Are they concordant? J Interv Card Electrophysiol 4JanSuppl, 2000.
2. Dahlof B, Pennert K, Hansson L: Reversal of left ventricular hypertrophy in hypertensive patients: A meta-analysis of 109 treatment studies. Am J Hypertens 5:95–110, 1992.
3. Eagle KA, DeSanctis RW: Diseases of the aorta. In Braunwald E (ed): Heart Disease: A Textbook of Cardiovascular Medicine, 5th ed. Philadelphia, W.B. Saunders, 1997.
4. Kuck K, Cappato R, et al: Randomized comparison of antiarrhythmic drug therapy with transplantable defibrillators in cardiac arrest. The Cardiac Arrest Study–Hamburg (CASH). Circulation 102:748–754, 2000.
5. Landsberg L, Young JB: Pheochromocytoma. In Wilson JD, Braunwald E, Isselbacher KJ (eds): Harrison's Principles of Internal Medicine, 13th ed. New York, McGraw-Hill, 1994, pp 1976-1979.
6. Morimoto S, Shimizu K, Yamada K, et al: Can beta-blocker therapy be withdrawn from patients with dilated cardiomyopathy? Am Heart J 138(3 pt 1):456–459, 1999.
7. Nademanee K, Taylor R, Bailey W, et al: Treating electrical storm. Circulation 102:742–747, 2000.
8. Pinski SL, Yao Q, Epstein AE, et al: Determinants of outcome in patients with sustained ventricular tachyarrhythmias: The antiarrhythmics versus implantable defibrillators (AVID) study registry. Am Heart J 139(5):804–813, 2000.
9. Sharma S, Kini A, et al: Cardioprotective effect of prior b-blocker therapy in reducing creatine kinase-MB elevation after coronary intervention. Circulation 102:166–172, 2000.
10. Sra JS, Anderson AJ, Sheikh SH, et al: Unexplained syncope evaluated by electrophysiologic studies and head-up tilt testing. Ann Intern Med 114:1013–1019, 1991.
11. Steinbeck G, Andresen D, Bach P, et al: A comparison of electrophysiologically guided antiarrhythmic drug therapy with beta-blocker therapy in patients with symptomatic, sustained ventricular tachyarrhythmias. N Engl J Med 327:987–992, 1992.

49. ANTICOAGULANT AND ANTIPLATELET DRUGS

Madeline Jean White, M.D.

1. What anticoagulant and antiplatelet agents are commonly used in cardiology?

The main anticoagulants are aspirin and warfarin, given orally, and heparin, given intravenously or subcutaneously. Low–molecular-weight heparin (LMWH) has proven benefit in unstable angina, but the lack of reversibility has raised some concern about its use in patients who may be undergoing intervention. This problem will be solved as soon as rapid laboratory testing for factor Xa activity becomes available.

Antiplatelet drugs include aspirin, the thienopyridines, and the glycoprotein IIb/IIIa antagonists. Glycoprotein IIb/IIIa antagonists are now standard treatment during coronary interventions and are of proven benefit in high-risk patients with unstable angina.

The American College of Cardiology and the American Heart Association have published guidelines for the interplay of the various agents.

2. How does warfarin work?

The synthesis of several clotting factors (prothrombin, factors VII, IX, and X) depends on the availability of the hydroquinone form of vitamin K for the final carboxylation. Without carboxylation, the factors are biologically inactive. Warfarin is able to inhibit enzymes in the recycling process of vitamin K, thereby decreasing levels of the required hydroquinone form. The anticoagulation effect of warfarin results from the decline and depletion of carboxylated clotting factors. Because synthesis and clearance play a role, it takes 4–5 days to achieve a therapeutic level, in contrast to heparin's instantaneous effect.

3. What is the INR value?

In the past, warfarin therapy was monitored with the prothrombin time (PT). Problems with standardization of anticoagulant intensity arose because the thromboplastin used in the PT test varied among batches in its ability to facilitate coagulation. Now, commercial producers assign each lot an ISI (International Sensitivity Index), which relates the preparation's activity to that of an international reference thromboplastin. Individual laboratories then calculate an INR value (International Normalized Ratio) to relate the patient's PT to the intensity of actual anticoagulation:

$$INR = \left(\frac{\text{Patient PT}}{\text{Mean Normal PT}} \right)^{ISI}$$

Results are reported with both the PT (in seconds) and INR value. The INR is variable in the initial stages of treatment and is most useful once stable dosing is achieved.

4. Which factor level drops the fastest with warfarin therapy?

Factor VII has the shortest half-life (6 hrs) and falls the fastest. Factors X and IX have half-lives of about 24 hours. Thus, the PT/INR may prolong before all the critical clotting factors have fallen and before full anticoagulation is achieved.

5. List the guidelines for starting and following warfarin therapy.

Many indications for chronic anticoagulation are being developed. Maintain sanity by sticking with a few rules:

1. Start with 5 mg orally each day.
2. Large loading doses are not recommended. Use 10 mg for 1–2 days if there is some urgency.
3. Check the PT/INR daily until a therapeutic level is reached for that clinical setting.
4. After 4–6 days, the dosage may need adjusting as the individual's sensitivity to warfarin is established.

5. Monitor the PT/INR twice weekly for 2 weeks, then weekly for 2 months.

6. Once the dose is stable, check the PT/INR every 4–6 weeks.

7. Never go > 8 weeks without a PT/INR check for therapeutic doses. Many factors can influence the anticoagulant intensity and increase the risk of bleeding unpredictably.

8. For patient convenience, if the patient needs < 1 tablet on a given day of the week, make it $\frac{1}{2}$ or 0 tablets, not $\frac{1}{4}$.

9. If the patient is on dose "x" on certain days of the week and dose "y" on the rest, always use dose "x" on the same days. For example:

Dose "x mg" once a week—Monday

Dose "x mg" twice a week—Monday and Friday

Dose "x mg" three times a week—Monday, Wednesday, and Friday

10. To make adjustments, look at the total weekly warfarin dose. Go up or down by $\frac{1}{7}$ of the total weekly dose distributed over the week. For example, if the week's dose will be decreased by 1 tablet, reduce the Mondays and Fridays by $\frac{1}{2}$ tablet rather than eliminate 1 tablet on Mondays.

11. If the dose is adjusted, check the PT/INR at 2–3 weeks depending on the magnitude of the change.

6. How do you avoid the possible development of relative protein C deficiency?

Because protein C, a clot inhibitor protein, has a short half-life, a relative deficiency can result on the first few days of warfarin use. Most warfarin is started concurrently with intravenous heparin, so the concern for relative protein C deficiency is addressed. If the use of warfarin is planned without full heparin anticoagulation (i.e., in atrial fibrillation), the first 5–7 days should be covered with subcutaneous heparin or LMWH.

7. List some drugs that alter the PT.

Drugs the Alter Prothrombin Time by Interacting with Warfarin

PHARMACOKINETIC (Drugs that change warfarin levels)	PHARMACODYNAMIC (Drugs that do not change warfarin levels)	MECHANISM UNKNOWN (Drugs whose effect on warfarin levels is unknown)
Prolongs prothrombin time	**Prolongs prothrombin time**	**Prolongs prothrombin time**
Stereoselective inhibition of	Inhibits cyclic interconversion	Evidence for interaction
S isomer clearance*	of vitamin K (2nd- and 3rd-	convincing
Phenylbutazone	generation cephalosporins)	Erythromycin
Metronidazole	Other mechanisms	Anabolic steroids
Sulfinpyrazone	Clofibrate	Evidence for interaction less
Trimethoprim-sulfamethoxazole	Inhibits blood coagulation	convincing
Disulfiram	Heparin	Ketoconazole
Stereoselective inhibition of	Increases metabolism of	Fluconazole
R isomer clearance	coagulation factors	Isoniazid
Cimetidine†	Thyroxine	Piroxicam
Omeprazole†		Tamoxifen
Nonstereoselective inhibitions of	**Inhibits platelet function**	Quinidine
R and S isomers clearance	Aspirin	Vitamin E (megadose)
Amiodarone	Other nonsteroidal anti-inflam-	Phenytoin
	matory drugs	
Reduces prothrombin time	Ticlopidine	**Reduces prothrombin time**
Reduces absorption	Moxalactam	Penicillins
Cholestyramine	Carbenicillin and high doses of	Griseofulvin‡
	other penicillins	
Increases metabolic clearance		
Barbiturates		
Rifampin		
Griseofulvin		
Carbamazepine		

* Warfarin is a racemic mixture of *S* and *R* isomers, which have different metabolisms.

† Causes minimal prolongation of the prothrombin time.

‡ May cause increased metabolic clearance.

Adapted from Hirsh J: Oral anticoagulant drugs. N Engl J Med 324:1865–1875, 1991.

8. What clinical conditions can alter warfarin effects?

High vitamin K intake with diets rich in green vegetables or food supplements can antagonize warfarin's action. Situations that decrease vitamin K availability, such as fat malabsorption and starvation, can enhance the drug's effect. Increased catabolism with fever or hyperthyroidism causes increased clearance of clotting factors, and hepatic dysfunction can reduce synthesis— both of these situations increase sensitivity to warfarin. Elders may be more sensitive to warfarin effects than younger individuals are.

9. What are the recommended INR ranges?

Once the PT/INR has reached therapeutic levels for a specific clinical situation, the dose of warfarin should be adjusted to keep within the INR ranges recommended. For most conditions of anticoagulation, INR values of 2.0–3.0 are adequate. High-risk situations may call for greater intensity:

> **INR 2.5–3.5**
>   Mechanical prosthetic valves (high risk)[9]
>   Prevention of recurrent myocardial infarction

10. How long should anticoagulation be maintained?

In situations in which the risk of embolization is **chronic**, such as mechanical valves, atrial fibrillation, dilated cardiomyopathy with heart failure, and recurrent deep venous thrombosis, anticoagulation should be lifelong unless contraindications exist.

Duration after **acute events** (pulmonary embolism, deep venous thrombosis, acute anterior myocardial infarction) is controversial, but most clinicians maintain therapy for at least 6 months. **Prophylactic** use usually covers just the period of risk.

11. What factors increase the risk of bleeding during warfarin therapy?

Intensity of dose: INR values > 3.0 have increased risk.

Age: Risk rises with increased age, but some find age *not* to be an independent risk factor.

Duration of therapy: The risk of bleeding is highest in the first several weeks of therapy: 3% risk in the first month, 0.8% risk per month in the first year, and 0.3% risk monthly for subsequent years. Cumulative risk increases with the duration of therapy.

Comorbid conditions: Cerebrovascular, renal, heart, and liver disease are associated with more bleeding complications.

Concurrent medications: Some drugs can predictably alter the PT/INR, but variability is the norm. When adding any new chronic medication, increase monitoring of PT/INR until a stable state is achieved.

Compliance: Safe, effective, outpatient warfarin use demands regular monitoring and systematic dose adjustments. Patient compliance is critical.

12. How does heparin work?

Heparin is a highly sulfated, natural glycosaminoglycan. Commercial preparations are derived from porcine intestine or bovine lung. Its anticoagulant affect is mediated through antithrombin III, which has a native ability to inhibit thrombin, activated factor X (Xa), and activated factor IX (IXa). Once heparin binds to antithrombin III, this inhibition is increased up to 1000 times. Anticoagulation is almost instantaneous. LMWH, with its smaller size, has less binding capacity for thrombin, platelets, plasma proteins, and endothelial cells. It inactivates factor X_a, has good bioavailability, demonstrates increased plasma half-life, and is renally cleared.

13. Before starting therapy with heparin, what baseline tests should you obtain?

Hematocrit, platelet count, activated partial thromboplastin time (aPTT), and prothrombin time (PT—with INR). The aPTT serves as a baseline value to gauge the therapeutic dose of heparin; the PT/INR is the baseline for anticipated warfarin therapy. The hematocrit and platelet count provide pretreatment values if complications arise. For LMWH, a baseline coagulation panel is a good precaution, even though aPTT is not used to monitor therapy.

14. How do you achieve and monitor the therapeutic level of heparin?

Heparin therapy is very empirical, and there are many patterns for initiating and monitoring it. Most clinicians give an **intravenous** bolus of 80 U/kg, then start a continuous infusion of 18 U/kg/hr. The aPTT is checked at 4–6 hours. If it is not within the goal of 1.5–2.3 times baseline, the rate is adjusted up or down (2–4 U/kg/hr). Minimally prolonged aPTT may require a rebolus of 80 U/kg and an increase in rate of 4 U/kg/hr. It the aPTT is markedly prolonged, the infusion is held for 1 hour and then a reduced rate resumed. The aPTT is rechecked at 4–6 hours.

The body-weight dosing schedule reaches the therapeutic threshold (aPTT 1.5 times control) in more cases (90% vs. 77%) than the standard dosing schedule. In life-threatening situations, achieving a therapeutic level promptly is very important. With interpatient variability, the clinician must be alert and *not* assume that the dose selected is correct without laboratory confirmation. Once an adequate rate is achieved, the aPTT should be checked each day.

Brill-Edwards et al. have pointed out a considerable variation among aPTT reagents. A therapeutic range using protamine titrated heparin levels of 0.2–0.4 U/ml would be more accurate than relying on prolongation of aPTT versus control.

Subcutaneous heparin, used prophylactically, is started at 5000 U every 8–12 hours. It is not monitored because therapeutic goals are achieved at levels that may not prolong the aPTT.

Weight-based dosing of LMWH does not need lab monitoring, but antifactor X_a activity can be measured in cases of renal failure.

15. What are the complications of heparin therapy?

In any anticoagulant therapy, the major risk is bleeding. Estimates range from 0.8% per day to about 5% overall in recent surveys. Dose seems to be the most important factor, hence the vigilance regarding the aPTT. Bleeding risk also increases with intermittent subcutaneous use, duration of therapy, and concurrent use of anti-platelet and thrombolytic agents.

Heparin can cause mild or severe **thrombocytopenia**. The mild form is due to heparin-induced platelet aggregation and occurs after 2 days to 2 weeks of full-dose heparin in about 15–25% of cases. The platelet counts usually stabilize above 100,000/μl, even with continued heparin therapy. In the severe form, immune mechanisms cause a marked fall in platelet count (< 50,000/μl) and arterial thrombi can occur. Bovine-derived heparin is more commonly involved than the porcine product. Platelet counts should be checked daily; if they drop below 100,000, heparin should be discontinued. Ongoing antithrombotic therapy may include agents such as danaparoid, hirudin, and argatroban. Plasmapheresis or intravenous immunoglobulin also can be used adjunctively. LMWHs cross-react with heparin and are not safe substitutes.

At 5–10 days of therapy, transient abnormalities of **liver function** tests can occur. Rarely, anaphylaxis, skin necrosis, local urticaria, or hyperkalemia is seen. Long-term heparin use can cause osteoporosis. LMWH may cause less osteoporosis and heparin-induced thrombocytopenia.

16. What are some contraindications to heparin therapy?

Contraindications

    Severe active bleeding
    Allergic reactions
    Heparin-induced thrombocytopenia and thrombosis

Relative contraindications

Central nervous system hemorrhage	Endocarditis
Intracranial metastases	Recent surgery
Severe hypertension	Trauma
Retinopathy	
Pericarditis	

17. Is heparin "resistance" real?
Massive pulmonary embolism can be associated with increased clearance of heparin, giving a picture of relative resistance. Antithrombin III, which is required for heparin's action, can be the key to heparin "resistance." Congenital antithrombin III deficiencies usually reduce antithrombin III levels to 40–60%, sufficient for anticoagulation with heparin. In acquired deficiencies from hepatic cirrhosis, nephrotic syndrome, or disseminated intravascular coagulation, antithrombin III levels can fall to lower levels (< 25%), where heparin activity is impaired.

18. If long-term anticoagulation is anticipated, how do you combine heparin and warfarin?
Start warfarin on day 1 of heparin therapy. This allows depletion of vitamin K-dependent factors while the patient is fully anticoagulated with heparin. After 5–6 days of heparin and with at least 2 days of a therapeutic PT/INR, heparin can be discontinued. A minor decrease in PT/INR may be seen as the heparin effect wanes. Overlapping therapy is also needed if LMWH is used.

19. How do aspirin and the thienopyridines work?
Aspirin acetylates platelet cyclo-oxygenase irreversibly, thereby inhibiting the formation of thromboxane A_2. Platelet reactivity is diminished. Aspirin also inhibits the endothelium's production of prostaglandin I_2, which decreases platelet aggregation and induces vasodilatation. The thienopyridines act as adenosine diphosphate (ADP) antagonists, which inhibit ADP-mediated activation of the glycoprotein IIb/IIIa complex. Platelet aggregation is impaired.

20. Are any baseline studies needed before starting aspirin or the thienopyridines?
A good history is needed to evaluate possible allergies, ulcer tendencies, coagulation disorders, and medication interactions. Risk–benefit issues guide the clinician's decision regarding use, dose, and enteric coating. Specific laboratory tests are not routinely needed.

21. Should the effect of aspirin or the thienopyridines be monitored?
For aspirin, no. Clinical trials have used outcomes (morbidity and mortality) to evaluate aspirin's benefit in populations. Platelet function tests are not followed in the individual patient. There is a risk of severe neutropenia and thrombotic thrombocytopenic purpura with the thienopyridines, so some practitioners do monitor blood counts.

22. How do glycoprotein IIb/IIIa receptor antagonists interfere with platelet function?
The primary ligand of the glycoprotein IIb/IIIa receptor on the platelet membrane is fibrinogen. Fibrinogen simultaneously binds receptors on two separate platelets. Platelet cross-linking occurs leading to aggregation. The antagonist occupies the binding site and blunts the final common pathway of platelet aggregation.

BIBLIOGRAPHY

1. Braunwald E, Antman EM, Beasley JW, et al: ACC/AHA guidelines for the management of patients with unstable angina and non-ST-segment elevation myocardial infarction. Executive summary and recommendations: A report of the American College of Cardiology/American Heart Association Task Force on Practice Guidelines (Committee on Management of Patients With Unstable Angina). Circulation 102:1193–1209, 2000.
2. Chew DP, Moliterno DJ: A critical appraisal of platelet glycoprotein IIb/IIIa inhibition. J Am Coll Cardiol 36:2028–2035, 2000.
3. Clinical Practice Statement: The use of oral anticoagulants (warfarin) in older people. J Am Geriatr Soc 44:1112, 1996.
4. Hirsh J: Oral anticoagulant drugs. N Engl J Med 324:1865–1875, 1991.
5. Hirsh J, Dalen JE, Anderson D, et al: Oral anticoagulants: Mechanism of action, clinical effectiveness, and optimal therapeutic range. Chest 114(5 Suppl):445S–469S, 1998.
6. Hirsh J, Warkentin TE, Raschke R, et al: Heparin and low-molecular-weight heparin: Mechanisms of action, pharmacokinetics, dosing considerations, monitoring, efficacy, and safety. Chest 114(5 Suppl):489S–510S, 1998.

7. Hoffman R, Benz EJ, Shattil SJ, et al (eds): Hematology: Basic Principles and Practice. New York, Churchill Livingstone, 1999.
8. Levine M, Raskob GE, Landefeld S, et al: Hemorrhagic complications of anticoagulant treatment. Chest 114(5 Suppl):511S–523S, 1998.
9. Miescher PA, Jaffé ER, Beris P, Young NS: Heparin-induced thrombocytopenia: Pathophysiology and clinical management. Semin Hematol 36:1S, 1999.
10. Patrono C, Coller BAS, Dalen JE, et al: Platelet-active drugs: The relationship among dose, effectiveness, and side effects. Chest 114(5 Suppl):470S–488S, 1998.
11. Stein PD, Alpert JS, Dalen JE, et al: Antithrombotic therapy in patients with mechanical and biological prosthetic heart valves. Chest 114(5 Suppl):602S–610S, 1998.
12. Vorchheimer DA, Badimon JJ, Fuster V: Platelet glycoprotein IIb/IIIa receptor antagonists in cardiovascular disease. JAMA 281:1407–1414, 1999.

50. DIURETICS AND NITRATES

Jennifer L. Calagan, M.D., David T. Schachter, M.D., Mitchel Kruger, M.D.,
Robert W. Cameron, M.D., and Catalin Loghin, M.D.

1. Discuss the mechanism of action of the five groups of diuretics.

All diuretics interfere with sodium chloride resorption, but each class of diuretics has a distinct site of action in the nephron. The site of inhibition of sodium chloride resorption partially dictates the efficacy and side effects of each drug class.

Mechanism of Action of the Diuretics

CLASS	DRUGS	SITE OF ACTION
Thiazide diuretics	Hydrochlorothiazide Indapamide Chlorthalidone	Cortical thick ascending loop of Henle Cortical diluting segment
Loop diuretics	Furosemide Bumetanide Ethacrynic acid	Medullary and cortical portions of the thick ascending limb of loop of Henle
Osmotic diuretics	Mannitol	Proximal tubule Loop of Henle Distal tubule Collecting tubule
Potassium-sparing diuretics	Spironolactone Triamterene Amiloride	Distal tubule
Carbonic anhydrase inhibitors	Acetazolamide	Proximal tubule

2. A patient presented to the emergency department with pulmonary edema and was treated with intravenous furosemide and oxygen, with clinical improvement. The pulmonary congestive symptoms were alleviated without a significant increase in urine output. Can you explain why this patient improved?

This early effect of furosemide is believed to be due to direct pulmonary venous dilation. It may also redistribute pulmonary blood flow away from fluid-filled alveoli to well-aerated alveoli. This improves blood oxygen saturation and alleviates symptoms of congestive heart failure. Taken orally, furosemide has an onset of action within 1 hour, and its diuretic effect lasts for 6–8 hours. Administered intravenously, it has a diuretic effect beginning within minutes and lasting approximately 2 hours.

3. What are some adverse metabolic effects of diuretics?

Thiazide and loop diuretics cause **hyperglycemia**. The exact mechanism is unknown, but two theories are proposed. One states that diuretic-induced hypokalemia impairs insulin release from the pancreas. Correction of hypokalemia in some patients improves carbohydrate tolerance. The other theory is that diuretics cause peripheral insulin resistance. This may explain why serum insulin levels are increased in patients taking diuretics.

Diuretics elevate serum **cholesterol** and **triglycerides**. The mechanism for this might be a reduced insulin sensitivity which causes an increased hepatic production of cholesterol. The elevation is mild and can be overcome by maintaining a diet low in saturated fat and cholesterol. α-antagonists such as prazosin appear to block or reverse the hyperlipidemic effects of thiazides.

However, current evidence supports the finding that low doses of thiazides, even in association with beta-blockers, result in minimal changes to the lipid profile. These changes do not offset the beneficial effects of these drugs in treating hypertension.

All diuretics cause **hyperuricemia** by inhibition of the organic acid secretory pathway in the proximal tubule and by enhanced resorption of uric acid in the proximal and distal tubules.

4. Do diuretics have an effect on calcium excretion?

Yes. Thiazide diuretics increase serum calcium concentrations by promoting tubular resorption of calcium. They are contraindicated in acute hypercalcemic states. Thiazides are useful in preventing calcium-containing renal calculi or urolithiasis since they diminish the calcium concentration of urine. Thiazides may cause hypercalcemia in patients with renal insufficiency who take calcium-containing medications or vitamin D.

5. What complications of diuretic use are potentially life-threatening?

The thiazide diuretics and loop diuretics can cause **pancreatitis**. With loop diuretics, the mechanism is unknown but may involve excessive pancreatic secretion because of amplified secretin release. With thiazides, the inciting factor is thought to be hypercalcemia caused by the medication. Diuretic-induced pancreatitis is uncommon.

In patients prone to **ventricular arrhythmias**, such as those with congestive heart failure, hypokalemia may help precipitate ventricular tachycardia or ventricular fibrillation. This is especially important when digoxin is being used concurrently.

6. Diabetes insipidus is characterized by an inappropriate increase in urine production. Why are diuretics used to treat this disorder?

Thiazide drugs, by inducing mild sodium and extracellular volume depletion, invoke a compensatory increase in proximal tubule sodium and water resorption. The amount of filtrate delivered to the distal diluting segment is thereby reduced and urine output is diminished.

7. A patient is vacationing in Colorado to ski. On prior trips, he experienced headaches, nausea, and insomnia. His doctors advised him to take a "water pill" prior to skiing, but he forgot the medication and cannot remember its name. What medication would you prescribe?

This patient's history and symptoms are consistent with high-altitude sickness. Acetazolamide, a carbonic anhydrase inhibitor, has been used to treat this condition. Its mechanism of action is the induction of a metabolic acidosis which stimulates the respiratory drive and diminishes altitude-induced hypoxemia. It cannot, however, be relied upon to prevent the life-threatening complications of pulmonary or cerebral edema or reduce the incidence of retinal hemorrhage. Descent is the only effective treatment for these problems.

8. What is the role of diuretics in treating hypertension?

Thiazides frequently are still a first-choice therapy for hypertension, especially when cost and compliance are important. They are also effective in the elderly with isolated systolic hypertension. Diuretics are often still required in controlling severe hypertension when multiple classes of drugs at maximal doses are being used without complete success. Loop diuretics are effective in patients with renal failure, and in those with CHF or others in whom edema is a major complaint. The overall effect is mainly due to a long-term reduction of the peripheral vascular resistance and is translated in a reduced risk for hypertension complications: stokes, MI, and CHF.

9. What is the role of diuretics in treating heart failure?

Their major use is for the advanced stages of heart failure, by decreasing preload and providing symptomatic improvement and decreased hospitalization rates. For edematous patients and for those with impaired renal function, a loop diuretic, administered in two daily doses, is the first choice, either alone or in combination with spironolactone, metolazone, or thiazide.

Among loop diuretics for patients with right-sided heart failure, oral torsemide is preferred. Metolazone is reserved for refractory edema, once or twice weekly with careful monitoring of electrolytes.

Recently, a major trial studied the effects of spironolactone on the morbidity and mortality of patients with severe heart failure. The results clearly indicated that this drug, administered in conjunction with the standard therapy, reduces deaths (by 30%) and morbidity (by 35%) in this category of patients. Spironolactone can be used in conjunction with ACE inhibitors, which do not suppress the entire aldosterone production. Selective aldosterone receptor blockers, such as eplerenone, are to be further evaluated.

10. What are the indications for chronic nitrate therapy?

Nitrates are used to treat angina related to atherosclerotic coronary artery disease and coronary artery spasm. They also lessen symptoms of chronic congestive heart failure and, in combination with hydralazine, improve survival and delay progression of left ventricular dysfunction (though not as well as angiotensin-converting enzyme inhibitors).

11. How do nitrates achieve their antianginal affects?

Nitrates dilate epicardial coronary arteries and coronary resistance vessels. Atherosclerotic coronary arteries respond to nitroglycerin even in areas of significant stenosis. Collateral vessels also dilate. Both result in an increase in O_2 delivery to ischemic myocardium. There is no "steal phenomenon" described with nitrates, since they dilate both non-stenosed coronary arteries or stenosed vessels without circumferential calcifications.

Nitrates also affect systemic arteries and veins. Venodilation, by reducing preload, decreases diastolic volume, wall stress, and O_2 consumption. Dilatation of systemic arteries decreases myocardial O_2 consumption by decreasing afterload. Angina is relieved as O_2 delivery to ischemic regions is increased and O_2 consumption is decreased. In coronary spasm, nitrates relieve angina by their direct ability to dilate epicardial vessels at the sites of spasm.

Overall, nitrates improve myocardial oxygen supply and decrease the oxygen demand, resulting in their significant anti-ischemic effect.

12. By what additional mechanism may nitrates be beneficial in unstable angina or acute myocardial infarction?

Nitroglycerin has antiplatelet effects which inhibit thrombus formation. This antiplatelet effect may contribute to the improved survival seen when intravenous nitroglycerin is used during myocardial infarction, and it may decrease recurrent ischemic episodes in patients with unstable angina.

13. What kinds of nitrate therapy are available?

Nitroglycerin is available as a sublingual tablet or spray, a buccal preparation, long-acting oral tablets, topical preparations (ointment or patch) and intravenous preparations. **Isosorbide dinitrate** can be used sublingually or orally. **5-Isosorbide mononitrate** is available for oral administration only.

14. What are the mechanisms of action of organic nitrates on the cellular level?

Organic nitrates act as prodrugs which must be converted inside vascular smooth muscle cells to nitric oxide (also known as endothelium-derived relaxing factor). This conversion is accomplished by a reduction reaction using sulfhydryl groups from cysteine within the cytosol as follows:

$$NO_2 + 2 SH \rightarrow NO + S = S + H_2O$$
(nitrate + cysteine $\rightarrow$ nitric oxide)

Nitric oxide (NO) directly stimulates guanylate cyclase (GC), resulting in increased levels of intracellular cyclic GMP. GMP acts through phosphorylation of cellular proteins via protein kinases to decrease the availability of calcium to contractile proteins. This results in relaxation. NO is also involved in the control mechanisms of vascular growth and endothelial function, and plays a role in myocardial contractility. The current concept of endothelial dysfunction involves a reduced availability of NO.

15. How is nitrate tolerance manifested?

Tolerance was first noted nearly 100 years ago in munitions workers, who suffered headache, fatigue, and orthostatic symptoms on returning to work after short holidays. Their symptoms resolved after hours to days of continued exposure.

Tolerance today is manifested by loss of efficacy in treating symptoms of angina or congestive heart failure with long-acting preparations used without a nitrate-free interval. Tolerance is also seen when increasing doses of intravenous nitroglycerin are needed over time to achieve a specific hemodynamic response or antianginal effect. The molecular mechanism of tolerance is largely unknown. This phenomenon can be avoided by incorporating a nitrate-free interval, preferably during night hours. Such an interval is accomplished by using either a slow-release formulation or asymmetric twice-daily doses for short-acting nitrates.

16. A 64-year-old man with stable exertional angina has been doing well on isosorbide dinitrate, 20 mg twice daily. Recently, he increased his dose to four times daily, thinking "more is better." Soon after, he noted worsening angina. Why might this occur?

This patient could have worsening angina secondary to progression of his coronary artery disease or it may be the development of nitrate tolerance. Studies in patients with stable angina have shown persistent antianginal effects when a nitrate-free interval of 10–12 hours is provided. Many patients experience an attenuation or complete loss of anti-anginal effects when long-acting agents are used three or four times daily. Similarly, long-acting nitroglycerin patches should be removed for 10–12 hours daily.

17. Name some possible mechanisms of nitrate tolerance.

- Sulfhydryl depletion—Inadequate generation of sulfhydryl groups necessary for transformation of organic nitrates to nitric oxide.
- Chronic stimulation by nitric oxide causes desensitization of guanylate cyclase.
- Activation of counter-regulatory neurohumoral mechanisms—Increased catecholamines, arginine vasopressin, plasma renin, aldosterone, and angiotensin II.
- Increased intravascular volume—Starting forces favor net movement of fluid from tissues into the vascular space when capillary pressure is reduced by vasodilation.

18. How do nitroglycerin and heparin interact?

Nitroglycerin may interfere with the anticoagulant activity of heparin, necessitating increased heparin doses to achieve therapeutic results. When nitroglycerin is discontinued, excessive anticoagulation may occur.

19. A patient is admitted with unstable angina. Cardiac catheterization demonstrates triple-vessel coronary artery disease. Several episodes of chest pain develop at rest, and he is treated with increasingly high doses of intravenous nitroglycerin, calcium blockers, heparin, and aspirin. On rounds the following morning, he appears cyanotic and also complains of weakness, headache, and shortness of breath. His lungs are clear; he has no murmurs; and his chest x-ray is normal. How would you treat this syndrome? Are these findings related to his therapy?

High doses of nitroglycerin can result in clinically significant methemoglobinemia. Cyanosis occurs when the level of methemoglobin ($HbFe^{+3}$) exceeds 10%. When the level exceeds 35%, symptoms of dyspnea, headache, and weakness appear. The treatment for toxic methemoglobinemia is intravenous methylene blue at 2 mg/kg. Methemoglobin levels become significantly reduced, and symptoms substantially improve within 1 hour.

20. Which is the best preparation for delivering nitrate: the sublingual pill, spray, ointment, or patch?

Choice of nitrates depends on the clinical situation. For *acute* relief, a **sublingual tablet** provides the fastest absorption and response. The tablets must be kept in a dark bottle, and they should be replaced every 3 months. If more than three tablets are required to control an angina attack, it is best to seek immediate medical attention.

The **oral spray** is a viable alternative for treating acute anginal attacks, but its onset of action is slower. The spray has the advantage of staying active for up to 3 years.

The **ointment** can also be used in an acute situation. Compared to the sublingual tablet, the dose is harder to control, and the onset of action is slower. There is little evidence to support long-term usage of ointment.

The **patch** has been used for the last 20 years for *chronic* treatment of angina pectoris. Multiple studies have shown that tolerance can be avoided by using a 12-hours-on, 12-hours-off schedule.

The opinions and assertions contained herein are the private views of the authors and are not to be construed as official or reflecting the views of the U.S. Department of the Army or Department of Defense.

BIBLIOGRAPHY

1. Abrams J: Use of nitrates in ischemic heart disease. Curr Probl Cardiol 17:483–542, 1992.
2. Amsterdam EA: Rationale for intermittent nitrate therapy. Am J Cardiol 70:556–606, 1992.
3. Bell D: Insulin resistance. Postgrad Med 93:99–107, 1993.
4. Elkayam U, Mehra A, Avraham S, Osprzega E: Possible mechanisms of nitrate tolerance. Am J Cardiol 70:496–546, 1992.
5. Folts JD: Inhibition of platelet function in vivo or in vitro by organic nitrates. J Am Coll Cardiol 18:1537–1538, 1991.
6. Fung H, Chung S, Bauer J, et al: Biochemical mechanism of organic nitrate action. Am J Cardiol 70:4B–10B, 1992.
7. Gheorghiade M, et al: Current medical therapy for advanced heart failure. Heart Lung 29(1):16–32, 2000.
8. Greene MK, et al: Acetazolamide in prevention of acute mountain sickness: Double-blind controlled crossover study. BMJ 283:811–813, 1991.
9. Pitt B, et al: The effect of spironolactone on morbidity and mortality in patients with severe heart failure. New Engl J Med 341(10):709–717, 1999.
10. Smith TW, Braunwald E, Kelly R: The management of heart failure. In Braunwald E (ed): Heart Disease: A Textbook of Cardiovascular Medicine, 5th ed. Philadelphia, W.B. Saunders, 1997.
11. Weir MR, Moser M: Diuretics and beta-blockers: Is there a risk for dyslipidemia? Am Heart J 139(1):174–184, 2000.
12. Wood AJJ: Nitrate therapy for stable angina pectoris. New Engl J Med 338(8):520–531, 1998.

51. ANGIOTENSIN-CONVERTING ENZYME INHIBITORS AND OTHER VASODILATORS

Talley F. Culclasure, M.D., Christopher M. Kozlowski, M.D., William T. Highfill, M.D., and Catalin Loghin, M.D.

1. Which vasodilators are in common clinical use?

Vasodilators in Clinical Use

MECHANISM	DRUGS
Angiotensin-converting enzyme (ACE) inhibitors	Captopril, enalapril, lisinopril, quinapril, ramipril, benazepril, fosinopril
Angiotensin II receptor blockers (ARB)	Losartan, irbesartan, candesartan, telmisartan, valsartan, eprosartan
Direct smooth muscle relaxants	Nitroprusside, nitrates, hydralazine, minoxidil
Alpha-adrenergic blockers	Prazosin, terazosin, doxazosin
Calcium channel blockers	Nifedipine, isradipine, amlodipine, felodipine, nimodipine, verapamil

2. Why are vasodilators useful in congestive heart failure due to left ventricular systolic dysfunction?

In patients with low cardiac output, the arterial and venous beds are inappropriately constricted. This is the body's response to a low flow state, to maintain adequate blood flow to vital organs. Some **compensatory mechanisms** responsible for this constriction are increased catecholamine levels, increased sympathetic tone, and increased activity of the renin-angiotensin-aldosterone system. These compensatory mechanisms work against the failing heart, causing a vicious cycle of decreasing cardiac output and increasing vasoconstriction. Vasodilators break this cycle by decreasing vascular resistance, thus improving cardiac output. Along with beta-blockers, vasodilators constitute the main therapy for mild and moderate congestive heart failure (CHF).

3. What are the physiologic effects of the different classes of vasodilators on the kidney and renin-angiotensin-aldosterone (RAA) system?

Non-ACE inhibitor vasodilators are potent stimulators of the RAA system. This response is the result of lowering the mean systemic blood pressure and decreasing renal perfusion. Activation of the RAA system increases aldosterone levels which, in turn, act at the distal renal tubule to cause sodium resorption and water retention. The result of this process is increased intravascular volume and progressive edema.

ACE inhibitors, on the other hand, exert a direct effect on the RAA system by blocking the conversion of angiotensin I to angiotensin II. Because angiotensin II stimulates aldosterone production, circulating levels of aldosterone are reduced. Diminished aldosterone levels decrease sodium resorption and potassium secretion in the distal renal tubule. Thus, increased intravascular volume and edema are not side effects of ACE inhibition. Hyperkalemia can occur, and care should be taken when ACE inhibitors are used in conjunction with potassium-sparing diuretics or potassium supplements.

Angiotensin II receptor blockers (ARBs) have no influence on glomerular filtration rates, increase the renal blood flow, lead to a natriuretic effect, reduce urinary protein excretion, decrease filtration fraction, and reduce urinary albumin excretion.

The effects of blocking the RAA system are complex: antiproliferation and antimigration at the level of the arterial smooth muscle cells, neutrophils, and mononuclear cells; improvement of endothelial function; possible protection from atherosclerotic plaque rupture (see references), fibrinolysis, antiplatelet and antiatherogenic effects; reduction of the left ventricular (LV) mass in LV hypertrophy; improved balance between myocardial oxygen demand and supply (by decreasing LV afterload and preload), and increased insulin sensitivity.

Overall, ACE inhibitors and ARBs have a cardioprotective and vasculoprotective effect, and can decrease the progression rate of kidney failure. In contrast to ACE inhibitors, ARBs do not influence bradykinin, prostaglandins, and tissue plasminogen activator. In addition, they have a lower incidence of angioedema, do not produce cough, and might have less of a renal protective effect.

4. What are some other beneficial clinical effects of ACE inhibitors?
- In patients with reduced ejection fraction (< 40%) following myocardial infarction (MI), captopril reduces mortality by favorably altering LV remodeling, thus reducing LV dilation and hypertrophy.
- Many clinicians believe ACE inhibitors are more effective than other agents for reducing ventricular mass and improving diastolic dysfunction in patients with LV hypertrophy due to hypertension.
- Captopril provides more protection against decline in renal function in insulin-dependent diabetics than other antihypertensives provide.
- ACE inhibitors that contain a sulfhydryl group, such as captopril, may have a mild antiplatelet effect and may increase insulin receptor sensitivity.

5. Is there a role for the association between ARBs and ACE inhibitors?
Yes. ACE inhibitors do not prevent production of angiotensin II by enzymes other than ACE. The non-ACE produced angiotensin II can be blocked by an ARB at the receptor site. Using only an ARB would leave free circulating angiotensin II, capable of competing with the ARB at the receptor site. Therefore, the combination of the two drugs theoretically provides the maximum protection from angiotensin II.

Evidence shows that the addition of an ARB in patients with heart failure who are taking an ACE inhibitor leads to improved cardiovascular hemodynamics and symptomatology. However, the long-term effects of this association are still under debate. The ELITE II trial showed *no* benefit in mortality in subjects treated with ACE and ARB compared to ACE alone. This is the *opposite* of what the ELITE I trial suggested. Clearly, there is room for speculation. The combination of ARB and ACE inhibitor was observed to be beneficial for decreasing proteinuria in some patients with nephropathies of different etiologies. It is possible that the combination of the two drugs is also beneficial in acute MI.

6. Ten days after initiation of an ACE inhibitor for hypertension, a 71-year-old patient with a history of coronary disease returns complaining of malaise, progressive edema, diminished urine output, and a 15-lb weight gain. His serum creatinine has risen to 4.8 mg/dl. What happened?
ACE inhibitors can cause acute renal failure in patients with bilateral renal artery stenosis. ACE inhibition causes dilation of the efferent glomerular arterioles, resulting in decreased glomerular filtration and acute renal failure. Because of this potential complication, renal function should be evaluated prior to and monitored 1–2 weeks after the initiation of ACE inhibitors in high-risk patients. In this patient, the ACE inhibitor should be discontinued.

7. In the same patient, the ACE inhibitor was discontinued and renal function returned to baseline. What vasodilator regimen might now be substituted?
Hydralazine in combination with isosorbide dinitrate. Note that ARBs should not be tried in this situation, as their renal effects are very similar to ACE inhibitors.

8. A patient with CHF due to a dilated cardiomyopathy returns 1 month after the initiation of an ACE inhibitor complaining of a persistent, dry cough. Should the ACE inhibitor be discontinued?

Cough is a bothersome side effect in 10–20% of patients started on ACE inhibitors. The cough is almost invariably nonproductive and usually begins within 1–6 weeks after initiation of therapy. It is seen most frequently with longer-acting preparations. Changing to another ACE inhibitor is rarely helpful, though a trial of antitussive therapy may allow continuation in patients for whom ACE inhibition is essential. Occasionally, the cough is a manifestation of worsening heart failure. Changing to an ARB might be the best option.

9. What other side effects are seen with ACE inhibitors?

Other less common side effects of ACE inhibitors, most often seen with captopril, include rash, dysgeusia, angioedema, and reversible neutropenia.

10. ACE inhibitors and other vasodilators have been tried to slow or reverse LV dilation and systolic dysfunction in asymptomatic patients with severe, chronic LV volume overload lesions; aortic insufficiency; and mitral regurgitation. Some cardiologists have voiced concerns over the routine use of these agents for these conditions. Why?

Chronic LV volume overload lesions are typically well tolerated for many years, though about one-fourth of patients experience LV dysfunction prior to onset of symptoms. Once the ventricle begins to fail, 20–30% of patients continue to deteriorate despite valve repair. LV function is an important marker used to time valve repair. Vasodilators improve LV function, but there are few clinical data on how vasodilators might affect the timing of valve surgery. For example, if an asymptomatic patient with severe chronic aortic insufficiency would normally undergo valve replacement when the LV ejection fraction fell to 50%, at what ejection fraction should the valve be replaced in the same patient being managed with hydralazine? Conversely, aggressive vasodilation may improve the failing heart enough to allow valve repair in patients once thought to be inoperable. Vasodilators may be used in other nonsurgical candidates to relieve symptoms and postpone surgery indefinitely.

11. What are some cardiovascular diseases in which arterial vasodilators may be contraindicated?

Most contraindications to the use of arterial vasodilators are relative. For example, in **severe aortic stenosis**, blood pressure may be dependent on arterial vasoconstriction due to a relatively fixed stroke volume; thus, arterial vasodilators should be used cautiously. However, in patients with severe aortic stenosis and CHF who were not considered candidates for aortic valve replacement, careful use of arterial vasodilators has provided symptomatic improvement. Similar concerns apply in **hypertrophic cardiomyopathy** and **severe pulmonary hypertension**. Many patients with LV dysfunction are relatively hypotensive (systolic blood pressure < 100 mmHg); however, because this group of patients derives symptomatic and survival benefits from ACE inhibition, cautious use of ACE inhibitors is still indicated in such circumstances.

12. In which acute conditions can the prompt initiation of vasodilator therapy be life-saving?

Vasodilators can be life-saving in several situations that require acute afterload reduction and/or systemic blood pressure reduction.

Severe acute **mitral regurgitation** from any cause results in a sudden rise in left atrial and pulmonary venous pressure, leading to pulmonary edema. Emergent use of sodium nitroprusside lowers systemic blood pressure and afterload, which favors forward ejection of the LV volume, lowers the regurgitant volume, and reduces pulmonary venous pressure. Severe acute **aortic insufficiency** causes a sudden elevation in left ventricular diastolic pressure, leading to pulmonary congestion and systemic hypoperfusion. As in acute mitral regurgitation, the regurgitant volume can be reduced by lowering the systemic blood pressure by acute vasodilation with nitroprusside. Aggressive vasodilation in these instances can stabilize a significant number of patients and allow valve replacement under less emergent circumstances. **Hypertensive emergency** and **aortic dissection** are two other examples.

13. How are vasodilators used in the treatment of hypertensive crisis?

Hypertensive crisis requires rapid lowering of the systolic and diastolic blood pressure to prevent ongoing end-organ damage. Nitroprusside, a fast-acting intravenous drug with a short half-life, is the most-effective and easily-titrated drug for the treatment of this process. The initial dose is 0.5 µg/kg/min and is increased until blood pressure control is attained, usually at a systolic blood pressure of 140–160 mmHg. If hypotension occurs, the dose should be decreased or discontinued, and the patient should be placed in the Trendelenburg position. Prolonged use of high doses of nitroprusside can produce high thiocyanate levels which interfere with oxygen transport. Once blood pressure is controlled, oral antihypertensives should be initiated.

14. Which vasodilator was largely abandoned because of a specific side effect that later proved to be its major clinical indication?

Minoxidil (Rogaine) is a potent arterial vasodilator that is effective in patients with refractory hypertension. Minoxidil proved to have a unique side effect, hirsutism, which caused it to fall into disfavor, especially among female patients. Subsequently, minoxidil was introduced in a topical form to promote hair growth.

15. What is your initial management strategy for a patient with dissection of the descending thoracic aorta?

Although the definitive therapy for many types of aortic dissection remains controversial, most agree that the initial therapy for an uncomplicated dissection of the descending aorta should be medical. Aortic dissections are propagated by the absolute blood pressure and rate of pressure rise (dP/dt) in the aorta. Intravenous sodium nitroprusside allows rapid lowering of the systolic blood pressure to the desired level of 100–120 mmHg. Vasodilators lower the blood pressure but cause a significant rise in dP/dt; thus, concomitant use of beta blockers, initially intravenously, is recommended since beta blockers reduce dP/dt in the aorta.

16. What patient warning is necessary when initiating terazosin?

Terazosin and prazosin are arterial vasodilators that produce their antihypertensive effect through peripheral alpha-receptor blockade. Their use is complicated by significant first-dose hypotension and syncope, most commonly in the elderly. Patients taking this medication should be warned about this possibility, instructed to take the initial dose at bedtime, and to exercise extreme care should they need to get out of bed at night. These drugs are *not* first choices for hypertension treatment, and are best and typically used as third or fourth antihypertensive drugs in refractory hypertension.

The opinions and assertions contained herein are the private views of the authors and are not to be construed as official or reflecting the views of the U.S. Department of the Army or Department of Defense.

BIBLIOGRAPHY

1. Braunwald E: Aortic dissection. In Braunwald E (ed): Heart Disease: A Textbook of Cardiovascular Medicine, 5th ed. Philadelphia, W.B. Saunders, 1997.
2. Braunwald E: Vasodilators. In Braunwald E (ed): Heart Disease: A Textbook of Cardiovascular Medicine, 5th ed. Philadelphia, W.B. Saunders, 1997.
3. Burntet M, Brunner HR: Angiotensin II receptor antagonists. Lancet 355:637–645, 2000.
4. Califf RM, Cohn JN: Cardiac protection: Evolving role of angiotensin receptor blockers. Am Heart J 139(1):S15–S22, 2000.
5. Cohn JN, Johnson G, Ziesche S, et al: A comparison of enalapril with hydralazine-isosorbide dinitrate in the treatment of chronic congestive heart failure. N Engl J Med 325:303–310, 1991.
6. Grossman J, Messerh FH, Nentel JM: Angiotensin II receptor blockers: Equal of preferred substitutes for ACE inhibitors? Arch Intern Med 160: 1905–1911, 2000.
7. Lewis EJ, Hunsicker LG, Bain RP, et al: The effect of angiotensin-converting-enzyme inhibition on diabetic nephropathy. N Engl J Med 329:1456–1462, 1993.

8. Pfeffer MA, Braunwald E, Moyé LA, et al: Effect of captopril on mortality and morbidity in patients with left ventricular dysfunction after myocardial infarction: Results of the survival and ventricular enlargement trail. N Engl J Med 327:669–677, 1992.

9. Pratt RE: Angiotensin II and the control of cardiovascular structure. Am Heart J 132(1), 1996.

10. Schieffer B, Schieffer E, Hilfiker-Kleiner D, et al: Expression of angiotensin II and interleukin 6 in human coronary atherosclerotic plaques. Circulation 101:1372, 2000.

11. Schmieder RE, Schlaich MP: Comparison of therapeutic studies on regression of left ventricular hypertrophy. Adv Exp Med Biol 432:191–198, 1997.

12. Schmieder RE, Schlaich MP, Klingbeil AU, et al: Update on reversal of left ventricular hypertrophy in essential hypertension (a meta-analysis of all randomized double-blind studies until December 1996). Nephrol Dial Transplant 13(3):564–569, 1998.

13. Simon SR, Black HR, Moser M, Berland WE: Cough and ACE inhibitors. Arch Intern Med 152:1698–1700, 1992.

14. The SOLVD Investigators: Effect of enalapril on mortality and the development of heart failure in asymptomatic patients with reduced left ventricular ejection fractions. N Engl J Med 327:685–691, 1992.

15. Vaughan DE: AT(1) receptor blockade and atherosclerosis: Hopeful insights into vascular protection. Circulation 101(13):1496–1497, 2000.

52. DIGOXIN AND OTHER POSITIVE INOTROPIC DRUGS

Mohamed Chebaclo, M.D., and Catalin Loghin, M.D.

1. How many classes of inotropic agents are available clinically?

There are two classes of inotropic agents:
1. **Glycosides** include digoxin and digoxin-like agents.
2. **Nonglycosides** are divided into two large groups:
   - *Sympathomimetic amines* include dopamine, dobutamine, epinephrine, norepinephrine, isoproterenol, and methoxamine.
   - *Phosphodiesterase inhibitors* comprise amrinone and milrinone.

2. Do the classes of inotropic agents differ in their end-point effect?

No. They both increase the availability of Ca^{2+} to the contractile element at the time of excitation-contraction coupling, although the end-point effect is reached through different mechanisms.

3. What is the mechanism of action of the glycosides at the cellular level?

Digoxin and other glycosides increase inotropy at the cellular level by inhibiting the Na^+-K^+ ATPase pump. The glycosides bind to the Na^+-K^+ ATPase pump, which is responsible for active transport of Na^+ across the myocardial cell membrane. This blockage leads to an increase in intracellular Na^+ which, in turn, enhances Na^+-Ca^{2+} exchange. This leads to an increase in intracellular Ca^{2+}, which, in turn, contributes to an increase in inotropy.

4. By what mechanism do the beta-adrenergic sympathomimetic drugs increase calcium that leads to increased inotropy?

The beta-adrenergic agents stimulate adenylate cyclase, which results in an increase in cyclic AMP. cAMP phosphorylates a protein kinase which, in turn, increases the Ca^{2+} influx through the calcium channel.

5. Does the positive inotropic action of digoxin persist in the presence of full beta-adrenergic blockade?

Yes. The inotropic functions of digoxin are not mediated by catecholamine release or through increased sensitivity to catecholamines. Adenylate cyclase activity, which is responsible for the positive inotropic effects of beta-adrenoreceptor agents, is not influenced by digoxin.

6. Does the same increase in oxygen consumption during the use of an inotropic agent like digoxin occur in the failing heart as well?

No. Digoxin decreases heart size when administered to a patient in congestive heart failure. There is a reduction in oxygen consumption, heart size, and wall tension, as explained by Laplace's law.

7. How is digoxin excreted?

Digoxin is excreted through the kidney. Its half-life is 35–48 hours in the normally functioning kidney, so that one-third of the stores are excreted daily. Renal excretion is proportional to the glomerular filtration rate.

8. Do patients with digoxin toxicity benefit from dialysis?

Dialysis is not effective because of the high tissue binding of digoxin.

9. Should the digoxin maintenance dose be changed if amiodarone is added?

Yes. Amiodarone administration will increase the serum digoxin concentration; hence digoxin dosing should be reduced (cut in half) when administration of amiodarone begins.

10. What happens to the inotropic effect of digoxin in doses above its therapeutic range?

The therapeutic range for digoxin 1.5–2 ng/ml, but we usually titrate it in our patients. The inotropic effect of digoxin increases in a graded manner with increasing doses, nevertheless, above 2 ng/ml, the risk of toxicity becomes far greater than the additional therapeutic benefit for patients in congestive heart failure and sinus rhythm.

Remember that digoxin levels do not necessarily correlate with toxicity. Toxicity may occur at "therapeutic" levels of digoxin. Factors associated with increased incidence of arrhythmia include hypoxia, acidosis, and dilated hearts with severely depressed systolic function. Therefore, digoxin levels should be interpreted in the clinical context of each particular patient. EKG may be, on occasion, a better tool in evaluating for digitalis toxicity. Digoxin remains a drug with a narrow therapeutic range; thus, it should be used with appropriate caution.

11. Is digoxin indicated in every patient with heart failure?

No. Congestive heart failure (CHF) with dilated left ventricle, impaired systolic function, and an S_3 gallop are the prime candidates. CHF due to diastolic dysfunction and preserved systolic function are not candidates unless atrial fibrillation is a concomitant problem. The effect of digoxin is cumulative on the effect of angiotensin-converting enzyme inhibitors and diuretics, and therefore an added benefit can be seen with their combination. Digoxin is contraindicated in patients with hypertrophic cardiomyopathy presenting with heart failure.

A recent trial addressed the old, controversial issue of risks versus benefits when using digoxin in CHF. The results indicated a significant decrease in the risk of hospitalization and a trend toward a reduction in death from heart failure, in particular in patients with ejection fractions < 25%. However, since the mainstay of therapy appears to be beta-blockers, it is difficult to arrive at a definitive conclusion on the role of digoxin in the future.

12. Is digoxin indicated and safe in acute myocardial infarction?

This issue has been long debated. There appears to be no convincing evidence for an increased incidence of arrhythmias complicating digitalis use in patients with acute myocardial infarction (MI) when serum levels do not exceed the conventional therapeutic range. Still, the clearest indication for digoxin is atrial fibrillation with fast response. Electrical cardioversion is preferred for other supraventricular arrhythmias or atrial fibrillation in hemodynamically unstable patients. The available data do not support the assertion that digoxin therapy is excessively hazardous after infarction. However, a randomized study is not available to confirm this belief. In summary, digoxin use has no place in MI without CHF or supraventricular arrhythmias.

13. What are the electrocardiographic (ECG) findings in digoxin toxicity?

An array of ventricular and supraventricular arrhythmias and blocks can result from digoxin toxicity—e.g., atrial, ventricular, atrioventricular (AV) node arrhythmias, AV junctional escape, nonparoxysmal AV junctional tachycardia, paroxysmal atrial tachycardia, ventricular tachycardia, sinus arrest, Mobitz type I and II block. Most commonly seen are premature ventricular contractions.

An ECG rhythm combining increased automaticity and escape ectopic pacemakers with impaired conduction suggests digoxin toxicity. A typical example is paroxysmal atrial tachycardia with atrioventricular block.

Note that IV administration of calcium in patients loaded with digoxin may provoke lethal ventricular arrhythmias, in the absence of any sign of digoxin toxicity.

14. What are some of the clinical symptoms of digoxin toxicity?
- Gastrointestinal symptoms: nausea and vomiting
- Neurologic symptoms: headache, fatigue, confusion
- Visual symptoms: scotomas, halos, change in color perception

15. How do you treat digoxin toxicity?
- There is no role for dialysis in treating digoxin toxicity.
- For ventricular arrhythmias, phenytoin and lidocaine are helpful.
- Correction of hypokalemia is vital.
- Beta-blockers are useful for ventricular or supraventricular arrhythmias, especially short-acting beta-blockers like esmolol, which are easy to titrate.
- On occasion, direct countershock is necessary in hemodynamically unstable arrhythmias.
- For potentially life-threatening arrhythmias, Digibind, an Fab-specific digoxin antibody, is helpful.

16. What would you do for a digoxin level of 56 ng/ml after Digibind?
Nothing. The typical scenario is a patient who has runs of ventricular tachycardia and episodes of high-grade AV block with a digoxin level of 56. The use of Digibind would success-fully control the arrhythmias and AV block, but a repeat digoxin measurement would remain above 50. No therapy is needed, because digoxin levels are usually elevated after Digibind due to the binding of Fab to digoxin from body stores which has not yet been excreted by the kidney. The digoxin is not active in this bound state. Digoxin levels measured post-Digibind are not clin-ically helpful and should not be obtained.

17. On what receptors are the sympathetic amines active? What is their effect?
Sympathetic amines exert effects on four different receptors:
1. **Alpha-receptors** provoke vasoconstriction of peripheral arteries when stimulated.
2. **Beta-receptors** increase atrial and ventricular contraction, increase heart rate by stimu-lating the sinus node, and enhance AV conduction.
3. **Beta$_2$-receptors** promote bronchodilation and vasodilation.
4. **Dopaminergic receptors**, found in various tissues including blood vessels and nervous system tissues, are of two types: The activation of dopamine-1 receptors causes vasodilation in coronary, renal, mesenteric, and cerebral vascular beds, by stimulating adenylate cyclase and in-creasing cAMP. The activation of dopamine-2 receptors causes vasodilation, but by inhibiting transmission of sympathetic nerve endings.

18. What amines are alpha or beta selective?
Isoproterenol has practically no alpha-stimulating effect, with relatively pure beta-stimula-tion. It is clinically valuable in stimulating the sinus node and enhancing AV conduction in brad-yarrhythmias. Its limitation in this setting is its hypotensive effect through its beta$_2$ properties.
Methoxamine is a practically a pure alpha-stimulant, helpful in hypotension in the cardiac catheterization laboratory.
Norepinephrine is predominantly alpha- and beta-stimulant and is valuable in cardiogenic shock following bypass surgery for stunned myocardium, and in hypotension.

19. What are the effects of dopamine at different dosages?
Dopamine has different effects at different dosages, which can create a conflicting clinical response if not known.
$\leq$ **2 µg/kg/min**. Stimulate the dopamine receptors; promote renal perfusion; and promote cerebral, coronary, and mesenteric circulation.
2–5 µg/kg/min. Have a predominantly positive inotropic effect manifested by an increase in cardiac output and cardiac contractility with little change in heart rate.
5–10 µg/kg/min. Increase in blood pressure, peripheral vascular resistance, and heart rate; and a decrease in renal blood flow.

20. How do you reduce the vasoconstrictive effect of high-dose dopamine in patients with shock?
When high doses of dopamine are required for inotropic effects it may be infused together with nitroprusside or nitroglycerin to counteract the vasoconstrictive action.

21. How does prolonged administration of sympathomimetic drugs affect the failing myocardium?

Myocardium obtained from patients with congestive heart failure demonstrate marked reduction in beta-adrenoreceptor density and in myocardial contractility. This is consistent with an increase in norepinephrine that downregulates beta-receptors. The decrease in receptor density is proportional to the severity of heart failure and involves $beta_1$, but not $beta_2$-receptors. This might be the basis for use of low doses of beta-blockers to reverse the downregulation of beta-receptors and restore responsiveness to adrenergic inotropic stimulation. In sum, the failing myocardium becomes tolerant to prolonged exposure to catecholamines.

22. What is the mechanism of action of the phosphodiesterase inhibitors?

This positive inotropic agent increases availability of Ca^{2+} to the intracellular compartment. The beta-adrenergic mimetic drugs stimulate adenylate cyclase that then increases cAMP. cAMP phosphorylates the protein kinase which, in turn, increases the Ca^{2+} influx through the calcium channel. The phosphodiesterase inhibitors inhibit the degradation of cAMP, thereby limiting Ca^{2+} influx through the calcium channel.

23. What are the indications for use of intravenous cardiotonic agents?

Intravenous infusions are indicated for treatment for CHF refractory to digoxin and furosemide and for post-myocardial depression, for left ventricular failure in MI, and in patients awaiting cardiac transplantation.

Aside from intravenous cardiotonic agents, a number of *oral* drugs have been studied. Despite initial great enthusiasm, later studies showed increased mortality rates associated with these drugs.

24. What are two intravenous cardiotonic agents currently in use?

Amrinone causes a dose-dependent increase in cardiac output and a decrease in right and left filling pressure and systemic vascular resistance. Its effects are similar, in ways, to a combination of sympathomimetics and vasodilators. The effect of amrinone is additive to the effect of digoxin and other mimetic agents, and there is no tolerance problem as seen in other amines.

Milrinone increases cardiac index without a significant change in heart rate or increase in myocardial oxygen consumption: this may represent a significant advantage over amrinone. Milrinone is being evaluated in a new trial, OPTIME CHF, and is currently included in ACC/AHA guidelines as a combination therapy along with dobutamine for patients with refractory heart failure. Milrinone dosage needs to be adjusted according to the renal clearance.

25. Are there any risks to long-term use of these cardiotonic agents?

Yes. Current evidence suggests that long-term usage of amrinone or milrinone, in oral preparations, is associated with increased mortality. This phenomenon may be due to the presence of stunned or hibernating myocardium. Chronic stimulation of ischemic areas of myocardium may induce necrosis by triggering myocyte apoptosis. Evaluate for the presence of ischemic (stunned or hibernating) myocardium prior to starting therapy with these drugs. OPTIME CHF results will answer the question of whether or not short-term IV administration of milrinone is leading to an increased long-term clinical risk.

BIBLIOGRAPHY

1. Akerman GL, et al: Peritoneal dialysis and hemodialysis of tritiated digoxin. Ann Intern Med 67:718, 1967.
2. Braunwald E: Effects of digitalis on the normal and the failing heart. J Am Coll Cardiol 5(5 Suppl A):51A–59A, 1985.
3. Braunwald E: A symposium: Amrinone. Introduction. Am J Cardiol 56:1B–2B, 1985.
4. Cuffe SM, et al: Rationale and design of the OPTIME CHF trial. Outcomes of a prospective trial of intravenous milrinone for exacerbations of chronic heart failure. Am Heart J 139:15–22, 2000.

5. Gheorghiade M, et al: Current medical therapy for advanced heart failure. Heart Lung 29(1):16–32, 2000.
6. Hauptman PJ, Kelly RA: Digitalis. Circulation 99(9):1265–1270, 1999.
7. Heilbrunn S, Shah P, Bristow MR, et al: Increased beta-receptor density and improved hemodynamic response to catecholamine stimulation during long-term metoprolol: Therapy in heart failure from dilated cardiomyopathy. Circulation 79:483–490, 1989.
8. Maskin CS, Ocken S, Chadwick B, LeJemtel TH: Comparative systemic and renal effects of dopamine and angiotensin converting enzyme inhibition with enalapril in patients with heart failure. Circulation 72:846–852, 1985.
9. Muller JE, Turi ZG, Stone PH, et al: Digoxin therapy and mortality after myocardial infarction: Experience in the MILIS Study. N Engl J Med 314:265–271, 1986.

53. CALCIUM CHANNEL ANTAGONISTS

Querubin P. Mendoza, M.D., and Catalin Loghin, M.D. *

1. What are some of the important pharmacologic properties of calcium channel antagonists?

There are important pharmacologic differences among calcium channel antagonists. Knowledge of these properties is helpful when selecting a drug for a given patient, and for avoiding potential toxicities.

Pharmacologic Properties of Calcium Channel Antagonists

	VERAPAMIL	NIFEDIPINE (AND OTHER DIHYDROPYRIDINES)	DILTIAZEM
Heart rate	↓↓	↑	↓
AV nodal conduction	↓↓	—	↓
Myocardial contractility	↓↓	↓	↓
Arterial vasodilatation	↑↑	↑↑↑	↑

2. Are the calcium channel antagonists interchangeable?

No. Although they belong to the same broad category, there are distinct subclassifications. The major approved indications for these agents are summarized in the table below. The sustained-release preparations often do not have the same indications as the shorter-acting preparations.

Therapeutic Uses of Calcium Channel Blockers

CHEMICAL CLASS DRUG	VASOSPASTIC	ANGINA STABLE	UNSTABLE	HTN	ATRIAL FIBRILLATION OR FLUTTER	PSVT
Diphenylalkylamine Verapamil	+	+	+	+	+	+
Benzothiazepine Diltiazem	+	+	+	+	+	+
Dihydropyridine Nifedipine	+	+	+	+		
Amlodipine	+	+	+	+		
Nicardipine	+	+	+	+		
Other Bepridil				+		

HTN = hypertension; PSVT = paroxysmal supraventricular tachycardia

3. Name some contraindications to the use of calcium channel antagonists.

In addition to known hypersensitivity reactions, contraindications are related to the pharmacologic properties of the various subclasses, including hypotension, congestive heart failure, sick-sinus syndrome, and second- or third-degree atrioventricular (AV) block. Because of significant vasodilatation and lowering of vascular resistance, the dihydropyridine subclass is avoided in patients with severe aortic stenosis and hypertrophic cardiomyopathy. Bepridil prolongs QT intervals, is contraindicated in patients with a history of serious ventricular arrhythmias, and is reserved for patients with angina that does not respond to other medications.

---

* The authors acknowledge Arvo J. Oopik, M.D., whose text from the first edition is incorporated in this chapter.

4. What is the role of calcium channel antagonists in treating angina pectoris?

In the U.S., amlodipine, diltiazem, nicardipine, nifedipine, and verapamil are approved for treating classic and variant angina in combination with nitrates and beta-blockers. Calcium channel antagonists should not be used alone to treat angina, unless there is a clear contraindication for beta-blockers or nitrates. Rapid-acting preparations, which may worsen angina, should be avoided. Most often, dihydropiridines are used in conjunction with a beta-blocker, to compensate for the induced tachycardia. Since they can induce significant bradycardia, verapamil and diltiazem are to be used with caution if a beta-blocker is part of the regimen, and they are better associated with nitrates.

5. Why is nifedipine potentially deleterious when used in unstable angina?

By lowering arterial pressure with subsequent reflex tachycardia, nifedipine may aggravate angina. This problem can be avoided with simultaneous use of beta-blockers. Withdrawal of beta blockade in some patients taking nifedipine may worsen angina.

6. What are some of the important drug interactions of calcium channel antagonists?

Drug Interactions of Calcium Channel Antagonists

INTERACTION WITH	RESULT
Beta-adrenergic blockers	Negative inotropic and chronotropic effects; heart block
Digoxin	Increased plasma digoxin levels
Alpha blockers (prazosin)	Excessive hypotension
Quinidine	Hypotension, bradycardia, decreased quinidine level
Carbamazepine	Increased carbamazepine levels
Cimetidine	Increased plasma level of calcium channel antagonist
Cyclosporine	Increased cyclosporine levels
Enzyme inducers (rifampin, sulfinpyrazone, phenobarbital)	Decreased effects of calcium channel antagonists

7. What are the signs and symptoms of calcium channel antagonist toxicity?

The most common toxic effects are hypotension and bradydysrhythmias. Of the latter, most common are AV block and sinus bradycardia with junctional escape rhythms. Rarely, one sees a slow idioventricular rhythm and prolonged QRS duration.

8. Aside from discontinuation of the drug, how are these toxicities treated?

Treatment is primarily supportive. For severe cardiotoxicity, such as seen with large ingestions in suicide attempts, catecholamines with chronotropic activity (dopamine, epinephrine, norepinephrine) should be used. Isoproterenol is effective in this regard, but may potentiate vasodilation. Atropine is inconsistently effective. Temporary pacing should be considered. Whereas intravenous administration of calcium may improve contractility, this maneuver is less effective in managing heart block or excessive vasodilation. Oral charcoal should be given for acute ingestion. Hemoperfusion, however, is ineffective in clearing these drugs because of their large volume of distribution and high endogenous clearance. Glucagon has been useful in a few cases. The mechanism is thought to be improvement in myocardial contractility through increased cyclic AMP in myocardial cells.

9. Are calcium channel antagonists indicated in patients with acute Q-wave myocardial infarctions?

No. Most studies of the calcium channel antagonists have not demonstrated any definitive benefits in patients with acute MI. In a meta-analysis of 22 trials, no improvement in mortality, reduction of infarct size, or reduction in incidence of reinfarction was documented. One trial that explored administration of verapamil starting 1 week after the acute event showed a significant reduction in mortality. In another trial, nifedipine was associated with increased mortality and re-infarction rate.

10. Are calcium antagonists indicated in non-Q-wave myocardial infarctions?

Calcium channel antagonists may have a role in patients without evidence of left ventricular failure. Diltiazem decreases the short-term reinfarction rate and the incidence of postinfarction angina, but does not improve overall survival. In patients with pulmonary congestion, however, use of diltiazem was associated with increased mortality.

11. Is there a role for calcium-channel antagonists in the treatment of heart failure due to left ventricular systolic dysfunction?

Dihydropyridines, on short-term administration (3 months), have beneficial effects by rais-ing cardiac output and decreasing vascular resistance. However, on long-term treatment (12 months), these effects are either no longer apparent or the hemodynamic profile worsens (V-HeFT III trial). These results are contradicted by other trials.

Similarly, evaluation of exercise tolerance and overall quality of life of CHF patients treated with calcium channel antagonists yielded conflicting results. Survival is improved in nonis-chemic patients, but is not siginificantly influenced in ischemic cases of heart failure. There is no reduction in the number of hospitalizations and the incidence of worsening CHF—not even in patients treated with second-generation dihydropyridines.

The above consideration concerns patients with systolic dysfunction of the left ventricle. Calcium channel antagonists are acceptable for treatment of diastolic dysfunction, but their effi-cacy in terms of a clinically relevant effect remains to be seen. Overall, the role played by these drugs in CHF treatment is limited; they may be most useful as an adjuvant therapy, particularly for patients with angina pectoris of hypertension.

12. Do patients with hypertrophic cardiomyopathy benefit from calcium channel antagonists?

Yes. Most experience has been with verapamil. By depressing myocardial contractility, vera-pamil can decrease the left ventricular outflow gradient. It also improves diastolic filling by im-proving myocardial relaxation. Exercise capacity and overall symptoms often improve.

13. Are calcium channel blockers useful in the reduction of left ventricular (LV) hypertro-phy caused by hypertension?

Yes. Numerous studies have shown that calcium channel antagonists reduce LV mass and improve pathophysiologic sequelae, such as ventricular dysrhythmias, impaired ventricular fill-ing, and coronary reserve, while maintaining LV pump function. It remains to be seen, however, whether a reduction in the degree of LV hypertrophy will ultimately reduce the risks of sudden death, acute MI, and CHF associated with hypertensive heart disease.

14. Why are calcium channel antagonists frequently used in patients undergoing percuta-neous transluminal coronary angioplasty (PTCA)?

Calcium channel antagonists may prevent coronary spasm, which is frequently seen during and shortly after PTCA and other percutaneous coronary interventions. They have not been shown, however, to reduce the incidence of restenosis, which usually occurs within the first 6 months after PTCA.

15. Are there any studies suggesting benefit of calcium channel antagonists in the preven-tion of coronary atherosclerosis?

Yes. Some preliminary information suggests that calcium blockers may affect the atheroscle-rotic process. The Montreal Heart Institute Trial with nicardipine showed less progression of stenotic lesions that are ≤ 20% in severity. In the International Nifedipine Trial on Antiatherosclerotic

Therapy (INTACT), nifedipine reduced the rate of appearance of new coronary lesions. In both trials, however, no effect was seen on the overall progression or regression of atherosclerosis. Other preliminary data also suggest that diltiazem may slow the development of accelerated coronary atherosclerosis often seen in heart transplant recipients. At this time, there is not general agreement on the use of calcium channel blockers for this indication.

16. Do the calcium channel antagonists have long-term benefits in patients with primary (unexplained) pulmonary hypertension?

Maybe. High doses of nifedipine or diltiazem produce reductions in pulmonary artery pressure and pulmonary vascular resistance in some patients. However, no clinical trial of calcium channel antagonists in primary pulmonary hypertension has demonstrated a survival benefit.

17. A patient with known Wolff-Parkinson-White syndrome presents with atrial fibrillation and a rapid ventricular response. He is given intravenous verapamil, but then becomes hypotensive, and ventricular fibrillation develops. What is the likely mechanism for this deterioration?

This case illustrates the potential danger of using calcium channel antagonists in patients with accessory bypass tracts who present with atrial fibrillation. Calcium channel antagonists may depress conduction through the AV node and enhance conduction through accessory bypass tracts, resulting in acceleration of the ventricular response. Very rapid ventricular rates may lead to hypotension and syncope and may cause rhythm degeneration to ventricular fibrillation.

The opinions and assertions contained herein are the private views of the authors and are not to be construed as official or reflecting the views of the Department of the Army or Department of Defense.

BIBLIOGRAPHY

1. Abernathy DR, Schwartz JB: Drug therapy: Calcium antagonist drugs. New Engl J Med 341(19): 1447–1457, 1999.
2. Cohn BA, Ziesche SM, Smith R: Effect of the calcium antagonist felodipine as supplementary vasodilator therapy in patients with chronic heart failure treated with enalapril: V-HeFTIII. Circulation 96:856–863, 1997.
3. Hermans WRM, Rensing BJ, Strauss BH, Serruys PW: Prevention of restenosis after percutaneous transluminal coronary angioplasty: The search for a "magic bullet." Am Heart J 122:171–187, 1991.
4. Messerli FH, Aristizabal D, Soria F: Reduction of left ventricular hypertrophy: How beneficial? Am Heart J 125:1520–1524, 1993.
5. Morris AD, Meredith PA, Reid JL: Pharmacokinetics of calcium antagonists: Implications for therapy. In Epstein M (ed): Calcium Antagonists in Clinical Medicine. Philadelphia, Hanley & Belfus, 1992, pp 49–67.
6. Multicenter Diltiazem Postinfarction Trial Research Group: The effect of diltiazem on mortality and reinfarction after myocardial infarction. N Engl J Med 319:385–392, 1988.
7. Pentel PR, Salerno DM: Cardiac drug toxicity: Digitalis glycosides and calcium-channel and beta-blocking agents. Med J Aust 152:88–94, 1990.
8. Rutherford JD, Braunwald E. Chronic Ischemic heart disease. In Braunwald E (ed): Heart Disease: A Textbook of Cardiovascular Medicine, 4th ed. Philadelphia, W.B. Saunders, 1992, pp 1310–1316.
9. deVries RM, et al: Efficacy and safety of calcium channel blockers in heart failure: Focus on recent trials with second-generation dihydropyridines. Am Heart J 139(2):185–194, 2000.
10. Waters D, Lesperance J: Interventions that beneficially influence the evolution of coronary atherosclerosis: The case for calcium channel blockers. Circulation 86(Suppl III):III-111–III-116, 1992.

54. THROMBOLYTIC AGENTS

George M. Pachello, M.D., James C. Lafferty, M.D., Donald A. McCord, M.D., and Ali R. Homayuni, M.D.

1. Describe the usual pathogenesis of acute myocardial infarction.

Most acute myocardial infarctions are caused by the occlusion of a coronary artery by a thrombus at the site of a ruptured atheromatous plaque. Total occlusion of an infarct-related artery has been seen in up to 87% of patients undergoing cardiac catheterization within 4–6 hours of acute myocardial infarction.

2. What is the final common pathway in the development of thrombosis?

Whatever the initiating cause, the final pathway involves the conversion of prothrombin to thrombin. Thrombin subsequently converts fibrinogen into fibrin which, together with red blood cells, platelets, and plasminogen, can produce a thrombus.

3. Describe the final common pathway in thrombolysis.

The endogenous thrombolytic system can be activated by thrombus and endogenous or exogenous plasminogen activators. The activation proceeds by converting plasminogen into plasmin. Plasmin, in turn, lyses stable fibrin clots and degrades circulating fibrinogen, both of which result in the formation of fibrinogen split products which further inhibit fibrin formation. This process may also be termed **fibrinolysis**.

4. Why would lysing a thrombus potentially alleviate the effect of a myocardial infarction?

A myocardial infarction is not an all-or-nothing phenomenon. Instead, it is a dynamic process known as a wave-front phenomenon that generally progresses over several hours. Thus, there is a window of opportunity to lyse a thrombus and restore flow to the jeopardized myocardium and potentially limit infarct size.

5. Does the endogenous fibrinolytic system play a role in spontaneous fibrinolysis to produce reperfusion?

Yes. This was demonstrated by DeWood and others who noted that the incidence of total occlusion of an infarct-related artery tends to decrease the longer the time from the development of a myocardial infarction to the time of catheterization. This spontaneous process generally appears to fall outside the window of opportunity for myocardial salvage. For this reason, activating agents have been developed to accelerate the course of thrombolysis.

6. What are the thrombolytic agents available, and how do they differ?

Thrombolytic Agents

	SOURCE	ROUTE
Tissue plasminogen activator (tPA)	Endogenous (human)	Intravenous
Urokinase	Endogenous (human)	Intracoronary
Streptokinase	Exogenous	Intravenous, intracoronary
APSAC*	Exogenous	Intravenous
Retavase (reteplase)	Altered form of tPA	Intravenous, bolus
Tenecreplase (TNKase)	Altered form of tPA	Intravenous, bolus

* APSAC = anisoylated plasminogen-streptokinase activator complex.

Streptokinase acts indirectly by combining with plasminogen for form an activation complex which, in turn, converts plasminogen to plasmin both at the site of a thrombosis and systemically. Streptokinase is antigenic and can cause an early anaphylactic or late serum sickness-like reaction. It has a 50–60% infarct artery patency rate when used intravenously. It is the cheapest agent available and has the lowest incidence of intracerebral bleeds.

tPA directly converts plasminogen to plasmin but only in the presence of fibrin. This allows for increased, but not absolute, clot specificity. It is the most expensive agent but has the highest patency rates (75–85%). It also carries a mildly increased risk for intracerebral bleeding.

APSAC is inactive (due to the acyl group) until exposed to fibrin, when decylation occurs and culminates in an activity similar to that of streptokinase. The patency rates and antigenic activity are similar to that of streptokinase. The acyl group only mildly improves the drug's clot-specific activity. APSAC is very similar to streptokinase but also more expensive.

7. Does the use of thrombolytic agents translate into improved clinical results?

Yes. Early mortality (within the first few weeks) after Q-wave myocardial infarction has been reduced by 33%, from 10–15% to approximately 5–10%. Thrombolytic agents often lead to better recovery of left ventricular function, less ventricular dilatation or remodeling, fewer arrhythmias, and presumably improved long-term survival.

8. What are the indications for intravenous thrombolytic agents?

They are used to treat, within 6 hours of onset, newly developed chest pain consistent with **acute myocardial infarction**, along with ST elevations > 0.1 mV in at least two contiguous leads or the development of a new left bundle branch block. Administration between 6 and 12 hours after onset may show less benefit but is still deemed important. Time frames > 12 hours but < 24 hours yield diminishing benefits but may be useful in certain situations.

Thrombolytic agents may also be considered with ST-segment depression in leads V_2 and V_3; along with the development of an R wave in similar leads, that are thought to represent a **posterior wall myocardial infarction** and not unstable angina.

9. What are the contraindications to thrombolysis?

Absolute Contraindications

Active internal bleeding
Suspected aortic dissection
Known intracranial neoplasm
History of any hemorrhagic CVA ever, or other cerebrovascular event < 1 year

Relative Contraindications

Prolonged or traumatic CPR (> 10 min)
Severe hypertension on presentation (BP > 180/110)
History of chronic severe hypertension
History of prior CVA or other intracranial pathology
Recent trauma (< 2–4 weeks) or major surgery (< 3 weeks)
Non-compressible vascular punctures
Recent internal bleeding (< 2–4 weeks)
For SK/APSAC, prior exposure or allergy (use tPA)
Known bleeding diathesis or current INR > 2–3

AHA/ACC Guidelines for Treatment of Myocardial Infarction, updated 1996.

10. How are bleeding complications managed?

Bleeding is a major drawback to thrombolytic therapy. It is usually mild and easily treatable, but occasionally it can be devastating, especially intracerebral bleeding, which occurs in 0.2–0.6% of cases. Age, hypertension, prior stroke and prior use of tPA may predispose to bleeding.

Most bleeding occurs at vascular puncture sites, so the initial management is wound compression. If bleeding cannot be controlled or if it involves an intracranial site, all thrombolytic agents, heparin, and aspirin should be discontinued. Protamine can be given to reverse heparin's effects. Because thrombolytic agents cause a depletion of clotting factors, cryoprecipitate infusion can replace fibrinogen and fresh frozen plasma can replace factors V and VIII. Aspirin causes platelet dysfunction, and a platelet infusion may be considered. Additional antifibrinolytic agents, such as ε-amino caproic acid, that prevent the binding of tPA and plasmin to fibrin may be useful. Even with this management, intracerebral bleeding still yields a poor prognosis.

11. What are the markers of reperfusion?

The gold standard for measuring reperfusion or coronary artery patency is coronary angiography. Bedside markers of reperfusion include the resolution of chest pain, reduction in ST-segment elevations, reperfusion arrhythmia, and early peaking creatine phosphokinase level. These markers, however, are extremely insensitive and lack specificity unless all occur together. Other available tests include early myoglobin peaking, thallium or sestamibi redistribution, improvement of wall motion abnormality on echocardiography, gated blood pool or magnetic resonance imaging, as well as signal average parameters and ultrasound tissue characterization. These tests have different availabilities, various advantages, and disadvantages. Their usefulness may depend on the institution as well as the clinical setting.

12. Does any thrombolytic agent confer improved survival benefit over the others?

Although tPA has higher patency rates than streptokinase or APSAC, there were no differences noted in survival until the GUSTO trial. This trial, using an accelerated tPA dosing schedule along with intravenous heparin, provided an approximately 14% survival benefit when compared to streptokinase combined with subcutaneous heparin, intravenous heparin, or tPA. A mildly increased risk of intracerebral bleeding also was noted in the tPA group.

13. What adjunctive therapies are used to prevent reocclusion and potentiate thrombolysis?

Antiplatelet therapy with aspirin is an essential adjunct and has been recommended ever since ISIS II demonstrated its efficacy with or without a thrombolytic agent. Agents that bind or competitively inhibit glycoprotein receptors (glycoprotein IIB–IIIA) and prevent platelet cross-linking are under investigation. Inhibitors or the binding site for von Willebrand factor are also under investigation. Heparin accelerates the formation of antithrombin III complexes which, in turn, impede thrombin activity. Hirudin is a more specific direct inhibitor of thrombin and is currently being evaluated in the GUSTO II trial.

14. Do thrombolytic agents work in unstable angina?

Because coronary thrombosis plays a role in unstable angina, one would expect lytic agents to be useful in unstable angina. Although this makes sense intuitively, thrombolytic agents do not improve outcome in unstable angina. In fact there is evidence that they may *worsen* unstable angina. There are several postulated reasons why this might be true. One is that in unstable angina, the thrombus may be largely below the fibrous cap of the atheromatous lesion, making it difficult for the thrombolytic agent to reach the thrombus. Another is that thrombolytic agents promote the production of thrombin, which ultimately may lead to development of thrombus. This clearly is a problem in MI as well, since it is known, based on angiographic findings, that arteries initially opened by thrombolytic agents later may reclose.

15. Compare the benefit of immediate angioplasty versus intravenous thrombolytic therapy.

Contraindications may prevent the use of intravenous thrombolytic therapy in 60–70% of patients presenting with acute myocardial infarction. Clearly, in this group, direct angioplasty presents a therapeutic option.

Many studies have now compared direct angioplasty to thrombolytic agents and found that direct angioplasty results in a better outcome. This is also true in the era of stents. Recently, a trial comparing coronary stenting with adjunctive glycoprotein IIb/IIIa inhibition (using abcix-imab) showed improved myocardial salvage and better clinical outcome using the combined measure of death, reinfarction, or stroke at 6 months. In the coronary stent group, this composite outcome occurred in 8.5% vs. 23.5% in the group that received thrombolysis (p = 0.02). Note that the thrombolytic regimen was accelerated tPA.

16. What are glycoprotein 2B-3A receptors?

The GP2B-3A receptor is the most abundant protein on the platelet surface. It is the primary receptor mediating platelet aggregation, a process central to acute arterial thrombosis and to he-mostasis. This receptor is tightly packed on the platelet cell surface, with approximately 80,000 receptors per platelet.

17. What are GP2B-3A receptor inhibitors?

Antagonists that block the binding of adhesive proteins to the GP2B-3A receptor, thus prevent-ing platelet aggregation and consequent thrombus formation. There are currently three available.

Brand Name	Type
Reopro (abciximab)	monoclonal antibody
Aggrastat (tirofiban)	non-peptide
Integrilin (eptifibitide)	peptide

18. Where are GP2B-3As used in clinical practice?

Percutaneous coronary intervention (PCI)
Coronary stents
Unstable angina pre-PCI
Unstable angina medical stabilization

19. How are GP2B-3A inhibitors used in combination with fibrinolysis?

There are several studies supporting combination use:

SPEED Trial (The GUSTO IV Pilot Trial)

Conclusion: Adding reteplase to abciximab treatment of acute MI versus reteplase alone en-hances the incidence of early complete reperfusion after the initiation of therapy in the emer-gency department.

TIMI 14

Conclusion: Combination therapy with abciximab and reduced-dose tPA improves myocar-dial reperfusion, as reflected in greater ST-segment resolution, in addition to epicardial flow. This finding may translate into improved clinical outcomes by enhancing myocardial salvage.

GUSTO IV-AMI: Conclusion: Combination therapy with abciximab plus one-half dose rPA (retavase) resulted in a reperfusion rate similar to that achieved with tPA alone. The risk of intracerebral hemorrhage trended lower compared to tPA alone.

20. How are thrombolytics classified? How are they usually administered?

1st Generation:
  • Streptokinase
  • Eminase (anistreplase—streptokinase derivative)
2nd Generation:
  • Retavase (reteplase)—*non-weight-based*, 10 + 10U double bolus injection, 30 minutes apart (nonglycosylated recombinant plasminogen activator)
  • Tenecreplase(TNKase)—weight-based, single bolus injection (recombinant tissue plas-minogen activator)

21. How do the thrombolytics compare?

Gusto 1: Compared the effects of (tPA), streptokinase, or both on reducing mortality pa-tients with acute myocardial infarction.

Results: Accelerated dose tPA and IV heparin resulted in a significant 14% relative reduction in total 30-day mortality compared with SK and IV or SC heparin. Accelerated tPA was associated with a significantly higher incidence of hemorrhagic stroke compared to SK. Accelerated tPA led to an actual survival benefit of 10 additional lives saved per 1,000 patients treated when compared with SK.

Gusto 3: Compared the effects of non-weight adjusted Retavase to weight-adjusted Alteplase on reducing mortality rate at 30 days after acute infarction.

Results: Efficacy and safety were found to be comparable—in terms of 30-day mortality, hemorrhagic stroke, the combined end point of death and stroke, and bleeding complications; the results of Retavase therapy were similar to those of alteplase therapy.

Assent 2: Compared 30-day mortality rates of an IV bolus dose of TNKase or an accelerated infusion of Alteplase.

Results: Tenecteplase and alteplase were equivalent for 30-day mortality.

BIBLIOGRAPHY

1. Anderson HV, Willerson JT: Thrombolysis in acute myocardial infarction. N Engl J Med 329:703–709, 1993.
2. Arnold AZ, Topol EJ: Assessment of reperfusion after thrombolytic therapy for myocardial infarction. Am Heart J 124:441–447, 1992.
3. Bar FW, Verheught FW, Col J, et al: Thrombolysis in patients with unstable angina improves the angiographic but not clinical outcome. Circulation 86:131–137, 1992.
4. de Lemos, et al: TIMI 14. Circulation 101:239–242, 2000.
5. Fry TA, Sobel BE: Coronary thrombolysis. In Zipes DP (ed): Progress in Cardiology. Philadelphia, Lea & Febiger, 1990.
6. Fuster V: Coronary thrombolysis—A perspective for the practicing physician. N Engl J Med 329:723–725, 1993.
7. Grimes CL, et al: A comparison of immediate angioplasty with thrombolytic therapy for acute myocardial infarction. N Engl J Med 328:673–691, 1993.
8. GUSTO Investigators: An international randomized trial comparing four thrombolytic strategies for acute myocardial infarction. N Engl J Med 329:673–682, 1993.
9. Handin RI, Loscalzo J: Thrombolytic therapy. In Braunwald E (ed): Heart Disease: A Textbook of Cardiovascular Disease. Philadelphia, W.B. Saunders, 1992.
10. Lincoff, Topol: Platelet GP2B/3A inhibitors in cardiovascular disease. Contemp Cardiol 1999.
11. Ohman, et al: SPEED Trial—The Gusto IV Pilot Trial. Circulation 101:2788–2794, 2000.
12. Pasternak RC, Braunwald E: Coronary thrombolysis. In Braunwald E (ed): Heart Disease, 5th ed. Philadelphia, W.B. Saunders, 1997.
13. Schomig A, Kastrati A, Dirschinger J, et al: Coronary stenting plus platelet glycoprotein IIb/IIIa blockade compared with tissue plasminogen activator in acute myocardial infarction. N Engl J Med 343:385–391, 2000.

VII. Other Medical Conditions with Associated Cardiac Involvement

55. HEART DISEASE IN PREGNANCY

Kimberly A. Schleman, M.D., and Jeffrey Pickard, M.D.

1. What changes in cardiovascular physiology occur during normal pregnancy?

Cardiac output starts to rise by about 10 weeks' gestation and plateaus at about 40% above baseline during the second trimester. Blood volume increases to nearly 50% above baseline by around 32 weeks, while erythrocyte mass increases to about 30% above baseline. This accounts for the "physiologic anemia" of pregnancy. Despite the significant increase in cardiac output, blood pressure falls because of a marked diminution in systemic vascular resistance. Pulmonary vascular resistance also decreases. At the time of delivery, cardiac output can be up to 180% of prepregnancy levels.

2. How is this increase in cardiac output distributed to various organs?

The most dramatic increase in blood flow is to the uterus, which receives about 10 times the normal flow. However, this still accounts for a small proportion of the overall increase. Flow to the kidneys increases 20–30% above baseline, the skin receives 2–3 times its normal flow, and the breasts receive 3–5 times their normal flow.

3. What are some of the cardiac signs and physical symptoms seen during normal pregnancy?

On physical exam normal pregnant women may have increased jugular venous pressure, a prominent first heart sound, and splitting of the second heart sound. An S_3 is present a majority of the time. An early peaking systolic murmur is almost always present (90%) and usually represents a pulmonary outflow murmur.

Other symptoms are dyspnea, chest pain, fatigue, palpitations, dizziness, and even syncope. In fact, young women who are not known to be pregnant who present with syncope should have a B-HCG checked. Depending on the clinical picture, syncope evaluation may require further work-up, including Holter monitor or echocardiogram.

4. What is peripartum cardiomyopathy?

Congestive heart failure with LV systolic dysfunction that occurs during the last trimester of pregnancy or within 6 months after delivery. It is characterized by heart failure symptoms such as fatigue, dyspnea, edema, cough, or jugular venous distention. It is most commonly diagnosed during the first month postpartum. The cause is unknown. The prognosis is variable; 50% of women recover their left ventricular function within 6 months. Recurrence with subsequent pregnancies is common. Because the risk of recurrence is greater in women with persistent left ventricular dysfunction, further pregnancies are contraindicated in this subgroup. Treatment is a standard heart failure regimen including diuretics for symptoms, afterload reduction, probably digoxin, and beta blocker therapy.

5. Which cardiac medications can be used during pregnancy?

Diuretics (thiazides are class B): This class crosses the placenta. No teratogenic effects have been reported, but there are reported cases of neonatal thrombocytopenia, jaundice, and hyponatremia. Because of the possible impairment of uterine blood flow and placental hypoperfusion, diuretics are not usually begun during pregnancy but are often continued during pregnancy in patients who are taking them chronically.

Calcium channel blockers (most are class C): There is little experience with this class so the effects on the fetus are not well known. However, this class has been used to treat tachyarrhythmias in pregnant patients and fetal tachycardia in utero without adverse effects.[12]

Beta-blockers (most are class C although atenolol is class D): This class, with the exception of atenolol, is relatively safe. These agents may cause uterine contractions, intrauterine growth retardation, bradycardia, and hypoglycemia.

Angiotensin-converting enzyme (ACE) inhibitors (most are class D for the 2nd and 3rd trimesters): This class should be avoided during pregnancy. They are associated with oligohydramnios, neonatal renal failure, and premature delivery. Angiotensin receptor blockers are contraindicated as well.

Hydralazine (class C): No fetal adverse effects reported. Used often in hypertensive patients.

Methyldopa (class B): Used often to treat chronic hypertension in pregnant women. No significant adverse fetal effects have been reported.

6. What is the most common form of cardiac disease in pregnant women in the United States?

Congenital heart disease has surpassed rheumatic heart disease. This includes ASD, VSD, PDA, bicuspid aortic stenosis, coarctation, tetralogy of Fallot, and transposition of the great vessels. Also, because women are trending toward pregnancy later in life, the incidence of ischemic heart disease is increasing.

The overall risk of congenital heart disease in the children of these patients is about 5% (versus 1% in the general population). Therefore, fetal echocardiography is recommended in these women to diagnose congenital heart disease prenatally.

7. What cardiac lesions are well tolerated during pregnancy?
- **Mitral valve prolapse** is not adversely affected. Endocarditis prophylaxis is not necessary with vaginal deliveries, unless there is evidence of ongoing infection or a history of endocarditis.
- Regurgitant lesions such as **aortic insufficiency** or **mitral regurgitation**, especially if symptoms were mild at the patient's prepregnancy baseline.
- **Tricuspid regurgitation** and **pulmonic insufficiency**.
- **Atrial septal defect**, **ventricular septal defect**, and **patent ductus arteriosus** if corrected without evidence of large left-to-right shunt or pulmonary hypertension.

8. Which cardiac conditions are contraindications to pregnancy?
- Pulmonary hypertension (PA pressure > 75% of systemic pressure)
- Eisenmenger's syndrome
- Cardiomyopathy with New York Heart Association (NYHA) class III–IV
- Severely obstructive valvular disease; mitral stenosis, aortic stenosis, pulmonary stenosis, coarctation, hypertrophic obstructive cardiomyopathy
- Marfan's syndrome with aortic root > 40 mm
- Severe cyanosis
- A history of peripartum cardiomyopathy with persistent left ventricular dysfunction

9. How do you assess maternal mortality in the pregnant patient with cardiac disease?

Mortality is related to the underlying cardiac lesion and the patient's NYHA functional class at baseline prior to pregnancy. Work-up should include an echocardiogram, arterial oxygen saturation, and hematocrit to check for erythrocytosis. Right-to-left shunting, cyanosis, and a hematocrit > 65% all portend high maternal and fetal mortality (25–50%). NYHA class III–IV mitral stenosis or aortic stenosis is a moderate risk (10–15% mortality).

10. What risks are associated with mitral stenosis during pregnancy?

Ideally, significant mitral stenosis should be repaired prior to pregnancy.

Mitral stenosis accounts for almost 90% of rheumatic heart disease during pregnancy. Approximately 25% of women with mitral stenosis have their first symptoms during pregnancy.

As blood volume, heart rate, and cardiac output increase during pregnancy, there is an increased relative obstruction to flow across the stenosed mitral valve. This increases pulmonary venous congestion, which can lead to overt pulmonary edema.

Medical management includes loop diuretics if necessary, possibly beta blockers if tachycardic, and bed rest. If the patient is in atrial fibrillation, digoxin can be used to slow the ventricular rate, or direct current cardioversion can be used safely to cardiovert back to sinus rhythm.

If medical therapy fails, a balloon valvuloplasty should be considered. If this fails, mitral valve replacement has been done with reportedly low fetal mortality.

During labor, patients may require a Swan-Ganz catheter to monitor their hemodynamics. (The pulmonary capillary wedge pressure in this case does not reflect left ventricular filling pressure, so cardiac output must be measured.) During delivery, the maternal circulation receives a 500 cc "autotransfusion" from the placenta, which can precipitate pulmonary edema. Also, a Valsalva maneuver may decrease preload, causing cardiac output to drop.

11. Which cardiac lesions necessitate endocarditis prophylaxis during delivery?

The consensus statement of the American Heart Association (AHA) does not recommend routine antibiotic prophylaxis in patients with valvular heart disease undergoing uncomplicated vaginal delivery or cesarean section unless infection is suspected. However, antibiotics are optional, and often used, in patients with prosthetic heart valves, a prior history of endocarditis, complex congenital heart disease, or a surgically constructed systemic-pulmonary shunt.

12. How is anticoagulation managed in patients with prosthetic valves?

Maternal risks are increased because of thromboembolic events or hemorrhagic complications from anticoagulation. Prophylaxis against valve thrombosis must be maintained throughout pregnancy. Although the ACC/AHA guidelines state that warfarin can be used during weeks 13–35 of gestation, this is controversial because of the substantial risk of embryopathy, spontaneous abortion, and stillbirth. Most advocate heparin therapy with goal aPTTs 2–3 times normal. Antifactor Xa levels should be kept between 0.2 and 0.4 IU/ml. Although some advocate placing porcine heterograft valves in women wanting to become pregnant, pregnancy seems to increase the risk of premature bioprosthetic valve failure.

13. Can a women breast-feed while taking a cardiac medication?

In almost all cases, breast-feeding women should be encouraged to continue. Only an estimated 2% of the maternal dose of a drug is ingested by the baby and is rarely of clinical significance. If necessary, drug levels can be monitored in breast-feeding infants.

Heparin does not get into breast milk, and the amount of warfarin ingested by the baby is too small to affect coagulation. Therefore, women taking warfarin may breast-feed their babies without concern.

Continue to avoid ACE inhibitors during breast-feeding.

BIBLIOGRAPHY

1. American College of Cardiology/American Heart Association: ACC/AHA guidelines for the management of patients with valvular heart disease. J Am Coll Cardiol 32:1486–1588, 1998.
2. Carson MP, Rosene-Montella KR: Managing the pregnant patient with heart disease. IM 19:14–27, 1998.
3. Lubbe WF: Use of diltiazem during pregnancy. N Z Med J 100:121, 1987.
4. Mariani P: Pharmacotherapy of pregnancy-related supraventricular tachycardia. Ann Emerg Med 21:229–230, 1992.
5. Sibai BM: Treatment of hypertension in pregnant women. N Engl J Med 335:257–265, 1996.

56. HEART DISEASE AND CHEMOTHERAPY

Astrid Andreescu, M.D., and Marie Wood, M.D.

1. What conditions need to be considered when a cancer patient presents with heart failure?
Potential etiologies of congestive heart failure (CHF) in these individuals include:
- Superior vena caval obstruction or portal hypertension
- Lymphangitic spread of the primary tumor to the lung
- Cardiomyopathy, either intrinsic or drug-induced
- Pericardial disease: effusion or restrictive/constrictive pericarditis
- Infectious disease, such as tuberculosis or coxsackie B–induced pericarditis
- Autoimmune diseases, uremia, or hypothyroidism

2. Which chemotherapy drugs most frequently cause CHF?
The drug most commonly associated with CHF is doxorubicin. Daunorubicin, another anthracycline, also causes CHF but is used less frequently. The newer anthracyclines, mitoxantrone and idarubicin, are less cardiotoxic but may cause CHF at high total doses. Interferon and 5-fluorouracil also cause CHF. Herceptin, a novel monoclonal antibody against the HER-2/neu receptor that is used in the treatment of advanced breast cancer, has also been found to cause CHF by an unknown mechanism. The cardiotoxicity of Herceptin is exacerbated by prior or concomitant treatment with doxorubicin.

3. How do the anthracyclines cause CHF?
The anthracycline (doxorubicin in experimental models) binds to cardiolipin in myocytes. This binding appears to have two consequences: (1) adenosine triphosphate (ATP) synthesis is disrupted, leading to decreased contractility, and (2) free radicals are generated by the anthracycline-cardiolipin complex. Free radical lipid peroxidation occurs and is believed to cause myocyte damage.

In addition, doxorubicin administration is associated with a decrease in the amount of endogenous antioxidants that scavenge free radicals. The decrease in antioxidants and the increase in free radicals (oxidants) cause an increase in oxidative stress that leads to cardiomyopathy and CHF.

4. What increases anthracycline damage?
The most important factor is **dose**. Thirty percent of individuals treated with > 450–550 mg/m^2 develop CHF. Also important is the **route** of administration. When the **dosing schedule** was changed from large doses given once every 3 weeks to weekly dosing or continuous infusion over 24–72 hours, the incidence of toxicity decreased. Thus, fewer people developed CHF when given smaller doses more frequently.

Other factors that contribute to anthracycline-induced CHF include older age, concomitant drugs (mitomycin C may increase risk), prior or subsequent radiation therapy to the heart, preexisting cardiac conditions (i.e., hypertension or myocardial infarction), hypertension, liver disease, and whole-body hyperthermia. The iron status of the individual may be important, because iron-deficient individuals tolerate more anthracycline.

5. How can you monitor for or diagnose anthracycline-induced cardiomyopathy?
The gold standard is **endomyocardial biopsy**, which can identify damage prior to the appearance of clinical symptoms. This technique is a very expensive, as well as invasive, way to diagnose cardiomyopathy. Other studies that may be helpful include **echocardiogram** and **radionuclide cardiac angiography** (MUGA). Generally, the anthracycline should be withheld if

the left ventricular ejection fraction (LVEF) drops below 50% or decreases 10% during therapy. This is usually evaluated by a gated blood pool scan at rest. There are still some cases where stress-gated scans are also used.

6. How is anthracycline-induced cardiomyopathy treated?

Essentially the same as any other type of CHF: inotropic support and afterload reduction. Other than stopping the anthracycline, there are no special methods of treating this type of CHF.

7. Describe the natural history of anthracycline-induced cardiomyopathy.

Anthracycline-induced cardiomyopathy can present acutely (within days), subacutely (up to 30 months after the last dose), or late (6–20 years after the last dose). Most patients show symptomatic improvement with conventional treatment. If diagnosed early, symptoms may completely resolve.

8. How can anthracycline-induced cardiomyopathy be prevented?

Currently, close monitoring of the total dose and LVEF is the primary means of prevention. The drug should be stopped if the LVEF decreases 10% or to < 50% during a course of therapy. Monitoring of total dose and LVEF is critical. Understanding factors that increase the incidence of cardiotoxicity such as age and comorbid diseases is important. Use of a prolonged infusion will decrease the likelihood of cardiotoxicity by decreasing peak plasma concentrations. Clinical trials are now addressing the use of liposomal doxorubicin, which alters the pharmacokinetic properties of doxorubicin, such as a decrease in the free drug concentration in plasma, and prolonged drug circulation. Cardioprotection against oxidative damage with dexrazoxane, an iron chelator, is currently being used in certain regimens but has been associated with side effects and is not yet clearly useful for prevention of late cardiac toxicity.

9. Besides CHF, what other cardiac problems does chemotherapy cause?

1. Myocardial ischemia (from ST-T wave changes to infarction)
2. Arrhythmias (atrial and ventricular)
3. Pericardial effusions
4. Myocardial hemorrhage (very rarely)

10. When should chest pain be considered a complication of chemotherapy?

Chest pain and myocardial injury do not commonly occur with chemotherapy, but either can be seen with the vinca alkaloids (vincristine, vinblastine, and vinorelbine) as well as 5-fluorouracil and paclitaxel. However, cancer patients can have myocardial infarctions, just like other individuals with typical cardiac risk factors. Myocardial injury due to the hypercoagulable state or Trousseau's syndrome is an important diagnosis to consider, because the treatment differs from that of other causes of myocardial injury (i.e., chronic heparinization). Pericardial effusion, usually secondary to the cancer or infection, also should be considered, and an echocardiogram ordered to rule it out. Pericarditis is also part of the differential diagnosis.

11. What chemotherapeutic agents cause pericardial effusions?

Cyclophosphamide can cause a serosanguinous pericardial effusion. This is seen at very high doses when acute cardiac hemorrhage develops. Retinoic acid, interleukin-2 (IL-2), and other biologic agents can cause pericardial effusions as part of a syndrome of fever, dyspnea, edema, and pleural effusions.

12. Does radiation therapy damage the heart?

Yes. The development of shielding techniques has greatly reduced cardiac toxicity associated with mediastinal or lung radiation. Nevertheless, toxicity still occurs, especially when radiation is given along with certain chemotherapeutic agents. Among a host of cardiac abnormalities are pericardial disease, valvular disease, coronary artery disease, conduction abnormalities, and myocardial dysfunction. Prior to the development of shielding techniques, pericarditis and pleural effusions were more common complications. Now, coronary artery disease is the most common problem.

13. How does radiation therapy cause coronary artery disease?

Radiation appears to cause atherosclerotic lesions as well as an increase in coronary spasm. Atherosclerotic plaques develop with the usual cardiac risk factors and histologically have more fibrosis. The circumflex coronary artery tends to be spared in radiation-induced coronary artery disease.

CONTROVERSIES

14. Should all patients receiving anthracyclines have LVEF determined before chemotherapy?

For: Any individual is at risk to decrease the LVEF with anthracyclines; if caught early, severe toxicity may be prevented.

Against: Determination of LVEF may be an unnecessary cost to patients, especially if they are young or are going to receive < 450 mg/m^2 of doxorubicin.

15. Should patients receive endomyocardial biopsy to diagnose anthracycline-induced cardiomyopathy?

For: It is the best test. Endomyocardial biopsy is much more sensitive and specific than echocardiography or MUGA scan.

Against: Endomyocardial biopsy is expensive. It is an invasive procedure with a risk of myocardial perforation, which can be a morbid complication.

16. Should all patients receiving anthracycline chemotherapy also receive the cardioprotective agent dexrazoxane?

For: It protects the heart, especially from the early anthracycline toxicity.

Against: It may also "protect" the tumor, making the therapy less effective. It also has side effects such as myelosuppression.

BIBLIOGRAPHY

1. Arsenian MA: Heart disease after mediastinal radiotherapy. Postgrad Med 91:211, 1992.
2. Braverman AC, Antin JH, Plappert MT, et al: Cyclophosphamide cardiotoxicity in bone marrow transplantation: A prospective evaluation of new dosing regimens. J Clin Oncol 9:1215–1223, 1991.
3. Freeman NJ, Costanza ME: 5-Fluorouracil-associated cardiotoxicity. Cancer 61:36–45, 1998.
4. Hancock SL, Tucker MA, Hoppe RT: Factors affecting late mortality from heart disease after treatment of Hodgkin's disease. JAMA 270:1949–1959, 1993.
5. Klein P, Muggia FM: Cytoprotection: Shelter from the storm. Oncologist 4:112–121, 1999.
6. Naschitz JE, Yeshurun D, Abrahamson J, et al: Ischemic heart disease precipitated by occult cancer. Cancer 69:2712, 1992.
7. Rowinsky EK, McGuire WP, Garner T, et al: Cardiac disturbances during the administration of taxol. J Clin Oncol 9:1704–1712, 1991.
8. Singal PK, Iliskovic N: Doxorubicin-induced cardiomyopathy. N Engl J Med 339:900–905, 1998.
9. Sonnenblick M, Rosin A: Cardiotoxicity of interferon: A review of 44 cases. Chest 99:557, 1991.

57. RENAL DISEASE AND THE HEART

June Y. Scott, M.D., and Harmeet Singh, M.D.

1. What renal complications can occur from cardiac catheterization?

- **Contrast nephrotoxicity:** acute renal failure occurring within 2–5 days of the procedure, due to nephrotoxic effects of contrast dyes. It is especially common in patients with preexisting chronic renal insufficiency and diabetes mellitus (> 60% incidence when ≥ 30 ml of dye was used).
- **Atheroembolic renal disease:** mechanical disruption of aortic atheroma by the catheter and subsequent microembolization into the kidneys. Clinically, it is characterized by a sudden or slow increase in serum creatinine level, which is usually not completely reversible and occasionally may be associated with eosinophilia, thrombocytopenia, and transient decreases in serum complement levels. Urinary abnormalities may range from benign sediment to hematuria, proteinuria, eosinophiluria, or red cell casts. Embolization to other organs may occur (e.g., livedo reticularis, peripheral cyanosis, bowel ischemia).

2. What precautions can be taken to prevent or minimize contrast nephrotoxicity?

Recognize high-risk individuals prone to this complication (i.e., those with diabetes mellitus and chronic renal insufficiency).

Volume replete, because hypovolemic patients are at much higher risk. In patients without congestive heart failure (CHF) or overt signs of volume excess, diuretics should be stopped at least 1–2 days before the procedure, and intravenous fluids should be started several hours before the test.

The concept of giving mannitol (or furosemide) before and after a procedure to prevent contrast-induced nephropathy is dated and has been shown to be ineffective in a randomized trial. The only intervention that reduces contrast-induced nephropathy is hydration using normal saline.

3. Does nonionic, low-osmolality contrast media cause less contrast nephrotoxicity than conventional high-osmolality contrast media?

Low-osmolality agents have a lower adverse profile; in particular, allergic reactions are less. Whether nephrotoxicity is less is still controversial, but a meta-analysis has shown lower risk of nephrotoxicity. Most would now agree that patients with increased risk of nephrotoxicity, particularly diabetics, should receive low-osmolality contrast agents.

4. What are the lipid abnormalities associated with renal disease?

In **nephrotic syndrome**, elevation of total and low-density lipoprotein (LDL) cholesterol is a result of increased hepatic synthesis of lipoprotein B, most likely due to hypoalbuminemia. The hypercholesterol~emia is usually severe.

In **chronic renal failure**, hypertriglyceridemia is seen in 30% of patients. The defect may be due to the reduced lipolysis of triglyceride-rich lipoproteins (mainly very low density lipoproteins).

5. Should these lipid abnormalities be treated?

The rationale for lowering lipid levels is to reduce the risk for coronary artery disease (CAD). The evidence for the independent role of lipids in causing progression of renal disease is largely experimental and *not* a rationale to lower lipid levels in renal disease.

The **hypercholesterolemia of nephrotic syndrome** should be treated, and because of its severity, dietary therapy alone is not sufficient. The drugs of choice are the HMG-CoA reductase inhibitors, which can reduce LDL cholesterol levels by 40–80 mg/dl. If another drug is needed, a bile acid sequestrant (cholestyramine) is the best choice for combination therapy.

For the **hypertriglyceridemia of chronic renal failure**, there is no scientific evidence to support the use of triglyceride-lowering agents in lowering the CAD risk, but there is ample evidence of a higher incidence of adverse reactions to these agents in this population.

6. Describe the cardiac complications seen after renal transplantation.

CAD is a major cause of morbidity and mortality in the post-renal transplant period. An accelerated atherosclerosis occurs after renal transplant that has a multifactorial basis. These patients already have a high incidence of asymptomatic CAD (diabetes mellitus and renal insufficiency), and the use of steroids and cyclosporine, both of which cause lipid abnormalities, hastens atherosclerosis. These patients may have hypercholesterolemia, hypertriglyceridemia, or mixed hyperlipidemia.

Other factors that contribute to the atherosclerotic risk and independent CAD risk are post-transplant hypertension, which is very common, and possibly post-transplant erythrocytosis, which may predispose to vascular thrombosis.

7. What should be done to prevent post-transplant CAD?

Preexisting CAD is an important predictor of post-transplant ischemic events, and aggressive attempts should be made to identify and treat (medically and surgically) pre-transplant patients with CAD. In diabetic patients there is a high incidence of silent ischemia, and pre-transplant stress testing should be done. Aggressive pre-transplant treatment improves the patient survival in this group.

After transplantion, patients with known CAD should have regular follow-up, and diagnostic evaluation should be instituted on appearance of the first symptom related to coronary ischemia. Other means of treatment include:

Lowering lipid levels:
- Achieve ideal body weight.
- Eliminate medications that alter lipids (i.e., beta blockers, diuretics).
- Decrease prednisone and cyclosporine dose if possible.
- Use cholesterol-lowering agents. Be cautious with HMG-CoA inhibitors because of their high risk of complications in the post-transplant population.

Modifying other risk factors:
- Smoking cessation
- Exercise program
- Blood pressure reduction
- Improved glycemic control

8. Describe the common causes of azotemia seen in congestive heart failure.

Patients with CHF frequently show elevated blood urea nitrogen (BUN) and creatinine (Cr) levels.

Prerenal azotemia is the most important cause of acute increases in BUN and Cr in patients with CHF and is secondary to reduced renal perfusion resulting either from true volume contraction due to diuretic use or from decreased cardiac output. It is manifested by an increased BUN/Cr ratio (normally < 10:1), benign urinary sediment, low urine sodium (< 20 mEq/L), and a low fractional excretion of sodium (< 1%).

Acute tubular necrosis results from a prolonged prerenal state resulting in ischemic renal tubular injury with increased BUN and Cr, a normal BUN/Cr ratio, granular casts and renal epithelial cells in urine, high urine sodium (> 20 mEq/L), and elevated fractional excretion of sodium (> 1%). This is a reversible insult.

Ischemic nephropathy is characterized by subacute or chronic deterioration of renal function in patients with CHF and atherosclerotic disease with or without hypertension. The underlying renal lesion is bilateral renal artery stenosis.

9. Does the use of angiotension-converting enzyme (ACE) inhibitors in heart failure carry any associated risks?

Yes. Clearly, the ACE inhibitors are the agents of choice in patients with CHF because they improve survival. However, ACE inhibitors also can cause renal insufficiency in severe CHF.

In CHF, renal hypoperfusion results in elevated renin and angiotensin II levels. Angiotensin II causes efferent more than afferent vasoconstriction and helps maintain the glomerular filtration rate (GFR). Because ACE inhibitors block angiotensin II synthesis, the protective effect of angiotensin II to maintain GFR is lost as a result of efferent vasodilatation. This is a reversible phenomenon.

Sometimes the use of ACE inhibitors results in a small increase in creatinine, which then stabilizes; in these patients, ACE inhibitors may be continued. The survival benefits from the ACE inhibitors outweigh the minor increases in serum creatinine.

10. What are the electrocardiographic (EKG) abnormalities seen in various electrolyte disturbances?

- Hypokalemia: flattened T waves, U waves, ST depression, arrhythmias (atrial and ventricular arrhythmias), prolonged QT intervals
- Hyperkalemia: tall, peaked T waves in precordial leads, followed by decreased amplitude of R waves, widened QRS complex, prolonged PR interval, and decreased amplitude and disappearance of P wave; arrhythmias
- Hypocalcemia: prolonged QT interval, arrhythmias
- Hypercalcemia: shortened QT interval, arrhythmias
- Hypermagnesemia: bradycardia, heart block (various degrees)
- Hypomagnesemia: arrhythmias, prolonged QT interval

11. Are there any risks in using nonsteroidal anti-inflammatory drugs (NSAIDs) in patients with CHF?

Yes. In congestive cardiac failure, decreased renal blood flow results from low cardiac output. There are adaptive attempts to maintain renal blood flow and GFR through various mechanisms, both intrinsic and extrinsic to the kidney (such as circulating hormones, e.g., adrenergic system, renin angiotensin system). An important intrinsic adaptation by the kidney is the release of vasodilator prostaglandins (PGE_2, PGI_2), which maintain renal blood flow and GFR by afferent arteriolar vasodilation. Hence, NSAID use in this setting counteracts this physiologic adaptation by inhibiting the production of vasodilator prostaglandins, thereby decreasing GFR.

12. What is uremic pericarditis?

In end-stage renal disease, there are two types of pericarditis. **Uremic pericarditis** occurs prior to initiation of dialysis, and **dialysis pericarditis** is seen in patients on stable maintenance hemodialysis. The pathogenesis of uremic pericarditis seems to relate to uremic toxins, since it improves with dialysis. The causative factors for dialysis pericarditis are unclear. Fluid overload may contribute to both forms of pericarditis.

13. What are clinical features of uremic pericarditis?

Physical findings
    Chest pain (60–70%)
    Pericardial rub (> 90%)
    Fever (60–90%)
    Hypotension

Laboratory abnormalities
    ECG changes
    Leukocytosis
    Abnormal chest x-ray
    Demonstration of pericardial fluid on echocardiogram

Systemic features and cardiac tamponade are more common in dialysis pericarditis. The pericardial fluid can range from serous, serosanguineous, to hemorrhagic.

14. How is uremic pericarditis treated?

The presence of uremic pericarditis in patients with end-stage renal disease is an absolute indication to **initiate dialysis**. Even in dialysis pericarditis, increasing intensity of dialysis (frequency and duration) should be the first step, as this results in resolution of disease in many patients. Pericardiocentesis is reserved for patients with hemodynamic compromise secondary to cardiac tamponade. These patients eventually need either pericardiotomy or pericardiectomy. NSAIDs and steroids are generally not beneficial in treating uremic pericarditis.

15. What is uremic cardiomyopathy?

Uremic cardiomyopathy is a broad term used to describe abnormal left ventricular function seen in patients with end-stage renal disease. The etiology of heart failure in these patients is multifactorial. Hypertension, CAD, and volume overload seem to be the major causative factors. Others include anemia, arteriovenous fistula, acid-base and electrolyte abnormalities, secondary hyperparathyroidism, nutritional deficiencies, β_2-microglobulin, and uremic toxins.

16. Name the cardiovascular consequences of hemodialysis.

- Hypotension. This is the most common side effect of hemodialysis, and the etiology is multifactorial.
- Electrolyte disturbance. Rapid changes of serum, potassium, calcium, magnesium, and pH occur which affect cell membrane potential and may lead to cardiac arrhythmias.
- Arteriovenous fistula. A fistula is an area of low resistance that leads to increased cardiac output and workload, which can cause heart failure.

17. List the renal diseases seen in infective endocarditis.

Renal emboli
Acute tubular necrosis (secondary to renal ischemia)
Interstitial nephritis (a complication of antibiotics used)
Immune-mediated glomerulonephritis (due to immune complex deposition in the kidney)

18. Describe the common electrolyte disorders seen in CHF.

Hyponatremia. *Hyper*volemic hyponatremia occurs in the face of excess total body sodium and reflects excessive water retention. *Hypo*volemic hyponatremia occurs in aggressively treated patients on diuretics and is due to true volume depletion from excessive diuresis leading to antidiuretic hormone release. Urinary analysis in both the types of hyponatremia shows low urine sodium (< 20 mEq/L), low fractional excretion of sodium (< 1%), and elevated urine osmolality.

Hypokalemia. Excessive urinary K losses are a result of elevated aldosterone concentrations, due to poor renal perfusion or diuretic use.

Hyperkalemia. This can occur from low urinary K excretion or use of ACE inhibitors.

Hypomagnesemia. This results from diuretic use, especially loop diuretics, which cause urinary magnesium losses.

19. What acid-base abnormalities are seen in CHF?

- Respiratory alkalosis (due to hyperventilation from hypoxemia)
- Metabolic acidosis (poor tissue perfusion resulting in anaerobic metabolism
- Metabolic alkalosis (excessive diuretic use and hypovolemia)
- Respiratory acidosis (rare except in severe CHF, when after prolonged hyperventilation, there is respiratory muscle fatigue and elevation of PCO_2)

20. Do angiotensin receptor blockers (ARBs) carry the same risks as ACE inhibitors?

Perhaps not. ARBs seem to have the same beneficial effects as ACE inhibitors, but some studies show a decreased incidence of acute renal failure and hyperkalemia with ARBs.

21. How does CHF impact morbidity and mortality in patients with end-stage renal disease?

In a recent study, 37% of patients starting therapy for end-stage renal disease had a history of CHF. The median survival of patients with CHF at or before starting this therapy was 36 months, compared to 62 months in patients without CHF. The independent significant predictors of CHF in those patients starting the therapy were: older age, diabetes mellitus, ischemic heart disease, systolic dysfunction on echocardiogram, and hypoalbuminemia.

BIBLIOGRAPHY

1. Barret BJ, Parfrey PS: Prevention of nephrotoxicity induced by radiocontrast agents. N Engl J Med 331:1449–1450, 1994.
1a. Barrett BJ, Carlisle EJ: Meta-analysis of the relative nephrotoxicity of high- and low-osmolality iodinated contrast media. Radiology 188:171–178, 1993.
2. Case records of the Massachusetts General Hospital (case #34-1991). N Engl J Med 325:563, 1991.
3. Daugirdas JT: Dialysis hypotension: A hemodynamic analysis. Kidney Int 33:233, 1991. 3. Grundy SM: Management of hyperlipidemia of kidney disease. Kidney Int 37:847, 1990.
4. Harnett JD, et al: Congestive heart failure in dialysis patients: Prevalence, incidence, prognosis, and risk factors. Kidney International 47:884, 1995.
5. Hirshfield JW: Low osmolality contrast agents: Who needs them? N Engl J Med 326:482, 1992.
6. Manske CL, Sprafka MJ, Strony JT, Wang Y: Contrast nephrography in azotemic diabetic patients undergoing coronary angiography. Am J Med 89:615, 1990.
7. Pastan SO, Braunwald E: Renal disorders and heart disease. In Braunwald E: Heart Disease, 5th ed. Philadelphia, W.B. Saunders, 1997.
8. Schrier RW, Gottschalk CW. Diseases of the Kidney, 6th ed. Boston, Little, Brown, 1997.
9. Solomon R, Werner C, Mann D, et al: The effects of saline, mannitol, and furosemide on acute decreases in renal function induced by radiocontrast agents. N Engl J Med 331:1416–1420, 1994.
10. Veelken R, Hilgers KF, Mann JF: The acute renal effects of angiotensin II receptor blockers. Nephrology, Dialysis, and Transplantation 13(8):1928–1929, 1998.

58. ENDOCRINE AND NUTRITIONAL DISORDERS

Olivia V. Adair, M.D., Jane Reusch, M.D., and Fred D. Hofeldt, M.D.

1. In acromegaly, what associated cardiac diseases may be seen?

Coexisting cardiovascular diseases are common in acromegaly and are the most common cause of death in untreated acromegalic individuals. Evidence for cardiac enlargement, hypertrophy, diastolic filling abnormalities, congestive heart failure (CHF), arrhythmias, myocardiopathy, arterial hypertension, aortic and mitral valve disease, and advanced atherosclerotic diseases (including coronary artery disease [CAD]) are seen. Diabetes mellitus with associated hyperinsulinism contributes to the increased atherosclerotic occurrence, morbidity, and mortality.

2. What hemodynamic changes are seen in hyperthyroidism?

Patients with hyperthyroidism have a high cardiac output state, characterized by increased stroke volume and increased pulse rate. There is a decreased peripheral vascular resistance, increased blood volume, increased pulse pressure, and a hyperdynamic precordium, resulting from increasing cardiac contractility.

3. What cardiac manifestations may be seen in hyperthyroidism?

- Hypertension (particularly isolated systolic hypertension)
- Sinus tachycardia
- Premature atrial contractions
- Paroxysmal atrial tachycardia
- Atrial fibrillation
- Conduction disturbances (varying degrees)
- High output heart failure (with cardiomyopathy)
- Low output failure (with underlying compromised left ventricular function)
- Mitral valve prolapse
- Ischemic heart disease with angina and coronary insufficiency

4. How is atrial fibrillation managed in hyperthyroidism?

Hyperthryroid patients with atrial fibrillation are at an increased risk for peripheral thromboembolism. Anticoagulation is recommended. These patients may be resistant to the usual dosage of digitalis. Beta blockers are frequently helpful.

5. Describe the cardiac hemodynamic changes in hypothyroidism.

The hypothyroid patient has decreased cardiac contractility and presents with increased peripheral vascular resistance, decreased blood volume, decreased cardiac output, decreased heart rate, and decreased pulse pressure.

6. What are the cardiovascular presentations of hypothyroidism?

The cardiovascular manifestations of hypothyroidism may include bradycardia, a quiet precordium, diastolic hypertension, and a dilated cardiac silhouette on chest x-ray. Patients may have pericardial effusions accounting for the cardiac enlargement. However, worsening CHF occurs in the hypothyroid state as thyroid hormone deficiency leads to decreased myocardial contractility. Some patients present with noncardiac chest pain and elevations in creatinine kinase, with elevation of the MM fraction ruling out myocardial infarction (MI). Electrocardiographic (EKG) abnormalities typically include sinus bradycardia, nonspecific ST-T wave abnormalities, and low voltage. Hypothyroidism has been seen in association with ventricular arrhythmias, including torsade de pointes. Hypothyroid patients have increased prevalence of atherosclerotic heart disease, which may be related to the dyslipidemia accompanying hypothyroidism.

7. What consideration is needed in hypertensive patients with low potassium?

Excess adrenal mineralocorticoids cause hypertension in < 1% of the population. However, they may be implicated when the hypertension is associated with hypokalemia, particularly in the patient who has a high salt intake or may not be taking diuretics.

8. Which mineralocorticoids cause hypertension?

Aldosterone, 11-desoxycorticosterone (DOC), and corticosterone.

9. Which laboratory tests exclude the diagnosis of Cushing's syndrome?

Frequently, a simple overnight **dexamethasone suppression test** will assist in evaluating the patient with suspected Cushing's syndrome. The patient is given 1 mg of dexamethasone at 11 p.m., and the plasma cortisol is measured at 8 a.m. the following morning. Values less than 5 µg/dl indicate normal suppression; values between 5 and 10 µg/dl are borderline; and values > 10 µg/dl are abnormal.

An equally helpful test is a 24-hour urine measurement for **free cortisol**. Patients with elevated urinary free cortisol or nonsuppressible cortisol values should be evaluated for Cushing's syndrome.

10. Which laboratory tests are used to characterize Cushing's disease?

A failure to suppress to 1-mg **overnight dexamethasone** (or its equivalent test, 0.5 mg of dexamethasone administered every 6 hours for 2 days) or an elevated **24-hour urine free cortisol** is seen in patients with Cushing's *syndrome*. Cushing's *disease* (hypothalamic-pituitary Cushing's) is distinguished from the other causes of Cushing's syndrome by a 50% reduction in the plasma cortisol value after an 8-mg overnight dexamethasone suppression or a similar 50% suppression in urinary cortisol metabolites (17-hydroxycorticosteroids or free cortisol) with the long suppression test of 2 mg of dexamethasone every 6 hours for 2 days.

Patients with pituitary Cushing's disease have normal to slightly elevated plasma ACTH levels. They show enhanced responsiveness to **corticotropin-releasing factor** (CRF) testing, which helps distinguish them from patients with adrenal forms of Cushing's syndrome and ectopic Cushing's syndrome, where there is usually no ACTH response to CRF testing. Localization of pituitary Cushing's disease is achieved by inferior petrosal sinus sampling for ACTH during a CRF infusion.

11. List the clinical features that suggest the presence of pheochromocytoma in a hypertensive patient.

- Headache, which is characteristically, but not always, pounding and severe
- Palpitations with or without tachycardia
- Excessive, inappropriate perspiration

12. How is pheochromocytoma best diagnosed?

For screening purposes, a 24-hour urine collection for vanillylmandelic acid, total catecholamines (epinephrine, norepinephrine), and metanephrine, normetanephrine, and creatinine typically establishes the diagnosis in the hypertensive patient. Occasionally, urinary catecholamines and their metabolities collected during a typical "spell" are helpful in diagnosing the patient with episodic disease.

In patients requiring further evaluation, plasma catecholamines can be measured under standardized conditions; patients with pheochromocytoma have plasma catecholamine values > 950 pg/ml (5.62 nmol/L). These values do not suppress on the clonidine suppression test.

Note that provocative stimulation tests for pheochromocytoma such as glucagon, histamine, and tyramine are considered dangerous and should be avoided.

13. What is syndrome X?

This *multimetabolic* syndrome describes the association of certain clinical features and risk factors predictive of CAD: abdominal obesity (waist/hip > 0.85), hypertension, carbohydrate intolerance or type II diabetes mellitus, and dyslipidemia (hypertriglyceridemia and low high-density lipoprotein levels). The unifying associations with these clinical states are hyperinsulinemia and insulin resistance. Other related findings in these patients include hyperuricemia, physical inactivity, and aging.

In contrast to this metabolic syndrome X, a *cardiac* syndrome X exists in which patients have anginal symptoms and normal coronary arteries on catheterization studies, but small, more distal occlusive disease (microvascular angina). Both syndromes may coexist in the same patient.

14. How common is CAD in patients with diabetes mellitus?

CAD is the most common cause of morbidity and mortality in diabetic individuals, being 1.2–6.6 times more prevalent than in the nondiabetic population. Its predominance is even greater in individuals with non-insulin-dependent diabetes and in diabetic females. Seventy-seven percent of all diabetic hospitalizations are related to CAD.

15. What are the risk factors for CAD in diabetic patients?

Diabetes alone is an independent cardiovascular risk factor, along with the classic cardiac risk factors of advancing age, male gender, postmenopausal status in females, cigarette smoking, hypertension, family history of CAD, and dyslipidemia. Diabetes has been noted to amplify the effects of these classic risk factors for CAD. In patients with insulin-dependent diabetes mellitus, hypertension and proteinuria are the strongest risk factors associated with CAD. In individuals with non-insulin-dependent diabetes, hypertriglyceridemia and proteinuria are the most potent risk factors.

16. How is proteinuria implicated?

Proteinuria is the strongest predictor of cardiovascular mortality in all individuals with diabetes mellitus. It is frequently associated with hypertension and is a marker of renal disease. It is also associated with increased fibrinogen and increased platelet aggregability, as well as abnormalities in lipid profiles.

17. What is the role of fibrinolysis?

Abnormally slow fibrinolysis is a recently established independent risk factor for CAD. In individuals with non-insulin-dependent diabetes mellitus, there is an increase in plasma-activating inhibitor-1 activity (PAI-1 activity). This has been associated with insulin resistance, and there is a direct correlation between hyperinsulinemia and an increase in PAI-1 activity.

18. Is it true that in diabetic patients, the atherosclerotic disease is more diffuse and seldom operable?

No. It has long been assumed that diffuse coronary atherosclerosis is associated with diabetes mellitus, implying that these patients have an inoperable disease. Recent data have failed to show any true incidence of more diffuse CAD in diabetic individuals compared with non-diabetics. This observation is important when considering revascularization by coronary artery bypass graft. The vessels do appear to be similarly operable in both groups.

19. Is there a difference in success rate for coronary artery bypass grafting in diabetic versus non-diabetic patients?

No. Although diabetics have a higher risk of perioperative groin and sternal wound infections, as well as renal insufficiency, the late follow-up after surgery shows a similar survival and symptom-free interval for diabetics compared to non-diabetics. One study suggested a slower flow rate in the grafts of individuals with diabetes, but this has not been confirmed in subsequent studies. Overall, the two groups behave similarly.

20. What is diabetic cardiomyopathy?

Diabetic cardiomyopathy is abnormal cardiac function leading to CHF symptoms in individuals without CAD, valvular disease, rheumatic fever, or other known cardiac disease. Hence, individuals with diabetic cardiomyopathy have classic symptoms of CHF (i.e., paroxysmal nocturnal dyspnea, orthopnea, edema, dyspnea on exertion) in the absence of any obvious cause for their cardiomyopathy besides diabetes mellitus. Pathologically, patients have a dilated cardiomegaly and interstitial fibrosis. Some reports have described an interstitial deposition of a periodic acid–Schiff-positive material.

Approximately 15% of the individuals with diabetes and CHF in the Framingham study were believed to have diabetic cardiomyopathy. It is a common clinical entity.

21. Is angina a reliable marker of ischemic disease in diabetics?

No. Classically, many individuals with diabetes have been thought to have silent ischemia. Individuals with diabetic autonomic neuropathy clearly have an increased incidence of silent MI secondary to abnormal enervation of the heart. However, despite a plethora of studies, it has not been shown conclusively whether silent ischemia is more common in diabetics without autonomic neuropathy.

Because there is a significant incidence of autonomic neuropathy that could impair angina or anginal equivalents in individuals with diabetes, it is important to do an aggressive work-up of nonspecific symptoms or those of early CHF, especially in individuals with long-standing diabetes.

22. In acute MI, what are the implications of concurrent diabetes?

Overall, individuals with diabetes do significantly worse than non-diabetics in the setting of acute MI. They suffer from an increased frequency of events during their initial hospitalization as well as long-term.

In the acute setting, individuals with diabetes are more prone to develop shock, CHF, myocardial rupture, and reinfarction, all of which are associated with increased mortality. Because of the increased catecholamine surge associated with acute MI, a transient increase in glucose concentration frequently develops.

Delayed complications of acute MI are also more common among diabetics. The survival following MI at 1, 2, and 5 years is 82%, 78%, and 58% in diabetics compared with 94%, 92%, and 82% in non-diabetics. Although beta-blockers are relatively contraindicated in diabetes, they are of benefit after MI and should be given. An associated asymptomatic hypoglycemia may be present and requires frequent monitoring in patients on insulin and oral agents.

23. What is beriberi? Who gets it?

Beriberi is a thiamine deficiency that is relatively uncommon in the United States. *Wet beriberi* is seen in the Middle East and Asia, among people who wash their rice before they eat it. They develop a thiamine deficiency while replete in other vitamins. Both wet and dry beriberi are characterized by malaise and fatigue, an increased cardiac output secondary to decreased systemic vascular resistance and increased venous return, and edema with enlarged cardiac silhouettes and pulmonary effusions. Patients respond very well to thiamine replacement.

Dry beriberi is thiamine deficiency in generalized protein calorie malnutrition and is more commonly seen in the U.S. Individuals with poor caloric intake that is relatively high in carbohydrates, e.g., alcoholics, are at risk. The usual clinical picture is an elevated heart rate with warm hands (representing the decreased systemic vascular resistance), and a generalized neuropathy (including motor deficits and decreased reflexes). This can be associated with a nutritional cirrhosis or paresthesias of the extremities. Treatment is with thiamine replacement, but may include early digitalis and diuretics.

24. Are there any cardiac effects of parathyroid disease or increased parathyroid hormone (PTH)?

Both cardiac arrhythmias and hypertension are associated with increased PTH. Also, hypertrophy is more frequent in patients with hyperparathyroidism—even without hypertension. The cause is most likely secondary to a change in extracellular calcium, but PTH also has a direct positive inotropic and positive chronotropic effect, likely related to increased calcium entry into cardiac cells and PTH increasing myocardial release of endogenous norepinephrine. Chronic hypercalcemia with increased deposition of calcium may be a risk factor for atherosclerosis.

25. Are diabetics at greater risk of cardiac events?

CAD is a major factor responsible for increased mortality, 30% greater risk by age 55, and 50% greater risk of sudden cardiac death in diabetic men. The risk of sudden cardiac death is 300% greater in diabetic women than in matched non-diabetic men and women.

26. Why is there a difference in diabetics' mortality and morbidity after MI?

Multivessel CAD and a greater amount of disease per vessel have been thought to be largely responsible for the difference in outcome. Recent studies correcting for the extent of CAD still show greater acute coronary events in diabetics. There is increased platelet aggregation, impaired fibrinolysis, and enhanced coagulability, all of which may increase the chance of thrombosis. Also, the autonomic nervous system dysfunction present in diabetics may contribute to plaque disruption and thrombosis. Parasympathetic dysfunction may lead to tachycardia and hypertension, resulting in increasing myocardial oxygen demand.

BIBLIOGRAPHY

1. Donahue RP, Orchard TJ: Diabetes mellitus and macrovascular complications: an epidemiological perspective. Diabetes Care 15:1141–1155, 1992.
2. Fuh MM, Jeng C, Young M, et al: Insulin resistance, glucose intolerance and hyperinsulinemia in a patient with microvascular angina. Metabolism 42:1090–1092, 1993.
3. Ganda OP, Arkin CF: Hyperfibrinogenemia: An important risk factor for vascular complications in diabetes. Diabetes Care 15:1245–1250, 1992.
4. Garratt KN, et al: Sulfonylurea drugs increase early mortality in patients with diabetes mellitus after direct angioplasty for acute myocardial infarction. J Am Coll Cardiology 38(1):119, 1999.
5. Jarrett RJ: Risk factors for coronary heart disease in diabetes mellitus. Diabetes 41:1–3, 1992.
6. Koskinen P, Mänttäri M, Manninen V, et al: Coronary heart disease incidence in NIDDM patients in the Helsinki Heart Study. Diabetes Care 15:820–825, 1992.
7. Liao Y, Cooper RS, Ghali JK, Lansky D, Cao G, Lee J: Sex differences in the impact of coexistent diabetes on survival in patients with coronary heart disease. Diabetes Care 16:708–713, 1993.
8. Malmberg K, Norhammer A, et al: Glycometabolic state at admission: Important risk marker of mortality in conventionally treated patients with diabetes mellitus and acute myocardial infarction. Long term results from Diabetes and Insulin-Glucose Infusion in Acute Myocardial Infarction (DIGAM) study. Circulation 99(20):2626, 1999.
9. Nesto RW, Benzaquen L: Optimizing the treatment of coronary artery disease and myocardial infarction. Diabetes Update. Intern Med 21(3):21–28, 2000.
10. Nesto RW, Zarich S: Acute myocardial infarction in diabetes mellitus: Lessons to be learned from ACE inhibitors. Circulation 97(1):12, 1998.
11. Schneider DJ, Nordt TK, Sobel BE: Attenuated fibrinolysis and accelerated atherogenesis in Type II diabetic patients. Diabetes 42:1–7, 1993.
12. Sniderman A, Michel C, Racine N: Heart disease in patients with diabetes mellitus. In Draznin B, Eckel R (eds): Diabetes and Atherosclerosis: Molecular Basis and Clinical Aspects. New York, Elsevier, 1993, pp 255–274.
13. Stamler J, Vaccaro O, Neaton JD, Wentworth D: Diabetes, other risk factors, and 12-yr cardiovascular mortality for men screened in the Multiple Risk Factor Intervention Trial. Diabetes Care 16:434–444, 1993.
14. Williams GH, Braunwald E: Endocrine and nutritional disorders and heart disease. In Braunwald E (ed): Heart Disease: A Textbook of Cardiovascular Medicine, 5th ed. Philadelphia, W.B. Saunders, 1997.

59. CARDIAC MANIFESTATIONS OF RHEUMATOLOGIC DISORDERS

Richard W. Erickson, M.D., Mark Malyak, M.D., and David H. Collier, M.D.

1. What is Marfan syndrome?

Marfan syndrome is an example of an heritable disorder of connective tissue that may have cardiovascular manifestations. It is an autosomal dominant disease that in many cases appears to be due to a mutation in the gene encoding for fibrillin, a component of the connective tissue microfibril. The characteristic skeletal abnormalities of the classic form of Marfan syndrome include increased limb length, pectus excavatum or carinatum, spinal deformities, and arachnodactyly. Excessive height is due to long lower extremities; therefore, the ratio of upper segment (top of head to pubis) to lower segment (pubis to heel) is abnormally low. Ocular abnormalities include subluxation of the lens and myopia.

2. Describe the cardiovascular manifestations of Marfan syndrome.

Cardiovascular abnormalities, particularly sequelae of dilatation of the ascending aorta, are responsible for the majority of excessive deaths in Marfan syndrome. Aortic insufficiency results primarily from dilatation of the annulus and the ascending aorta. Compared with the mitral valve, myxomatous degeneration of the aortic valve leaflets probably plays only a minor role.

The most feared complication of Marfan syndrome is acute dissection or rupture of the aorta, which often results in the patient's death. The **degree of ascending aorta dilatation** appears to correlate with the risk of aortic regurgitation, aortic dissection, and aortic rupture.

Mitral valve prolapse potentially leading to severe mitral regurgitation is also commonly seen in patients with Marfan syndrome. As opposed to aortic insufficiency, the primary pathologic process occurs within the mitral valve leaflets themselves, termed myxomatous degeneration.

3. How is aortic dilatation best assessed?

Simple bedside examination, chest radiography, and electrocardiography are insufficiently sensitive to diagnose and assess the degree of aortic dilatation, the best predictor of impending acute aortic dissection or rupture. Therefore, annual **echocardiography** is recommended in all patients with Marfan syndrome. Once the diameter of the aortic root reaches 45–50 mm, it is reasonable to assess the patient every 3 months.

4. Summarize treatment options for cardiovascular disorders resulting from Marfan syndrome.

Once the aortic diameter reaches 50 mm in patients with Marfan syndrome, consider prophylactic surgery. Pharmacologic beta-adrenergic antagonism may be beneficial in patients with dilated aortic roots who are not yet candidates for surgery. Isometric exercise should be avoided. In addition to assessment of the aorta and aortic valve, echocardiography allows evaluation of the mitral valve. Antibiotic prophylaxis for infective endocarditis is necessary in patients with mitral or aortic regurgitation.

5. What other heritable disorders of connective tissue may result in cardiovascular abnormalities?

Ehlers-Danlos syndrome
Osteogenesis imperfecta
Homocystinuria

6. What is polyarteritis nodosa?

Polyarteritis nodosa (PAN) is a primary vasculitis syndrome that results in necrotizing vasculitis of medium and small-sized muscular arteries. Though by no means definite, immune complex deposition within vessel walls is likely responsible. In certain patients the antigen has been identified, and in such cases it is most commonly hepatitis B surface antigen (HBsAg).

7. Polyarteritis nodosa causes what cardiac abnormalities?

The manifestations of the disease result from systemic inflammation (constitutional symptoms such as fatigue, malaise, anorexia, and weight loss that are likely manifestations of circulating cytokines) and focal tissue ischemia and infarction as a consequence of vascular compromise resulting from the vasculitic process. Focal aneurysms of vessels may occur and occasionally rupture.

Involvement of the renal vasculature commonly results in hyper-reninemic hypertension, which may lead to secondary cardiovascular disease. Primary involvement of the heart is also common in PAN, usually due to vasculitis of the medium and small-sized muscular arteries. The vessels involved are usually smaller and more distal than those involved in atherosclerotic heart disease. Occlusion of these vessels due to vasculitis may result in recurrent and usually small myocardial infarctions (MIs), leading to patchy myocardial fibrosis on pathologic examination. The vasculitis may manifest clinically as angina pectoris, acute MI, sudden death, dysrhythmias, or congestive heart failure (CHF).

Fibrinous pericarditis due to the underlying inflammatory disease may occur, but is more commonly due to uremia. Finally, conduction defects may occur as a result of ischemia/infarction or inflammation extending beyond vessels into the SA and AV nodes.

8. What is the treatment for polyarteritis nodosa?

The treatment for PAN includes high-dose glucocorticoids and often cytotoxic therapy, particularly the administration of daily, oral cyclophosphamide. A subgroup of patients with PAN associated with hepatitis B may benefit from alpha-interferon and ribavirin therapy.

9. What other primary vasculitic syndrome may affect the cardiovascular system?

Allergic angiitis and granulomatosis (Churg-Strauss syndrome)
Hypersensitivity vasculitis syndromes
Wegener's granulomatosis
Giant cell arteritis (temporal arteritis)
Takayasu's arteritis
Behçet's disease
Kawasaki disease

10. Can subacute bacterial endocarditis mimic a primary arthritic condition?

Yes. Extracardiac manifestations of subacute bacterial endocarditis (SBE) may be due to circulating cytokines, deposition of immune complexes, or embolic phenomena. Since SBE is an inflammatory process, cytokines may be elaborated into the circulation and result in symptoms such as fever, fatigue, malaise, anorexia, and weight loss—findings common in primary rheumatologic disorders. Circulating immune complexes due to the chronic antigenemia are common; these may deposit in a variety of end organs, such as the kidney, where they can lead to acute glomerulonephritis—also a common finding in a variety of rheumatologic disorders.

This mechanism likely also contributes to the arthritis which may be present in SBE. Additionally, direct infection of joints (septic arthritis) may occur secondary to the chronic bacteremia. Embolic disease may result in infarction of a variety of end organs, including the brain and heart. To make the situation even more confusing, 24–50% of patients with SBE are rheumatoid-factor positive due to the chronic antigenemia. Therefore, blood cultures should be obtained in every patient with fever and arthritis to exclude the possibility of SBE.

11. What is rheumatoid arthritis?

Rheumatoid arthritis (RA) is a systemic autoimmune disease of unknown etiology that manifests predominantly as a chronic, symmetric, inflammatory synovitis of the peripheral joints. Extra-articular manifestations are quite variable and usually mild but occasionally severe and life-threatening. They are usually due to vasculitis of small blood vessels or to granulomatous infiltration in end organs.

12. True or false: Rheumatoid arthritis rarely affects the heart.

False. Although only 2% of patients with RA manifest symptoms of pericarditis, evaluation of patients by echocardiography or during postmortem examination reveals evidence of pericardial inflammation in approximately 30% of patients. Most patients with symptomatic pericarditis respond to treatment with nonsteroidal anti-inflammatory drugs (NSAIDs). Pericardial tamponade and constrictive pericarditis are unusual but well-described complications.

Like pericarditis, focal or diffuse granulomatous infiltration of the myocardium, endocardium, and valves is a fairly common pathologic finding that rarely manifests clinically. Microscopically, this finding resembles the rheumatoid nodule, with which it likely shares a common pathologic origin. Clinical manifestations, when they occur, include CHF, valvular dysfunction, and dysrhythmias.

Inflammation of the coronary arteries is demonstrable in approximately 20% of patients on postmortem examination but, like the other cardiac manifestations of RA, rarely manifests clinically as myocardial ischemia.

13. Define systemic lupus erythematosus.

Systemic lupus erythematosus (SLE) is a systemic autoimmune disease of unknown etiology characterized by the production of various autoantibodies, including antibodies directed against nucleic acids and (deoxy)ribonucleoproteins, cell membrane epitopes (blood cells, neurons), and phospholipids. Clinical manifestations result from deposition of immune complexes or through the interaction of antibodies that directly interfere with cellular or coagulation function.

14. How may systemic lupus erythematosus affect the heart?

The most common cardiac manifestation of SLE is **pericarditis**, which is found in up to 80% of postmortem examinations. Clinical manifestations of pericarditis, either characteristic pain or an auditory rub on auscultation, may be present at some time in up to 50% of patients. SLE tends to be an episodic disorder characterized by remissions and exacerbations; pericarditis associated with SLE tends to follow this general rule. Cardiac compression due to large effusions or to constrictive pericarditis has been reported but is unusual.

CHF in the patient with SLE may be secondary to various extracardiac causes, including renal failure and hypertension. Occasionally, myocarditis due to infiltration of the myocardium by inflammatory cells may manifest clinically as CHF or dysrhythmias.

Endocarditis caused by Libman-Sacks vegetations is present in up to 75% of patients with SLE on postmortem examination. These small 1- to 4-mm lesions are found on the edge of the mitral and aortic valves most commonly but occasionally involve the right-sided valves, valve rings, papillary muscles, and endocardium. They are usually clinically silent but occasionally may lead to valvular compromise, embolic phenomenon, and bacterial endocarditis.

Premature coronary artery disease due to atherosclerosis is becoming a common problem as patients with SLE survive longer. Potential causes of this premature atherosclerosis include hypertension, glucocorticoid therapy, and chronic immune complex deposition within coronary artery walls.

Finally, patients with SLE and **antiphospholipid antibodies** may have the same manifestations as patients with primary antiphospholipid antibody disease (see Questions 20 and 21).

15. What is the neonatal lupus syndrome?

The neonatal lupus syndrome is a disease of the fetus and neonate that likely results from maternal transfer of the autoantibodies anti-Ro (SS-A) and/or anti-La (SS-B) to the fetal circulation. Clinical manifestations are variable and include dermatitis, hepatitis, hemolytic anemia, and thrombocytopenia. The most common cardiac manifestation of the neonatal lupus syndrome is complete congenital heart block; this lesion is responsible for the major morbidity and mortality of this disorder. Many patients require permanent pacemaker therapy.

16. Describe polymyositis and dermatomyositis.

Both polymyositis and dermatomyositis are autoimmune disorders of unknown etiology; their primary clinical manifestation is weakness due to inflammation and necrosis of **skeletal muscle**. Helpful clinical findings include proximal muscle weakness, elevated serum enzymes (such as creatine phosphokinase), and characteristic electromyographic and biopsy abnormalities. Dermatomyositis is characterized by dermatologic findings in addition to myositis.

17. Is cardiac muscle ever involved in polymyositis and dermatomyositis?

Up to 40% of patients with polymyositis and dermatomyositis have cardiac abnormalities. Supraventricular tachyarrhythmias are most common. Various degrees of conduction defects and ventricular tachyarrhythmias also have been noted. An inflammatory myopathy of cardiac muscle resulting in CHF has occasionally been observed. Finally, pericarditis with varying degrees of effusion may occur. Coronary arteritis and valvular lesions are unusual.

18. What is systemic sclerosis?

Systemic sclerosis is an autoimmune disorder of unknown etiology that results in a diffuse bland vasculopathy and variable fibrosis of skin and various end organs, particularly the heart, lungs, kidneys, and gastrointestinal tract. The diffuse vasculopathy may lead to varying degrees of ischemia and infarction in the skin and various end organs; the consequence of these diffuse ischemic events may be the characteristic fibrosis of the disease.

Two major subcategories are often recognized. The first is systemic sclerosis with limited cutaneous scleroderma or CREST syndrome (calcinosis, Raynaud's phenomenon, esophageal dysmotility, sclerodactyly, and telangiectasia). The other is systemic sclerosis with diffuse cutaneous scleroderma.

19. What are the cardiac manifestations of scleroderma (systemic sclerosis)?

The heart may be involved directly, in the form of myocardial fibrosis, or indirectly, as a result of pulmonary or renal involvement. Clinical features include CHF, supraventricular and ventricular tachyarrhythmias, conduction disturbances, and syndromes of myocardial ischemia, including angina, acute MI, and sudden death. Pericarditis also may be present, either as a primary manifestation or secondary to uremia.

Pulmonary hypertension is seen in 10–20% of patients with limited systemic sclerosis. These patients may present with dyspnea on exertion and/or pedal edema. They are commonly found to have tricuspid regurgitation and may eventually develop right heart failure.

20. Describe the cardiac abnormalities that can occur in ankylosing spondylitis.

Cardiac abnormalities can occur in patients with severe and long-standing ankylosing spondylitis. Aortitis of the ascending aorta, causing dilatation of the aortic ring and aortic valve incompetence, can develop. Cardiac conduction abnormalities may occur from involvement of the His bundle or the atrioventricular node. Some patients experience complete heart block, causing Stokes-Adams attacks—this necessitates a cardiac pacemaker. Rarely, the anterior leaflet of the mitral valve is involved, causing mitral valve incompetence.

21. What is the antiphospholipid antibody syndrome?

The antiphospholipid antibody syndrome (APS) is a disorder characterized by circulating antiphospholipid antibodies and manifesting clinically as variable degrees of recurrent arterial and venous thromboses, recurrent spontaneous abortions, and thrombocytopenia. The disease may be primary, or associated with another disorder such as SLE. It remains unclear how the antiphospholipid antibodies result in clinical expression.

Antiphospholipid antibodies may be recognized by the presence of the lupus anticoagulant (elevated partial thromboplastin time not corrected by addition of normal sera and not due to antibodies directed against specific clotting factors), a false-positive serologic test for syphilis, or the presence of anticardiolipin antibodies as determined by enzyme-linked immunosorbent assay.

22. Describe the cardiac manifestations of the antiphospholipid antibody syndrome.

Cardiac manifestations of APS include thromboses of the coronary arteries that lead to myocardial ischemia and/or infarction. Cardiac valvular abnormalities also may be present, including sterile vegetations and aortic and mitral regurgitation. Such lesions can occur in patients with primary APS, as well as in those with APS associated with SLE.

23. What is drug-induced lupus? How does it differ from systemic lupus erythematosus (SLE)?

Drug-induced lupus is a constellation of problems, including fever, myalgias, arthralgias/arthritis, and pleuritis. About one-third of patients have pulmonary infiltrates. All the patients are antinuclear antibody (ANA)–positive, and many have anti-histone antibodies.

Patients with SLE have more rashes, such as malar rash or discoid lesions, much more nephritis (about 40–50% of SLE patients) and central nervous system involvement (seizures, strokes, organic brain syndrome, or psychosis), and fewer pulmonary infiltrates. SLE patients may have antibodies to double-stranded DNA or the Smith antigen, which is not seen in drug-induced lupus.

24. What cardiovascular drugs are associated with drug-induced lupus?

Drugs *definitely* associated with positive ANA and lupus-like disease: procainamide, hydralazine, methyldopa.

Drugs *possibly* associated with positive ANA and lupus-like disease: beta-adrenergic blocking agents, quinidine, simvastatin, captopril.

Note that only a select list of drugs may induce this disorder, and many are cardiac drugs.

25. Are drugs that can induce lupus contraindicated in SLE? Can they exacerbate disease activity in a patient with SLE?

No and no. The two populations at risk appear to be quite different in age, race, and genetic background. There is no evidence that using a drug that can cause drug-induced lupus exacerbates disease activity in patients who already have SLE. However, it is prudent to use an alternative drug if available, so that a flare of the SLE will not be confused with drug-induced illness.

26. Do the selective cyclo-oxygenase-2 (COX-2) inhibitors offer an advantage over the traditional NSAIDs in patients with cardiovascular disease?

Yes. Traditional NSAIDs inhibit cyclo-oxygenase-1 (COX-1) and COX-2. There are now two selective COX-2 inhbitors available, Celecoxib and Rofecoxib, with more on the way. They have significant advantage over traditional NSAIDs in decreasing gastrointestinal (GI) effects. **COX-1** products, specifically prostaglandin E2 in the gut, induce mucus and bicarbonate and increase blood flow in stomach mucosal cells. This protects the stomach from gastritis and ulcers. Inhibiting COX-1 by traditional NSAIDs increases the incidence of gastritis and gastric ulcers.

COX-2 selective inhibitors do not induce gastritis or gastric ulcers beyond which are seen in patients taking placebos. More recently, selective COX-2 inhibitors have shown significantly less GI bleeds, perforations, and obstructions as compared to traditional NSAIDs. Selective COX-2 inhibitors may even be more GI-tolerable than traditional NSAIDs. Patients with systemic diseases are at more risk for GI bleeds, and a selective COX-2 inhibitor would be advantageous for them.

27. What other advantage does the COX-2 inhibitor offer?

Selective COX-2 inhibitors do not inhibit platelet aggregation and can be used with anticoagulants such as warfarin. It is **controversial** whether selective COX-2 inhibitors have fewer renal effects. Traditional NSAIDs can block sodium excretion, induce edema, and increase hypertension in patients with borderline heart failure, hypovolemia, or chronic renal insufficiency. They can block hypotensive effects of diuretics, angiotensin-converting enzyme inhibitors, and beta-adrenergic blockers. COX-2 has been found in the glomerulous podocytes and afferent arteriole of the human kidney.

In general, the use of selective COX-2 inhibitors causes the same incidence of edema and increase in blood pressure as traditional NSAIDs. However, recent data from the Celecoxib Long-Term Arthritis Safety Study (CLASS) demonstrated small, but statistically significant, blood pressure elevations with traditional NSAIDs as compared to Celecoxib. Use over time will tell whether this is a clinically useful effect.

28. How do COX-2 inhibitors and NSAIDs differ regarding myocardial infarction?

In general, there is no difference in MI in patients on selective COX-2 inhibitors versus traditional NSAIDs. However, a recent, large study on rofecoxib demonstrated a slight increase in MIs in patients taking this drug, as compared to patients taking naproxen. Since the selective COX-2 inhibitors do not affect platelets, patients with significant coronary artery disease taking a COX-2 inhibitor should be on some aspirin or platelet inhibitor prophylactically—provided there is no contraindication to taking aspirin. However, aspirin increases the patient's risk for GI side effects.

BIBLIOGRAPHY

 1. Bombardier C, Laine L, Rekin A, et al: Comparison of upper gastrointestinal toxicity of rofecoxib and naproxen in patients with rheumatoid arthritis. N Engl J Med 343:1520–1528, 2000.
 2. Follansbee WP: Organ involvement: Cardiac. In Clements PJ, Furst DE (eds): Systemic Sclerosis. Baltimore, Williams & Wilkins, 1996, pp 333–364.
 3. Godfrey M: The Marfan syndrome. In Breighton P (ed): McKusick's Heritable Disorders of Connective Tissue, 5th ed. St. Louis, Mosby, 1993, pp 51–135.
 4. Khan MA: Ankylosing spondylitis: Clinical Aspect. In Calin A, Taurog JD (eds): The Spondylarthritides. Oxford, Oxford University Press, 1998, pp 27–40.
 5. Klippel JH, Dieppe PA (eds): Rheumatology. St. Louis, Mosby, 1994.
 6. Le Goff P, Saraux A: Drug induced lupus. Rev Rhum Engl Ed 66:40–45, 1999.
 7. Quismorio FP: Cardiac abnormalities in systemic lupus erythematosus. In Wallace DJ, Hahn BH (eds): Dubois' Lupus Erythematosus, 5th ed. Baltimore, Williams & Wilkins, 1997, pp 653–671.
 8. Rubin RL: Etiology and mechanism of drug-induced lupus. Curr Opin Rheumatolol 11:357–363, 1999.
 9. Schlant RC, Alexander RW (eds): Hurst's The Heart: Arteries and Veins, 8th ed. New York, McGraw-Hill, 1994.
10. Swan SK, Rudy DW, Lasseter KC, et al: Effect of cyclooxygenase-2 inhibition on renal function in elderly persons receiving a low-salt diet. A randomized control trial. Ann Intern Med 133:1–9, 2000.
11. Whelton A: Nephrotoxicity of nonsteroidal anti-inflammatory drugs: Physiologic foundations and clinical implications. Am J Med 106:13S–24S, 1999.

60. SUBSTANCE ABUSE AND THE HEART

Olivia V. Adair, M.D.

1. When should alcohol cardiomyopathy be suspected?

All patients with dilated cardiomyopathy should be asked about alcohol consumption. In addition, macrocytosis is a good indicator of chronic alcohol abuse, even when liver function tests are normal. Susceptibility to the adverse effects of alcohol on the heart is apparently individual. Susceptibility is demonstrated by the presence of immunoglobin A on the sarcolemma and muscle of small blood vessels at biopsy of patients with alcoholic cardiomyopathy.

2. Does the type of alcoholic drink influence the effect on the heart?

No. Studies show no difference in the abnormalities observed in patients using predominantly wine, beer, or whiskey. Moreover, no consistent pattern of drinking is associated with heart failure. Possible additives in home brew and/or moonshine alcoholic substances may cause additional toxic damage.

3. Describe the presentation of patients who develop myocardial damage secondary to chronic alcoholism.

Alcohol abuse causes the diffuse myocardial damage seen in other primary myocardial diseases. However, fewer than one-half of patients present with symptoms of congestive heart failure (CHF), whereas in other primary myocardial diseases CHF is the predominant feature. A significant number of patients with alcoholic cardiomyopathy present with arrhythmias and chest pain.

4. Are specific electrocardiographic (EKG) changes associated with alcoholic cardiomyopathy?

The EKG of patients with alcoholic cardiomyopathy may be normal or display nonspecific changes. As disease of the ventricle progresses, poor R wave progression is common, reflecting conduction delay. In addition, enlargement of the left ventricle and left and/or right atrium is common, whereas left or right bundle branch block is seen in 10% of patients.

5. What common arrhythmias are associated with alcohol ingestion?

Supraventricular arrhythmias predominate in patients without overt cardiomyopathy and in patients with acute intoxication; atrial fibrillation is the most prominent. The etiology appears to be moderate delays in conduction, which cause acute arrhythmias or "holiday heart." Acute arrhythmias are seen in heavy, binge drinking, in chronic abuse, or in special circumstances (e.g., prolonged sleeplessness) without chronic abuse. The risk of supraventricular arrhythmias with 6 or more drinks/day is increased by 2.6. Atrial flutter also is common.

Treatment includes hydration, magnesium IV, and beta blockers. Check electrolytes and thyroid function. Conversion is usually within 24 hours. Anticoagulants generally are not needed, but the patient may well require thiamine and folate.

6. Are the arrhythmias seen during withdrawal the same as acute intoxication arrhythmias?

During withdrawal, concentrations of plasma catecholamines are high, and patients may have frequent ventricular ectopy. Ventricular ectopy may help to explain the sudden deaths in young and middle-aged alcoholics without coronary artery disease (CAD). The threshold for ventricular fibrillation is reduced, and moderate alcohol levels suggest a declining blood level at the time of cardiac arrest.

7. What is the prognosis in alcoholic cardiomyopathy?

The prognosis is variable, depending on the extent of cardiac involvement. If the patient continues to drink, the prognosis is particularly grave. In one study, patients who remained abstinent over a 4-year period experienced a 9% mortality rate, whereas > 50% of those who continued to drink died during the same 4 years. Unfortunately, the recovery rate with abstinence is not as great as previously reported; earlier studies probably observed and reported cases of milder cardiac involvement. Only a minority of patients with moderate-to-severe alcoholic cardiomyopathy show clinical improvement with abstinence; after a certain stage of disease, the prognosis most likely continues to be poor, regardless of abstinence or therapy.

8. Can alchohol consumption cause syncope?

Yes. A recent study on alcohol and syncope found that short-term alcohol consumption elicits hypotension with orthostatic stress due to impairment of vasoconstriction. As a result, the decrease in systolic pressure doubles, compared to placebo intake. In the typical dehydrated state of the drinker, this chain of events may be heightened.

9. Are alcoholic cardiomyopathies reversible?

Yes, if the cardiomyopathy is a genuine effect of alcoholism. Termination of alcohol use, good nutrition, and thiamine are effective. A recent study suggests that chronic alcoholic cardiomyopathy may be related to a viral myocarditis: mice given a myotropic virus plus alcohol developed more frequent and more severe dilated cardiomyopathy than mice not given alcohol but given the myotropic virus. These results indicate that additional examination of the alcoholic cardiomyopathies is warranted. Note that even if alcohol is only a component, thiamine therapy should be initiated.

10. Is there a risk of stroke associated with alcohol consumption?

Yes. Recent heavy drinking was found to be an independent risk in patients 16–60 years old being evaluated for etiology of stroke. Drinking 150–300 g of alcohol the week preceding the stroke markedly increased cardioembolic and cryptogenic factors, approximately five fold. Patients with large-artery atherosclerosis and acute drinking of intoxicating amounts have a 7.7% increased risk. It has been concluded that heavy drinking may trigger the onset of embolic stroke in patients with a source of thrombus in the heart or large arteries (e.g., the aorta).

11. How common is cocaine use in the United States? Why is it important in cardiac problems?

An estimated 8 million people regularly use cocaine in the U.S., by inhalation, smoking, or intravenous injection. Recent surveys show that the number of hard-core cocaine users has increased. The mean age of hard-core cocaine users is rising as addicts age. Older or aging cocaine users experience a higher incidence of cardiac abnormalities.

12. How is cocaine use diagnosed as the cause of a specific cardiac problem?

All patients presenting with CAD syndrome, cardiac arrhythmias, myocardial dysfunction, myocarditis, or endocarditis should be questioned about use of cocaine and other drugs. The age, gender, and social status of the patient are *not* determining factors; grandmothers, executives, and all sorts of people use illicit drugs. Examine patients for marks from intravenous use, nasal redness, nasal septum irritation, or other physical signs of use. Analyze urine for metabolites of cocaine if there is a concern, as the urine remains positive for 1–2 and even sometimes several days, whereas plasma half-life is approximately 50–90 minutes.

13. How does cocaine affect the heart?

The cardiovascular effects of cocaine are multifactoral and complex. Cocaine has been shown to cause or to be associated with cardiomyopathy, myocarditis, endocarditis (in IV drug users), ventricular arrhythmias, myocardial infarction, coronary artery spasm and angina, and sudden death. Cocaine inhibits the neuronal or presynaptic reuptake of norepinephrine and the neuronal uptake of catecholamine hormones. This pharmacologic action increases the synaptic cleft concentration of norepinephrine and the circulating levels of both norepinephrine and epinephrine.

Cardiovascular Complications of Cocaine

Sudden death

Acute myocardial infarction

Chest pain without myocardial infarction

Acute, reversible myocarditis

Irreversible heart muscle disease

Acute, severe hypertension

Acute aortic dissection, rupture

Electrocardiographic changes: sinus tachycardia, premature ventricular complexes, Wolff-Parkinson-White arrhythmias, ventricular tachycardia, torsade de pointes, ventricular fibrillation, prolongation of QTc, and early repolarization (ST segment) changes

Pneumopericardium

Stroke

Subarachnoid hemorrhage

Accelerated coronary atherosclerosis

Intimal hyperplasia of coronary vessels

From Crawley IS, Schlant RC: Effect of noncardiac drugs, electricity, poisons, and radiation on the heart. In Schlant RC, Alexander RW (eds): Hurst's The Heart, 8th ed. New York, McGraw-Hill, 1994, with permission.

14. What is the most common clinical presentation in cocaine abuse?

Chest pain is the most common symptom, and acute myocardial infarction (MI) is the most common clinical presentation.

15. How does cocaine abuse cause an acute MI?

Cocaine affects the heart in multiple ways, both directly and indirectly. Cocaine abuse may result in MI in patients with normal coronary arteries, coronary artery spasm, or previous CAD. The **mechanisms include: (1)** increased oxygen demand (secondary to increases in heart rate and blood pressure), **(2)** decreased coronary artery blood flow (secondary to vasospasm or thrombosis with increased platelet aggregation), and **(3)** myocarditis (secondary to toxic effect or hypersensitivity). Cocaine use also promotes intimal proliferation in coronary arteries.

16. How significant is the cardiomyopathy associated with cocaine use?

The link between cocaine and the development of cardiomyopathy has been supported by animal studies that show the drug's depressant effect on cardiac function. Acute as well as chronic left ventricular (LV) dilatation and dysfunction may lead to significantly depressed cardiac function. Other causes of cardiomyopathy, such as ischemia or cardiomyopathy associated with acquired immunodeficiency syndrome (AIDS), should be ruled out. Patients may present with significant cardiomyopathy and heart failure. In a large study at the University of Colorado, 13% of a young population (mean age 36 years) of cocaine users had LV dysfunction or ejection fraction < 50%.

With symptoms of shortness of breath and fatigue, the diagnosis may be missed. All cocaine users with symptoms suggestive of CHF should be examined by echocardiogram for cocaine-induced cardiomyopathy. In a significant number of patients (7%, according to one study) asymptomatic cardiomyopathy may promote arrhythmias.

17. What electrophysiologic abnormalities are seen in cocaine users?

Cocaine blocks the fast sodium channels in the myocardium, thus depressing depolarization and slowing conduction velocity. The refractoriness of the atrial and ventricular muscle is also prolonged. Cocaine is similar in its electrophysiologic properties to class 1 antiarrhythmic agents, and QT prolongation and ventricular arrhythmias, including torsade de pointes, occur. Transient heart block of the second and third degrees also has been reported. Heart block as well as arrhythmias may respond to correction of acidosis, hypokalemia, and hypomagnesemia.

18. What EKG changes are seen in cocaine users?

A study of cocaine users presenting to an emergency department (ED) found significant EKG abnormalities in 50% of patients. The major abnormalities were prolonged PR, QRS, and QT intervals (with an increase in atrial and ventricular refractoriness); tachycardias or bradycardias; increased QRS voltage; poor R wave progression; nonspecific ST-T wave changes; early repolarization and ST elevation (with possible ischemia); and ventricular and atrial arrhythmias. Another study of asymptomatic cocaine users found abnormal EKGs in up to 29%. During the first weeks of withdrawal, cocaine abusers frequently develop silent myocardial ischemia, manifested as ST elevation during ambulatory EKG monitoring. These changes are believed to be associated with coronary vasospasm.

19. How should patients with cocaine-induced chest pain be evaluated? Should they be admitted to the hospital?

The etiology of chest pain after cocaine use is most likely multifactoral; myocardial ischemia, infarction, and aortic dissection must not be overlooked. Consider **chest radiographs** to rule out cocaine-induced pneumomediastinum, pneumothorax, and widened mediastinum. **Prompt EKG** is important to evaluate patients with ischemia because of the common occurrence of early repolarization. The creatinine kinase level may be elevated as a result of rhabdomyolysis; although the pattern is different from that in acute MI, the distinction is not helpful in the ED.

In one study, angina was ruled out in 101 consecutive cocaine users presenting to the ED with suggestive chest pain, but there was no work-up for cardiac risk. Another study looked at risk stratification in cocaine users (mean age 37 years) presenting with chest pain and found a significant amount of CAD (40% with > 70% stenosis and 21% with ≤ 70% stenosis). Young cocaine users, therefore, seem to be predisposed to myocardial ischemia, CAD, and MI. As a result, admission to a coronary care unit or monitored bed is advisable for cocaine users who present with typical or atypical chest pain, if MI is suspected. Even hours after cocaine use, coronary spasm and arrhythmias may occur.

20. Is endocarditis frequently seen in cocaine users?

Yes. Intravenous cocaine abuse has a strong association with endocarditis; *Staphylococcus aureus* is the most commonly isolated organism. Unfortunately, because the staphylococci may be resistant, drug sensitivity must be established. Moreover, rare organisms may be the culprit. In intravenous users, the tricuspid valve is more commonly involved in the endocarditis, patients are prone to develop paravalvular abscess, which may require transesophageal echocardiography.

21. Which arrhythmias are most commonly seen with cocaine abuse?

The most common arrhythmias are tachycardia and premature ventricular beats, which are usually transient and do not require treatment. Cocaine-induced supraventricular tachycardia, ventricular tachycardia, and ventricular fibrillation are also seen; management depends on etiology and hemodynamic status of the patient. The underlying problems may be MI or ischemia, QT interval prolongation, reperfusion after coronary spasm, or electrolyte imbalance. Bradycardia also has been reported in the absence of infarction, but it is transient.

22. What arrhythmia is likely in syncope in a cocaine user presenting to the ED?

Though ventricular arrhythmias are induced by cocaine, bradyarrhythmias also may occur, especially in younger patients (see Castro and Nacht).

23. Describe problems among potential heart donors, related to the large demand for donor hearts and the prevalent use of cocaine?

Recently, a heart recipient died of acute right ventricular failure. The donor had a history of binge drinking and cocaine abuse. The donor had died of traumatic brain death, and his serum was positive for cocaine prior to transplant. The autopsy of the patient receiving the transplant revealed findings consistent with cocaine cardiomyopathy.

This case (and others) is leading to intensified focus on obtaining toxicology screens and accurate histories from donors. Cocaine users may no longer be considered as donors, especially in traumatic brain death.

24. A 24-year-old bodybuilder presents to the ED with symptomatic atrial fibrillation. What should the work-up include?

A complete history on any drug use or stimulants, an EKG, and an echocardiogram to evaluate for hypertrophy associated with weight-lifting. Toxicology may need to be drawn to rule out substance/drug abuse. This patient admitted to ingesting large doses of anabolic steroids. Echocardiogram revealed mild concentric hypertrophy without obstruction.

Anabolic steroids have been associated with hypertension, ischemic heart disease, hypertrophic cardiomyopathy, and sudden death.

BIBLIOGRAPHY

1. Adair OV, Rainguet S, Pearson T, et al: Echocardiography abnormalities in chronic cocaine users [abstract]. Circulation 23 (Suppl):150A, 1994.
2. Balfour D, Benowitz N, et al: Diagnosis and treatment of nicotine dependence with emphasis on nicotine replacement therapy. A status report. Eur Heart J 21(6):438–445, 2000.
3. Baumann BM, Perrone J, et al: Cardiac and hemodynamic assessment of patients with cocaine-associated chest pain syndromes. J Toxicol Clin Toxicol 38(3):283–290, 2000.
4. Bertolet BD, Freund G, Martin CA, et al: Unrecognized left ventricular dysfunction in an apparent healthy cocaine abuse population. Clin Cardiol 13:323–328, 1990.
5. Castro VJ, Nacht R: Cocaine-induced bradyarrhythmia: An unsuspected cause of syncope. Chest 117(1):275–277, 2000.
6. Chakko S, Fernandez A, Mellman TA, et al: Cardiac manifestations of cocaine abuse: A cross-sectional study of asymptomatic men with history of long-term abuse of "crack" cocaine. J Am Coll Cardiol 20:1168–1174, 1992.
7. Cregler LL: Cocaine: The newest risk factor for cardiovascular disease. Clin Cardiol 14:449–456, 1991.
8. Hillbom M, Numminen H, Juvela S: Recent heavy drinking of alcohol and embolic stroke. Stroke 30(11):2307–2312, 1999.
9. Houser SL, MacGillivray T, Aretz HT: The impact of cocaine on the donor heart: A case report. J Heart Lung Transplant 19(6):609, 2000.
10. Kupari M, Koskinen P, Suokas A, Ventila M: Left ventricular filling impairment in asymptomatic chronic alcoholics. Am J Cardiol 661:1473–1477, 1990.
11. Lange RA, Cigarroa RG, Yancy CW, et al: Cocaine-induced coronary artery vasoconstriction. N Engl J Med 321:1577, 1989.
12. Nademanee K, Adair O, Havranek E, et al: A prospective study of cocaine related cardiovascular morbidity and mortality: Chronic cocaine users vs post-angioplasty patients. Circulation (abstract) 1994.
13. Nademanee K: The cardiovascular toxicity of cocaine. Primary Cardiol 17(3):40–49, 1991.
14. Narkiewicz K, Cooley RL, Somers VK: Alcohol potentiates orthostatic hypotension: Implications for alcohol-related syncope. Circulation 101(4):398–402, 2000.
15. Om A: Cardiovascular complications of cocaine. Am J Med Sci 303:333–339, 1992.
16. Om A, Ellaham S, DiSciascio G: Management of cocaine-induced cardiovascular complications. Am Heart J. 125:471, 1993.
17. Patel R, McArdle JJ, Regan TJ: Increased ventricular vulnerability in a chronic ethanol model despite reduced electrophysiologic responses to catecholamines. Alcohol Clin Exp Res 15:785–789, 1991.
18. Sullivan ML, Martinez CM, Gallagher EJ: Atrial fibrillation and anabolic steroids. J Emerg Med 17(5):851–857, 1999.

61. CARDIAC MANIFESTATIONS OF AIDS

Olivia V. Adair, M.D.

1. How commonly is the heart affected in patients with AIDS?
Cardiac involvement has been reported in 25–50% of patients with AIDS, as defined by echocardiographic, endomyocardial biopsy, or autopsy findings. This involvement may cause clinically apparent manifestations in only 10–25% of patients, depending on the stage of disease and whether the patients are hospitalized.

2. List the common lesions in cardiac involvement in AIDS.
- Metastatic or primary involvement of Kaposi's sarcoma or other malignant lymphomas involving the myocardium, epicardium, or pericardium
- Myocarditis (infectious, viral, lymphocytic, noninfectious), endocarditis, or pericarditis
- Pericardial effusions
- Cardiomyopathy (right, left, or biventricular)
- Vasculitis
- Toxic effects of drugs used against infectious complications or anti-HIV drugs

3. What are the most common clinical manifestations of AIDS when there is heart involvement?
- Myocarditis (40–52%)
- Pericarditis (in up to 15% of cases, with an effusion in 18–40%)
- Congestive heart failure due to left ventricular dilatation and dysfunction (10–42%)

These lesions may present as angina, dyspnea, fatigue, and dyspnea on exertion. Also ventricular arrhythmias, endocarditis, and right-heart failure may be presenting abnormalities. Anderson and Virman proposed the use of four clinical categories of AIDS heart disease: (1) endocardial disease, (2) myocardial disease, (3) pericardial disease, and (4) neoplasms.

4. When a patient with HIV infection presents with dyspnea, should I be concerned about a cardiac etiology?
Yes. AIDS patients have multiple symptoms for which the system involved may be unclear. For example, chest pain, dyspnea, fatigue, edema, and palpitations are general symptoms which may have multi-system etiologies. Because these patients may not have overt clinical evidence for cardiac disease, only through a heightened awareness of the frequent involvement of the heart will correct diagnosis and management be initiated.

5. Describe the diagnostic work-up for the AIDS patient with dyspnea.
The physical examination may help implicate a pulmonary or cardiac etiology. However, usually this is not sufficient, and a chest x-ray may be inconclusive since old and/or new pulmonary infiltrates do not rule out a cardiac problem. An echo-Doppler study, however, may be very helpful in evaluating a patient for pericardial effusion, tamponade, cardiomyopathy, valve disease, (especially tricuspid regurgitation secondary to pulmonary hypertension), or segmental wall motion abnormalities. Many of these patients also may have risk factors for coronary artery disease (i.e., male smokers) and ischemia or infarction should be considered; therefore, an electrocardiogram should be routinely obtained.

6. Why is it important to perform an echocardiogram on an AIDS patient with chest pain or shortness of breath?
Because there may be specific findings on the echocardiogram that will change the management, improve the quality of life, and provide symptomatic improvement for the patient. For

example, if the patient has a cardiomyopathy, diuretics and angiotensin-converting enzyme (ACE)-inhibitors may markedly alleviate the shortness of breath not otherwise treated if the patient is diagnosed as having a chronic pulmonary infection. Also, specific antibiotics are indicated for infectious myocarditis and pericarditis, as well as antineoplastic therapy for specific neoplasms. When a pericardial effusion is present, arrangements need to be made for pericardiocentesis and possibly biopsy for specific diagnosis. Tuberculous pericarditis often presents with tamponade and requires urgent drainage.

7. How common is pericarditis in AIDS? What are the common etiologies?

Pericarditis occurs in 5–15% of patients with AIDS and usually presents as chest pain. The causes may be viral disease, bacterial infection, tuberculosis, neoplasm, or fungal infection.

8. Does the patient's clinical status affect the likelihood of cardiac abnormalities?

Only a few studies have looked at this issue. Patients with more advanced disease, i.e., AIDS, had more cardiac abnormalities on echo-Doppler than patients who were HIV-positive but pre-AIDS. Also, patients with $CD4^+$ lymphocyte counts $\leq 100/mm^3$ had a higher prevalence of abnormalities on echo-Doppler compared to patients with higher $CD4^+$ counts. The presence of an active opportunistic infection, however, did not correlate with the presence of abnormalities. One study showed an association of opportunistic infection with more cardiac abnormalities, but no association with left ventricular dysfunction. The highest relationship with a low $CD4^+$ count was pericardial effusion.

9. How common is endocarditis in AIDS patients?

Endocarditis is not a common finding in AIDS patients. Because most of the larger studies have been done in centers where the major HIV-positive population is not intravenous drug abusers though, this may be an unidentified area of concern. We (see ref. 1) have reported frequent valve abnormalities (67%) in a study of a large group of patients who were HIV-positive and intravenous drug abusers. However, only 7% of the patients had active endocarditis at the time of evaluation.

10. Which patients develop cardiomyopathy and poor left ventricular function?

This is controversial. One study showed a correlation between the $CD4^+$ counts of $\leq 100/mm^3$ and the presence of left ventricular (LV) dysfunction. Levy et al. showed that patients with $CD4^+$ counts $\leq 100/mm^3$ and AIDS had the most cases (55%) of LV dysfunction, whereas those with a $CD4^+$ count $> 100/mm^3$ and active AIDS or pre-AIDS had approximately the same percentage of cases of LV dysfunction (17% and 16%, respectively). However, in a young population, even these numbers are unexpectedly high. These findings suggest that HIV itself, directly or indirectly, influences the cardiac pathology.

11. What are the suggested therapies for dilated cardiomyopathy and heart failure in HIV-positive patients? What is their prognosis?

Unfortunately, congestive heart failure in HIV-positive patients has been reported to have a rapidly progressive downward course. Despite the poor outcome, however, the heart failure initially responds to conventional therapy with ACE inhibitors and diuretics. Zidovudine therapy does not appear to change the poor outcome or prevent the development of dilated cardiomyopathy.

12. What are the major cardiac malignancies in AIDS?

Two types of malignancies affecting the heart have been described in AIDS/Kaposi's sarcoma and malignant lymphoma, with Kaposi's sarcoma being the more common. **Kaposi's sarcoma** is found mostly in HIV-positive male homosexuals. Kaposi's sarcoma may involve the epicardium (a common location), myocardium, and/or pericardium.

Malignant cardiac lymphoma may be primary or secondary and is usually high-grade, with Burkitt-like cells (small and noncleaved) or large-cell immunoblastic plasmacytoid types. In most cases, they appear to originate from B cells.

13. Do cardiac abnormalities improve in AIDS patients?

There have been few specific follow-up studies of AIDS-related cardiac findings. In one study, Blanchard et al. reported approximately 1 year's follow-up data on AIDS and asymptomatic HIV-positive patients. Over the follow-up, 44% of the AIDS patients and only 5% of the asymptomatic HIV-positive patients died. Echocardiographic abnormalities were common in both groups, but persistent LV dysfunction was more prevalent in the AIDS group and had the grim prognosis of 100% mortality in 1 year. Resolution of cardiac abnormalities was seen with LV dysfunction in 43%, right ventricular enlargement in 44%, and without specific intervention, pericardial effusion resolution in 42%.

14. Why are the cardiac lesions occasionally transient?

This issue needs further study, but it is possible that infectious myocarditis may be the major cause of LV dysfunction and pericarditis and that there is transient occurrence of these cardiopathic agents. The right ventricular transient changes are most likely due to changes in pulmonary hypertension associated with opportunistic pulmonary infections. Therefore, it is important to have patients re-evaluated, especially if symptoms change, as medications may need frequent adjustments. Perform echo-Doppler studies on AIDS patients as symptoms dictate, or electively every year if patients have significant cardiac involvement or advanced disease.

15. What are the clinical manifestations of AIDS myocarditis?

The clinical manifestations of AIDS myocarditis depend on the severity of the inflammatory process, i.e., focal or diffuse, and/or the location of the lesion. For example, if the focus is in the His bundle, the patient presents with conduction abnormalities; diffuse disease presents with full-blown congestive heart failure or with chest pain, shortness of breath, or significant arrhythmias. Most patients have no clinical manifestations or only subtle clinical findings.

16. Do the new drugs for HIV therapy cause additional cardiac side effects?

Yes, the new, highly active antiretroviral therapy (HAART), which has been found to achieve a durable, undetectable viral load, has some physicians worried about drug toxicity. There is special concern about increased risk for hyperlipidemia, diabetes, heart disease, and angina.

The concerns are heightened with the assumption that the patient will be on HAART for life. Research now shows that an earlier start is better to achieve the desired HIV levels. Moreover, the side effects are cumulative, with lipid changes being progressive as with fat distribution. Premature atherosclerosis appears to be a side effect, and we should see more clinical evidence of angina and infarction.

BIBLIOGRAPHY

1. Adair OV, Mendoza RE, Chebaclo M, Vacarrino R: A prospective study of 67 acquired immunodeficiency syndrome patients for evaluation of cardiac abnormalities. Clin Res 38(2):361A, 1990.
2. Blanchard DG, Hagenhoff C, Chow LC, et al: Reversibility of cardiac abnormalities in human immunodeficiency virus (HIV)-infected individuals: A serial echocardiography study. J Am Coll Cardiol 17:1270–1276, 1991.
3. Cotton P: AIDS giving rise to cardiac problems. JAMA 263(16):2149, 1990.
4. Freedberg KA, Samet JH: Think HIV: Why physicians should lower their threshold for HIV testing. Arch Intern Med 139(17):1994–2003, 1999.
5. Klima M, Esudier SM: Pathologic findings in the hearts of patients with acquired immunodeficiency syndrome. Texas Heart Inst J 18:116–121, 1991.
6. Levy WS, Simon GL, Rios JC, Ross AM: Prevalence of cardiac abnormalities in human immunodeficiency virus infection. Am J Cardiol 63:86–89, 1989.
7. Lewis W, Grody WW: AIDS and the heart: Review and consideration of pathogenetic mechanisms. Cardiovasc Pathol 1:53–64, 1992.
8. Schiezer J: Earlier is better for starting HAART. Intern Med World Report 15(3):34, 2000.

62. EXERCISE AND THE HEART

Fernando Boccalandro, M.D.

1. Describe the general physiologic changes that occur during exercise.

Which physiologic processes are engaged to allow us to adapt to exercise depends on the type of exercise—specifically, the intensity, and the amount of muscle mass involved that requires increased oxygen. In a purely *dynamic* exercise (e.g., running, bicycling, walking), the individual experiences an increase in pre-load due to an increase in cardiac output and heart rate without substantial changes in blood pressure. In a purely *static* exercise (e.g., weight lifting) there is mainly an after-load increase, which is reflected in blood pressure. In most activities, a combination of both types of exercises results in a mixed physiologic response.

A complex series of events that occurs during dynamic exercise can be summarized as an increase in heart rate due to a decrease in vagal tone and an increase in sympathetic tone. Increase in stroke volume and cardiac output, increase in systolic blood pressure, and a slight decrease in diastolic blood pressure with an increase in contractility occur as well. The vascular beds undergo vasoconstriction, except for in the brain, heart, and skeletal muscles used during exercise. The oxygen extraction of the peripheral tissues used during physical activity also increases.

2. What is a metabolic equivalent?

Metabolic equivalent (MET) is the resting oxygen consumed by a 40-year-old man weighing 70 kg. It is the equivalent to 3.5 ml of oxygen/minute/kg of body weight and is used to calculate the amount of work done during different activities. This gauge is also very useful to determine exercise prescriptions and disability, and to report workloads. Average, normal daily activities involve about 4–5 METs.

3. What benefits are derived from exercise?

Inactivity is a risk factor for coronary artery disease (CAD). Regular aerobic exercise increases exercise capacity and plays a role in both primary and secondary prevention of cardiovascular disease (CVD). Exercise also improves an individual's lipid profile, lowers blood pressure, decreases insulin requirements, and contributes to weight control and general psychological well being.

4. Can patients with coronary artery disease exercise?

Stable patients with CAD receive a significant benefit from exercise. Training can induce a decreased demand for myocardial oxygen for the same level of work, permitting higher levels of activity without inducing ischemia. Some studies have also shown that exercise decreased mortality in patients after a myocardial infarction. Coronary patients can benefit from cardiac rehabilitation programs that slowly, progressively, and under supervision train the patient to achieve higher levels of aerobic capacity.

5. Can patients with heart failure exercise?

Training increases maximum ventilatory oxygen uptake by increasing both maximum cardiac output and oxygen extraction. Beneficial changes in hemodynamic, hormonal, metabolic, neurological, and respiratory function occur with increased exercise capacity. These changes can also benefit persons with impaired left ventricular function, in whom most adaptations to exercise training appear to be peripheral and which occur with low exercise intensity.

6. What amount of exercise is needed to achieve cardiovascular benefits?

A dose:response relation between the amount of exercise that expends 700–2000 kcal of energy per week, and all-cause mortality and CVD mortality in middle-aged and elderly populations, has been reported. Most effects of physical activity on CVD mortality are attained through moderate to intense activity with an approximate 50–60% of maximal oxygen uptake. This level of activity can be accomplished through formal training or leisure-time physical activities. Studies comparing structured exercise programs with daily activities have failed to show significant differences in terms of cardiovascular benefit.

7. Does the benefit from exercise differ by age or sex?

Most studies have been undertaken in the male population, but recent evidence indicates that the same benefits are obtained by women as well as the elderly.

8. What are the risks of exercise?

Risks are minimal, as evidenced by sudden cardiac death rates at 100,000 hours of exercise: 0–2 in the general population, and 0.13–0.61 in cardiac rehabilitation programs. Studies have also demonstrated the cardiovascular safety of maximum strength testing and training in healthy adults and low-risk cardiac patients. Falls and joint injuries, which can be minimized with low-impact forms of exercise, are additional risks associated with physical activity.

9. How much exercise is recommended for primary and secondary prevention?

Based on current evidence, the ACC/AHA guidelines recommend dynamic exercise of the large muscles for 30–60 minutes, three to six times weekly. This activity may include short periods of moderate intensity (60–75% of maximal capacity for approximately 5–10 minutes).

Resistance training using 8 to 10 different exercise sets with 10 to 15 repetitions each (e.g., arms, shoulders, chest, trunk, back, hips, and legs) at a moderate to high intensity (e.g., 10 to 15 pounds of free weight) for a minimum of 2 days per week is also recommended.

10. What is the most important factor in achieving sustained cardiovascular benefit from exercise?

Adherence is indeed the most important factor to achieve long-term cardiovascular benefit from exercise. Only 50% of individuals who initiate an exercise program continue the habit for more than 6 months. The benefits of exercise are only obtained if it is maintained for extended periods of time. Thus, strategies and education for habit formation are important tasks in the primary and secondary prevention of CVDs.

11. What are the benefits of resistance training?

The benefits of resistance training have only recently been clarified. Resistance training improves strength, power, endurance, muscle mass, and bone mineral density, and helps in the maintenance of independence and basal metabolic rate. Resistance training decreases myocardial demands during daily activities, which helps the ischemic patient. It also benefits individuals who have a low risk for CVD. But for individuals with high risk and difficulty controlling hypertension or left ventricular dysfunction, the benefits of resistance training are still to be determined, and such training cannot be recommended without further study.

Note that resistance training is *contraindicated* in moderate aortic insufficiency.

12. What are the cardiovascular contraindications for competitive sports?
- Hypertrophic cardiomyopathy
- Marfan's syndrome
- Aortic stenosis with a degree worse then mild
- Suspected congenital or acquired CAD
- Uncontrolled hypertension

13. What is an athletic heart?

Constant exercise causes the heart to undergo an adaptive process that has been evidenced on echocardiography and electrocardiography. Individuals may have a left ventricular (LV) thickness in the upper limits of normal (usually < 1.3 cm), uniform hypertrophy, normal septum to free wall ratio, proportional papillary muscle hypertrophy, normal LV outflow dimensions, normal left atrial size, normal systolic function, absence of valvular disease, and normal mitral filling pattern. The EKG may show sinus bradycardia, first degree A-V block, wandering pacemaker, Wenckebach Mobitz I block, LV hypertrophy, vertical axis, early repolarization, and T-waves inversion.

BIBLIOGRAPHY

1. Blair SN, Kohl HW III, Paffenbarger RS Jr, et al: Physical fitness and all-cause mortality: A prospective study of healthy men and women. JAMA 262:2395–2401, 1989.
2. Blumenthal JA, Sherwood A, Gullette EC, et al: Exercise and weight loss reduce blood pressure in men and women with mild hypertension: Effects on cardiovascular, metabolic, and hemodynamic functioning. Arch Intern Med 160(13):1947–58, 2000.
3. Braith RW, Pollock ML, Lowenthal DT, et al: Moderate- and high-intensity exercise lowers blood pressure in normotensive subjects 60 to 79 years of age. Am J Cardiol 73:1124–1128, 1994.
4. Donker FJ: Cardiac rehabilitation: A review of current developments. Clin Psychol Rev 20(7):923-43, 2000.
5. Elliott PM, Poloniecki J, Dickie S, et al: Sudden death in hypertrophic cardiomyopathy: Identification of high-risk patients. J Am Coll Cardiol 36(7):2212–8, 2000.
6. Fletcher GF, Balady G, Froelicher VF, et al: Exercise standards: A statement for healthcare professionals from the American Heart Association. Circulation 86:340–344, 1992.
7. Fletcher GF, Balady G, Blair SN, et al: Statement on exercise: Benefits and recommendations for physical activity programs for all Americans: A statement for health professionals by the Committee on Exercise and Cardiac Rehabilitation of the Council on Clinical Cardiology, American Heart Association. Circulation 94:857–862, 1996.
8. Hambrecht R, Niebauer J, Fiehn E, et al: Physical training in patients with stable chronic heart failure: Effects on cardiorespiratory fitness and ultrastructural abnormalities of leg muscles. J Am Coll Cardiol 25:1239–1249, 1995.
9. Jager EH: Formulas for dynamic exercise heart rate and blood pressure. Cardiology 94(1):66–7, 2000.
10. Kobashigawa JA, Leaf DA, Gleeson MP, et al: Benefit of cardiac rehabilitation in heart transplant patients: A randomized trial. [abstract] J Heart Lung Transplant 90:S77, 1994.
11. Lee IM, Hsieh CC, Paffenbarger RS Jr: Exercise intensity and longevity in men: The Harvard Alumni Health Study. JAMA 273:1179–1184, 1995.
12. Lamaitre RN, Siscovick DS, Raghunathan TE, et al: Leisure-time physical activity and the risk of primary cardiac arrest. Arch Intern Med 159(7):686–90, 1999.
13. Morris JN, Clayton DG, Everitt MG, et al: Exercise in leisure time: Coronary attack and death rates. Br Heart J 63:325–334, 1990.
14. Oka RK, De Marco T, Haskell WL, et al: Impact of a home-based walking and resistance training program on quality of life in patients with heart failure. Am J Cardiol 85(3):365–9, 2000.
15. Pollock ML, Franklin BA, Balady GJ, et al: AHA Science Advisory. Resistance exercise in individuals with and without cardiovascular disease: Benefits, rationale, safety, and prescription. An advisory from the Committee on Exercise, Rehabilitation, and Prevention, Council on Clinical Cardiology, American Heart Association. Position paper endorsed by the American College of Sports Medicine. Circulation 101(7):828–833, 2000.
16. Tanaka H, Monahan KD, Seals DR: Age-predicted maximal heart rate revisited. J Am Coll Cardiol 37(1):153–156, 2001.
17. Weir MR, Maibach EW, Bakris GL, et al: Implications of a healthy lifestyle and medication analysis for imiproving hypertension control. Arch Intern Med 160(4):481–90, 2000.

INDEX

Page numbers in **boldface type** indicate complete chapters.

Joyful Living: Build Yourself a Great Life!

Joyful Living is a step-by-step, easy to read recipe that stirs the soul and awakens the spirit. Amidst the many examples and touching stories, Pelger asks that you not be passive, but actively participate to discover yourself, chart your own destiny, and find joy in your life.

I now realize one of the best ways to relate to my kids on a non-superficial level; I must open up and share my experiences, my life, that they might find it within themselves to share theirs.

Ray DeStephen, P.E., president, Schnabel Engineering

…it made me laugh and cry as I considered some of my own life experiences…**Joyful Living** is not just a book to be read, but a book to be worked. In the exercise of completing the worksheets, in demanding of oneself the truth from within, the refining process begins.

Mike Sharpe, founder of Suzy's Soup

Pelger has more guts than I do to admit being "de-pantsed" in front of 80,000 people. His honesty, bluntness, desire for excellence, and refreshing humor are invigorating.

John Hess, hog farmer

"Most people don't know how to transcend the circumstances life hands them. This victim mentality is especially prevalent today. **Joyful Living** not only points out that we can choose our level of joy, but it provides a method for doing it."

Carl Ginder, director, United Zion Retirement Community

"A very human story, told well, which extends personal experience into spiritual guidance and fulfillment…quite an accomplishment."

Robert S. Walker, former US Congressman

I'm impressed with Pelger's deep understanding of the nitty-gritty of life.

Dr. J. Calvin Wenger

Joyful Living affords the reader an opportunity to examine life in a way that will provide a much deeper understanding of who they are and why they make those moment-to-moment choices. The real life examples made me feel very connected to the book.
Dr. Joe Narkiewicz, school principal

A wonderful road map to the difficult journey we take every day.
Mike Bingeman, CPA

Easy to read and applicable to anyone who desires to work toward a more joyful life.
Phil Geyer, construction superintendent

We really appreciate Pelger's unique approach to this material... so practical and full of common sense, which sad to say, is greatly lacking nowadays.
Fran and Leland Paris, directors, Youth with a Mission

Pelger produces a compelling blueprint for our social destiny, our voice of conscience, our raison d'etre for self-determination and spiritual evolution.
Dr. Mark Mentzer, scientist and musician

An outstanding book that should be read by every member of the family and then discussed.
Robert Beers, AIA architect

Pelger writes with the seriousness of a scholar, the precision of an engineer, the lightheartedness of a humorist, and the wisdom of a sage.
Paul Brubaker, banker

...a wonderful handbook for self evaluation, it's quite a resource.
George Rettew, P.E., president, Rettew Associates

Joyful Living:

Build Yourself a Great Life!

Ned Pelger, P.E.

**ATA Publishing Company
Lititz, PA**

ATA Publishing Company
507 W. 28th Division Hwy.
Lititz, PA 17543

EDITORS: SHARON AND JOHN CHARLES
COVER DESIGN: EVELYN AND BARNEY EPSTEIN
PRINTING: BANG PRINTING CO.

LIBRARY OF CONGRESS CARD NUMBER: 00-190062

ISBN # 0-9624569-8-5

Additional copies of this publication may be purchased from ATA Publishing Company. For information, please call toll free to 888-627-7744 or fax a request to 717-626-6222. Also see our website at www.pelger.com for free software downloads or to order additional copies.

Dedication

I dedicate this book to you, the reader. The principles presented here can change your life. Since many people give me guidance and love, I want to pass some of that help along to you. I hope you will enjoy my effort.

Acknowledgements

I sat in the office of John and Sharon Charles, discussing my manuscript. Prior to becoming my editors, they had reviewed the book and felt the editing would consist of a "light dusting" of grammatical corrections and word usage improvements. After four years of writing and many reviews by others, I thought there couldn't be too much more to revise. As usual, I was wrong.

After carefully reading the first few chapters, they asked to meet with me. John leaned back in his chair, looked in my eyes for several seconds without blinking, and said, "Well, Ned, we think you should cut about a third to a half of the material from the book." I felt sick. Then I thought, "How could I have chosen such obviously misguided people for my editors?" But I said, "You're the experts. Do what you think is best."

They didn't cut quite that much, but they did cut plenty and the book improved substantially. Thank you, John and Sharon, for your struggles, your guidance and your integrity.

While John and Sharon came into the project near the end, Evelyn and Barney Epstein critiqued and encouraged me from the beginning. They helped me stay true to the concept of the work. We had so many discussions, and contemplated so many changes. In particular, they designed the cover.

We disagreed on some issues, yet always retained respect for the beliefs of the other. I'll always cherish our friendship. Thank you, Evelyn and Barney, for challenging and encouraging me in many ways.

To my best friend and wife, Debby…what can I say? You have been there for 25 years, listening, gently directing, stubbornly refusing, whatever it took to move us in the right direction. I love you more than any words can say.

Alexey, Anna, and Tessa---we have so much fun together. Sorry if I embarrass you by sharing some of it here. But, if you've learned nothing else from me, you know that, "it builds character!" You have taught me so much about relationships and love. I'm proud of each of you.

I'm blessed to have a large group of friends and family to look to for guidance and direction. Thank you to the following people for reviewing manuscripts, providing comments, and encouraging me through this long process of writing and rewriting: Mima Adams, Bob Beers, David Billington, Mike Bingeman, John Bomberger, John Bonfield, Geneva and Bob Brandt, Mike Brubaker, Paul Brubaker, Skip Clair, Debby DeBord, Ray DeStephen, Jill and Shawn Erb, Gail Funk, Colleen and Phil Geyer, Carl Ginder, Belinda Graybill, Pam and Terry Griffe, Gene Griffith, Ken Groff, Donna Hammond, Martha and John Hess, Beth Hibshman, Sarah Holt, Bruce Jackson, Lehman Kaylor, Carol Kline, Nevin Kraybill, Dan Leaman, Anita Lipkowski, Sharon and Dennis Martin, Judy and Paul Martin, John Matarazzi, John May, Mark Mentzer, Joe Narciewicz, Lynn Neidermyer, Patty Owens, Fran and Leland Paris, Chris and Ed Pelger, Jim Pelger, George Rettew, Dawn Risser, Shelley and Mike Sharpe, Jeff Sholly, Jim Singer, Steve Slaby, Bruce Spicer, Cindy Sullivan, Wendy and Steve Terry, George Travis, Joe Wagman, Bob Walker, Sally Watkins, Calvin Wenger, Kristen Worley, and, finally, all the people that have taken my courses and provided feedback, teaching me as I taught.

Table of Contents

Appendixes

Getting Started

Do you want more out of life? You may be an active young mother with a loving husband and children, but you lack joy. You wonder, "Is this all there is?" You may be a divorced father loving your children in your own way, but unsuccessfully trying to make sense out of life. You wonder, "What's the purpose of all this?" You may be a grandmother who has dedicated your life to your family, but now feels unappreciated. You wonder, "How can I change now?"

A simple truth exists: each of us has the ability to choose the level of joy in our lives! Regardless of where we are right now, we can attain much more joy. Each of us can have a joyous, amazing life!

The key to experiencing this level of joy lies in one word --- **UNDERSTANDING**. We must strive to understand ourselves and our world. We must examine our past, the lives of those who came before us, how we live now and what we believe. When we do so, we will discover sparkling gems of understanding.

This book exists to help you build a collection of those gems of understanding – which will provide a solid foundation for a meaningful life. You will then have the stability to reach for more: more love, more joy, more acceptance, more achievement.

As an engineer designs a building to withstand the anticipated forces of nature, so you can design your life to withstand and joyfully overcome the inevitable problems you will face. A solid foundation of understanding allows you to reach for more with little risk of toppling over or failing. As you work through this book, you will expand your understanding of yourself, thereby strengthening your life foundation and allowing you to reach for more.

You may be wondering, "Who is this guy and why should I believe him?" I wonder that myself from time to time. Perhaps this story will tell you a little bit about me...

I sat in a panic, poring over my freshman physics mid-term exam. I was living my recurring childhood nightmare in which I would begin taking a test and then realize that I knew none of the answers. (At least I was not sitting there in just my underwear, which was another variation of the dream.) This was my first major test in my first year at Princeton University and I was completely overwhelmed.

Let me give you some background information on how I even ended up at a place like Princeton. I had not been much of a student in high school. I spent most of my time playing and partying. I talked my way into a work-release program to skip classes in the afternoon and spent those hours fooling around with wood-working equipment in my grandfather's garage. Not only was I not planning to go to college, I was not planning anything. My days just floated along.

The one discipline I had was high school wrestling. I enjoyed the head-to-head competition, the direct challenge and the fact that I was reasonably good at it. We got a new wrestling coach in the fall of my senior year and he stopped by my locker one day. I remember the conversation clearly.

"Hi, I'm Mr. McDonald, I'm the new wrestling coach."
"Yeah, I heard that."
"So, I understand you made it to States last year and won a match up there."
"Yeah, I was lucky."
"Where are you planning to go to college?"
"I don't think I'm going to college."
"Well, I talked to some of the other teachers about you and I think you would really enjoy Princeton. I've known the wrestling coaches there for years. I teach at their summer camps. I could talk with them about helping you get accepted. I think you would really like it."
"I've heard of Princeton. Where is it?"
"It's in New Jersey."

Over the next few months, Coach McDonald talked me into sending an application to Princeton; it was the only school I applied to because I was not planning to go to college. Due to some significant help from the wrestling coaches, I received a letter of acceptance. Many people told me what an honor it was to be accepted at Princeton and that I would be crazy not to go and give it a try. Hence, I found myself sitting in a freshman physics mid-term exam in turmoil.

As I read question after question, I became more overwhelmed. Most of the course had been focused on things like motion and force, mechanics and energy. In the last lecture before the mid-term exam, the professor had talked a few minutes about Einstein and the theory of relativity. Yet all the questions on this exam were about the theory of relativity ... questions about being on trains moving at the speed of light, and such. I tried to answer each question, but I just didn't have a clue.

The exam was to last one and one half hours. Within 45 minutes I had reached the end of the exam booklet since there were so many questions I couldn't answer. Reluctantly I turned back to the front cover, thinking that I would try to plow through it again. There on the top corner of the cover page I noticed the course title, "Physics 114." I was taking "Physics 101!" I was in the wrong room!

I was both embarrassed and relieved! Due to Princeton's honor code, there were no proctors in the exam room. Deciding to make the best of a bad situation, I put a big smile on my face, stood up, picked up my umbrella and my exam booklet and walked out of the room to panicked whispers of, "Oh my god, he's done already!" In the next room I explained my predicament to the professors, who had a great laugh and told me I could take a make-up exam.

I did make it through Physics 101 (I never did take Physics 114) and eventually graduated with an engineering degree. An engineer learns to solve a large, difficult problem by breaking it down into smaller, manageable-sized problems. The engineer then tackles the smaller problems one at a time. Eventually the large, difficult problem no longer seems overwhelming. For example, designing the structure for a five-story building may seem formidable. In practice, though, one works at it piece by piece. With patience and persistence (and probably some discussions with others about assumptions and methods) the design is completed. This problem-solving method was the most valuable thing I learned in my formal education.

Over the years, I have designed and constructed many buildings by working one step at a time. I have addressed many issues in my personal life using the same method. Remember the old question, "How do you eat an elephant?" The answer is, of course, "One bite at a time." **We can solve seemingly insurmountable problems in our lives if we are willing to break the problems down to manageable chunks.**

Before continuing with this book, you should ask yourself, "Do I want more out of life and am I willing to work for it?" If you answer "yes," you've got the right book! If you are willing to put forth effort to examine and understand your life, I guarantee you will dramatically improve your sense of joy. Though I present no magic solutions nor incredible words of wisdom, I do offer a method which works.

Step by step, you will grow and change for the better. You will stop just reacting to events in your same old way and begin choosing appropriate life responses. This capability to choose your response will reward you with great power and deep joy.

Please notice: we are considering something quite different from the typical wishful New Year's resolution. I remember working in an aluminum foundry as a 16-year-old. The work was hard, dirty and hot. On breaks I listened to the older guys talk. Their conversations usually came around to money and how to get rich. There was plenty of wishing going on, but not much action for change (other than buying lottery tickets). Just wishing will not bring joy; we need commitment and effort.

As I think about the value of commitment and effort, the name of Bruce Springsteen comes to mind. I learned a lesson from him that I will never forget.

When I was 17 years old, I got a job setting up sound equipment for concert tours with Clair Brother's Audio. We traveled from city to city, either in trucks or in a tour bus, and set up an entire sound system almost every day. My first tour was with the group Yes in 1975. At one point on their tour, we went 14 days with a concert in a different city each night. The 17-hour workdays were long and hard, but the money was good (it enabled me to pay most of my way through college).

In 1978 I took a year off from college to earn some money (and to find some direction), and I was put on the Bruce Springsteen tour. As you might imagine, most of the people that work on these tours are cynical. Everyone is too "cool" to be impressed with the artist. The first show was in Buffalo, NY and Bruce played for almost four hours. The rigger, a man named George Travis, said to me after the show. "Who is this guy? That was the best show I have ever seen in my life! He gives it all to the audience!" I completely agreed.

We toured the country for six months, constantly amazed at the energy and effort Bruce put into every show. During the afternoon rehearsals and sound checks, Bruce, the sound engineer and I walked the entire arena. Springsteen demanded that everyone who paid to see his show would enjoy a good view and excellent sound. We often added speakers or rearranged the sound system if a section of seats did not have adequate sight lines or audio coverage. Bruce Springsteen was committed to providing the absolute best show that was within his power to deliver. He always went the extra mile; the additional effort never seemed a problem for him.

Bruce learned the names of everyone on the crew in the first week. That was quite a rarity for a superstar performing artist. As I observed him on that six-month tour, I became more impressed with the integrity, commitment, and effort he put forth in his work. He cared deeply about his audience and required that everything about his shows be done well.

One evening in Portland, Oregon, a few days before Christmas, Bruce added the song "Santa Claus is Coming to Town" to the set. We were all getting in the Christmas spirit. George Travis, who was always lots of fun, had the idea that we should surprise Bruce with a fake snowstorm during that song. George bought several bags of pillow feathers to use as snow and arranged for the guys on the lighting truss above the stage to throw the feathers when the song started. As the feathers floated down, it truly did look like a snowstorm on stage. The effect was great! We all laughed at the surprised look on Bruce's face.

Unfortunately, there was one thing none of us had considered. After several hours of hard playing, Bruce was covered with sweat. The feathers that hit his face and arms stayed there. Others got stuck in his guitar strings. Feathers were everywhere! He must have felt like a big chicken out there on stage, and he was ticked! The crew reacted quickly with towels, brooms, and fans; we were all on feather clean-up duty. Later Bruce did laugh about it, but warned us to never pull such a stunt again!

Bruce Springsteen made an impression on me. He was the best at what he did, and not just due to God-given talent. Bruce worked hard and cared deeply about his performances. Years later, as I work at improving myself, I continue to be challenged by Bruce's example of commitment and effort.

So… do I live every moment with an intense level of commitment and effort? Of course not! I try, but I fail every day. I am sure Bruce Springsteen fails every day too! Realistically, we will never be totally satisfied with how we live our lives. But step by step, decision by decision, we can grow more joy and purpose and meaning in our lives. We can move toward becoming the person we want to be.

The key to moving in that direction lies in the "learning-by-doing" approach. Observing the experiences of others can be challenging and enlightening, but not a substitute for learning from our own experiences. **Examples from the lives of others are not as helpful as the lessons we learn from our own personal experience.**

The problem for most of us is that we don't recall all our personal experiences and lessons. Our life encompasses too much to keep clear in our head at one time. So when we try to choose a course of action for a specific situation, we do not get the full value of our prior experiences.

The solution is simple. **We have to write things down!** The exercise of writing helps us to learn. Therefore, this book utilizes a workbook approach. You can read through the text, fill in the worksheets with your own experiences, and (at your own pace) draw your conclusions. Since clearly understanding a problem usually creates a strong sense of purpose, the exercises in this book will help transform your life.

Begin with the following question, "Whom do I know that I respect and admire?" The accompanying questions in Worksheet #1 expand that thought, helping you look more deeply at specific characteristics. Remember, you don't need to choose someone who is perfect, simply someone you respect and admire.

When I'm asked about someone I admire, Aunt Mid comes to mind. Aunt Mid was the kindest, most compassionate person I ever knew. Her life was difficult. She never married, feeling responsible to take care of her aging parents until they died. Then she took care of a series of elderly folks. About every five years, Aunt Mid suffered through a brutal bout of depression.

Since she had neither money nor insurance, she was hospitalized in a state mental institution and given electro-shock therapy. In the early days no sedatives were used. The hospital beds were lined up in a big room and the doctor moved down the line from patient to patient, holding the electrodes against both temples for the big zap! Can you imagine the horror, lying there waiting for your turn? Aunt Mid suffered greatly through her times of mental illness and was so ashamed of them. Yet, Aunt Mid gave all she had all the time and loved those around her unconditionally.

As I stood in the cemetery after her funeral, my father commented to me, "That casket is by far the most expensive thing she ever owned." The humility, courage, and honor that Aunt Mid exhibited in her life inspire me. Her example continues to challenge me. Her pictures (on the front cover in a bathing suit to the right of my grandmother and on the back cover holding our daughter Tessa) allow you to put a face to the story.

As you think about Worksheet #1 and the people who inspire you, consider some basics about these Worksheets. My learning increases when I see an example. Therefore I include example Worksheets based on a fictional character named John Miller. If you find examples helpful, study the John Miller example Worksheets. If you find these example Worksheets confusing, please ignore them.

Blank Worksheets are available to you in several ways, described in Appendix A. You may want to read the book prior to filling in the Worksheets (most people prefer this method). Or you could complete the Worksheets during your first read through the book. Either way, I strongly encourage you to take the time to complete the Worksheets.

Name: *John Miller*   Worksheet #1   Date: *3-1-00*
Whom do I respect and admire?

1. Who comes to mind when I think about someone I personally know, respect, and admire?
    Grandma Miller

2. What do I like about this person?
    She is very kind and loving. I feel good when I talk with her.

3. How has this person affected my life?
    She has been the one person who always loved me, no matter what. She is a role model for how to treat others.

4. What seems to motivate this person?
    Making other people feel good.

5. What outstanding characteristics does he/she have?
    Selflessness, tolerance, kindness, unconditional love

6. Does this person have a sense of purpose?
    She seems to.

7. Does he/she exhibit joy?
    Absolutely. She has a great sense of humor, and even in sad times she has a quiet joy.

> As John read the first question, he immediately thought of his grandmother. He pictured her many acts of kindness. When he thinks of a truly good person, he always thinks of her.

8. Would I desire to be more like this individual? In what ways?
    Yes, to care more about others

9. What event, or situation, involving this person, illustrates why I respect and admire him/her?
    She always remembered my birthday and other special occasions with a card and a few dollars (even though she never had much money).

Filling out the Worksheets takes you on a guided tour of your life. A few instructions will help the process go smoother.

Reserve a certain time each day to study. Perhaps 15 or 30 minutes a day will be appropriate. If you are a morning person, work in the morning. If you are a night person, work in the evening. Use your best time of day for this study.

Try to use the same place, a place where you are comfortable and mostly uninterrupted. I have actually never been able to find such a place for myself, but I imagine it would be quite a good thing!

Most importantly, make a commitment to yourself; decide to put forth the effort required to work through this book.

Please be realistic and understand that you will be working on these (or similar) issues for the rest of your life. So don't get discouraged and don't set your initial expectations too high. We gather gems of understanding in a step-by-step process. Remember, though, **good organization and looking in the right direction is 80% of success.**

As you begin this work, you will struggle with the need for honest self-evaluation. Honestly examining your life is always difficult. Putting those observations on paper becomes even more difficult. What if someone should read those thoughts and conclude you are foolish? One of Dostoevsky's characters said, "Above all things, I don't want to appear ridiculous." I believe we all share that fear.

Therefore, you may wish to use a 3-ring binder for the worksheets, and keep the binder in a private place. If you complete the Worksheets on the computer, you could password protect your files. You might even want to use your own personal "shorthand" for certain sections that you wish to keep confidential.

If, as a child, you were raised with a "Don't feel!" attitude, it may seem unnatural to think about your feelings, much less write about them. But you are reading this book because you want to move your life in the right direction. You want joy and you want purpose. **When you record personal experiences and insights in a logical, rational sequence, you build personal understanding. REMEMBER, no examples are as effective as the ones we create for ourselves.** So please, take the risk — write! It will be worth the effort!

"Life is like playing a violin solo in public," wrote Samuel Butler, "and learning the instrument as one goes along." I feel foolish and ridiculous often in my life, as do we all. In spite of those embarrassing moments, I continue to struggle toward joyful living. You must remember that finding joy requires courage. In order to succeed with this process, you need to consider, "Do I want to be a person of courage?" You may not be a person of courage at this moment, but you must desire to become one.

If you desire to be a person of courage and will take small steps in that direction, I guarantee that you will find more and more joy. In fact, I will make that a money-back guarantee. If you work through this book and are not satisfied, send me a note, and I will send back to you the cost of the book. I believe in what I'm doing.

A final sensitive issue to discuss in this Getting Started section concerns spiritual matters. To understand our life's purpose, we must consider the spiritual component. To avoid discussing spiritual matters parallels trying to fix a stalled car without checking the fuel. If the car does not start, we need to wonder whether gas is getting to the engine. If your life is not filled with joy, you need to examine possible spiritual factors.

Whether you are a Mormon, an Orthodox Jew, an evangelical Christian or not associated with any religion --- you can reflect on spiritual matters. Focus on your relationship with God. Your religious affiliation tells little of your relationship with God. I'm not interested in debating theological doctrines. I have discovered that, as I focus on seeking truth about my own life, I make sound decisions about religion.

I encourage you to examine all my ideas, spiritual or not, with a healthy skepticism. I think I have some right ideas and I'm sure I have some wrong ones as well. **You will be wise to choose your beliefs carefully.**

I assume most people reading this book grew up, as I did, in the Judeo-Christian culture. We learned about God in the context of that culture. I was raised in a Protestant home, so I learned about God from the writings in the Bible. I will refer to stories from the Bible because it is most familiar to me.

To end this introduction, let me tell you the story behind one of my favorite Bible quotes. As mother of the child Jesus, Mary experienced a confusing series of events. She was a young woman who loved God and knew her place in society. Then her life went crazy. She had a meeting with an angel. She became pregnant. Her elderly cousin pronounced her most blessed of all women. When her baby was born, shepherds arrived, telling of a sky full of angels proclaiming Jesus as king. A group of astronomers also visited, bringing incredibly expensive gifts. When Jesus was only twelve, he astounded religious leaders in Jerusalem with his amazing knowledge and insight.

How could Mary make sense of all this? The Bible explains in Luke 2:19, *"Mary treasured up all these things and pondered them in her heart."*

We all experience confusion; there are times in all our lives when we simply do not understand what's going on. We can learn a great lesson from Mary. We must treasure our experiences, both past and present, and think about them and learn from them. We must "treasure up these things and ponder them in our hearts." This can be the foundation for changing your life. Let's get to it!

CHAPTER 1

What Makes You Unique

Sitting in my office at High Construction, I received a call from my wife, Debby. I'd never heard her so agitated! She kept saying something about the donkeys being in the basement, but I was only half listening since I was making a construction schedule and preparing for a project meeting. Eventually I discerned that our two full size donkeys had managed to get into our daylight basement sunroom and had apparently spent the night there. The donkeys had deposited the usual large animal messes all over our nice brick floor and new braided carpets.

Debby's agitation stemmed from those messes. This was early in our marriage and I was at least a little stupider than I am now. I told Debby that I was busy with an "important meeting" and she would just have to deal with the situation herself. When I arrived home that evening (I was lucky Debby hadn't changed the locks), I learned the rest of the story.

The previous evening I had been reading on the porch and thought I heard glass breaking, but ignored it. We live in the country and hear plenty of strange noises. Apparently our donkeys, Jeremiah and Zechariah, had been curiously nosing around our basement door. Our fenced pasture bordered the front and side of the house so the donkeys could walk right up to the basement door. One of the children must have left the door partially open and the donkeys walked right into the basement sunroom. The breaking glass I heard must have been Jeremiah shoving his nose through a window pane in the door, inadvertently pushing the door shut. The donkeys were trapped in the sunroom!

When Debby got up the next morning, she heard strange noises coming from downstairs. She opened the basement stair door and saw the two donkeys standing at the bottom of the steps, staring forlornly up at her. When Debby went downstairs she found a foul mess of donkey droppings, urine and blood (from Jeremiah's injured nose). She spent most of the day cleaning up the mess.

So I came home to a clean basement and an extremely irritated wife. All Debby would say to me was, "Do not make a joke, this will NEVER be funny." So I didn't joke about it (at least not in front of Debby) for about a year. Eventually she came to see the humor in the situation and our "donkeys in the basement" story became one more life experience we enjoy laughing about.

Sometimes I wonder why I have donkeys and sheep and other miscellaneous critters around. They have caused me hundreds of hours of work and more than a little aggravation. Why do I bother?

Perhaps for various reasons…I believe our children benefit from being around animals. The children love to see the new lambs born in the spring. The children also observe the natural cycles of birth and death and that seems to be a healthy, if sometimes difficult, experience. I also enjoy the fact that hundreds of people drive by our property and regularly look to see "what those cute donkeys are up to." Besides providing a pleasant diversion, I find the presence of the animals to be somehow comforting.

I am willing to build the fences, buy the feed, chase the miserable critters when they escape back into the woods and do the other bothersome chores because the benefits outweigh the aggravations. Having the animals around just feels right to me. It is simply one of the interests that makes me unique.

Discovering Your Own Uniqueness

The thousands of people I've known over the years have one thing in common: each one is unique. Think of all the people you know; are any two completely alike? We all are different from each other. Each person is unique.

This concept of uniqueness may make us uncomfortable. Since most of us tend to be herd creatures by nature, we like the idea of blending into the group. The group provides safety. But to progress in our search for joy, we must recognize we are not simply clones. We exist as unique individuals, even if we don't fully understand our uniqueness. Hence the purpose of this first chapter...to discover some of the things that make you unique.

For starters, consider the areas in which you have talents and abilities. Worksheet #2 challenges you to think about things you are good at. Most of us do not allow ourselves that luxury very often. In fact, most people have a difficult time naming their strengths because they spend so little time thinking about themselves in an objective way.

Perhaps you dread the thought of doing such a worksheet. The idea of naming your talents and abilities might not feel comfortable to you. But rather than getting anxious about it, just take a deep breath, read the questions and write down the first answers that come to mind. Don't over-analyze these early worksheets; just get some thoughts on paper and keep on going. Later worksheets will provide opportunity for review and modifications can be made at that time.

Name: *John Miller*   Worksheet #2   Date: *3-2-00*

Knowing My Talents and Abilities

1. What are some things I enjoy doing? Consider the various areas of my life such as work, home, friends, church, family, hobbies, interests, etc.
    a. *Working as a construction superintendent, being "The Man" on a complicated building project.*
    b. *Rebuilding my old Triumph Spitfire.*
    c. *Making love with Rachel.*
    d. *Drawing and sketching, though I don't take much time to do this anymore.*

2. What are some things that other people have told me I'm good at?
    a. *Drawing – my school teachers*
    b. *Understanding details on a building project – my project manager Bill is always amazed at how I can see tricky details and get them built right.*
    c. *Settling conflicts fairly on the jobsite.*

> John Miller wrote the answers to Worksheet #2 quickly. He didn't spend much time agonizing over the questions. As he read the answers the next day, however, he was surprised that his greatest strength was the ability to see and understand details clearly. If someone had asked him in conversation to name his greatest strength, he would have been at a loss to answer. As he reviewed his answers on Worksheet #2, he realized he had jotted down something true about himself that was not previously obvious to him. It seemed to him that this small piece of information could be helpful to him in the future.

3. Considering the items above, which can I become so absorbed in that I lose track of time?
    When I am working on a set of difficult shop drawings on a project, I really get into it. Sometimes I will look up and notice that hours have passed and I didn't even realize it.

4. Without being conceited, just simply being honest with myself, what do I think my strengths are? Does one seem to be a predominant talent or ability?
    The ability to see and understand details clearly.

5. How has this talent or ability benefited me in the past?
    Getting promoted to superintendent at such a young age.

It is not necessary to interpret the significance of every answer, either. Hopefully some of the worksheets will provide an "AHA" experience, but most will not produce any instant illumination of your life. The value of this process tends to build as you progress through the book.

Worksheet #2 will help you identify your talents and abilities. It is a huge asset to know your outstanding gifts. You can excel if you know what to focus on. When you identify your highest potential, you become motivated to work harder on improving it. We all love to do the things we're good at. Knowing your strengths also helps you see what makes you unique.

Since an area of failing balances every talent, you also need to consider your most significant weakness. It's usually easier to name our weaknesses than to identify our strengths. Worksheet #3 quizzes you on areas of failing that hurt the most.

As I filled in this worksheet, I was not surprised by the results. My main area of failing involves not paying attention to things going on around me. I often get so involved in my own mind, running through different possibilities and scenarios, that I forget to pay any attention to what is actually happening. Consequently, my actions can look pretty silly at times.

Just last week I was cutting off a tree limb with a chain saw and thinking about a number of things. Somehow I forgot that the law of gravity would most likely be in effect that day as I stood on the stepladder and sawed through the branch. At the moment the freshly sawed end of the large branch fell, hit me in the mouth and knocked me off the ladder, I realized that I was again not paying attention. As I rubbed my mouth to check for missing teeth, I glanced to the garage to see my co-worker staring in disbelief. His look clearly said to me, "How can you be that stupid?" I chose not to answer.

Name: *John Miller*   Worksheet #3   Date: *3-2-00*

Knowing My Areas of Failing

1. What are some things I dislike doing? What are some things I do not do well? Consider the various areas of my life such as work, home, friends, church, families, hobbies, interests, etc.

    a. *I don't like going to pointless, stupid meetings at work. I hate to have my time wasted.*

    b. *I don't like fighting with Rachel.*

    c. *I am not good at showing or explaining my feelings very well.*

    d. *Don't particularly like going to church, just doesn't seem real to me.*

    e. *Not good at saying "No," especially at work.*

2. What are some areas that other people have told me I need to improve?

    a. *My boss told me I need to communicate better.*

    b. *Rachel told me she needs to know what I'm thinking more.*

> John Miller names poor communication skills as his main area of failing. This was no surprise to John, since both his wife and his boss have told him that he needs to communicate better. He may not really believe it, but he is certainly aware of this criticism.

3. Which of the items above causes the most damage in my life? Which prevent me from living the way I would like to live?

    I guess my problems in communicating cause me the most difficulty. I can tell a guy what job to do and how to do it with no problem. I seem to have a problem more in the non-technical stuff.

4. What habits or characteristics do I think are my weaknesses? Does one seem to surface as my predominant area of failing?

    The ability to clearly communicate about things I care about.

5. How has this area of failing hurt me in the past?

    I guess in fights with Rachel and in not being as close to the kids as I ought to be. Probably at work too.

Unfortunately, my life is full of examples of not paying attention. Here's another example you may enjoy...I had spent the afternoon negotiating the closeout details on a building project. It had been a difficult project and I was pleased we were able to resolve the problems in an amicable way. Wanting to reward myself, I stopped to get an ice cream cone.

I truly love ice cream and it felt great to stop in the middle of the afternoon to grab a cone. As I drove away from the ice cream shop, I realized something was wrong. The ice cream tasted terrible, and the more I ate the worse it got. Contrary to every part of my ice cream loving nature, I decided to throw away the rest of the cone. I was driving on a four-lane highway and decided it would not be littering to throw the cone out the window. After all, it was organic and the ants would devour it completely in a few days. I wanted to make sure it landed in the grass but I certainly could not stop the car since that would not have been efficient use of time (I get sort of nutty about maximum efficiency).

So I pulled into the right lane, checked for traffic and threw the ice cream cone toward the grass at the edge of the road. It seemed eerie to me how the ice cream cone just hung in the air, almost as if time had stopped. Then I realized the ice cream cone really *was* hanging in the air! I had forgotten to roll down the passenger side window. The ice cream cone was stuck right there on the glass with the cone pointing back at me. For a few moments it hung there and then it plopped to the seat. By then I was laughing so hard I couldn't drive and had to pull over, park and laugh.

I wish all my cases of not paying attention were as funny and cost me so little aggravation. In reality I have made many significant mistakes because of not paying attention. I have damaged relationships, put others and myself in danger and simply screwed things up by this weakness. It is, nevertheless, one of the things that make me unique.

I work on paying better attention and have made some improvement over the years. However, I don't expect this will ever become an area of strength. I will be content to improve to a level where I cause less significant problems for me and those around me. We will discuss how to do this in later chapters.

Why Goal Setting Rarely Works

Identifying areas of failing leads to goal setting. New Year's resolutions are prime examples. Imagine that you look in the mirror and see about 15 pounds more than you previously saw. You are not real happy about that and you understand that the extra weight came from a weakness of yours (i.e. eating like a hog over the holidays). When the new year arrives, you think, "Now is the time to lose those extra pounds!" So you make a New Year's resolution to lose the weight. The goal is set and the dieting begins.

The first few days of dieting go OK, but then you begin to sow the seeds of failure... a little cheating here and a little cheating there. You resolve to do better. And for a while, you succeed. Then comes the fall. For some people, it's a gradual decline. Others fall off the wagon with a thud, as in, "Forget this diet; let's go for banana splits!" (My personal favorite.)

Most of us can relate to this experience. We make and break our New Year's resolutions. Why does this type of goal setting usually fail? Because we lack an understanding of the problem. Our goal setting is simply wishful thinking.

A few percent of the population love to set goals. They can set a goal, work hard and achieve results. Successful sales people often fall into this group. If you are a natural goal setter, have at it...the world awaits.

For the rest of us, though, simple goal setting programs don't work. We start with enthusiasm, but since we lack a real understanding of the problem, we lose motivation and fail. After a few failures, we don't have much desire to try again. There are plenty of goal setting books on the market, but this is not one of them. We must first understand ourselves before making plans to improve.

The Need for Hope in Your Life

Most of us dislike setting goals, but we enjoy dreaming about possibilities. There is great benefit in thinking about our hopes, dreams and wishes for the future. Relax and take some time to ponder how you would like your life to be different. Think about what you would like to do or have. The value of writing those hopes, dreams and wishes (see Worksheet #4) can be significant. Perhaps one of those dreams will provide the motivation to help change your life.

Most of us spend little time contemplating the future. We are conditioned to live in the here and now and not "waste time" dreaming about things that may never happen. We have learned to be practical, and that means not dreaming.

I believe we need to dream. We need to consider how we would like our lives to be different. We need to let our minds soar. Don't worry about being practical or the probability of achieving your dreams. Just write what you wish you could do, have, or be in the future.

In this first chapter, you named some things that make you unique. By looking at your talents and abilities, your areas of failing and your hopes, dreams and wishes, you got a sense of what makes you a unique individual. Hopefully you also caught a glimpse of the person you are capable of becoming.

That glimpse provides motivation to continue this process. Joyful living, here you come! So why work through the rest of the book? Remember the words of Lily Tomlin, "I always wanted to be somebody, but I should have been more specific."

Name: *John Miller*   Worksheet #4   Date: *3-4-00*

Hopes, Dreams and Wishes
(Don't be too practical; let yourself soar!)

1. What would I like to achieve in my lifetime?

a. *Build a 4 story building*
b. *Make $50,000/year*
c. *Build a church*
d. *Stay married to Rachel*

2. What things would I like to possess in my lifetime?

a. *House paid off*
b. *Harley*
c.

3. What character traits would I like to develop?

a. *Known as a very fair and honest man*
b. *Have courage*
c.

4. What other hopes, dreams and wishes come to mind?

a. *The kids to be happy and healthy*
b. *To be able to say what I mean/feel*
c. *Make a true peace with my dad*
d.

As John Miller worked on this particular worksheet, he struggled. He prided himself on being a realist who did not have time for foolishness. Wishes for the future seemed like foolishness to him. On the other hand he was accustomed to completing tasks he did not particularly enjoy so he got started. He was surprised when he wrote the last two items. While he had thought of both many times before, he had never put either on paper. It was odd to see these thoughts in writing.

CHAPTER 2

Understanding Who You Are

"There comes a time in the affairs of a man when he must take the bull by the tail and face the situation."
W.C. Fields

Most of us are not very perceptive about ourselves. We may be perceptive about other people yet have a blind spot when it comes to understanding our own lives. We need to investigate our basic nature. We need to stop pretending that, "Everything is just fine," and take a look at who we really are.

Will Rodgers said, "It is not so much what we don't know that gives us trouble, it's what we know that ain't so." We need to approach self-evaluation with honesty and a desire to know the truth. A good sense of humor helps too.

This chapter provides several basic tools to help understand ourselves better. Any tradesman knows the benefit of using the right tool for the job. In fact, one can often determine a tradesman's productivity by simply looking in his or her toolbox. Let's work through these exercises and add some new tools to our toolboxes.

Optimists and Pessimists

Did you ever notice how some people are incredible optimists? It seems no matter what happens, they have a positive outlook. If these wild optimists get a ton of cow manure dropped on them, they are delighted about all the free fertilizer for their garden. The optimist always seems to find the silver lining in the clouds, even when there is none.

The pessimist occupies the other side of the coin. These folks never saw a gift horse whose mouth did not need looking into. When they win the lottery, they lament the amount that has to be paid in taxes. The pessimist always looks for, and finds, the negative in any situation.

I heard a story of a father with twin boys; the one boy was ultra pessimistic and the other was a real optimist. The father decided that both sons would benefit by moving toward middle ground, so he decided to "cure" them one Christmas. He bought the pessimistic son a beautiful new train set and filled the optimistic son's Christmas stocking with horse manure. The boys rushed down Christmas morning and opened their gifts. The father gave them a few minutes and then asked what Santa Claus had brought them.

"I got a train set," said the pessimistic son in a gloomy voice, "but it's going to take me forever to put it together and then it probably will break within a week."

This was not the response the father had hoped for, but he was sure that the other boy would learn a good lesson. Just then, the optimistic son came running into the room, all excited and exclaimed, "Guess what Dad? I got a pony for Christmas! Only I haven't found him yet!"

So if we want to live with joy, should we be an optimist or a pessimist? The positive-thinking gurus tell us to simply adopt an optimistic mental attitude. Then we'll be happy. Yet most of us recognize that doesn't work. We know people who see only the good in every situation and are fools. They see what they want to see and ignore the truth. They have not found joy, they have deceived themselves.

Our happiness does not depend on our optimism or our pessimism. Our happiness depends on our ability to understand our tendencies and to develop strategies to help us live.

For example, my friend Bruce happens to be a pessimist by nature. He always sees the danger where I see the fun. We have built several house additions together, and the difference in our natures consistently emerges. I always assume the board I am about to cut will fit "just right" and Bruce always figures it will not fit at all. Of course, I do make more mis-cuts than he does, but he spends more time measuring and agonizing than I do.

An optimist and a pessimist often make a good team. My optimistic enthusiasm, ("Oh this will be simple, we'll be done in no time!") combined with Bruce's attention to likely pitfalls, tends to get projects done well and with lots of fun. I have grown to appreciate his cautious nature, and Bruce now enjoys (I think) the glee with which I attack a task.

What makes an optimist or a pessimist? We must evaluate ourselves by our ability to accurately predict the outcome of an event. Imagine you are planning a trip to the zoo in a nearby city. As you consider the trip, you may think about the drive to the zoo. That becomes the anticipated event, and your expectations reveal your degree of optimism or pessimism.

You could have a variety of predictions regarding the outcome of the event: "Everything will go fine," "We'll have car trouble," "We'll get lost," "We'll get car jacked," etc. An optimist tends to think everything will go well and a pessimist tends to think everything will go badly. If you do drive to the zoo, though, things will go a certain way (whatever that happens to be). So we have an anticipated event, expectations for that event and how things actually go.

In order to tell if you are an optimist or a pessimist, consider how many times your expectation of an event matches the actual outcome. If actual events usually turn out to be worse than you anticipated, you are an optimist. If events usually turn out to be better than you anticipated, you are a pessimist. If outcomes usually match your expectations, you are a realist.

Do you consider yourself an optimist, realist or pessimist? Worksheet #5 quizzes you on this topic.

Discovering my own tendencies helped me choose my career. As a young man I worked in a consulting engineering office. Most of the time I was behind a desk performing architectural or structural engineering designs. The design aspect of the work was enjoyable, but I struggled when I needed to go out in the field as an inspector. The role of an inspector is to point out problems (items of work that were not in accordance with the intent of the drawings and specifications). I was not supposed to solve the problems because that was the contractor's job.

I thoroughly disliked being an inspector. I loved solving problems, but I hated having to tell other people they had a problem and then walking away. As I considered why I disliked this part of my job, I realized that I was an optimist. It was more natural for me to see the positive and focus on solutions, not the problems.

> As John Miller reviewed this worksheet, he saw himself mostly as a pessimist, but did not like the word "pessimist." He preferred to think of himself as "just realistic." It was clear to him, though, that he almost always saw the difficulty in an upcoming task or the potential pain or embarrassment that was on his horizon.

Name: *John Miller*   Worksheet#5   Date: *3-7-00*

Do I Tend To Be an Optimist or a Pessimist?

1. My boss unexpectedly says, "We need to talk, please come into my office." My immediate response is:

| Mostly Pessimistic | (Somewhat Pessimistic) | Realistic | Somewhat Optimistic | Mostly Optimistic |

2. My five-year old daughter, while riding bike in the driveway, crashes to the pavement. My first response is:

| Mostly Pessimistic | (Somewhat Pessimistic) | Realistic | Somewhat Optimistic | Mostly Optimistic |

3. I have a romantic dinner date with my spouse tonight. As I think about how things will go, I am:

| Mostly Pessimistic | Somewhat Pessimistic | (Realistic) | Somewhat Optimistic | Mostly Optimistic |

4. I am about to walk across a one-way street. The old saying is, "A pessimist looks both ways when crossing a one-way street." I am:

| (Mostly Pessimistic) | Somewhat Pessimistic | Realistic | Somewhat Optimistic | Mostly Optimistic |

5. While driving my car near the speed limit on the highway, I hear the siren and see the flashing lights of a police car behind me. My reaction is:

| (Mostly Pessimistic) | Somewhat Pessimistic | Realistic | Somewhat Optimistic | Mostly Optimistic |

6. I get a telephone call informing me that I have won $5,000 in a sweepstakes that I entered. I am:

| Mostly Pessimistic | (Somewhat Pessimistic) | Realistic | Somewhat Optimistic | Mostly Optimistic |

7. During a routine physical with my doctor, she comes in with a grave look and says, "We found a lump that concerns us. We would like to schedule you for a test to take a sample for a biopsy." After the initial shock, my reaction is:

| (Mostly Pessimistic) | Somewhat Pessimistic | Realistic | Somewhat Optimistic | Mostly Optimistic |

8. Considering all the above, my nature is probably:

| (Mostly Pessimistic) | Somewhat Pessimistic | Realistic | Somewhat Optimistic | Mostly Optimistic |

I decided to take another job as a project manager for a contractor. There, I found all the problems were mine to solve and I loved it! I was fortunate to find work that suited my nature and my particular set of talents. That decision to enter construction project management was based on recognition of my optimistic nature. This was truly a helpful tool in my life.

Many self-help books take a single concept (positive thinking, birth order, time management, etc.) and attempt to create a tool to solve our problems. These programs fail because we live in a complex world. While I benefited in my job change described above by understanding my optimism, most of the decisions in my life have nothing to do with optimism or pessimism. I believe there are, ultimately, some simple answers for our lives, but we must obtain an understanding of our complexity before we get to the simple answers.

The Values You Live

The next exercise involves understanding our personal values. We all have values by which we live. Most of us never take the time to consider what these things are and how they drive our lives. Not being aware of their importance does not lessen their influence.

Values are defined as our beliefs or our standards, those things that we believe have worth.   I like to think of our values as the attributes we highly prize. For example, many people value compassion. If you are a compassionate person, you are attuned to the pain of others. Perhaps you have no idea why you have this strong sense of caring; it is just there and you consider it valuable.

We all have qualities that we value. Whether we were born with these traits or we developed them while growing up doesn't matter here. What does matter is discovering what we currently value.

The characteristics we value can work for good or move us toward destruction. Loyalty, for example, may seem noble. Consider a motorcycle gang that values loyalty above all else. Loyalty becomes its code of ethics. Any gang member involved in a fight can count on all the other members present to jump into the fight. In this case, loyalty could result in the brutal beating of an innocent person. As we identify the standards and beliefs we live by, we gain insight into ourselves.

In my life, I value a sense of humor. While growing up, a sense of humor was essential in my family, and we all learned to give and take.

One particular family trip stands out in my memory. We were on a 12-hour drive from Pennsylvania to New Hampshire, and there were five of us in the car: my father, my mother, my younger brother Jim, my then girlfriend Debby and me.

We were getting a little silly by hour 10, when Jim threw a used piece of chewing gum out the rear, driver's side window. A minute or two later my father said, "What in the world...?" and was moving his foot on and off the gas pedal. After a short distance he pulled over to the side of the highway saying, "I don't know what's going on here, my foot is sticking to the accelerator!"

Well, the rest of us had a pretty good idea of what was going on and were trying hard not to laugh (my father always hated being sticky and was quite irritated at this point). As Dad was leaning down, trying to figure out what was making his foot stick to the gas pedal, a police car pulled up behind us. The policeman approached the driver's window and asked, "What seems to be the problem, sir?"

To which my father replied, "Uh... I just... uh... have some chewing gum on my sock." At this point the rest of us could no longer contain ourselves and broke out in hysterical laughter. We laughed so hard that tears ran down our faces. Then we would tell the story to each other and laugh some more. Almost 20 years later, we still tell the story and laugh as if it just happened.

Although I did not think about it at the time, dad's response to that situation was significant for me and for our family. Even though Dad was sticky (which he hates) and embarrassed (which he also hates) he was laughing about the situation within minutes. Clearly, he valued his sense of humor.

As we consider our own valued attributes, we sometimes draw a mental blank. Perhaps we are not accustomed to thinking in these terms. Therefore Table 1 provides a list of attributes we may value. Of course, this list is not all-inclusive, so feel free to add to it.

As you read through the list of valued attributes, which seem to matter most to you? Be careful to focus on what you now value, not those attributes you think you ought to value. What attributes do you show, by your actions, to be important to you?

You need to be honest, but not overly hard, with yourself. Mother Teresa is not the only person in the world who could list compassion as a valued attribute. On Worksheet #6, list the attributes that you value. Please recognize, though, that you must oversimplify for this exercise. We are all complex human beings. We are never all one thing or all another. However, we make better decisions when we know our values.

Emerson wrote, "What you are shouts so loudly in my ears I cannot hear what you say." Look at what your life shouts into the ears of those around you and write your responses. Be as honest as you can.

As I consider my own valued attributes, I check my honesty level by considering how I would respond in certain circumstances. Since I consider integrity a valued attribute, I envision a situation in which I get pulled over for speeding by a policeman. Now, how am I going to respond? If I know I really was speeding, do I tell the truth? Or do I try and finesse my way out of it.

The true answer, of course, is, "It depends." The specific circumstances, my mood and many other factors affect how I respond to a given situation. Worksheet #7 offers several potential situations to consider for a "reality check" on the answers in Worksheet #6.

Table #1

List of Valued Attributes

1. Comfort
2. Caution
3. Commitment
4. Common sense
5. Compassion
6. Courage
7. Drive
8. Easy going
9. Encouragement
10. Excellence
11. Equality
12. Fairness
13. Faith
14. Forgiveness
15. Free-spirited
16. Gentleness
17. Goodness
18. Grace
19. Honesty
20. Honor
21. Hope
22. Human dignity
23. Human potential
24. Humility
25. Integrity
26. Intelligence
27. Introspection
28. Joy
29. Knowledge
30. Love
31. Morality
32. Patience
33. Paying attention
34. Peace
35. Power
36. Physical beauty
37. Perseverance
38. Pride
39. Punctuality
40. Purity
41. Responsibility
42. Risk taking
43. Revenge
44. Restraint
45. Self discipline
46. Self esteem
47. Sense of humor
48. Strength
49. Service
50. Sincerity
51. Trust
52. Wisdom

Name: *John Miller*   Worksheet #6   Date: *3-7-00*

Valued Attributes

What are my four most valued attributes? (Refer to Table #1 for ideas.)
  a. Why do I value this attribute?
  b. When have I been strong in demonstrating this attribute?
  c. When have I been weak in demonstrating this attribute?

Valued Attributes

1. *Compassion* _____ Why? *I am very sensitive to the pain of others.*

   When strong? *Hate to see animals abused or mistreated.*
   I once punched a guy in the mouth for whipping his dog.
   When weak? *Way too impatient with our 2 kids.*

2. *Fairness* _____ Why? *Cause Dad was never fair at home & I promised myself I would always try to be fair.*
   When strong? *I am known for settling disputes fairly on the job site.*
   When weak? *Can't think of any examples.*

3. *Perseverance* _____ Why? *It just seems to come natural to me.*

   When strong? *When I am in a tough situation, I just put my nose to the grindstone and keep on going.*
   When weak? *Sometimes with Rachel I want to give up.*

4. *Competence* _____ Why? *From when I was little, I always wanted to know how things worked and how to do things.*
   When strong? *My skills as a craftsman.*

   When weak? *My skills as a husband & father.*

Name: *John Miller*   Worksheet #7   Date: *3-7-00*
Valued Attribute Scenarios

Imagine the following situations and think, "How would I respond?" Consider the attributes listed in Table #1, your responses from Worksheet #6 or anything else that comes to mind.

1. When driving a car, someone inadvertently cuts me off and I just miss being in an accident.

> *I usually don't get mad. I mostly am assessing the specifics of the situation, trying to figure out exactly what happened and why.*

2. My child plays a sport and is often treated unfairly by the coach.

> *I have gotten right in a coach's face already over this. I hate unfairness.*

3. I get a small finance charge for a late payment I think I mailed on time.

> *I just tell Rachel, "Pay it and forget about it, it isn't worth the hassle."*

4. I am ready to park my car and another car zooms in and steals my space.

> *This happened to me 3 years ago and I went wild. I jumped out of my car and started yelling at the guy who stole my spot. At some point I told him (who was sitting in his car with his windows rolled up and doors locked) either he moves his car or I smash all his headlights and taillights. He moved but I wasn't real proud of my behavior.*

5. A co-worker tells me, face-to-face and without much tact, that I failed to keep a commitment.

> *I know it would probably tick me off at first, but after I cooled down, I would know the person was probably right and be glad for their gumption to tell me.*

After completing this worksheet, go back and look at Worksheet #6. Were your answers there honest and accurate? Write down any thoughts as notes to Worksheet #6.

U.S. Marine Corps training provides a good example of how influential values can be. Marine training stresses the values of honor, courage and commitment. These are constantly drummed into the young person's head: **honor, courage and commitment!** The trainee repeatedly hears that it takes honor, courage and commitment to be a Marine. The power of those clearly focused values is amazing. When the Marine has to make a hard decision, those are the values that come to mind. Many young men trained in this manner have retained these values for the rest of their lives.

Our American culture, on the other hand, tends to highly value physical beauty and intelligence. A child with beauty or high intelligence starts with a huge advantage in our society. Conversely, a child who is neither attractive nor bright, struggles through our school system and our culture. Even though this doesn't seem fair, it indicates the power of personal values in our lives and the lives of others.

Think about a person you highly respect and see if you can pick out the key values that they live by. I know a man who has done a wonderful job raising his family and living his life. He based his life on integrity, love and joy. I also know people who highly value revenge. Nothing matters as much as righting a perceived wrong. There are others who live their whole lives striving to be easygoing. Whatever is easiest is best. We can spot the values of others by observing how they live.

Your Central Focus

I first came across the idea of central focus from Steve Covey's excellent book, <u>The Seven Habits of Highly Effective People</u>. As I studied the concept, I found it to be helpful in understanding myself and others. Asking the simple question, "By the way I live, what do I care about most?" can provide valuable gems of understanding.

For example, I have a friend, Joe, whose central focus is clearly his work. While Joe has a nice, loving family, attends church, has friends and generally a full life, work matters most. He runs a successful family business and was brought up viewing work as his greatest priority. Joe enjoys his job, and he spends most of his time thinking about work. When a family crisis hit Joe's life, he came face-to-face with the reality of a life not based on the best foundation. If he desires more joy in his life, Joe will need to admit that work has been his central focus. Sometimes simply admitting our central focus provides the motivation for us to begin the process of change.

Consider someone who puts personal pleasure first. Pleasure becomes the measuring stick by which all decisions are made. Vacations, hobbies, sports and recreation become the strongest areas of interest.

We probably all know a mother who has made her family the central focus of her life. She lives for her husband and her children. Every decision she makes is based on the question, "How will this affect my family?" She will put the family needs ahead of her own needs in almost every case.

At this point we are not making value judgments. We are not trying to determine whether our central focus is good or bad. We are trying to recognize how we are presently living. For this exercise, forget about all the psychological terms (workaholic, co-dependent, etc.) and simply concentrate on how you live and what matters most to you. The following list may be helpful in determining your central focus.

Work	Family
Money	Self
Church	Pleasure
Spouse	Possessions
Friend	Enemy
Health	Principles
God	

As you read through the list, did any items seem to jump out at you? Think about where you spend your time. Consider your thoughts as you fall asleep, what you dream about, and what you think about as you wake up each morning. Remember, focus can change, so don't think that writing "possessions" as your central focus makes you a terrible person. J. Pierre Pont Morgan said, "A person usually has two reasons for what they do: the one that sounds good and the real one." Try to look at the real reasons for what you do and the real things you do. Worksheet #8 will help you gain some insight about your central focus.

Personality Styles

My high school yearbook lists my likes as "sex and money" and my dislikes as "promiscuity and materialism." I still laugh when I read that and consider how well it describes my personality. Apart from being a wise guy (which apparently I'm not going to grow out of), I still struggle with the way I am vs. the way I ought to be. By studying personality styles, though, I gain some clues as to why I act the way I act.

Over the years I examined many different personality systems, such as "The DISC Personality Profile," "Myers-Briggs Type Indicator," Get a Life Without the Strife by Fred and Florence Littauer, The Six Thinking Hats by Edward deBono, etc. I developed my own simple Basic Personality guidelines for your use based on the DISC model.

A Type D personality (Demanding Driver) pushes to get things done. Type D's dominate relationships; they usually have a strong sense of what needs to be done and move boldly to accomplish the goal. Stubborn and impatient, Type D's don't have time to fool around. They want things done and they want things done NOW! The hard-nosed boss is a classic Type D personality.

The Type I personality (Invigorating Influencer) concerns himself less with what gets done and more with having a good time doing it. The Type I is the people person, the social director of any group. With spirit and enthusiasm, Type I personalities

Name: *John Miller*   Worksheet #8   Date: *3-10-00*
Central Focus

1. The central focus of my life would be... *Work*

2. Why? *I spend most of my time thinking about it. I guess I don't want to fail at it.*

3. If I had trouble identifying just one clear focus, what are other possible candidates for central focus in my life? *family, possessions*

4. Why? *I love Rachel & the kids. I also love working on classic cars & cycles.*

5. If I explained this concept of central focus to the following people, what would they say was the central focus in my life? Why?

> a. Grandparents *Family, because I spend time with my kids.*

b. Parents *Family, they think I am a great dad.*

c. Siblings *Probably work since that's important to both my brothers.*

d. Children *Work*

e. Bosses *Doubt they think about it or would even care.*

f. Co-workers *Work, because I am pretty good at it.*

> As John Miller contemplated his central focus, he gained some valuable insights. He had never previously realized how important work was to him. He knew he liked work and was good at it, but never admitted it was the most important thing in his life. In fact, he still was not really sure work was his central focus, though even the possibility that it might be was sobering to him. John also surprised himself by writing that he did not really have any close friends. Some of the previous worksheets did not particularly connect with John. This one did.

g. Close friends *Don't really have any.*

want to have fun and usually expect the best of others. The downside of a Type I personality is the tendency to be naïve, haphazard and unpredictable. The successful salesperson is a classic Type I personality.

The Type S personality (Sensitive Sustainer) wants everyone to be happy and stress-free. They are often the nice people in our lives, the people who care about the feelings of others. Gentle and cautious, the Type S personality generally is also a good listener. Type S people have a tendency to worry and to be timid. The caring counselor is a classic Type S personality.

The Type C personality (Calculating Controller) wants things to be clear and precise. They want everything to be done properly. An analytical group, Type C's love details and accuracy. They have a tendency to be fussy, suspicious of those not like them, and overly-critical. The engineer or accountant is a classic Type C personality.

Think about how people make decisions. A Type D (Demanding Driver) person makes quick decisions, based on gut-feelings. The Type I (Invigorating Influencer) person considers which option will be the most fun; the decisions also tend to be intuitive. The Type S (Sensitive Sustainer) person must be sure how the decision will affect everyone else; no one must be hurt by the decision. The Type C (Calculating Controller) person wants more information and more data; decisions are careful, deductive and slow.

As an engineer and building contractor, I routinely work with many different building owners. I've learned to pay attention to the building owner's personality type as I struggle to obtain the many decisions to design and construct a building. When working with a Type D (Demanding Driver) owner, I have all the information summarized and quickly explain the options. Usually, I do not even write it down because they don't want to take the time to read. I can count on a quick decision from a Type D and know he will stand behind it.

With a Type I (Invigorating Influencer) owner, the presentation counts for much more. The Type I owner wants to see enthusiasm for the recommended option. It is easy to get a quick decision from a Type I; the problem is that it is just as easy for them to change their minds in the future.

The Type S (Sensitive Sustainer) owner tends to agonize over every decision in order to keep everybody happy. I have learned to expect Type S owners to get the opinions of others on most decisions, so I am prepared with information that is simple to pass on.

The Type C (Calculating Controller) owner wants all the available data to analyze for every single decision. When I need a decision from a Type C owner, I come prepared with a written analysis and every performance chart and graph I can find. I then expect to wait for all this information to be digested and more information to be requested.

So how can you use this concept in your life? First, determine your own personality type. Quickly read through Worksheets #9 and #10 and go with your first response on the answers. Determine if you strongly fit one of the four personality types or if you tend to be a combination of two or three of them. Write your thoughts in the margin. Next, consider the personality types of a few people you know well. You will remember the personality types better if you can think of someone who is a good example of each.

Let's consider a situation where knowing personality styles could help you. Perhaps your boss drives you crazy. Nothing you do meets his standards, and you find him to be picky, inefficient and irritating. You strive to do your job well, and you see your boss as a hindrance. An understanding of personality styles could go far in actually resolving your problem. (Remember, your options are: 1. continue to be miserable. 2. find another job. or 3. solve the problem.)

In reading the personality profiles above, you determine that you are a Type D (Demanding Driver). You look to do things efficiently, quickly and move on to the next task. You are good at what you do, and you know it; you just want to do your job. Your boss, on the other hand, clearly acts like a Type C (Calculating

Controller). Everything has to be perfect, and he always wants more details.

Can you see the steps that would diffuse the situation? As a Type D employee, you are struggling to get along with your Type C boss. The solution involves redefining what a completed task means to you. In order to have a completed task, you must provide the level of detail that satisfies your boss. By defining your job tasks from the beginning in a way that will satisfy your boss, you will probably resolve this problem without major effort or aggravation.

To summarize, if you want to get along with your boss, just understand that he needs more detail than you do. With little effort or aggravation, you can provide your boss with the extra information. As so often happens, the problem can be solved easily after it is understood clearly.

Since I have been paying attention to personality types for years, I can attest to their usefulness in day-to-day living. When you identify an individual's personality profile, you can better predict how that person will react in different situations. You gain a higher level of understanding in that relationship.

On the other hand, some people simply do not fit the personality profiles. For example, artistic people tend not to fit any of the categories. Please don't try to label every person with a personality type, for you will have gone beyond the usefulness of the concept. Use the personality types where they seem to fit. Used wisely this tool will be valuable in your own life and as you relate to others.

Name: *John Miller*   Worksheet #9   Date: *3-11-00*

My Basic Personality – Part 1
(Circle items that best describe you, X items that least describe you)

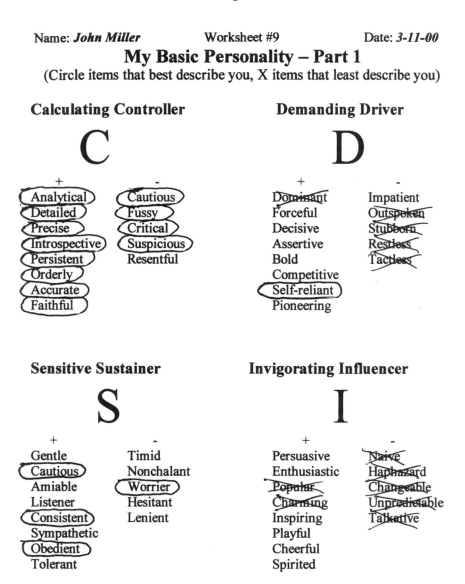

Calculating Controller

C

+	-
(Analytical)	(Cautious)
(Detailed)	(Fussy)
(Precise)	(Critical)
(Introspective)	(Suspicious)
(Persistent)	Resentful
(Orderly)	
(Accurate)	
(Faithful)	

Demanding Driver

D

+	-
~~Dominant~~	Impatient
Forceful	~~Outspoken~~
Decisive	~~Stubborn~~
Assertive	~~Restless~~
Bold	~~Tactless~~
Competitive	
(Self-reliant)	
Pioneering	

Sensitive Sustainer

S

+	-
Gentle	Timid
(Cautious)	Nonchalant
Amiable	(Worrier)
Listener	Hesitant
(Consistent)	Lenient
Sympathetic	
(Obedient)	
Tolerant	

Invigorating Influencer

I

+	-
Persuasive	~~Naive~~
Enthusiastic	~~Haphazard~~
~~Popular~~	~~Changeable~~
~~Charming~~	~~Unpredictable~~
Inspiring	~~Talkative~~
Playful	
Cheerful	
Spirited	

> As John Miller went through Worksheets #9 and #10, the answers came easily. No great insights came from these Worksheets, but the concept did seem interesting. He had no trouble thinking of examples of the various personality types.

Name: *John Miller*   Worksheet #10   Date: *3-11-00*

My Basic Personality – Part 2

1.   Which personality profile do I most strongly resemble? *Type C*

2.   Do I mostly fit one profile or am I more of a combination? Explain.
     I am fairly strong Type C, but I also have some of the Type S traits

3.   Who is the best example of a Type D person that I know? *Bill Jones
     (owner of Commersial Contractors)*

4.   What are his/her strengths? Weaknesses? *Decisive, gets things done,
     hard-nosed & efficient. He's a real jerk.*

5.   Who is the best example of a Type I person that I know? *Stan Hartman
     (a foreman I work with)*

6.   What are his/her strengths? Weaknesses? *Real funny, can get anyone to
     do anything. He goes in too many directions at one time.*

7.   Who is the best example of a Type S person that I know? *Pastor Toland*

8.   What are his/her strengths? Weaknesses? *Sensitive and seems kind.
     Timid, just kind of goes along.*

9.   Who is the best example of a Type C person that I know? *Grandpa Miller*

10. What are his/her strengths? Weaknesses? *He was so smart and detailed,
     he could figure out any kind of technical problem. He was so cau-
     tious, he never left farming, even though he would have liked to try
     some other type of work.*

11. What are the strengths of my personality and how do they help me?
     *I am analytical and detailed and get things done by staying at a
     task.*

12. What are the weaknesses of my personality and how do they hurt me?
     I am overly critical of others and not very trusting.

Love Languages

Did you ever think about the ways you show your love to another person? Gary Chapman, in his book, <u>The Five Love Languages</u>, examines that concept and discovers five different ways of showing love to another person:

- Words of Affirmation
- Quality Time
- Gifts
- Acts of Service
- Physical Touch

By learning about our Love Languages we gain another useful tool for understanding ourselves and others.

Gary Chapman spent years working with couples who were trying to save or improve their marriages. As he struggled to help, he discovered, again and again, the deep emotional need for love that most people have. As couples shared their secret pain, he would hear things like, "Our love is gone; our relationship is dead," or "We used to feel close, but not now," or "We no longer enjoy being with each other, we don't meet each other's needs." Many times husbands and wives had tried to meet each other's emotional needs, but not very successfully. It was like one spouse spoke Greek and the other spoke Russian.

Chapman then developed the concept of the five Love Languages. Stated simply, most of us tend to show our love, and want to receive love, in one or more of the five ways listed above. One of those ways will be most significant to us and is our primary Love Language. In our most intimate relationships (with our spouse, our parents, our children, our close friends, etc.), we will benefit greatly from an understanding of our own and our loved one's primary love language.

A person whose primary love language is *Words of Affirmation* wants verbal feedback. These people need to be told they are appreciated. "Thanks for cleaning up the dinner dishes," or "I really am glad you took the time to come to my ball game," are things this person will both say and like to hear. Complimentary, kind and loving words matter much to a person whose primary Love Language is *Words of Affirmation*. These words really register and make an impact. Conversely, someone who has *Words of Affirmation* as one of their lowest Love Languages will often disregard such statements or assume the words are said in order to manipulate them.

Quality Time is the primary Love Language of those who measure love not in words spoken but in time spent. A person whose primary Love Language is *Quality Time* simply needs to spend time, good focused time, with the people they love. The cry for help from these people will sound like, "We never do anything together," or "You are always too busy with the kids (or your work) to pay attention to me." A *Quality Time* person will tremendously appreciate an evening sitting together in front of the fireplace and chatting. On the other hand, someone who has *Quality Time* as one of their lowest Love Languages will view such an evening as, "Well we didn't really do anything; we just sat around."

We all know the person who has *Gifts* as their primary Love Language. These people are the ones who show up with a present and who seem never to miss a gift-giving opportunity. The person with *Gifts* as their primary Love Language feels special when giving or receiving gifts. It is not the size of the gift that matters; the sentiment behind the gift illustrates the love. A person for whom *Gifts* is the lowest Love Language tends to see gifts as manipulation.

One speaks the Love Language of *Acts of Service* by doing things for others. Washing the dishes, changing the baby (or a burned out light bulb), mowing the lawn or making a special meal are all examples of *Acts of Service*. With this primary Love Language, one feels truly loved only when another person puts forth the effort to perform helpful tasks. One who has *Acts of Service* as the lowest Love Language may tend to see all that activity as avoidance of the real issues.

Physical Touch is the Love Language that desires contact with the loved one. A *Physical Touch* person will value holding hands, hugs, playful punches on the arm and other physical contact. The handshake will be significant to this person, as will sexual intercourse (and I am willing to wager that's the first time you saw those two items tied together in one sentence). A *Physical Touch* person will place a high value on any type of touch and physical contact. Those who have *Physical Touch* as one of their lowest Love Languages tend to see the contact as insignificant.

To illustrate the usefulness of this concept, imagine a husband (Bill) and wife (Naomi) who are struggling in their marriage. Bill feels like he puts forth the bulk of the effort to keep the marriage going and resents Naomi for not trying harder. Naomi, of course, believes she puts most of the energy into their relationship and is angry at Bill for not noticing. Bill works all day at the telephone company and then comes home to mow the lawn, pull weeds, pick up the kids' toys, help with the laundry, do the dishes and coach a softball team. At the end of one of these busy days, when he feels a little frisky, Naomi rebuffs his romantic advances. Bill lies in bed and seethes, wondering why Naomi appreciates him so little and has become such a selfish witch (or sentiments to that effect).

Naomi, on the other hand, stays home with the three children in the mornings and works as a waitress many days at lunch and dinner. She tries to be a good mother by reading to each child and spending time with them; she does the bulk of the housework and she waitresses to bring in extra money. Naomi actually enjoys the waitressing because her regular customers tell her how wonderful she is, which she rarely hears at home any more. She falls into bed at night, exhausted physically and emotionally, and then Bill pouts when she does not feel like having sex. She wonders how she married such an insensitive dolt.

Do you see the Love Language clues in this scenario? They are right there in the open, as they are in most relationships. It is up to us to use the Love Languages as a tool to better understand and improve the situation.

Bill's primary Love Language is *Acts of Service* with *Physical Touch* being a close second. *Gifts* is in third place while *Words of Affirmation* and *Quality Time* are last. Bill works hard in the marriage by doing things other women complain their husbands never do. Bill feels that he puts forth so much effort and is not appreciated by Naomi, and he feels especially strongly about this issue at bedtime.

Naomi's primary Love Languages are *Quality Time* and *Words of Affirmation. Physical Touch, Acts of Service* and *Gifts* are not especially important to Naomi. When Bill comes home from work and rushes right out to mow the lawn or throws in a load of laundry, Naomi wishes he would just sit down with her for a while and talk about the day. Naomi knows she should appreciate all the work Bill does, but instead she finds herself resenting the work and Bill. Then she feels guilty. She knows they are growing apart, and it scares her.

Like many married couples, Bill and Naomi have different Love Languages. If they don't address this issue, they will probably continue to drift apart. Perhaps Bill will find temporary comfort in the arms of a co-worker or a softball team mom, and then the marriage will go down in flames. Perhaps nothing dramatic will happen, but their sense of love and closeness will just fizzle away to nothing. However, Bill and Naomi could decide to take action and turn their marriage around.

When Bill realizes that time and encouraging words truly matter to Naomi, he will begin to see his sitting and talking with her or giving her a compliment as an act of service and not as a waste of precious time. These efforts on Bill's part will be emotionally rewarding for both of them. Naomi will be hearing the Love Language she understands, and Bill will see the effort as an act of service, a Love Language he relates to.

Naomi will strive to do those little extra things for Bill that she knows he appreciates. She may still get more compliments as a waitress than she gets at home, but she knows Bill is trying and that helps her feel loved. Their love-making improves as their love grows and this aspect of their marriage motivates Bill more than Naomi can ever imagine. Understanding and using the Love Language concept can help produce strong, happy, enduring relationships.

In reviewing this book, our niece Wendy became intrigued with the Love Language concept (having never heard it before) and decided to try it. Her husband had a week of vacation in which he planned to get some things done around their house. Wendy correctly guessed that *Words of Affirmation* were quite important to her husband Steve, although they were not that important to her. Wendy spoke encouraging words to Steve each day when opportunities presented themselves.

After only a few days Steve commented how much he appreciated Wendy's encouragement. As a couple they had nourished their love. A strong marriage just grew a little stronger.

Worksheet #11 gives you an opportunity to think about Love Languages in your life and in the lives of a few other people. Many folks will find this Worksheet challenging. Please just take your best guess and move on. This Worksheet introduces you to the concept of Love Languages and helps you think about them.

Name: *John Miller*   Worksheet #11   Date: *3-12-00*

Love Languages

- Words of Affirmation
- Quality Time
- Gifts
- Acts of Service
- Physical Touch

List your Love Languages from most important (#1) to least important (#5) for yourself and three other people that you care about deeply. This is a highly subjective exercise, so just make your best guess.

1.   For myself, my Love Languages are:
   1. *Physical Touch*
   2. *Acts of Service*
   3. *Receiving Gifts*
   4. *Quality Time*
   5. *Words of Affirmation*

2.   For *Rachel Miller   (Wife)*   , his/her Love Languages are:
   1. *Words of Affirmation*
   2. *Quality Time*
   3. *Receiving Gifts*
   4. *Physical Touch*
   5. *Acts of Service*

3.   For *July Miller   (Mom)*   , his/her Love Languages are:
   1. *Words of Affirmation*
   2. *Quality Time*
   3. *Receiving Gifts*
   4. *Acts of Service*
   5. *Physical Touch*

4.   For *Samuel Miller   (Dad)*   , his/her Love Languages are:
   1. *Receiving Gifts*
   2. *Physical Touch*
   3. *Acts of Service*
   4. *Quality Time*
   5. *Words of Affirmation*

CHAPTER 3

Understanding & Managing Emotions

"If we want to discover the keys to our own motivation, we must look to our emotions. Thinking stirs feeling and feeling triggers action."
A.W. Tozer

If given my druthers, I would avoid this entire discussion of emotions. By nature, I gravitate toward concrete solutions to problems. I believe in "pulling one's self up by one's own bootstraps." Nevertheless, I find these tricky, difficult-to-understand emotions often control our choices. In order to understand why we do the things we do, we must begin to understand our emotions.

I was teaching a class based on **Joyful Living** a few years ago. I found the classroom give-and-take enjoyable and helpful. As we discussed one of the worksheets, a woman asked why I had not included any questions about the emotional side of the issue. It was a good question, and I made a note to throw in a few questions about emotions.

Another woman in the class challenged me much more deeply. She said little, but there was something about her. Her eyes haunted me; she seemed so intense. I discovered she was a survivor of incest; she had suffered horrible sexual abuse by her father throughout her childhood years. As I thought and prayed about my teaching and writing, I knew I must be sure about my material. I had to be certain the things I said were in fact true.

I read the 200-page curriculum I had developed and concluded it wasn't good enough. I decided to reconsider all my ideas. As I reviewed the section of the course about memories, I got bogged down. I believed it would be a good thing to record our clearest memories. Accessible memories, I reasoned, could help us better understand ourselves. But I had never actually tried it myself.

I started recording memories and was amazed at the amount of information that surfaced. I was also amazed at the amount of time I spent. While I felt foolish taking that much time to record my memories, I persevered and ended up with a large collection.

Due to my student's comment about emotions, I listed the strongest emotion associated with each memory. Debby and I put these stories, along with the corresponding emotions and dates, in a computer database. I wanted to know if this information would prove to be useful. I was to find out shortly.

As I was preparing to go to sleep one night, I found a letter on our bed from our then nine-year-old daughter Tessa. Written in childish handwriting, the letter floored me:

Dear Mom and Dad,
Today is the last day I will be around here. Let's stop fooling each other, I just don't belong in this family. Either tonight or after

school tomorrow I am leaving. Please don't try and find me because you never will. We have tried but it is just not working. I don't know where I will go but it will be away from here. I love you very, very, very much.

Tessa

I felt half sick. I knew this letter was more than a youngster's idle threat to "run away from home." She had not written it in anger. I knew this was extremely important and needed to be handled properly; I had almost no idea what was going on or what I should do.

Debby was away that evening so I went alone to talk with Tess. We talked, but on a superficial level. I did get a promise from her not to do anything until we had a chance to come up with a plan. When Debby got home, she spoke with Tess and got more information (Debby's a much better listener than I am). She discovered Tess had gone into the school bathroom to cry several times in the past weeks and was feeling sad much of the time. Tess, Debby and I felt we should talk with a psychologist.

In the following days, as I tried to process this new information, things just did not make sense. Tessa was a rambunctious, popular kid who excelled in her school work. In fact, most things came easily for her. I thought about my nightly ritual of going into each child's room and talking, telling stories and saying prayers. I realized these conversations were different with each child.

Alexey, who is four and one-half years older than Tessa, was easy to talk with. We had so many similarities and were so close that our conversations flowed from one topic to another. We laughed often and wholeheartedly. We also talked about many spiritual issues. Our bond of love and friendship seemed to grow deeper every day. Lex certainly could be a challenging child and often pushed the limits, but we were both able to put those conflicts behind us quickly. I treasured those nightly conversations with Lex as times to both teach and learn.

Anna, who is two years older than Tess, was quite different from Lex. Anna was like her mother in many ways; she was sensitive and kind and more intuitive than logical (which made things like math a challenge). Anna had an easy way of getting along with people. When I put her to bed each night, she chattered on about her day and the things she was thinking about lately. She was both funny and had a deep spiritual side. Anna and I were different in many ways yet I felt very close to her.

Tessa was like me in many ways, but she had an odd combination of a strong will and a sensitive nature (which was not like me). Our nightly bedtime routine turned into a battle of wills. There always seemed to be something to disagree over, and our discussions tended to be superficial. I certainly loved her and she loved me, yet our relationship was strained. I tried a bit harder with Tess, because I wanted to improve our emotional closeness.

The day after the letter, we made an appointment with a psychologist. When the day for the appointment came, we were all a bit nervous as we drove into Lancaster City. Dr. Mary Lindsey quickly made us feel comfortable. She spoke with Tess for about 40 minutes, then asked to speak with all of us. As we neared the end of our time, Dr. Lindsey gave us her initial evaluation. "It seems Tessa feels she's getting lost. Tessa feels like she's wandering further and further from the rest of the family and getting quite scared that she will not be able to find her way back."

Dr. Lindsey's comments immediately clicked with me. I had been lost in the woods already; I knew that panicky, sometimes irrational, feeling that sweeps over. I realized that Tess, in her strong-willed way, felt "lost in the woods" while the rest of our family went about our normal routines. Now that I had identified the problem, I prayed for a solution.

I sensed that Tess and I needed to connect on a much more emotional level. When I had recorded my memories (which we will discuss in the next chapter) I had categorized them according to eight basic emotions: anger, joy, fear, love, sadness, surprise, shame, and disgust. I decided to make a notebook entitled "Tessa's Stories" with tabs for each emotion.

I asked Tess if she would be interested in trying a little experiment. When I put her to bed at night, she would pick a card that had one primary emotion written on it. I would then check my list of memories and tell her a story about a time when I strongly felt that emotion. Then Tess would tell me when she had experienced that emotion, with as much detail as possible, and I would record her story in her notebook.

The results were amazing! After a day of superficial interaction, Tess and I would settle in for our story time. Tess would pick a card and we would see which emotion we were to talk about that night. Perhaps it would be fear or surprise or joy or whatever. I would look over my list of memories and tell her a story with as much detail as I could recall. Many of my memories were humorous to Tessa.

But something else began to happen. When Tess told her story, I realized we were suddenly communicating much more deeply. The petty games were gone, and we were connecting at a deep and loving level. It was truly wonderful! I began to see the strong artistic side of Tessa's personality and to understand her better.

We continued to see Dr. Lindsey for a few months. Things did not change overnight, but they did change. My relationship with Tess grew consistently stronger. Debby and I were thankful we had faced this when Tess was only nine years old. If we had hit this crisis with a teenager, we probably would have endured a much more difficult challenge.

No event from my life more clearly illustrates the value of emotions. When we learn to understand our emotions and use them in our lives, we discover our own personal "buried treasures." In this chapter, we will help develop that simple, working knowledge of our emotions.

Eight Primary Emotions

For many years, psychologists studied emotions and disagreed on how to categorize them. The hundreds of human emotions overlap and do not easily group together. Rather than tackling all the complexity of a complete model of emotions, we can obtain value from a simple, common-sense approach. We will use a basic model of eight primary emotions:

- Anger
- Joy
- Fear
- Love
- Sadness
- Surprise
- Shame
- Disgust

The first letter for each emotion can be remembered by the following saying, "**A** **J**olly **F**armer **L**oves **S**inging **S**ome **S**illy **D**itties." Anger, Joy, Fear, Love, Sadness, Surprise, Shame and Disgust.

Thinking about emotions in theory bores most of us. Recalling some of our own powerful emotions, on the other hand, can be fascinating. Worksheet #12 provides the opportunity to recall some of your most vivid emotions. As you fill in Worksheet #12, struggle to recall the power of past emotions.

As I thought about my various emotions, I remembered a funny incident which included almost every emotion. Alexey suggested we go on a Saturday afternoon bicycle ride, so away we pedaled on a beautiful, sunny day. We were speeding down a steep hill with the wind in our faces. I could coast much faster than he could, so I got up over the crest of the next hill and lost sight of him briefly. What I did see, however, was a big, old dead groundhog lying in the middle of the road with all four legs sticking up in the air. I had an idea! Jumping off my bike, I laid down next to that groundhog and assumed a similar "dead groundhog position."

Lex rode over the crest of the hill and saw me lying on the road, on my back with my legs in the air. "Dad, are you alright?" he gasped. Then he looked at the groundhog. Then he looked at me again. Then he understood! He burst out laughing, as did I. He said, "Man, I was worried when I first came over that hill and saw you. I didn't know what happened." We continued to laugh as we enjoyed the rest of our long bicycle ride.

Can you see some of the emotions in the story? I remember the sense of joy as we rode down the steep hill with the wind and sun on our faces. When I saw the dead groundhog, I experienced surprise and disgust in quick succession. Then I felt the joy of my prank. Lex feared for me upon first sight, then felt the mixed emotions of surprise, disgust, joy and love. I was a little ashamed that my prank had worried Lex, but mostly we both felt this strong bond of love. When I feel that love for our children, I also feel sadness, knowing how relationships change with time.

Worksheet #12 challenges you to recall the emotions in your life. Everyone experiences these emotions, yet few think about them. Be one of the few!

Rational vs. Emotional Thinking

Think about a time that you based a decision primarily on logic. Perhaps your refrigerator had stopped working, and the re-pairperson said it was not worth fixing. Most of us solve this type of problem in a rational way. We talk to friends and relatives about where they got their refrigerators; we go to a new appliance store and compare values; we look in the newspaper for used re-frigerators. Then we choose the option that best meets our needs.

Name: *John Miller*   Worksheet #12   Date: *3-17-00*

Emotions Remembered
(When did I strongly feel each of the following emotions?)

1. Anger: *When Rachel and I get into an argument, I get so mad I feel like I could kill her.*

2. Joy: *The most joy I ever felt was the moment Nate was born and the moment Katie was born. It was amazing.*

3. Fear: *When we went down to Orlando and Katie got lost at Sea World. She was about 3 years old.*

> When John Miller first looked at this Worksheet he basically drew a blank. He was not accustomed to thinking about emotions. After a few minutes of brooding over the Worksheet, however, he was amazed how his responses just popped out.

4. Love: *When Rachel and I make love.*

5. Sadness: *I was 14 years old when our dog Barney died and the sadness just blew me away. It felt like I cried for days.*

6. Surprise: *When Bill Jones came out to the job site and told me they wanted me to be a Project Superintendent. I had no idea. I thought I'd work as a carpenter my whole life like Dad did.*

7. Shame: *Before I met Rachel, I once had sex with my best friend's girl friend. We were both a little drunk, but I felt so ashamed and embarrassed. Things were never the same again with either of them.*

8. Disgust: *When I found that Uncle Bill had molested two of my younger cousins.*

Your method may be more or less exhaustive, but most of us go through some similar approach to procure a refrigerator. In a rational approach, we gather facts and information, process that information using our intellect and make a decision. Some of the information may have an emotional component, such as, "I don't want a used refrigerator because we always bought used stuff when I was growing up and I always felt ashamed." Nevertheless, the decision to buy a refrigerator is generally made in a rational, logical way.

Emotional thinking operates differently. Our emotions give us a quick response. They are our "gut feelings" and tend to be quite intense. Think about some rational thinking process you went through in the past, such as the refrigerator example above. Do you have strong feelings about that process? Probably not. You may clearly recall the steps you went through, but it doesn't move you as a powerful memory.

Now think about a "gut feeling" you had recently. Perhaps you met someone to whom you took an instant dislike. This type of emotional thinking is difficult to understand. Yet these emotional "gut feelings" often surprise us with their accuracy. Our emotional thinking system includes this intuition as well as the emotions considered previously.

We must realize that our emotional thinking is reactive. Both our intuition and our emotional responses are always reactions to some stimulus. Our emotional thinking system can provide us with some amazingly quick information, which we can use to make decisions. For example, when we meet someone for the first time and our intuition strongly warns us to be cautious, we do well to take heed.

On the other hand, we need to test our emotional thinking since it sometimes sacrifices accuracy for speed. Using our rational thinking system, we can scrutinize our emotional responses. For example, we can rationally explain that bad "gut feeling" we had about the person we just met. We recall all the verbal and nonverbal clues that the person gave. Which of those clues seemed significant?

Obviously this sounds like too much work. And many times it's unnecessary. If the bad feeling is about a person on the bus, you just choose to sit somewhere else and that's that. If you have the bad feeling about the woman your brother just introduced as the love of his life, you will want to analyze that intuition. We make a mistake when we totally ignore or totally trust our intuition.

So, our emotional thinking system reacts to the stimulus in our life and gives us quick, often powerful, information. We need to be wary of the accuracy of this information and sometimes use our rational thinking system to test it. Our rational thinking system works more slowly and logically. We can trace the line of thinking and even write it down. Our rational thinking system doesn't need to be reactive; we can choose to think about things outside our current circumstances.

Another difference between the two types of thinking lies in the degree of certainty of the conclusions. Emotional thinking gives clear, quick direction. Answers tend to be black or white, such as "Run!" or "Fight!" or "Get Angry! You've been insulted!" In contrast, rational thinking allows us to work toward various, detailed conclusions.

Everyone I've ever met utilizes both their emotional and their rational thinking systems. At this point, it is not important to know which system you use most. It is important simply to understand that both supply us with information from which we choose our actions.

Emotions, Moods and Temperament

As we seek to better understand our basic emotions and intuition, we come to the topic of moods. Figure #1 helps illustrate the relationship between emotions, moods and temperament. Personality style (discussed in the previous chapter) can also be called temperament. Most of us naturally demonstrate one type of temperament or another. I noticed this phenomenon with each of our children. Their personalities seemed to be in place from the time they were born.

For most of us, our temperament is rather consistent. Moods, on the other hand, can vary greatly. Some days I wake up feeling the world is wonderful and created just to make me happy. On other days, the entire universe seems to be conspiring to make my life as miserable as possible. The main difference between those two days is my mood.

It is natural for us to have good moods, bad moods and many types of in-between moods. I strongly disagree with the positive-thinking gurus who tell us our key to happiness lies in manufacturing good moods. Ultimate happiness lies in our understanding of the truth, and that includes understanding our moods.

Certainly there are times we need to use our will to change our mood. For example, perhaps one day you happen to be in a particularly lousy mood at work, and you bring the mood home. Then you realize that your eight-year old daughter is having a slumber party at your house with six other girls. If you stay in your current mood, everyone is likely to be miserable. Or, you could use your will in that situation to "get in a good mood" and thereby have a less painful evening. We can all change our moods by using our wills from time to time.

Most important is that we learn from our moods. Rather than trying to make ourselves into a constantly happy person, we need to understand the dynamics of our moods. Ironically, it is often from our worst moods and most shameful behavior that we learn the most.

TEMPERAMENT

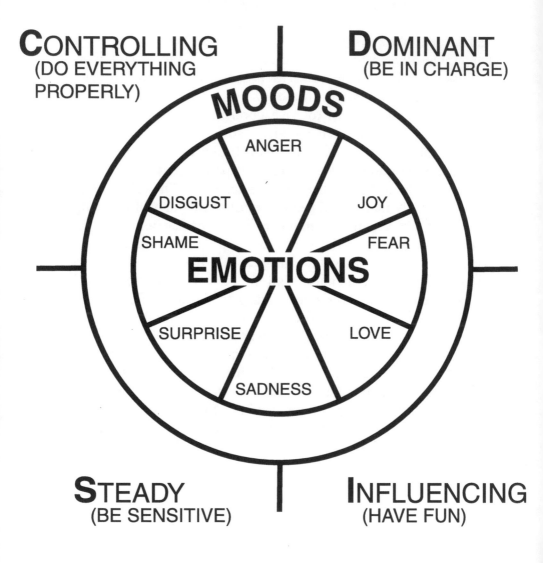

Emotions, Moods and Temperament
Figure #1

Emotional Hijackings

Debby, the kids and I drove from Pennsylvania to Atlanta to attend the 1996 Summer Olympics. We had planned the trip for two years and had a packed itinerary. The first leg of the trip was a nine-hour drive to the Great Smoky Mountain National Park in Tennessee. The children seemed to be constantly arguing, and I was stressed about all the details of the trip. On the second day, as we were driving through the magnificent beauty of the National Park, the kids were yelling and slapping at each other. I felt my lousy mood intensify. I bellowed, "That's enough!" at the top of my lungs as I slammed on the brakes and shoved the transmission into "park." Unfortunately, I put the vehicle into "park" while we were still moving and that only made me madder. I jumped out, ran around the minivan and jerked open the sliding door.

"I am sick and tired of your constant fighting and bickering! It ends and it ends now!" At that moment, Anna began to giggle, ever so slightly. I went nuts! "YOU THINK THIS IS FUNNY? ARE YOU TRYING TO MAKE A FOOL OUT OF ME?" I grabbed her arm and squeezed hard. Anna started to cry as the other two looked on in shock (this was not behavior they typically saw from Dad). Not a word was spoken as I got back into the car and drove to the motel.

As I drove, I calmed down, and my rational thinking began to work again. Anna's behavior that pushed me over the edge had not been a disrespectful laugh; it had been a nervous giggle. Anna was the sensitive, peacemaker of the group and did not deserve the treatment she had received. I did apologize, but we all knew I had allowed my bad mood to go too far.

The phrase "Emotional Hijacking" describes this type of behavior. I had allowed my strong emotions to take complete control of me for a short time. My rational thinking system seemed to just shut down, and I let my emotions totally dictate my actions. I did exactly what I felt like doing. And I was thoroughly ashamed of the result.

Most of us can relate to the concept of an emotional hijacking; we have experienced the rush of full-blown anger or fear or even joy. Most of us, at times, simply give in to a strong emotion and let it dictate our actions. Worksheet #13 quizzes you about emotional hijackings in your past.

I have known people who seemed to let their emotions completely control their responses in almost every situation. These folks are rarely boring, but can be a challenge. On the other hand, I have known people who seem to be devoid of emotions. They are always in control, but are deadly dull.

An over-reliance on our emotions leads to many life problems. When we give in to our emotional hijackings, we are rarely proud of our behavior. On the other hand, an under-reliance on emotions keeps us from living life to its fullest. To live without ever having experienced anger, joy, fear, love, sadness, surprise, shame and disgust is to barely live at all. So how do we find a happy medium? How do we obtain the maximum benefit from our emotions without going out of control?

Simply stated, we manage our thinking process just as we manage other areas of our lives. We need to learn to identify our emotions and use them productively. We can significantly improve our relationships with others by understanding and managing our own emotions.

Name: *John Miller*   Worksheet #13   Date: *3-17-00*

Emotional Hijackings

1. I recall the following incident when my emotions hijacked me:
    That time when the guy zoomed into the parking space in front of me and I went nuts on him. Threatening him with everything under the sun. I totally lost it.

2. My primary emotion in that incident was: ___*Anger*___.

3. Upon reflecting rationally on the incident, I recognize...
    I felt very foolish and embarrassed. I hope I never meet that guy again.

4. Did this incident change me in any way?
    In a way I think it did change me. I felt so foolish that I told myself I would never let something like that happen again. I have "lost it" many times since then, but never quite that totally.

5. What is the most recent emotional hijacking I can recall?
    When Nate sassed his mother just yesterday. I told him in no uncertain terms that he was not allowed to talk back to his mother, then he turned around and sassed me. I instantly was furious and started yelling at him and sent him to his room for the rest of the night.

6. My primary emotion in that incident was: *Anger*.

7. Upon reflecting rationally on the incident, I recognize...
    There was no reason for me to get so mad.

8. Overall, how do emotional hijackings affect my life?
    At work I keep things in pretty good control. If I have an outburst I usually know what I'm doing and use it for my advantage on the job. But at home I get angry with the kids more than I should. I need to do better with that.

CHAPTER 4

Your Memories

I have a great question for you. What is your earliest memory? Twelve year-old Alexey and I were talking one night before bedtime. I asked him his earliest memory and he quickly responded, "I remember coming down a long, dark tunnel with a bright light at the end." We both cracked-up laughing! His actual first memory wasn't so funny. He remembers being transported in an ambulance after being hit by a car (he was three years old). He remembers the darkness as the woman from the ambulance crew covered his eyes (he had a nasty gash near his eye). He was yelling and thrashing around, and the paramedics had to hold him down so he didn't aggravate his injuries. He remembers his arm hurting as they held him still.

Earliest Memory

My own earliest memory contrasts with Alexey's. I am three or four years old and playing outside on the sidewalk with my childhood pal Mike Bingeman (who is now a CPA and does our taxes). The sun shines brightly in a clear blue sky on this warm summer day. I just got up from a nap and am wearing only underwear and a tee shirt. Bingy is pedaling like mad on his tricycle as I stand on the back. The memory is like a short, vivid film clip which exudes peacefulness and pleasantness. Indeed in this memory, the world appears to be an inviting place.

Part of the value in recalling one's earliest memory comes from the overall feeling it evokes. People whose earliest memory is harsh, scary, etc. tend to perceive the world as a dangerous place. On the other hand, those who recall a happy, carefree memory tend to see the world as friendly and affirming. There is no right (or even preferred) type of earliest memory; the memories we have are those we have. By recalling and contemplating our earliest memories, we gain a clue about who we are and why we respond the way we do.

My own earliest memory accurately reflects my general view of the world. I tend to see goodness and affirmation even when it's not there. As I became an adult, I developed a slightly more realistic view of the world. Alexey being hit by a car as a toddler was a major event, causing me to see the world as a more dangerous place. It is ironic that this accident became Alexey's earliest memory. But then, this world is a strange place.

Just close your eyes and picture your first memory. What do you see? Can you recall how you felt during this event? Consider even the smallest details. If the memory is your own (as opposed to an incident you have been shown in a photo or told about) you will probably remember some odd, incidental details. Write down even the smallest details from this first memory. You can utilize the questions at the top of Worksheet #14 to assist in recording information about the memory.

Name: *John Miller*   Worksheet #14   Date: *3-19-00*
Earliest Childhood Memories
When recalling memories, ask, "Who?" "What?"
"Where?" "When?" "Why?" and "How?"

For example: Who was with you? What did they look like? What were they
wearing? What were you wearing? What were you doing? What else was going on? When was it? Where were you? How was the weather? How did you
feel? How strong is the memory?

1. My earliest memory is: *When I was about 4 yrs. old, I remember banging
   on nails with a hammer outside my uncle and aunt's house. My uncle and aunt were there. They were old. My aunt had on a dress, my
   uncle had on short pants with high socks and a short sleeved shirt.
   I just had on shorts, no shirt and I was barefoot. I remember ham-
   mering nails and banging away on a block of wood. I remember hitting my thumb with the hammer and crying like crazy. My uncle
   laughed at me and called me a "sissy boy." Seemed like it would
   have been late morning. I was outside their door at their house near
   Denver, PA. It was a very sunny day. I felt humiliated and mad at
   my uncle for laughing at me. I remember feeling embarrassed for
   not being able to use the hammer right. It is a very strong, vivid
   memory.*

2. Other early memories:

Childhood Memories

What if you can't recall early memories? No big deal; try another direction. Think about your happiest childhood memory. Don't just say, "I was happy when I played outside." Try to recall specific events when you felt joy. Write as much information as you can remember. You will probably be surprised by some of the small details that are stuck in your mind. I encourage you to take the time to record this information in Worksheet #15.

Along with pleasant childhood memories, try to recall several of your more painful ones. For many of us, these are much more vivid. A word of warning is necessary here...if your past had significant trauma (severe abuse or humiliation), please proceed cautiously. Overwhelming feelings can be unleashed and drive an unprepared person into deep despair. Consider the use of a qualified counselor in such cases.

Memories, Memories, Memories

Finally, consider your entire life up until today. What are your most joyful memories? Which ones bring a smile? What are your most painful memories? When were you most hurt, embarrassed, or humiliated? How about memories of special days, family gatherings, or holidays? What was the best day and the worst day of your life? What about everyday, commonplace events?

It takes an investment of time to complete this exercise. I recommend that you gather mementos from your life prior to beginning. As you sit amidst your old yearbooks, report cards, family photos and other assorted memories, you may feel a strange mix of emotions. Don't worry, that's a good thing, there is power in those emotions.

Name: *John Miller*   Worksheet #15   Date: *3-19-00*

Strongest Childhood Memories

When recalling memories, ask, "Who?" "What?"
"Where?" "When?" "Why?" and "How?"

1. My three most pleasant childhood memories are:

   a.   *Getting ice cream after little league baseball games.*

   b.   *Driving with my dad and a bus full of people going down to see the Baltimore Orioles play.*

   c.   *Building dams in the creek with my best friend Jim.*

2. My three most painful childhood memories are:

   a.   *When Grandpa Long would get drunk and say real mean things to Mom.*

   b.   *When Tonto, our pet German Shepherd was run over and killed by a car.*

   c.   *When the kids in first and second grade made fun of me saying, "John, John, uses the John" over and over.*

> Since John tends to be a no-nonsense kind of guy, these Worksheets are somewhat annoying to him. He thinks, "Why waste my time on the past? I can't change anything in the past, so there's no use thinking about it." Yet even as he writes several of the memories, he feels some surprising emotions stirring him.

You can record your memories either low-tech or high-tech. If you choose the low-tech route, take a 3-ring notebook with plenty of paper and divider tabs. Organize it chronologically. For example, make tabs for "Infant/Toddler/Pre-School," "Elementary School," "Jr. High School," "Sr. High School," "Late Teen/Early 20's" and "Adult." As you look though your mementos and reflect on your past, write down what comes to mind.

The high tech method uses the Microsoft Office 2000 version of Access Database. The software (which you can download free from www.pelger.com) allows you to input your memories into a simple database. You can search and sort the memories based on dates, emotions, relationships, humor, key words, etc. If you have access to Access (sorry), I recommend you record your memories directly into the database. You will obtain a treasure for the future.

Regardless of whether you choose high tech or low tech, please take the time to embark on this process of recording memories. You won't regret it. You may, though, have trouble getting the memories to start flowing. Perhaps the following subjects will help jog your recollections.

1. Arts	10. Over-night experiences
2. Athletics	11. Parents/Siblings
3. Dreams	12. Pets
4. Dysfunctions	13. Proud moments
5. Embarrassing moments	14. Recess/lunch
6. Friends	15. Religious experiences
7. Grandparents	16. Sexual interests
8. Holidays	17. School
9. Humorous moments	18. Vacation

You may remember certain friends from elementary school that you have not thought about for years. A special teacher may come to mind. Perhaps a funny story will be recalled or a particularly embarrassing moment. Just jot down the ideas, in no special order, as they flow through your mind.

You may wonder, "Why spend all this time on something I can't change." True, we cannot change the past. However, past events shape us not only by what actually happened but also by our impressions, beliefs and memories of what happened. Remember though, memory of any past event is not necessarily absolute truth; it is simply our impression of the way things were.

Two illustrations from my own life may be helpful here. I loved sports as a child. So I decided to go out for midget baseball though I really didn't know much about it. The coach put me in right field (the location where the least number of balls are likely to be hit). I recall standing out there in right field with my hands hanging at my sides. I would be out there daydreaming when all of a sudden I would catch movement out of the top of my eyes and spring into my ball-catching position. Unfortunately, the movement I saw was normally a bird flying overhead. No memories of "Glory Days" here!

I also recall making an Appalachian dulcimer (stringed musical instrument) in my grandfather's wood shop when I was 17 years old. I loved the challenge of making the dulcimer, and it turned out very well. I spent hours over the next few years trying to learn to play. I practiced hour after hour and never became proficient. I had neither an ear for music nor any sense of timing. It took me years to reach the conclusion that I wasn't going to be a musician.

Recently, I thought about these two memories, along with several others, and observed a trend. I generally have a strong character trait for perseverance but often head off in directions where I have no aptitude. I have spent much time struggling to succeed in areas where an impartial observer could have easily told me that I had limited likelihood for success. This review of my past helped me uncover a personal "gem of understanding" -- I need to carefully consider my own strengths and weaknesses before heading off in a new direction.

This may seem like a trivial conclusion, but I benefited greatly from it. I now consciously consider my aptitude prior to undertaking a new direction. Often the simple discoveries help us most.

Don't worry if the memories you write seem insignificant or do not immediately make sense. It may take awhile for you to spot trends from your past. But remember --- you are embarking on a journey for truth, and only a fool would expect to find all the truth in a few weeks.

As you record these memories, try to recall the emotions you felt at that time. List a primary emotion with each memory. The combination of memories and emotions can provide great insights for your life.

Of course not all, nor even most, childhood memories will give you great insight. Go through the effort anyway! At the very least, you'll have assembled a fascinating bunch of stories. Perhaps one of those memories that doesn't seem significant now, may be quite helpful in several years. From a personal standpoint, I'm not sure of the significance of my earliest memory -- being chauffeured on a tricycle in my underwear by a future CPA -- but perhaps time will tell.

As I reviewed my list of memories, I discovered one you'll enjoy. Jim Singer was my best friend in high school. We acted goofy, like most 16 year-old boys. We were insensitive louts, with a dash of self-obsession and a bunch of hormones thrown in. We lived the motto, "If you can't laugh at other people, who can you laugh at?"

Speech class seemed an easy course, so we both took it. The teacher assigned a ten-minute prepared speech on any topic. I don't remember my speech but I surely recall the one Singer gave. "I had a dog," Singer began as he stood in front of the class. "His name was Spot. Spot ran away. Here Spot. Here Spot..." Singer kept repeating, "Here Spot" as he walked out the classroom door. I still remember his voice fading away as he walked down the hall. We waited silently, then we began to laugh. After ten minutes, we heard Singer coming back down the hall, "Here Spot, Here Spot, Here Spot..." He came back in the class and took his seat amidst cheers and laughter.

The teacher, of course, was not laughing. She was livid. She escorted Singer to the Principal's office. She wanted to flunk him for the entire year. The Principal tried to be supportive of the teacher, but couldn't keep the big smile off his face. Singer failed that speech and went on to become a computer programmer. And I get a good laugh every time I think about that story.

Take the time to record your memories! You'll remember things you haven't thought about for years and benefit from the effort.

Name: *John Miller*   Worksheet #16   Date: *3-19-00*

Recalling Memories: Infant/Toddler/Pre-school

When recalling memories, ask, "Who?" "What?"
"Where?" "When?" "Why?" and "How?"
(Anger, Joy, Fear, Love, Sadness, Surprise, Shame, Disgust)

l. Drawing pictures on the side walk with many different colors with my friend Bill. (Joy)

2. Making clay pots down by the stream and drying them in the sun. (Joy)

3. Getting in fights with my friend Bill and pulling each other's hair and kicking at about 5 yrs. old. (Anger)

4. Feeling afraid when my sister and I went to sleep upstairs because the attic door was in our bedroom. (Fear)

5. Having the little kid from down the street come visit and being a pain in the neck. (Disgust)

6. Grandpa Bob's big smelly face right next to mine at holidays and Grandma being real nervous and worried. (Shame)

Name: *John Miller*   Worksheet #17   Date: *3-19-00*

Recalling Memories: Elementary School
When recalling memories, ask, "Who?" "What?"
"Where?" "When?" "Why?" and "How?"
(Anger, Joy, Fear, Love, Sadness, Surprise, Shame, Disgust)

*l. My first day at first grade was a disaster. I got lost, I cried, I hated it.
(Shame)*

*2. I always hated going on the school bus. There were always a couple of
bully kids that made life miserable. (Fear)*

*3. I remember really liking art class every year in elementary school, cause I
could draw pictures better than anyone. (Joy)*

*4. I always liked gym class cause I was always one of the fastest runners.
(Joy)*

*5. My favorite teacher was in fourth grade, Miss Krebbs. Before I had her I
was really nervous because everyone called her "Crabby Krebbs," but she
was so kind and thoughtful and she really seemed to believe in me.
(Surprise)*

*6. I remember Dad coming home from work and Mom complaining how bad
we were that day. Dad would make us line up, pull down our pants and whip
us with his belt. Not just a slap or two, but real hard and over and over. The
anticipation was horrible. I hated him for being so unfair, for not even both-
ering to find out what actually happened. (Anger)*

Name: *John Miller*   Worksheet #18   Date: *3-19-00*

Recalling Memories: Junior High School
When recalling memories, ask, "Who?" "What?"
"Where?" "When?" "Why?" and "How?"
(Anger, Joy, Fear, Love, Sadness, Surprise, Shame, Disgust)

l. When I got to junior high, I really felt out of place. (Shame)

2. We took a family vacation to Disney World, which I don't remember that well, but it was a lot of fun. (Joy)

3. I was on the junior high track team. I ran sprints and I liked it. I didn't win too often but I was often in the race. (Joy)

4. I didn't have any girlfriends, but I did have Jim Long for a friend through that time. (Joy)

5. My older brothers (Bob and Steve) were in high school and sometimes would take me along to football games. It was great when they would take me. (Love)

Name: *John Miller*   Worksheet #19   Date: *3-19-00*
Recalling Memories: High School
When recalling memories, ask, "Who?" "What?"
"Where?" "When?" "Why?" and "How?"
(Anger, Joy, Fear, Love, Sadness, Surprise, Shame, Disgust)

l. Tenth grade was a major year of change for me. I started to drink beer and smoke pot. (Shame)

2. My first girlfriend, Linda Kime, was in the spring of 10th grade. I couldn't think of anything else. (Love)

3. I got my license in the summer and I bought an old 1963 Chevy Impala for $300. (Joy)

4. I worked at a restaurant as a busboy enough to pay my gas and insurance. (??)

5. I remember going to parties in my junior and senior years. We would get so drunk we could hardly stand. (Shame)

6. Stopped going to church somewhere in 11th grade. (Shame)

7. In 12th grade I realized I better start thinking about something to do after high school. I thought about college, but since nobody in our family ever went before, I didn't buck the trend. I was sick of school anyway, but I didn't know what I wanted to do. (Fear)

Name: *John Miller*   Worksheet #20   Date: *3-19-00*

Recalling Memories: Late Teen/Early 20's
When recalling memories, ask, "Who?" "What?"
"Where?" "When?" "Why?" and "How?"
(Anger, Joy, Fear, Love, Sadness, Surprise, Shame, Disgust)

1. After graduation, I got a job as a carpenter's helper at the construction company where Dad worked. I liked the work and was pretty good at it. I got along well with the guys and the foremen often tried to get me on their job (that was a nice feeling). I learned to be a real good carpenter. (Joy)

2. I partied a lot. Sometimes I'd work all day, drink all night and work the whole next day. (Joy)

3. I met Rachel at a party in July when I was 20. I clearly remember looking across the room and seeing her. My first thought was, "Man, I'd like to nail her!" Real romantic, huh? (Love)

4. We dated for 2 yrs, then she got pregnant with Nate and we got married. (Love)

5. I settled down pretty much after we got married. (Surprise)

Name: *John Miller*   Worksheet #21   Date: *3-19-00*

Recalling Memories: Adult
When recalling memories, ask, "Who?" "What?"
"Where?" "When?" "Why?" and "How?"
(Anger, Joy, Fear, Love, Sadness, Surprise, Shame, Disgust)

1. Nate and Katie being born were probably the 2 most important things that ever happened to me. (Love)

2. I still work for Commercial Contractors, Inc. and they made me a Project Superintendent 2 yrs ago (the same year I turned 30). (Surprise)

3. I remember the first time my dad came on my job as a carpenter. It felt kind of weird. (Surprise)

4. Rachel and I went to the Bahamas on an all expenses paid trip from a vinyl siding company. We had a great time -- laid around on the beach, snorkeled, and made love in the ocean. We really seemed connected down there. At home Rachel often complains that I am too "distant" from her and the kids. She says I work too much and when I'm not working, I am thinking about work. Maybe she's right. (Joy & Sadness)

CHAPTER 5

Understanding & Managing Relationships

"All happy families are alike, each unhappy family is unhappy in its own way."
  Leo Tolstoy's opening sentence in <u>Anna Karenina</u>

Reflecting on my memories has led me to a conclusion: my life would be empty without relationships. I treasure my relationships with my parents, children, siblings, extended family, friends, and co-workers. Even acquaintances from school, people that picked me up hitch-hiking, people I picked up hitch-hiking, waitresses, taxi drivers, people that gave me directions when I was lost (a rather large group), and so many more have enriched my life.

Our relationships connect us to the rest of the world. If we lack joy in our relationships, we will lack joy in life. Therefore, we must put forth the effort to understand and manage our relationships.

Relationship Bank Account

Before we look at specific relationships in our lives, let's consider a helpful tool. Steven Covey presented this concept in <u>The Seven Habits of Highly Effective People</u> and I found it useful. I call this simple concept the "relationship bank account."

Think about a particular relationship in your life, perhaps with your spouse. Imagine that every interaction you have is like a bank transaction. Some interactions are like deposits in the relationship bank account. Things like courtesy, kindness, honesty, and integrity, make deposits. Of course, you also have negative interactions, which are withdrawals in the relationship bank account. Withdrawals occur through acts of unkindness, harshness, not keeping commitments, etc. Many transactions are neither positive nor negative and do not affect the account balance.

If you awaken and whisper lovingly, "Good morning dear, you are so beautiful!" (and you mean it) you have made a deposit in the relationship bank account. If you growl, "Oh man, your breath stinks!" you have made a withdrawal. As we are kind, even in small ways, our relationships tend to improve. Trust grows.

On the other hand, as we act with disrespect and rudeness, interrupting others and slighting them, even in little ways, we are withdrawing from the account. When the balance reaches zero or goes into the red, trust is gone.

Several years ago, I supervised two employees who hated each other. They needed to work together, but because of some petty jealousies, problems with compensation, etc., they simply could not stand each other. We talked about their problems and discussed the relationship bank account concept. We agreed they could either learn to work together while hating each other or build some sort of positive relationship. They both decided they would try to keep track of the transactions in the relationship bank account.

It was amazing to see their relationship grow as they both became aware of extending small courtesies, keeping commitments, etc. Of course, there were times when they made withdrawals, when their emotional thinking system overrode the rational and they spoke quick, harsh words. However, because of their efforts, these brief battles did not escalate into a full-scale war. With effort on both their parts, they developed a fine working relationship. In fact, a mutual respect and a friendship grew that continued beyond the workplace.

Withdrawals tend to come naturally for most of us; I know they do for me. Perceived insults to my self-esteem make me want to strike back, to take my "deserved revenge." None of us needs lessons in how to make the withdrawals from our relationship bank accounts. Let's consider some actions, though, which can make valuable deposits.

1.   Keep your word. It's amazing how many times people make a commitment and don't follow through. Integrity precedes trust. That means we need to do what we say we are going to do. We need to strive to keep our word, even in the smallest things.

2. Show small courtesies. The little things in life always add up to be the big things. The small courtesies that cost very little can change everything. As we open the door, bring a small present, or say thank you, we connect with others more than we realize.

3. Make a serious effort to understand the other person. Few people know how to listen these days. Most people only wait for the other person to stop talking so they can jump in with the response they've been busy formulating. Focused listening makes a big deposit in the relationship bank account.

4. Apologize when you make a mistake. We're all going to make many mistakes. If we sincerely apologize, we can usually turn a withdrawal into a deposit.

Worksheet #22 asks about a relationship in your life. I think you'll agree the concept of a bank account works well to track the status of a relationship. The relationship deposits and withdrawals are monitored and tallied. Even if you don't keep track of the balance in the account (i.e. ignore the status of the relationship), the balance is a reality.

I remember in my earlier years I often overdrew my checking account. The bank would send an overdraft notice with a fifteen dollar service charge. I would be indignant about the charge and go to the bank to argue it away. I was too self-absorbed to realize it was my mistake. I needed to pay for my mistakes. When we become overdrawn in our relationships, we often have a similar response. We blame someone or something else; we try to maneuver out of the situation or we ignore it.

Since Debby took over our banking many years ago, we have fewer overdrafts. She also arranged for bank overdraft pro-tection, which provides automatic coverage in the event we spend more money than is in the account. Of course, this protection is only available because some level of trust has been established between the bank and us. Our relationship bank account operates much the same way. Trust is absolutely necessary.

Functional and Dysfunctional Families

Let's consider the relationship between parents and chil-dren. Most of us have first-hand knowledge about the parent-child relationship. We grew up in a family with one or two par-ents. Some families operate smoothly with lots of love while other families are constantly in crisis. What do you think helps create the "happy family" that Leo Tolstoy writes about in Anna Karenina? What separates functional families from dysfunctional families? A highly functional family encourages personal growth. Physical, intellectual, emotional, and spiritual needs are met.

Name: *John Miller*   Worksheet #22   Date: *3-25-00*

Relationship Bank Account

1. Choose a significant relationship.
    Spouse. Rachel and I.

2. In what ways have I made deposits into this relationship bank account?
    When I talk to her and tell her what I am thinking about.

2. In what ways have I made withdrawals from this relationship bank account?
    Brooding.
    Not bothering to call and tell her that I'll be late from work.

4. How has the other person made deposits into this account?
    Active lovemaking.
    When she cooks a special meal for me.

5. How has the other person made withdrawals from this account?
    Letting the house stay messy, just not getting her jobs done.

6. Overall, how would I describe this relationship account balance?
    (overdrawn, small balance, medium balance, large balance)
    Small balance.

Children are prepared to handle the responsibility that comes with adulthood. Most of us would agree there are not too many highly functional families. For the sake of discussion, let's say that 5% of families consistently operate in this manner.

Then there are the highly dysfunctional families. In these families, one's needs are not met, growth is not encouraged, and kindness seems to be non-existent. In the highly dysfunctional family, the parents tend to ignore or even show contempt to the child. In these families, abuse is so pervasive and evil so prevalent, it overwhelms. Perhaps 5% of families operate in a highly dysfunctional style.

The remaining 90% of the families (in which the vast majority of us grew up) operate somewhere in between. The degree to which needs are met in a family, or the degree of functionality, can be illustrated by a bell curve (See Figure #2).

The interesting thing about this bell curve is that most of us tend to see our own home situation as "normal." We may know better intellectually, but in our gut, we still see our own childhood as the norm from which to measure other families. Our emotions tend to override our rational thinking here. We benefit from realistically evaluating our family relationships and striving for objectivity.

M. Scott Peck uses an interesting example in The Road Less Traveled. Peck describes a situation where a six-year old child chatters away to a parent. The parent has several response options:

1. Forbid the child to talk.
2. Allow the child to talk but don't listen.
3. Pretend to listen, saying things like, "Uh-huh," "Umm," or "Yeah."
4. Selectively listen, i.e. pay attention if you hear a phrase that seems important.
5. Truly listen.

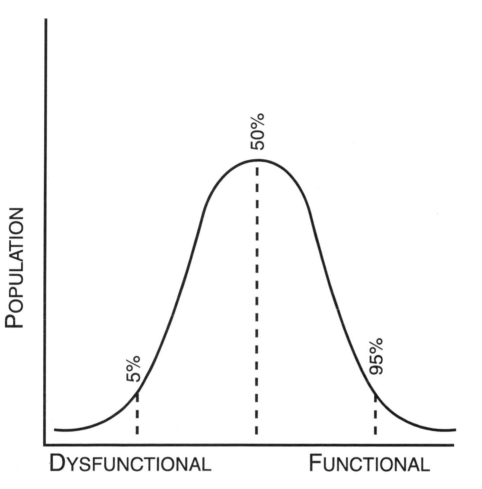

Bell Curve of Functional and Dysfunctional Families
Figure #2

Which of these methods is best? If you think #5 must be best, I challenge you to think again. Consider a circumstance which may make each of these methods appropriate. For example, if a friend calls you on the phone and threatens suicide, it would be most appropriate to forbid your child to talk so you could completely focus on the needs of your friend. Or, if you are driving a car during a blizzard, you may choose to simply let your child talk and not listen since you must focus totally on driving.

There are certainly times when I finish a difficult work day, sit down to relax and read the newspaper, and merely grunt my responses to the kids. I enjoy those few minutes of relaxation and the children don't seem permanently damaged. Perhaps as I relax, I pay more attention and pick up on an important phrase. Of course, in any healthy relationship, there must be times of true listening. However, a healthy relationship does not require constant listening. Humans cannot operate at that level all the time.

Many believe a highly functional parent-child relationship must have minimal conflict. We need to challenge that idea. A lack of conflict or a tensionless state rarely indicates a healthy relationship; it more likely indicates repressed emotions. Humans have natural conflicts. The way we deal with those conflicts determines the level of functionality of our relationship. A functional family doesn't always act, "nicey nice and kissy face." They encourage personal growth.

When I took our pre-school children to the park to play, each one of them wanted to climb on the large pieces of playground equipment. Other parents lifted their children onto the equipment, but I told our kids they needed to learn to climb up on their own. It was very difficult for me to watch our toddlers struggle and fail. They wanted to get up there and play and would get frustrated when they could not. I would encourage them and even try to show them how, but I would not lift them.

It would have been easier for me and for them if I had simply placed them on the equipment. It would certainly have seemed "nicer" on my part. However, I strongly believed (and still believe) that children benefit greatly by trying, failing, getting frustrated, and trying again. After they learned the tricks of climbing each piece of equipment, they scampered up and down like little monkeys. The children whose parents had lifted them onto the equipment were still requiring assistance.

The essence of successful parenting lies in this concept of allowing our children to make decisions, fail, deal with the failure, and try again. This process builds character. In a highly functional family, the children learn perseverance and hope from many different lessons. With these two traits, children are prepared to tackle other problems successfully in the world.

The parents in a highly functional family also strive to identify strengths, weaknesses and gifts of their children and help them find their best direction in life. These parents humbly put aside their own preconceived desires and choose instead to encourage their children in the direction that best fits their abilities and interests.

For example, a surgeon father who loves his vocation and loves his son, naturally wishes that the son would also choose to become a surgeon. The father knows the path is difficult, but the rewards are many, both financially and personally. He believes he could perhaps make the path a little easier for his son. And, of course, the father can envision a future time when he and his surgeon son will discuss cases and spend time together. These are normal, loving desires in a father.

However, in a highly functional family, the father must go beyond his natural hopes to an honest evaluation of the situation. Perhaps the son has no interest in medical things. From an early age he has loved to build things: tree houses for himself and his friends and complicated dams in the stream. And he has loved to take things apart and put them back together. He hates school. Learning has never come easily for him.

The father realizes, through careful observation, that it is unlikely his son will become a doctor. In fact, the father has to consciously struggle with his own pride (e.g. "All my children have attended the best colleges"). He concludes that carpentry training at a trade school would be best for his son, leading to his highest fulfillment, happiness and success. The path is obviously much different from the path the father preferred, but therein lies the lesson.

The highly functional family struggles to help its members find the course which best suits their gifts, nature, and personality. Abraham Lincoln said, "When I die, I want it said of me, 'He plucked a weed and planted a flower wherever he thought a flower would grow.'" Effective parenting requires more than just effort (plucking weeds and planting flowers), it involves determining where flowers will and will not grow and planting accordingly.

Parents in a highly functional family go beyond loving their children. Effective parents observe, study and play with their children in order to help them discover their talents, skills and abilities. A careful interaction with one's children provides clues and hints. Effective parenting requires effort to find how the child might distinguish and feel good about themselves. Through this, the child establishes his or her own positive identity.

Few families live up to the preceding descriptions of highly functional families. Think back to the bell curve; the highly functional family is the top 5% of all families. It is therefore unlikely that you grew up in such a family. The purpose of defining the highly functional family is not to make us feel bad; the purpose is to help us better evaluate our own family experiences.

The highly dysfunctional family is probably more familiar to most of us. We have seen families where the selfishness and laziness of the parents appall us. The children are treated with contempt (if they are noticed at all). Their potential is ignored and their capabilities are never considered. These parents abuse, neglect, and tyrannize their children. Being around a highly dysfunctional family makes my skin crawl. I just want to get away and breathe clean air again.

Worksheets #23 and #24 ask probing questions about our relationships with our parents and our children. I encourage you to take some time and deeply consider these Worksheets. Truly understanding our relationship with our parents and our children is foundational to understanding ourselves.

Relationships with Family and Friends

We considered relationship bank accounts and parent/child relationships. Now we move on to other relationships: friends, co-workers, siblings, other relatives, enemies, acquaintances, spouses, etc. Most of us have many significant relationships. These relationships are critical to our emotional health. I'm amazed how little effort we normally put into understanding our relationships.

I grew up in a family with three older sisters and a younger brother. My relationship with my brother Jim exemplifies how a relationship can change. Jim is seven years younger than I am, and we had an odd relationship while growing up. I don't recall playing with him very much. I usually played with kids my age or older. I mostly ignored Jim but occasionally paid attention to him in order to torment him…normal family stuff.

As I look back, I realize Jim had a troubled adolescence, although I was not paying much attention at the time. I vacillated between ignoring him and treating him harshly in order to help him "build character." We were both self-absorbed and not really close to each other. One amusing event stands out in my memory.

One cold winter day, Jim, our nephew Mick, and I were all out in the woods behind our house. An activity Jim and I enjoyed doing together was sapling climbing. The goal in sapling climbing is to pick a small tree (trunk diameter about 2" to 4") and climb up the trunk, hand over hand, as high as you can. At some height the sapling tree starts to bend. At that moment, you hold on tightly and throw your legs out to the side. As the tree bows, you get a ride back to the ground.

Name: *John Miller*   Worksheet #23   Date: *3-26-00*

My Relationship with My Parents

1. Thinking of my relationship with my parents when I was a child, I would describe it as:
    Things were kind of tense most of the time. We never knew when Dad was going to yell at us or smack us. His moods varied a lot. Mom tried to smooth things out.

2. Thinking of my relationship with my parents when I was an adolescent, I would describe it as:
    Dad stopped hitting me but he would belittle me when he was mad. I just tried to stay out of his way and away from home as much as possible.

3. Thinking of my relationship with my parents when I was an adult, I would describe it as:
    Better. Dad has mellowed some and I think he is proud of my success at work. Mom sure loves to spend time with her grandkids.

4. I am most grateful to my parents for:
    They provided for me.

5. What do I wish my parents had done differently?
    Dad's drinking, of course, but also I wish we had spent time together doing something.

6. How much fun and play occurred with my parents?
    Not much.

7. How was discipline handled in my home?
    Mom did none and Dad just reacted to his moods. To tell the truth, it was lousy.

8. What is the level of trust in this relationship?
    I guess at this point it is OK.

9. Overall, how do I rate the effectiveness of the family I grew up in?
    Mildly Dysfunctional

Highly Dysfunctional	Mostly Dysf.	Mildly Dysf.	Mildly Functional	Mostly Functional	Highly Functional

Name: *John Miller*   Worksheet #24   Date: *3-26-00*
My Relationship with My Children

1. Thinking of my relationship with my children when they were young, I would describe it as:
   I am more distant than I would like to be. I love them very much.

2. Thinking of my relationship with my children when they were adolescents, I would describe it as:
   NA

3. Thinking of my relationship with my children when they were adults, I would describe it as:
   NA

4. My children are most grateful to me for:
   They just seem to love me because I'm their Dad (which is a great feeling).

5. What do my children wish I had done differently?
   Spend more time with them, play with them more.

6. How much fun and play occurred with my children?
   Some, but not as much as there should be.

7. How was discipline handled in our home?
   Rachel and I mostly agreed on discipline. We spanked from the time they were toddlers, but never hit them any place except on the butt.

8. What is the level of trust in this relationship?
   Fairly high.

9. Overall, how do I rate the effectiveness of our family?
   Mildly Functional

Highly Dysfunctional	Mostly Dysf.	Mildly Dysf.	Mildly Functional	Mostly Functional	Highly Functional

If the tree is too small, it bows too soon and that's no fun. If the tree is too large, you have to climb very high and, if it just doesn't bend, you have to climb back down (to the ridicule of others). The right size tree, though, is truly wonderful. You climb higher and higher, begin to get afraid and then the tree bows and gives an exhilarating ride back to earth. Jim, Mick, and I loved to go sapling climbing.

This particular winter afternoon, we had tried a few saplings and had not had any really good rides. I spotted a tree I thought might be too thick, but decided to give it a try. As I climbed higher and higher, I felt fear in me. Jim and Mick were yelling, "Come on. Just a little more!" The tree started to bow and I was ready to throw my legs out to the side to ride down. But something happened different this time.

Since it was so cold, the sap was frozen and the tree trunk snapped at ground level. I didn't hear the snap and didn't get my feet pointed toward the ground. I fell quickly and landed flat on my back on the ground with a THUD (I remember the THUD!). As I immediately began to sit up, the tree trunk came down and hit me right in the middle of the forehead. At this point, Jim and Mick were rolling on the ground in laughter. They did manage to gasp out, "Are you OK?" I just lay there on that frozen ground trying to get my breath. It was not too long till we were all laughing at the improbability of that sapling trunk hitting me square in the forehead.

I am grateful that in my family we learned to laugh at ourselves and not take ourselves too seriously. Over the years, Jim and I laughed at that memory and at many other funny things that happened to us. As we became adults, our relationship grew in mutual respect. As we both struggled to become responsible men, we came to appreciate each other more and more. We now have a loving and affirming relationship (which still has plenty of laughter in it). Where there was no bond, there is now a relationship which gives us both great joy.

Jim and I changed our relationship slowly. Usually we weren't even aware of the changes. As we became adults, we both wanted a closer relationship, and both took some small steps in that direction. We made a point of staying in touch, we talked about work and family issues, we spent time together. I always loved my brother in a family sort of way; now I love him as a close friend.

As stated earlier in this chapter, we must find joy in our relationships in order to find joy in our lives. Worksheet #25 will quiz you about a relationship with a significant person in your life. It could be your spouse, a brother or sister, a co-worker, a friend or whomever.

Friendship is the glue that bonds relationships together. I have observed over the years that many people simply do not know how to be friends. Like many skills, though, we can both teach and learn it.

Building friendship requires that we become interested in the other person and desire their good. A man focused on himself cannot be a good friend. Ironically, a man focused on himself will not even be a good friend to himself.

Think about a friend whom you truly enjoy. That friend probably listens to you and appreciates you. We all love that! Con artists rely on this fact to ply their trade; they understand that people want to be listened to and appreciated. A con artist develops the ability to quickly endear himself to another person. Then, he uses that trust to take advantage of the other person. The con artist feigns friendship in order to selfishly manipulate others.

If we are going to cultivate friendships, we must become interested in the other person and desire their good. This idea sounds simple and natural, but my experience indicates that it is neither. Abiding friendships do not just happen. We need to work at them.

Name: *John Miller*   Worksheet #25   Date: *3-26-00*

My Relationship with Another Person

1. Choose an important relationship to examine:
    a. This relationship is with...   *Bobby Miller*
2. How did it begin? (When, where, why?)   *When I was born.*

3. How has it changed? (When, where, what, how much, why?) *As kids I would tag along whenever I could. I tried not to be a pain to him and usually he and his friends didn't mind me being around. I still look up to him.*
4. What has been the high point of this relationship? *One night about two years ago we went out for a few beers, he said how proud he was of how I was doing with my job and family.*
5. What has been the low point of this relationship? *When I was a senior in HS and he smashed his car and wanted to use mine. I wouldn't let him.*
6. What attributes does this person value? *Goodness, commitment, caution.*
7. What is the central focus of this person? *Work.*

7. What are the main needs in this relationship? Mine? His/hers? *Mine: to get approval and to be close. His: to help guide me and to be close.*
9. How well are the needs met? Mine? His/hers?   *Fair.*
10. Who has control in this relationship? *Bobby.*

11. What is the level of trust? *I'd say the trust level is high.*
12. What is the level of tolerance? *Neither of us is overly tolerant.*
13. Is there any fear of being abandoned? *I worry about him just leaving.*
14. What happens when someone screws up? *We just avoid each other for awhile.*
15. How much play & fun is in this relationship? *Some, but not that much. I wish there was more.*

> John Miller decided to examine his relationship with his older brother, Bob. While this was certainly an important relationship in his life, he was aware that he understood little about it, and knew it was not as strong as it should be. John had little contact with his oldest brother, Steve who had moved out of the area years ago, but John saw Bobby a few times a year.

16. Does this relationship help me grow as a person? *Yes.*

17. On a scale of 1-10, how do I rate this relationship?   *7*

My wife Debby and I now have a wonderful friendship which we both treasure. This was not always the case. In the early years of our marriage, we hit a time when we could barely tolerate each other. I remember the sense of drifting further apart and not really knowing what to do about it. I was playing one-on-one basketball with a good friend, Bruce Spicer, and we discussed the situation.

Bruce gave me some great advice: "Ned, when you're interacting with Debby and feeling angry, think about what you plan to do or say next, and then do the opposite." At first this seemed like nonsense; how could I benefit by doing the exact opposite of what I felt like doing? The idea seemed silly, but it did stick in my head.

The next few times Debby and I were having a skirmish (since she would never actually fight), I remembered Bruce's advice. If I felt like saying, "Fine!" and walking out of the room, I would stay and continue to talk. If I wanted to use logic to "prove" my point, I would try to just keep my mouth shut. The results were amazingly positive; our relationship improved almost immediately (although we still had a long way to go).

I've never really understood why this advice worked. Perhaps the mere act of stopping my natural response in the middle of a dispute and considering other options is a positive move. For whatever reason, that piece of advice helped Debby and me to get beyond the stage we were in and move toward a deep, abiding friendship.

If you have a loving relationship with your spouse, you are well aware of the great joy and peace that comes with that love. If you do not have that type of relationship, don't despair. Loving relationships do not spring up effortlessly; they come from understanding, working hard and taking emotional risks.

Relationship with Yourself

In order to build loving relationships with others, we need to have some understanding of our relationship with ourselves. To be a friend to others, as we discussed above, we must be interested in them and wish for their good. The same concepts apply in our relationship with ourselves.

It seems obvious that we would be interested in ourselves, that we would have an extraordinary level of interest in our own affairs. However many people do not appear to be very interested in their own lives. I think of the mother who slavishly devotes herself to her family, so no sacrifice is too much. The mother trades any interest in herself for an increased interest in her family's welfare.

I have seen many people who live with an apparent lack of interest in their own welfare. It reminds me of the saying, "She's a woman who truly lives for others, and you can tell the others by their hunted looks." If you do not have a reasonable amount of self-interest, you will be neither a friend to others nor a friend to yourself.

Of course, at the other side of the spectrum are those people who have an inordinate amount of self-interest. These folks consider every situation from the sole viewpoint of, "How does it affect me?" People that are completely self-absorbed are exasperating. To such narcissists, other people do not really matter. In fact, nothing really matters except the protection of their precious self-image.

Narcissists perpetrate many of horrible, evil acts in this world and often do not view their victims as fellow human beings. We have a friend who was raised by a narcissistic mother. Our friend endured a horrible childhood, at the hands of the one person who was supposed to love and protect her. She was forced to stand for hours with her face exactly 2 inches from the wall; when she moved she was beaten. When this mother became irritated with her daughter, she would grab scissors and chop off her hair. Narcissistic parents humiliate their children. For these parents, nothing seems to exist except themselves, their moods and their all-important self esteem.

If we live without paying any attention to our own needs, we err. If we live completely absorbed by our own needs (as a narcissist), we are also wrong. As in so many areas of life, the correct path appears to be the middle road.

As mentioned earlier, a strong, positive relationship needs two components. First, one needs an appropriate level of self interest. Next, one must wish for one's own good. One need not take the middle path when wishing for one's own good, though. People should be very interested in their own future good. You may think everyone would want their future to be full of good things, happiness, joy, etc. However this is not always the case.

Think about a person that seems to have so much going for them, yet always chooses relationships with people who have major problems. This person always dates a substance abuser or someone who is out of work ("although it's not their fault") or just someone who is creepy. I observe that many people choose relationships which an impartial observer (me, in this case) could easily point out will bring them sadness and hurt.

Why do some people choose to embark on relationships with those that will hurt them? I don't know the answer to that question; I do know these situations are common. Therefore, we need to consider the extent to which we wish our own happiness or unhappiness. Worksheet #26 examines this issue.

Relationship with God

We have examined our relationships with other people and our relationships with ourselves, now we investigate our relationship with God. We must understand this personal area of our lives to find the joy we desire. Let's start with an example...

Name: *John Miller*   Worksheet #26   Date: *3-29-00*

My Relationship with Myself

1. How interested am I in myself? On a scale from totally uninterested to totally narcissistic, where do I fall?
    I think I am fairly interested in myself and my own well being.

2. Describe a situation, event, or story that illustrates my level of self-interest.
    When I get a job performance evaluation (which isn't too often), I get very defensive about any criticism.

3. To what extent do I wish for my own good (my future happiness)?
    As I think about it, I don't really wish for my future happiness that strongly. I just am so busy with things of today.

4. Describe a situation, event, or story that illustrates how I desire my own good?
    I am so focused with my job on any given day that I rarely if ever even think about the future. It seems to take all the energy I have just to do a half decent job getting through the day.

5. Do I like myself? *Sometimes.*

6. What is my self-image?
    To be honest, I see myself as a failure in many areas.

7. Does this self-image seem consistent with the reality of my life?
    I do better than I give myself credit for, generally. I probably think of myself as worse than I actually am.

8. How well do I nurture my physical body and my mind?
    I have a good bit of self-control in my diet and staying in some kind of shape. I don't know what I do to nurture my mind.

9. How much responsibility do I take for myself and for the rest of the world?
    Too much.

10. On a scale of l-l0, how do I rate my relationship with myself? *5*

Most everyone has read about the tremendous struggles Abraham Lincoln had during his years in the White House. The Civil War was raging, soldiers were dying by the thousands, and everyone in the country seemed to want something different from him. President Lincoln worked one of the most challenging jobs during one of the most difficult times in history. Lincoln wrote about the way in which he faced those difficulties: "I must confess that I am driven to my knees by the overwhelming conviction that I have nowhere else to go. My wisdom and that of all about me is insufficient to meet the demands of the day."

Lincoln was a brilliant man who turned to God in prayer because the problems he faced were overwhelming. Now Abe Lincoln had not been a church-going man. He had been accused of infidelity to religion during one of his early political campaigns. He responded to the charge with the following, "That I am not a member of any Christian Church is true, but I have never denied the truth of the Scriptures; and I have never spoken with intentional disrespect of religion in general." This cagey response fended off the true charge that Abe did not go to church.

Abraham Lincoln matured as a person and turned to God for wisdom and direction because the answers he needed were not found anywhere else. While he often had quoted the Scriptures for political expediency, for years Lincoln appeared to not have much of a relationship with God. In his most difficult times, however, Lincoln learned to come to God for guidance and direction. Lincoln discovered and developed a personal relationship with God. The extent of that relationship was between him and God.

President Lincoln superbly met the demands of his day. Many people believe he was the most effective U.S. President in history. Yet, he was ridiculed and despised by many of his contemporaries. Abraham Lincoln appears to have struggled with God and man, yet he completed the task history laid upon him.

Few of us deal with issues the size of Abe Lincoln's. Nevertheless, our problems can seem insurmountable. We all confront difficult situations that seem to have no solutions. I have met thousands of people in my life and never met one who did not have problems that:

1. Seem large.
2. Have no simple solution.
3. Are a source of concern to them.

If you have such problems, then the concept of consulting God should at least be considered as an option.

What is your current relationship with God? Worksheet #27 quizzes you about this. Some of these questions you may have considered many times; others you may have never thought about. As you fill in the worksheet, I recommend writing the answer that first comes to mind. The purpose is to determine how you perceive God at this point in your life.

Name: *John Miller*   Worksheet #27   Date: *3-30-00*

My Relationship with God

1. When was I first aware of my relationship with God? (How, where, why?)
    I was about 10 or 11 years old and Mom   took us kids to Sunday School and church. I remember singing in the children's choir and feeling so close to God. I guess I really believed then.
2. How has this relationship with God changed? (When, where, what, how much, why?) *Just lost interest as I hit my teen years, too much other stuff going on. Rachel insists that we all go to church together now, but to be honest, it doesn't really mean much to me. It's just another obligation I have to fulfill. I wish it was different from that.*
3. What has been the high point? *When Nate and Katie were born, I truly felt how amazing God's creation is.*
4. What has been the low point? *I don't know that there is a low point, it seems I just kind of go along.*
5. How active is God in my life? *Not very, as far as I can tell.*
6. What does God expect from me? *I have no idea.*
7. What do I expect from God? *For things to be fair. (although I don't really know why I would expect that)*
8. What is the most terrible personal tragedy I can imagine? *For Rachel, Nate and Katie to be killed in a car accident.*
9. How would I view God if this tragedy occurred? *I would probably go off the deep end, take a rifle and start killing people.*
10. How much joy is there in my relationship with God? *Not much, since I don't relationship with God. I am just so busy, there isn't time for everything.*
11. On a scale of 1-10, how do I rate my relationship with God? *2*

> When John Miller filled out Worksheet #27 he did not like it one bit. He rarely thought about God. He did go to church with Rachel and the kids, but it was routine and didn't affect him much. He did not meditate on God as he sat in church, or at any other time. John was uncomfortable looking critically at his relationship with God and putting those observations on paper.
>
> John sees himself as a practical person who gets important things done. He sees most other people as ineffective boobs who don't get things done. The idea that his relationship with God may be an important thing that he is ignoring disturbs him. John wonders, "If I wanted to improve my relationship with God, how would I go about it?"

Was this worksheet difficult? Few of us spend much time talking or even thinking about our relationship with God. Nevertheless we probably have some sort of relationship with God and that leads us to the question, "If I were to try to improve my relationship with God, how would I go about it?"

One learns to know God better by the basics of study and prayer. This process has been called the inward journey. There are risks involved in this journey: we may discover our own shallowness or inadequacy or we might have to face our lack of commitment and hypocrisy.

We start by reading the Scriptures, we start by spending some time each day in prayer (even though it feels so very odd), and we start by thinking more about the nature of God. We really do not need any complicated plan, we merely need a desire to begin and a commitment to keep at it when it gets a bit difficult or boring.

To improve your relationship with God, some time should be spent with Him daily. Start by finding a book that you think may be enlightening (for me that would be the Bible) and read it for 10 minutes each day. Obviously, read longer if you have the time or inclination.

This discipline helps provide direction for our inward journey. The books we choose to study should challenge and make us think. Don't believe something just because someone you respect says it or you see it in print. Be critical and always analyze for the truth. So few people examine what they read for truth and thereby are deceived.

I recently saw a woman who had a look of misery in her eyes. I had known her well in happier times, when she found joy in her husband and small children. This woman had an interest in the inward journey and went to her minister for help. Unfortunately, her minister was a self-centered, evil man who was more interested in seducing this woman than leading her to truth. This minister fed her "feel-good lies" which ultimately destroyed the family unit. After the divorce, the minister dropped out of the picture, and all that was left was a big pile of misery where previously there had been love.

Please do not embark on the inward journey lightly, as some sort of lark that may prove to be interesting. If you choose to proceed with the inward journey, include study as part of your plan. Study utilizes both our rational thinking and our emotional thinking. Rational thinking allows us to critically analyze the accuracy of the material and decide whether we believe it or not. Our emotional thinking process utilizes our intuition and sensitivity to help us evaluate the practicality of a passage.

Over time, studying produces results. We strengthen our faith because we think it through. The different things we study and read build on each other to further our level of understanding.

The process of studying and learning about the nature of God must be more than just an intellectual experience, though. To truly learn about God, we must come to know God. If we want to get warm, we must stand near the fire. If we want to know God, we must spend time in prayer. During time in prayer, we communicate directly with God.

If you were not raised in a religious tradition or taught how to pray, the entire idea may seem foreign to you. Prayer really is quite simple. Take some time, quiet yourself, and begin to tell God the things that are important to you as you would to a good friend.

Don't expect prayer to instantly feel natural or soothing; it probably will not. When I decided to spend some time each day in prayer, I set the egg timer for 10 minutes and got down on my knees. Those were the longest 10 minutes in my life. This was a new experience and everything felt odd. In the first few weeks, my mind would wander, I would fall asleep, or the time would pass agonizingly slowly.

As I developed the habit of prayer, though, things began to change. The time began to pass quickly and I often felt a deep connection with God. Of course, my mind still wanders sometimes, and occasionally I fall asleep. But prayer has become a special time of connection with God, and I usually emerge from it refreshed and ready for the challenges of the day.

There are five basic types of prayer. You may want to keep these five categories in mind to help guide you through your time of prayer.

- Prayer asking for **forgiveness** for things you have done or have not done
- Prayer of **thanksgiving** for the blessings you have received
- Prayer of **intercession** asking God to help others
- Prayer of **petition** asking God to help you with your own problems
- Prayer of **praise** to God because He is God

Sometimes it seems that nothing happens when we pray. Everyone who prays experiences this feeling. When we persevere, though, we will look back and realize things have changed. Prayer, like discipline, can only be appreciated in retrospect.

Since prayer changes things, it carries one great risk: we will not remain the same. As we embark on this inward journey of study and prayer, we must be aware that it will change us. Remember the words of Oswald Chambers, "The battle is lost or won in the secret place of the will before God, never first in the external world." If we desire to have a relationship with God, we must start on this inward journey and anticipate changes.

The Psalmist wrote, "Be still and know that I am God." Our relationship with God can be nurtured and improved just as our relationship with our spouse, children, and friends can be. It takes effort and sincerity, but we can do it. We must work at it just as we would at getting our bodies in shape for an athletic competition. This inward journey requires our best effort.

Worksheet #28 asks specific questions concerning what you think about God. It will serve as a benchmark from which you can measure your changes or growth. Perhaps you never considered some of the questions before and you probably never gave written answers to them. Don't be overwhelmed by this worksheet, simply work through it and put in the answers that first occur to you.

This chapter on Understanding and Managing Relationships has covered a tremendous amount of material. Our relationship with others, ourselves and God are huge topics. Obviously we can not totally explore every aspect of these relationships. However, we can begin the process of gaining a better understanding of them.

The anticipated joy of improved relationships motivates us to change our lives. Later, we will return to the information in this chapter to further assist this process of change. But first, we need to consider a few more issues.

Name: *John Miller*   Worksheet #28   Date: *3-30-00*

How would I describe God?

1. Is God active in the world? *Yes, I think so.*
2. Is God active in my life? *Yes.*
3. Do I trust God to protect me? *No.*
4. Is God loving toward me or is God harsh? *Mostly harsh, I think.*
5. Is God judgmental of me? *Yes.*
6. Do I ever feel joy in my relationship with God? *Not really, not that I can think of.*
7. Do I ever feel a strong sense of belonging to God? *No.*
8. Do I clearly know right from wrong? *Absolutely.*
     a. Do I know what God wants from me? *No, not really much at all.*
   c. How do I know what God wants from me?

9. Is there a force of evil in the world? *There sure seems to be.*
10. What happens when people die? *I don't know, but I don't think we just stop existing.*
     a.   Is there a heaven? If so, how do people get there? *I think so. By being good.*
     b.   Is there a hell? If so, how do people get there? *Probably. By being bad.*
11. On a scale of 1-10, how would I rate my faith in God? *5*
12. On a scale of 1-10, how would I rate the certainty of my convictions? *1*
13. Which of my actions glorify God? *Treat Rachel and the kids well.*
14. Which of my actions show rebellion towards God? *Ignoring him, I guess.*

15. Do I pray? If so: *Not really.*
     a. Where do I pray?
     b. How often do I pray?
     c. How long do I pray?
     d. What do I think about the value of my prayers?
16. Do I study any religious text? What text? How often? *Not really.*
17. Do I believe God forgives my mistakes? *No.*
18. What do I give to God? *Some money in the church offering (not sure that gets to God!)*
19. What does God give to me? *Don't know.*
20. When I feel discouraged, how do I feel about God? *Lousy.*
21. When I am in a crisis, how do I feel about God? *Don't usually consider God.*
22. When I feel great, how do I feel about God? *Don't usually consider God.*

Story by Leo Tolstoy

"That Whereby Men Live"

Throughout this book, I include several paraphrased short stories written in the late 1800's by Leo Tolstoy, a Russian author. The stories are quite captivating! A great author manages to touch our soul and teach us more about ourselves.

If you don't enjoy reading fiction, skip to Chapter Six. On the other hand, if you take the time to read these stories, they will entertain and enlighten. The story that follows moves me every time I read it. It's truly amazing.

A shoemaker named Simon lived with his wife and children in a farmer's house. He did not have a house or land of his own and supported himself and his family by shoe cobbling. Since food was expensive and work was cheap, they barely made ends meet. The shoemaker and his wife had one sheepskin coat between them and it was a ragged one at that!

For two years, he had been saving up to buy a skin for a new one. By autumn, he had saved a small sum. He had three rubles and he was owed five rubles and 20 kopecks from farmers in the village. So one morning after breakfast, he got ready to go to the village to collect his money and to buy sheepskins. He thought to himself, "I'll get the five rubles I am owed by the farmers, add those to the three I have here, and buy sheepskins for a sheepskin coat."

As he went into the village, he stopped at one farmer's house. The farmer was not home, but his wife promised to send her husband with the money in a week. He went to the house of another and the farmer swore to God that he had no money. He gave him only 20 kopecks for mending his boots. The cobbler thought perhaps he could go to the fur dealer and buy the sheepskins on credit.

But the fur dealer had another idea. "Bring the money first," said he, "and then take what you like. We all know how debts mount up."

So the shoemaker did not get his coat nor collect his money. He only got the 20 kopecks for mending the boots and he took away another pair of old boots for resoling.

Depressed at the result, he went and spent the 20 kopecks for a drink of vodka and set off for home without his sheepskins. While he had been cold in the morning, he now felt quite warm, even without a fur coat. He walked along hitting the frozen snow clods with a long stick and swinging the boots by the laces with the other hand.

As he went, he talked to himself, "I'm warm without a sheepskin coat; I've drunk a thimbleful of vodka and it skips all through my veins. So a sheepskin coat is not necessary after all. Here I go and forget all my troubles. That's the sort of fellow I am. What do I have to worry about? I can get along without sheepskins. I don't need them. There's one thing though...that wife of mine will fret. She'll say, 'It's a shameful thing that you do a job for someone and then let him lead you by the nose."

He could imagine his wife telling him that they must have money to buy bread. "The farmer grinds his own flour to make bread," she will say. "They certainly can find the few rubles to pay us. Our bills go on no matter what."

The shoemaker went on until he came to a church. He looked at the church as he was passing by and saw something strange. "What is that? A stone?" he thought. "No, perhaps it's a cow." But it was not a cow either. It looked like a man, but it was all white. As he got closer, he saw that it was a man, sitting naked, leaning against the church. He could not tell if he was alive or dead. The shoemaker felt quite odd. He said to himself, "Robbers must have killed this man, taken his clothes and pitched him here; don't mix yourself up in this."

So the shoemaker went on. As he was passing by, though, he saw the man begin to move. The shoemaker became more afraid. "Should I go up to him or should I keep on walking?" he said to himself. "Oh some evil is going to come of this. Nothing good has brought him here. He'll probably leap at me and choke me and do me in. And even if he doesn't, what can I do with a naked man? I can't give him the last rags off my back. I just have to pass by, that's all." And the shoemaker quickly passed by.

Slowly, his conscience began to bother him and the shoemaker stopped in the middle of the road and looked back. "I wonder what it is with that fellow," he said to himself. "What are you doing, Simon? Here is a man, dying in misery and you get scared and run by. Have you grown so rich that you need to guard against having your valuables stolen? Shame on you Simon, this won't do!"

So he turned back and approached the man. As he did so, he saw he was a young man and in the prime of his life. He also saw that he had no marks of violence on his body. He just seemed very cold. As Simon reached him, the young man lifted his head and opened his eyes wide and looked at Simon's face. That made Simon feel better. Simon threw down the boots, unclasped his belt and began to take off his outer coat.

"Come, stand up," he said. "You must have something to put on," and he helped the man put on the coat and the boots. Simon thought about taking off his cap, but he looked at the man's full head of hair and thought, "I'm bald all over, I think I need this more than he does."

With the man thus clothed with the boots and the coat, Simon said to him, "Now brother, get up and walk and get yourself warm. Things like this can't be helped. Are you able to move?" The man looked at Simon in a friendly way, but said nothing. "Why don't you speak?" said the shoemaker. "We can't spend the winter here. We'll go home to my lodgings; take my stick to lean on if you feel weak. Come on, let's go."

The man started and walked easily enough without lagging behind. As they walked, Simon asked him, "Where are you from?"

"I'm not of this place," he said.

"So I see, because I know everyone who lives here. How did you come to be here?"

"I may not tell you," replied the man.

"I suppose the people here treated you badly."

"Nobody has treated me badly, but God has punished me."

"Yes, indeed. God is everywhere and he puts his hand upon us. But where would you like to go?"

"It doesn't matter to me," replied the man.

Simon was amazed. The man was gentle in speech, not like a robber and he would give no answers about himself. Simon thought, "One knows little of the things that go on in this world."

"Well, come to my lodgings and you can go on your way later," said Simon.

As they walked together, the stranger easily kept up. The wind was rising now and blowing through Simon's shirt and the drink had begun to wear off. Simon felt quite cold. As he wrapped his thin shirt around him he thought, "So, this is what my sheepskin trip has come to. I went out for sheepskins and am returning without even my coat and bringing back a naked man. Matrina will not be pleased, I'm afraid." But yet, when he looked at the stranger and remembered the look on his face when he first went to him, his heart somehow leapt for joy.

Simon's wife finished her duties early that day. She had chopped the firewood, brought in the water, fed the children, had something to eat herself and then began to think, "Should I make bread today or tomorrow? There is still a piece left. If," she thought, "Simon gets here for supper and doesn't eat much, the bread will last till tomorrow." She turned the piece over looking at it and finally decided, "I won't make bread today. There is only meal enough left for one loaf. We can last another day."

As she put the bread down and began to sew a patch on her husband's shirt, she wondered how he had made out getting sheepskins for the coat. "I do hope the sheepskin seller won't cheat him," she thought. "But that man of mine is so simple. He never cheats anyone himself, but he is like a little child in many ways. Eight rubles...that is no small amount of money. We should get a good sheepskin coat for that. I went through last winter the best I could without a sheepskin coat. I really couldn't go anywhere when it got cold. We were almost prisoners in the house. It's a long time coming for this coat. I hope Simon gets back soon. I hope nothing bad happened to him."

As Matrina was thinking over these things, she heard a noise outside. Someone was coming. Matrina stuck her needle in her work and went into the passage. She saw two people there: Simon and some sort of man without a cap and in felt boots. Matrina immediately noticed the breath of her husband. "Yes," she thought, "he's been drinking." And then, when she saw that he was without his long coat, in his shirt only and was carrying nothing in his hand, she got hot.

"He's drunk away the money," she thought. "He's been wandering around with some bum and now has brought him home with him." Matrina let them go into the room and looked at the stranger. He was young and the coat he had on was their own and he stood right where he first came in, neither moving nor raising his eyes.

Matrina thought, "He's not a good man. He's afraid."
Matrina just stood there and stared at them, wondering what they
would do next. Simon took off his hat, sat down on the bench as if
everything was fine.

"Well, Matrina, give us some supper, let's go!"

Matrina grumbled to herself, but kept standing by the oven
as if she never heard him.   First she looked at the one and then
she looked at the other, but she only shook her head.

Simon said to the stranger, "Sit down brother. We'll have
some supper." And the stranger sat on the bench next to Simon.
"Have you cooked anything that you could give us?" said Simon
to his wife.

Then temper got the better of Matrina. "Yes, I have cooked
something," she said, "but not for you. You, I can see, have
drunk your senses away. You go out to buy sheepskins and you
come home without even your coat. And with a naked bum in tow
as well. I have no supper for drunkards like you."

"Come, come Matrina. Don't talk so silly. You should have
first asked who this man is."

"Well suppose you tell me. What have you done with the
money?"

Simon took his coat, pulled the three rubles out and
unrolled them. "Here is our money," he said. "The farmers did
not have the money to pay me."

This only made Matrina madder. She snatched the money
from the table and ran to hide it. "I have no supper for you. I
can't feed every naked drunk who comes along."

"Now, now Matrina. Hold your tongue. Give people a
chance to explain."

"What sense is going to come from a drunken fool like
you," she replied. "I should have known better than to marry a
tipsy brute like you. My mother gave me some things and you
drank them all away. You go out to buy a sheepskin and you
drink that away too."

Simon tried hard to explain to his wife that he had only
drunk 20 kopecks worth and that he had found the stranger by the

church. But she interrupted him on every turn bringing up issues that were ten years old. She got madder and madder as she talked and finally grabbed his shirt and said, "Give me that. That's mine. I have nothing warm to wear. May you die of a fever!"

Simon took off the shirt and handed it to her. As Matrina went to go into the other room, she stopped. Her anger was subsiding and the truth is, she wanted to know who this man was. Therefore she said, "If the man was honest, he wouldn't be sitting there without a shirt on his back. And if you had been up to any good today, you would have told me at once where you picked up this friend of yours."

"Very well," said Simon, "I'll tell you now. As I was passing a chapel, I saw this man lying naked and frozen. It's not summer time, you know, that a man should go naked. I knew that he would die if I left him there. What could I do? Such things do not happen for nothing. I took him, clothed him and brought him here. That's all. Don't be mad, Matrina. To give way to it is sinful. Remember that we must all die someday."

Matrina was ready to burst out again when she glanced at the stranger and decided to remain silent. He was sitting there motionless, on the edge of the bench, with his hands clasped to his knees, his head sunk to his chest, his eyes closed.

"Matrina," went on Simon. "Is there nothing of God within you?"

When she heard these words, and glanced at the stranger again, she suddenly felt compassion. She turned to the door, got the teapot and the last piece of bread and served the men some food.

"Eat away," she said. Simon nudged the stranger. "Come up here," he said. "Let's have some food."

When Matrina saw the stranger's face, she had to smile. She felt a certain indescribable joy. After supper, as she washed up things, she asked him, "Where do you come from?"

"From somewhere other than here," he replied.

"Then how came you to fall by the wayside?"

"I cannot say."

"Who was it who took your clothes from you?"

"God was punishing me."

"But you were lying there naked?"

"Yes, I was lying there naked and frozen when Simon saw me and had compassion on me. He took his coat, put it over me and told me to come with him. And you have kindly given me food and drink. May God do so unto you also."

Matrina got up and went back to her sewing. "Here," she said, "since you have no shirt or pants, put on these."

As Matrina and her husband went to bed, she could not get the stranger from her thoughts. They had eaten their last crust of bread. They had nothing for tomorrow. She had given him shirt and trousers. In a way, she felt angry with herself but then she remembered the stranger's smile and her heart jumped within her. She lay there unable to sleep.

"Simon."

"Yes?"

"We have eaten our last piece of bread and I don't have anymore. What shall we do tomorrow? I must beg some of the neighbor."

"Oh, but we shall manage to live and have enough," said Simon.

For a little while, his wife lay there without speaking. "He seems a very fine young fellow," she said. "Only why does he tell us nothing about himself?"

"He cannot, I suppose."

"Simon."

"Yes."

"We give things away, but why does no one give to us?"

Simon was at a loss for an answer, but remarked, "We can talk of that another time," and he turned over and went to sleep.

In the morning when Simon awoke, the children were still asleep and his wife had gone out to borrow some bread. The stranger was sitting on the bench alone, dressed in the old shirt and trousers from yesterday with his face turned up. His face was even brighter than it had been the night before.

Simon said to him, "Well, my good friend, the stomach craves for some bread and the body for some clothes. We must work to earn it. Do you know any trade?"

"No, none," replied the stranger.

Simon was rather surprised at this and said, "But you would try, would you not? A man can learn anything if he tries."

"Yes, men work and so also will I."

"What is your name then?"

"Michael."

"Well Michael, you do not tell us anything about yourself and that is your own affair, but we must earn our living. If you work, I will teach you and we will feed you."

"The Lord be good to you. I will learn, only show me how."

So Simon began to show him the trade of shoemaking.

"The trade is not difficult," he said. "Watch me."

Michael watched and followed each step and understood immediately. By the third day, he was able to work as if he had been a cobbler all his life. He never made mistakes and he ate very little. Only at times, he would stop for a moment and silently look upwards. He never went outside, never spoke of his own affairs and never joked or laughed. Indeed the only time he had been seen to smile was on the first evening, when Matrina had got him some supper.

Day followed day and week followed week and soon a year had passed. Michael still lived with Simon and worked for him. It became known that Simon's workman could sew better than anyone. And so, Simon's business increased.

One cold winter day, Michael and Simon were sitting together working, when a three-horse sleigh came to them. The two shoemakers looked through the window and saw that the sleigh had stopped and a gentleman in a fur coat stepped out and walked towards Simon's dwelling.

Matrina ran to open the door and the gentleman bowed his head as he came in and his head nearly touched the ceiling, he was so tall. He seemed to fill the whole corner of the room. Simon rose to greet the man. The gentleman breathed hard, took off his fur coat and sat on the bench.

"Which of you is the master boot maker?"

Simon stepped forward saying, "I am your honor."

Then the gentleman shouted to his footman, "Hey, Vedka, bring me that leather here!" The footman entered with a parcel and laid it on the table.

"Untie it," he said. When the footman did so, he showed the leather to Simon. "Look here boot maker, do you see this?"

"Yes sir, I do," answered Simon.

"And do you know what it is?"

Simon felt it for a moment and said, "It is good leather."

"Good leather, indeed!" cried the gentleman. "You knothead, you have never seen such leather as this in your life. It is German leather and it cost 20 rubles."

Simon was intimidated by this. "Yes, well what chance do folks like us get to see such leather?" he answered.

"Could you make me a pair of boots out of it?"

"Perhaps, sir," stammered Simon.

"Perhaps! You must clearly understand what you're going to work on and what you're going to make of it. I want a pair of boots that will last a year, that will never tread over and not split at the seams. If you can make me such boots, then set out to work at once. But if you cannot do these things, tell me beforehand because if these boots split or tread over in a year, I'll throw you into prison. But if they do not fail, I will pay you 10 rubles for your work."

Simon hesitated and did not know what to say. He looked at Michael and asked him. "What do you think about it, brother?"

Michael nodded to say, "Yes, take the work."

So Simon obeyed Michael and undertook to make this pair of boots that would not tread over or split within a year. Simon went to measure the man's feet. He carefully marked it on a piece of paper so as not to spoil the gentleman's sock. He measured first the sole and then the in-step and was going to measure the *calf. But the strip of paper would not go around it for the muscle of the gentleman's leg was as thick as a beam.*

"Take care not to make them too tight in the leg," remarked the great man.

So Simon measured it carefully.

"Who is this you have with you?" the gentleman asked.

"This is my skilled workman who will sew your boots."

"Look you," said the gentleman to Michael, "and remember this. You are to sew them so that they will last a year."

Simon glanced at Michael and saw that he was not so much looking at the gentleman as staring into a corner behind him as though he was gazing at someone. Michael gazed and gazed till suddenly his face broke out into a smile and he brightened all over.

"What are you grinning at, you fool?" cried the gentleman. "You had better see to it that the boots are ready when I want them."

To which Michael replied, "They shall be ready whenever wanted."

"Very well." The gentleman put on his boot again, buttoned up his fur coat and headed for the door. He forgot to bend his head and smacked it against the lintel. He swore violently, grabbed his head, jumped into his sleigh and drove away.

"What a man!" remarked Simon. "He nearly knocked the lintel out of place with his head. Yet he hardly minded."

"How could he not get hardened with the life he leads," replied Matrina. "Even death itself could not take such a rock of a man."

"Well, we have taken the work now," said Simon to Michael "and we must take care not to make a mistake. This leather is valuable stuff and the gentleman is quick tempered. There must be no mistakes. You have the better eyes and the better skill in your fingers, so take the measures and cut the stuff while I finish my work."

Michael took the leather obediently and spread it out on the table, folded it in two and began to cut. Now Matrina happened to approach Michael and saw what he was doing. She was astonished. She was well acquainted with the shoemaking art and she realized he was not cutting the leather into an ordinary boot shape but into rounded pieces. She felt inclined to say something but thought to herself, "It must be I who doesn't understand how a gentleman's boots ought to be made. Michael must know better than I do so I won't interfere."

When Michael finished cutting the shapes, he began to thread them. Not in boot fashion but as you sew the shoes that you put on the feet of a corpse. Matrina was even more surprised at this but still said nothing. Michael went on sewing until suppertime. Then Simon arose and walked over to Michael's bench. He saw, that from the gentleman's leather, Michael had made a pair of shoes to put on the feet of a corpse.

Simon groaned. "How is it," he thought, "that Michael has lived with me a whole year without making a mistake and now he makes this mistake! The gentleman ordered heavy-soled boots. Michael has gone and made these and spoiled the leather. How shall I ever settle things with such a gentleman? One cannot get leather like that everyday."

Then he said aloud to Michael, "My good fellow, what have you done? You've ruined me. The gentleman ordered boots but you have gone and made these instead." Just as he was about to tear into Michael, someone arrived at the door. Simon saw that a man had arrived on horseback and was tying up his horse. Presently the door was open and a footman from the very gentleman himself came in.

"Good day to you," he said.

"Good day. What can we do for you?"

"My mistress has sent me about the boots."

"Yes, what about them?"

"This indeed, that my master will not want them now. He has been dead some time."

"What do you say?"

"Yes, it's true. He died in the sleigh on the way home from your shop. We reached home and were just going to help him *out; we saw that he had slipped to the floor like a flour bag and breathed his last. There he lay dead. And it was only with great difficulty that we got him out of the sleigh. Then my mistress sent me, "Tell the boot maker that the gentleman who called to order the boots will now need a pair of shoes to put on a corpse. Wait until they are made and bring them back with you." So I came here at once.*

Michael gathered up the cuttings of the leather from the table and rolled them in a coil. Then he took the shoes, wrapped them against each other, wiped them with his apron and gave them to the footman.

Another year passed and again two more until Michael was now completing his sixth year with Simon. He still lived as he had before. He never went out, never spoke of himself and smiled only twice since he came... first when Matrina had given him supper upon his arrival and second when the rich gentleman had been there. Simon was well pleased with his workman and never returned to the subject of where he had come from. Indeed, his biggest fear was that he would go away again.

One day, they were all sitting together at home, when a woman came in with children. The one child was lame. As soon as Michael saw the children, he threw down his work and looked at them. This surprised Simon because Michael, as a rule, did not pay much attention to the affairs of others.

"Good day to you," said the woman.

"Yes, what can we do for you," said Simon.

"I want a pair of boots for each of my little girls to wear in the spring."

"Very well, madam, we have never made such small sizes, but it can be done. You can have the boots either leather throughout or lined with linen. Here is Michael, my skilled workman."

As Simon looked at Michael, he saw that he was sitting with his eyes affixed on the little girls. Simon was astonished. It is true they were beautiful little girls with black hair, rosy round cheeks and cute little shawls and jackets, but he could not understand why Michael looked at them as though he knew them. However, Simon went on talking to the lady and arranging the terms.

After they settled the terms, he went about making the paper measure for the boots. The lady lifted the lame little girl to her knee and said, "take both sets of measures from this little girl and make the one boot for a crooked foot and then the other three ordinary ones. The two children take the exact same size for they are twins."

Simon took the measures, then asked about the little girl. "How did she come to be lame? She is such a pretty little girl. Was she born so?"

"No, she was laid upon by her mother."

Matrina, hearing this, stepped closer. "Then you are not their mother?"

"No, in fact I am no relation at all. I only adopted the children."

"You are not their mother but yet you seem so fond of them."

"How could I not be fond of them? I raised them both. I had a child of my own once but God took it unto Himself. But yet I could not be any fonder of my own child than I am of these two."

"And whose are they?"

Then the lady went on to tell the story. "Six years ago, it happened that these two little girls lost both their father and their mother in the same week. Their father was buried on a Tuesday and the mother died on the following Friday. At that time, my husband and I were living nearby. The father of these children worked cutting down trees. One day when a tree was cut, it fell on him and crushed him. He was carried home but died immediately.

"His wife delivered her twins that week, these two little ones here. Poverty and loneliness, that is what they were born to. For the mother had no woman to help her with the birth. She was alone when the twins were born and she died in that bed. The next morning, I went over by chance for a neighborly visit and I

found her there, the poor woman, already stiff and cold, laying on the one little girl having crushed and bent her foot.

"I sent for help, washed the corpse and laid it out. We made a coffin for her and buried her. The little girls were left for orphans. I alone of all the women in the neighborhood was suckling a child. My little one was eight weeks old, so I decided to take the twins also.

"I began by feeding the uninjured child only since I did not expect the other one to live. Then I thought to myself, 'Why should this little one's angel spirit be left to fade away?' So, filled with compassion, I nurtured the two as I did my other child. All three of them at the same breast. I was young and strong and able to feed well and God had given me much milk. I would feed two at once while the third lay waiting. Then they would all be satisfied.

"Yet God did not have it that I should nourish all three children. I buried my own little one in his second year and God has never given me another since. Now my means have been increased and I have a good income and live comfortably but I have no children of my own. So, how could I ever bear to live alone without these little ones? Or how could I ever rest without them to love and care for? I can't even think about it. They are to me as wax is to the candle."

The lady drew the lame child to her and wiped the tears from her cheeks. "Surely the old proverb is true, without father or mother we may live, but without God, never."

Thus they talked for a while, after which the lady got up to leave. Her host saw her to the door and then glanced at Michael. He was sitting with his hands folded and he gazed intently upwards with a smile.

Simon approached him. "What is it, Michael?" he said.

Michael rose from the bench, laid aside his work and bowed to his master and his wife. "Pardon me good master and mistress," he said. "God has pardoned me, do you also pardon me?"

Then Simon and his wife saw that light was proceeding from Michael and bowed low. "Michael, I see you are more than an ordinary man and that I can not detain nor question you. Only tell me one thing. Why is it that when I first found you and brought you home you were downcast, but you smiled immediately when my wife offered you supper and became brighter thereafter? And again, why did you smile the second time when the gentleman was ordering the boots and became brighter than before? And lastly, why did you smile the third time and become bright all over when the lady brought the little girls here? Tell me, Michael, why you smiled those three times? And why is this light shining from you now?"

Then Michael answered him, "The light is shining from me now because I have been punished and God has pardoned me. And I smiled those three times because it was laid upon me that I should learn three things from God. And those three things I have now learned. The first thing I learned was when your wife had compassion upon me. That is when I smiled the first time. The second thing I learned was when the rich man was ordering the boots. That is why I smiled the second time. And the third and last thing I learned was when I saw the little girls. That is why I smiled the third time."

Then Simon said, "Tell me also Michael, why God punished you and what those three things of God may be that I too may learn them."

Michael answered, "God punished me because I disobeyed him. I was an angel in Heaven and disobeyed God. He sent me down to earth to bear away the soul of a woman. To earth I flew and saw there the woman lying sick, just having delivered the twins. The children were there beside their mother and she did not have the strength to put them to her breast. She saw me and understood that God had sent me to take away her soul. Crying she said, 'Angel of God, they have just buried my husband who was killed by a tree in the forest. I have neither sister nor mother nor grandmother, so there is no one to bring up my little ones. Do not take away my soul but leave me to feed and raise my

*children and set them on their feet. Little children cannot live
without father and mother.'*

"So I listened to the mother, laid one child on her breast,
and gave the other one in her arms, and ascended again to God
in Heaven. I flew to God and said, 'I could not take away the soul
from that mother. The father had been killed by a tree and the
mother just delivered twins. She begged me not to take her soul
away, saying, 'let me raise my children, rear them, and set them
on their feet. Little children cannot live without father or mother.'
So I did not take away the mother's soul.'"

"Then God said to me, 'Go and fetch away the soul of that
mother and you will learn three things. You will learn that which
dwells in men, that which is not given to men and that whereby
men live. When now you have learned these things, return to
Heaven.'

So I flew back to earth and took away the soul of the
mother. The child slipped from her breast. And the dead body
rolled back upon the bed, crushing as it did one of the little one's
legs. Then I rose above the village and tried to bear the soul to
God. But a wind caught me so that my wings hung down and
were blown from me. The soul returned alone to God and I
myself fell to earth by the roadside."

Now Simon and Matrina understood at last who it was they
had clothed and fed and taken in. They wept with fear and joy.
But the angel went on, "Thus I was left naked and alone in an
open field. I'd never before known human need, never before
known cold nor hunger, yet now I was a man. I was freezing and
hungry and I did not know what to do.

"Then I saw by the roadside a church built for God. I
approached God's building, hoping to take refuge there. But it
was barred and locked and I could not enter. Then I sat down
behind it to protect myself from the wind. Evening came and I felt
cold and hungry and in pain all over.

Suddenly I heard a man coming up the road, carrying a
pair of boots in his hands and talking to himself. And then, for the
first time since I became a man, I saw a deathlike human face.

The face seemed horrible to me and I turned away from it. But as I did so, I heard the man talking to himself about how he should protect his body from the winter's cold and feed his wife and children. I thought to myself, 'here I am perishing of cold and hunger while he is thinking about how he should clothe his wife and himself in sheepskin and feed himself and his family with bread. Surely I can look to this man for help.

"*The man caught sight of me and became still more horrible as he passed by. I was in despair. Suddenly, however, I heard him returning. I looked and could scarcely recognize him as the same man. In his face before there had been death, but now the face had suddenly come to life. And in that face I saw God.*

"*The man came to me, clothed me and took me with him to his home. As I entered his home a woman came to him and began to speak. The woman seemed even more dreadful than the man. The breath from her mouth was that of a corpse. And I was almost choked with the odor of death. She wished to cast me into the cold again. And I knew that I would die if she did so.*

"*Then all at once her husband reminded her of God and in a moment she became changed. When she had given us supper and was sitting there gazing at me and I gazed at her in return, there was no longer death in her face but life. And in her I recognized God.*

"*I remembered the first word of God, 'You will learn what it is that dwells in men.' I knew that the thing which dwells in men is love and felt that God had seen fit to reveal that to me. So I smiled for the first time. But I still had more to learn. I still had to learn that which is not given to men and that whereby men live.*

"*So I dwelt with you for over a year when the gentleman came to order the boots. They were to be, 'boots which will last a year without treading over or splitting.' As I looked at the man, I saw my comrade, the angel of death. No one but I saw that angel. Yet I knew him and knew that the sun would not set before the soul of the rich man would be required of him. And I thought to myself, 'Here's this man, making provision for a year from now, not knowing that he will not live out the night.'*

"Then I suddenly remembered the second word of God, *'You will learn that which is not given to men.'* Already I learned that which dwells in men, now I also learned that which is not given to men. What is not given to men is to know their own needs. Then I smiled the second time. I rejoiced that I had seen my comrade angel and God had revealed to me His second word.

"Yet I still had more to learn. I still had to learn that whereby men live. So I lived on and waited for the time that God would reveal this to me. During my sixth year with you, there came the woman with the twin girls.

I recognized the little girls and knew that they had been preserved alive. As I recognized them, I thought to myself, 'The mother begged me for her children and I listened to her, thinking that without father or mother the little ones would die.' Yet this woman, a stranger, has fed them and raised them. When I saw the woman moved to pity for the children and shedding tears for them, I recognized in her the living God and understood that whereby men live. I knew that God revealed to me his third and last lesson and had pardoned me. Then, for the third time, I smiled."

Suddenly the angel's form became stripped of clothing and he was robed only in light, so that you could not bear to look upon him. His voice became more resonant as though not proceeding from his mouth but from Heaven itself.

The angel said, "Yes, I learned that every man lives not by talking and not by taking thought of himself, but by love. It was not given to the woman to know what was needed for the preservation of her children's lives. It was not given to the rich man to know what was needful for his body. Nor will any man know whether the setting sun will bring need of boots or death shoes. When I was a man, my life was saved for me, not by taking thought for myself, but by the love which dwelt in the passerby and his wife. So that they could feel for me pity and affection. Again the two orphans were preserved alive, not by any thought *which was taken for them, but by the love that dwelt in the heart of a strange woman. So that she could feel for them pity and affection. For indeed, all men live, not by the thought which they may take for themselves, but by the love which dwells in all mankind.*

"I had known before that God gave life to men and desires them to live. Now I understood another thing. I understood that God would not have men live apart from one another but God would have men live together in unity. Therefore, God made men dependent on one another.

"Yes, I last understood that men only appear to live by taking care of themselves. But in reality they live by love alone. He that dwells in love, dwells in God and God in him. For God is love."

Then the angel sang a hymn of praise to God and the hut trembled with the sound of his voice. The roof parted in the middle and a pillar of fire shot up from earth to heaven. Simon and his wife and children fell down upon their faces in adoration. As they did so, wings burst forth upon the angel's back and he soared away into the sky.

When Simon opened his eyes again, the hut was as it had been before. There was no one there but his own precious family.

Wow! What a truly amazing story! I must admit when I read that story, a wave of emotion sweeps over me. Its power captivates me. The thought of "entertaining angels unawares" fascinates me. Do you think you may have come across an angel in your day-to-day living and not been aware of it? It seems possible to me. I believe much goes on in this world that we don't understand, and a story like this helps awaken my mind to the possibilities.

Worksheet #29 asks for your impressions of this story. Some of your responses may prove helpful in examining your own life.

Name: *John Miller*   Worksheet #29   Date: *4-1-00*

"That Whereby Men Live"

1. My first impression of the story is... *it doesn't seem too realistic.*

3. I related to the following character because...
   the character of the impatient man reminded me of my boss.

4. The story motivated or moved me in what way?
   The part about the lady's love for her adopted children was pretty moving. I can relate to loving children that much. The idea that God or his angels are involved in our everyday affairs is also kind of interesting. There is so much that I don't understand, I wish that I did have a better understanding of God.

5. Other impressions?

CHAPTER 6

Your Ancestors

When I was 17 years old, I found some old woodworking tools in the attic above my grandfather's garage. There were a table saw, jointer, sander, jig saw and lathe. These old tools fascinated me, so I carried them downstairs and decided to get them back into working order. I learned to enjoy using the woodworking tools. I made candle holders, Appalachian dulcimers, jewelry boxes, and other items.

One day as I was doing some work on the lathe, my dad came in and told me the chisels needed to be sharpened in order to cut better. He mentioned that my Uncle John, a craftsman who built grandfather clocks as a hobby, knew how to sharpen knives and chisels. Since our family was not the visiting kind, I had only seen Uncle John on a few occasions in my life. I wanted to learn to sharpen knives, though, so I called Uncle John and set up a time to meet with him.

I felt nervous going to Uncle John and Aunt Anna's house that night. As he led me back to his woodshop, Uncle John seemed a bit uncomfortable too. We simply did not know each other. I could see the skill in his hands as he showed me the basics of tool sharpening. I looked around his shop at the projects he was working on and gained great respect for his talents as a craftsman.

Then a strange thing happened. Uncle John, feeling more comfortable with me and perhaps sensing my respect for him, began telling me stories about his past. It was fascinating to listen to his life stories and to hear about the events that helped make him who he was. He was not a famous man and they were not dramatic stories, but they were true accounts. He told me the places he had worked, the things he had done and the interests he had. He told me about his parents and his upbringing. He showed me mandolins he had serenaded his wife with as a young man, and spoke of his children with affection and pride.

One particular story about his parents amused me. They were hard-working people who saved enough money to buy a new television set in the early 1950's (when all television sets were new). His father sat in their living room in front of their new TV, fascinated with this new-fangled device. Uncle John's mother came walking into the room in her nightgown and sat down to watch. Her husband said, "Mother, get a robe on!" It seems he drew the obvious conclusion that since he could see people on the screen, they could also see him. He did not want those men staring at his wife in her nightgown!

Uncle John, Aunt Anna, and I laughed hard at that story and enjoyed many others. We began that evening as strangers and built a bond that lasted until his death. Since then, I have spent many hours listening to relatives tell the stories of their lives, and it has been time well spent.

Family Stories

The lives of our parents, grandparents, and great-grandparents provide many clues for understanding our own lives. We gain important knowledge by investigating those who came before us. By listening to our ancestors' stories, chronicling them, and taking some time to reflect on them, we discover truths about our family that we never saw before. It is amazing how many times characteristics of a family are obvious to any casual observer, but not noticed by the family members. By considering your family's past, you gain an objective perspective.

We are not creating a detailed genealogy here (which can be tedious and difficult), but rather a collection of stories and interesting events. It should be fun and enjoyable. Talk to family members that are available and make notes regarding ancestors' names, significant dates, occupations, characteristics, and interesting stories. Worksheets #30 to #44 will help you gather this family information.

If you are comfortable working with a spreadsheet program, I have these worksheets in Microsoft Excel. The advantage of the spreadsheet program is the ability to see all the family traits for a specific category in one location. For example, if you fill in the blank for personality type for each of the four generations, the spreadsheet produces a chart illustrating all the personality types in your direct lineage. You can discover trends by viewing the information in this way that you otherwise may never notice.

While this exercise takes a bit of effort, if you put in the time, you will be delighted with the results. Begin by filling out Worksheet #30 (which lists your family tree to the fourth generation) with all the information you know. Next, call someone who knows information about your family and arrange an interview. Use Worksheets #30 to #44 as a basis for your interview. Try to do some other interviews utilizing these worksheets. Talk with anyone who can provide information about your ancestors.

Good sources of information may be your mother, father, grandparents, great-grandparents, aunts, uncles, siblings, or friends. If you are older, you may not find many folks who remember much, but probably there are a few. If you are younger, you likely have many sources of information. Don't be shy! I guarantee you will learn some valuable things, and you will get the added benefit of documenting family stories, which are great to tell children, grandchildren, and others.

You may hesitate to start this exercise. You can't just sit by yourself and mull over your own ideas to accomplish this. You must get out and talk with people. It takes some effort to pull out stories about your ancestors. Utilize, "Who, What, When, Where, How, and How Much," along with the worksheet questions, and record as much as you can.

Be Aware of the Risks

Besides the difficulties mentioned above, this exercise also involves some risk. Most of us tend to picture our parents and grandparents "larger than life," almost superhuman. When we discover their strengths, weaknesses, fears, etc., we gain a different perspective. Perhaps their human frailties will become obvious. We need to see our parents and grandparents as fellow adults, fellow strugglers, if that's possible.

Another risk involves uncovering unpleasant information. Perhaps you discover that grandma actually was an alcoholic or that great-grandfather was a thief. It may be more comfortable to not know certain family information, but learning and understanding the truth goes with being an adult. You can choose your response to a situation much better when you know the truth.

For some people, reviewing the lives of parents and grandparents will cause pain. I feel great sorrow for children from an abusive, dysfunctional home environment. Wounds from those hurts go deep and are difficult to heal. One thing I know, however, is that discovering joy and purpose in your life requires you to "come to grips" with your past. If you had a terrible upbringing, this information can dramatically change your life.

In the Ten Commandments, God tells us to "Honor your father and your mother." There are no conditions given. It does not say "Honor your parents if they were good," or "Honor your parents if they did their job." Each of us must honor our parents, if only to accept them for what they were and move on.

Remember -- we are embarking upon a lifelong journey for truth. If you had loving, involved parents, you caught a break and get to start on the path at point Y. If you had selfish, lazy parents, you have some additional issues to work through and get to start on the path at point X. Where you start doesn't matter, how you travel and where you finish matters.

As I chatted with my parents about their lives and the lives of their parents and grandparents, I was amazed at how much I learned. They also seemed to enjoy the walk down memory lane. I was especially surprised to discover the occupations of my grandparents and great-grandparents. There were many salesmen among my relatives. Like many engineers, I never had much respect for salesmen. But with so many salesmen in my ancestry, I realized something about myself. In my career, I had repeatedly (and unconsciously) moved toward selling. With my ancestral discovery, I became much more comfortable with that career trend and, in fact, made it a clear objective.

Story of Naaman

Naaman was commander of the army of the King of Aram. He lived with integrity, was highly regarded by the king, and successful in his military career. But Naaman had leprosy. He heard about a great prophet in Israel named Elisha who could cure leprosy. Naaman, loaded with gifts and presents, traveled to Israel to be healed. Elisha would not even see Naaman. Elisha simply sent a message, "Go, wash yourself seven times in the Jordan River and you will be healed."

Naaman was furious! "I thought he would come, wave his hands over me, call on the Lord his God and heal me. Don't we have better rivers in my country than the muddy Jordan? Couldn't I wash in them and be cleansed?" So he went off in a rage.

Naaman's servants appealed to him, "Our father, if the prophet had told you to do some great thing, would you not have done it? How much more, then, when he tells you, 'Wash and be cleansed!'"

Naaman realized this was good advice and dipped himself in the Jordan River seven times. And he was healed! *(Note: the complete Biblical account of Naaman can be found in II Kings, chapter 5.)*

This story illustrates a crucial concept. We can sit around and whine about the status of our lives. Or we can choose to take the small steps required to move us forward. To paraphrase Helen Keller, "We can not do everything but we can do something." If you truly want to improve your life, take some time to investigate your past.

Name: *John Miller*   Worksheet #30   Date: *4-4-00*

Family Tree to 4th Generation

Gaylon Miller
Great Grandfather

Edward Miller
Grandfather

Virginia Sload
Great Grandmother

Samuel Miller
Father

Harrison Moseman
Great Grandfather

Gladys Moseman
Grandmother

Suzanna Burr
Great Grandmother

John Miller
Self

Howard Long
Great Grandfather

Robert Long
Grandfather

Deborah Dieterly
Great Grandmother

July Long
Mother

Stanley Schroeder
Great Grandfather

Leah Schroeder
Grandmother

Emma Steeley
Great Grandmother

John Miller filled out his family tree form to the fourth generation. He talked to his Mom and Dad and gathered any information he could. He also made a few telephone calls to some aunts and uncles who could give some additional information. While some of the stories were interesting, John was surprised at the difficulty he had writing about his parents. It was not easy for him to think about them as one adult thinks about an other adult. He persevered, however, and gained some insights into his background and himself.

Name: *John Miller*   Worksheet #31   Date: *4-8-00*

Father Profile

Father Name: *Samuel Tyler Miller*

Birth Info
   Date: *Sep 9, 1936 at home on the farm in Denver, PA*
   Where:
   How:

Childhood Info
   Siblings: *Mary Anne (4-17-1932), John Rob (7-4-1934)*
   Schools: *Suzanna Burr (11-19-1937) , Mildred Mae (5-18-1939)*
   Stories: *Denver Public School*

Adult Info
   Occupation: *Carpenter*
   Characteristics (Valued attributes? Personality type? Love Language?) &
   Stories:

   Loud, boisterous, quick-tempered, mean when drinking

   Loved the Army but got in trouble for fighting. Worked real hard on the farm as a kid. Called Hoffy's Tavern his 2nd home.

Death Info
   Date: *NA*
   Where:
   How:

Strengths: *Hard worker, never sick, can build anything*

Weaknesses: *Alcoholic, selfish*

What did this person care about the most (central focus)? *Self/Drinking*

Name: *John Miller*   Worksheet #32   Date: *4-8-00*
Mother Profile

Mother Name: *July Long*

Birth Info
> Date: *July 7, 1938*
> Where: *Trenton, NJ in a hospital*
> How:

Childhood Info
> Siblings: *Fred Michael (1-13-1937) William James (5-8-1940)*
> Schools: *PS 24, Then Trenton HS*
> Stories:

Adult Info
> Occupation: *Homemaker*

Characteristics (Valued attributes? Personality type? Love Language?) &
Stories:

> *Pretty, Patient, Somewhat timid*
> *Loved to play make-believe as a girl. Her father was real hard on*
> *the kids. Did not like school much. Met Dad when he came back*
> *from Korean War and was stationed at Fort Dix. They met at a bar*
> *near the base. Got married 6 mos later and moved to PA.*

Death Info
> Date: *NA*
> Where:
> How:

Strengths: *Loving, patient, long-suffering, kind*

Weaknesses: *Never stood up for herself (co-dependent?)*

What did this person care about the most (central focus)? *Family*

Name: *John Miller*   Worksheet #36   Date: *4-8-00*

Grandmother Profile (Mother's side)

Grandmother Name: *Leah Schroeder*

Birth Info
    Date: *July 1, 1908   Trenton, NJ*
    Where:
    How:

Childhood Info
    Siblings: *Michael Lloyd (1-10-1907)*
            Elizabeth Ann (9-25-1911), Gerald Roy (4-5-1913)
    Schools: *Thru 8th grade in Trenton*
    Stories:

Adult Info
    Occupation: *Homemaker*
    Characteristics (Valued attributes? Personality type? Love Language?) &
Stories:

        Strong willed, leader in the family
        As a little girl she was always in trouble for disobeying. She ran
        away from home at 15 to get married to a circus roustabout. She
        married Grandpa a few years later.

Death Info
    Date: *Aug. 14, 1979 in Trenton of a stroke*
    Where:
    How:

Strengths: *Perseverance*

Weaknesses: *Very harsh as a parent, pretty selfish*

What did this person care about the most (central focus)? *Self*

Name: *John Miller*   Worksheet #43   Date: *4-8-00*

Great-grandfather Profile (Mother's mother side)

Great-grandfather Name: *Stanley Schroeder*

Birth Info
   Date: *May 2, 1878 near Munich, Germany, in the home*
   Where:
   How:

Childhood Info
   Siblings: *Estelle Marie(12-12-1880)   Jonathon Brent (5-30-1883)*

   Schools: *not much schooling*
   Stories:

Adult Info
   Occupation: *Blacksmith*
   Characteristics (Valued attributes? Personality type? Love Language?) &
Stories:

         Strong, didn't say too much, skilled
         Came to USA thru Ellis Island at 25 yrs. old with only $20 in his
pocket. Started his own blacksmith shop near Trenton by 35.

Death Info
   Date: *1941 at home in Trenton. Don't know from what.*
   Where:
   How:

Strengths: *Skilled tradesman*

Weaknesses: *Heavy drinker*

What did this person care about the most (central focus)? *Work*

CHAPTER 7

Truths and Lies

"We are generally better persuaded by the reasons we discover ourselves than by those given to us by others."

Pascal

You have covered a tremendous amount of ground in the preceding pages. You have considered everything from whom you most admire... to your psychological make-up... to the lives of your ancestors. Perhaps you're wondering, "Does this book really go anywhere, or is it just a series of worksheets and ideas to make me think?" That's a reasonable question. I'll use a project management concept to explain how this information can change your life.

The Phases of a Project

Most of my career I managed projects, such as: setting up a sound system for a rock concert, designing and constructing buildings, or creating policies and procedures to turn around a company.

Every project needs an objective; without an objective, a project becomes aimless wandering. When I begin designing a building for an organization, I attempt to discover their objectives as early as possible. My degree of success on the project usually depends on how well I understand the organization's objectives. The objective of this book is to help you find greater joy in your life.

From the objective, we move to actually doing something. Most people struggle with how to begin. I start by identifying these necessary project phases:

1. Idea
2. Study
3. Analysis
4. Plan
5. Implementation

The idea phase on projects usually comes easily, "Wouldn't it be nice to have…" The idea phase of your project was as simple as obtaining this book and deciding to work through it. You liked the idea of gaining more joy in life and began moving in that direction.

The study phase involves the gathering of data to use in understanding the project. The preceding chapters are part of the study phase. Your completed worksheets now constitute a valuable body of data. But what can you do with it?

The analysis phase requires us to examine data and decide what is true, what is false, what is useful and what is not. In this chapter, we review the previous worksheets and decide what is

true and useful for our lives. We will also find some things that
are not true or that cause us problems.

After pinpointing basic truth and lies, you will be ready to
create a plan (see next chapter.) The implementation of the plan
is discussed in the "Living the Plan" chapter.

This organized approach may seem like overkill, but consider the alternatives. Most people desire a change, but don't
want to go through this amount of effort. They try to jump right
from *idea* to implement and usually fail. Keep putting forth the
effort. This project approach to a joyful life works!

Finding the Meaning of Life

We are ready to tackle the analysis phase. Let's start by
considering a question that seems to be at the heart of our culture,
"What is the meaning of life?"

It seems as if we ought to be able to identify a simple
meaning to life, but we cannot. There exists too much
complexity, suffering, pain and joy to summarize it in one
sentence. To break complex problems into simple solutions is
wisdom, but to grossly oversimplify is foolishness.

Victor Frankl, a psychiatrist who survived the horrors of
Nazi Germany concentration camps, stated, "The meaning of life
differs from man to man, from day to day and from hour to hour.
What matters, therefore, is not the meaning of life in general but
rather the specific meaning of a person's life at a given moment."

Frankl goes on to explain that asking, "What is the meaning
of life?" is not a reasonable question. It is like asking a chess
master, "What is the best move in chess?" Of course, there is no
one best move. The best move is determined in the context of the
game being played, the position of the chessmen, the nature of
your opponent, etc. In a given situation on a chessboard, there
may be a best move. However, there is no overall best move, just
as there is no simple answer to the meaning of life.

Finding Truths

Rather than tackling the overall meaning of life, which is too big a task, let's look for manageable chunks of truth. We need to know the truth and lies of our life.

In order to survive in this world, we all make judgments based on what we believe to be true. In short, we all have things we believe in. If not, we could not force ourselves out of bed in the morning. There would be too many uncertainties.

For example, think about walking on the sidewalk along a busy street. You walk without worrying that each passing car will drive onto the sidewalk and hit you. Why don't you worry? Because you understand that rules prohibit cars from driving on the sidewalk and hitting pedestrians. You can walk with unconcern because you believe the cars will stay on the road.

If you didn't believe this truth and many others like it, the world would seem too dangerous and scary; you would not venture out. Of course, some people do live this way, paralyzed by fear. Most of us, though, tend to "go with the odds" and accept the many norms of modern society. We accept things such as which side of the road to drive on, paying for things we want rather than stealing them, the availability of food for our next meal, and many other assumptions.

There is not much value in listing all these assumptions about how society operates. But there is value in contemplating and recording our foundational truths. These constitute our present world-view. Having knowledge of foundational beliefs provides a great advantage. Decision-making gets easier when you know your foundational truths.

Most of us spend little time considering our foundational truths; it feels odd to even try. I named eight of my personal truths to provide an example. I reviewed my previous worksheets and wrote statements I believe to be both true and significant to my life. They are concepts I don't have to re-think with each decision. I count on these truths for my day-to-day living.

Ned Pelger Truth #1: It is hard work to find the truth

One of my favorite quotes from Samuel Butler helps illustrate this: "Life is like playing a violin solo in public and learning the instrument as one goes on." I don't know why life contains so much struggle; I just know that it does. Life challenges us continuously. We can choose to whine and avoid or work and persevere.

We will not discover truth by lying in bed and waiting for it. Truth requires work. We must think about truth and not be too lazy to learn.

Many people put off consideration of the truth because they believe they need to have their mental affairs in order before starting. They think they need to attain an emotionally tensionless state prior to considering the truth. These ideas are wrong.

We must start from where we are; it's that simple. As we challenge ourselves, as we struggle toward some worthwhile goal of our own choosing, we will find bits of truth along the way. But we must set ourselves on a course and begin, we must be willing to work.

Helen Keller said, "So much has been given to me, I have no time to ponder over that which has been denied." She had neither sight nor hearing, yet she inspired millions of people with her world-wide lectures and other activities. She also traveled far on her journey toward truth. As a child, Helen lived in a self-absorbed world, full of luxury and ease. She existed, not seeing, hearing nor speaking, just roaming around on her parents' estate. She was willful and undisciplined. Her teacher, Anne Sullivan, broke through the communication barrier with Helen. The world became real and understandable as Helen worked to learn names of objects, to communicate through sign language and eventually to speak.

You and I pass through a similar process. We begin living in a self-absorbed, childlike way. Then we start paying attention to others, to our surroundings and to ourselves. We learn to truly see with our eyes, truly hear with our ears and truly pay attention to those things going on around us. This increased level of attention takes effort, but the effort produces gems of understanding that are ours to keep.

Ned Pelger Truth #2: We have the freedom to choose our response

Sometimes we can control what happens to us and sometimes we cannot. For example, if we are out for a walk with a friend and a tornado suddenly descends, we cannot remove the wind. While we cannot control the situation (the weather), we can choose our response. We can run for home immediately, curl up and try to hide, hold onto our friend, forget about our friend, totally panic, or any number of other things. We have the freedom to choose our response.

Action is a choice. It may not always be a conscious choice, we may just react at a subconscious level. Or, we could let our emotional thinking system choose our response. Many waste their whole lives defaulting to their emotions, not exercising their freedom to choose. We must remember the important truth, though, that whether we exercise it or not, we definitely have the freedom to choose our response in any situation.

This concept is well-illustrated by Victor Frankl. He wrote about life in the concentration camps where every dignity, every right, was stripped away. Even in that situation, with so much freedom lost, he states that one still had the freedom to choose one's response. We need to remember that in all situations we have that freedom.

If our child is diagnosed with cancer or our spouse is violently killed in an automobile accident or if we win the lottery, in each case we have the freedom to choose our response. We cannot always control what happens to us. However, we can control our response to every situation. This puts the responsibility on us.

My wife thinks I'm a little goofy because of my fascination with labor camps and concentration camps. Often when a difficulty arises in my life, I think of concentration camps. The comparison forces me to conclude that I have no major problems, just minor annoyances. The following accounts of life in labor camps have been a major influence:

- Man's Search for Meaning by Victor Frankl
- Alexander Dolgun's Story: An American in the Gulag by Alexander Dolgun
- This Way for the Gas, Ladies and Gentlemen by Tadeusz Borowski
- A Day in the Life of Ivan Denisovitch by Alexander Solzhenitsyn

One fascinating thread runs through all these stories. Even in the midst of such pain, suffering, and squalor, there was a working human society in existence in these prisons. Even though the people were stripped of almost everything, many retained their sense of humor and deep spiritual commitment.

Victor Frankl explains, "It is easy for the outsider to get the wrong conception of camp life, a conception mingled with sentiment and pity. Little does he know of the hard fight for existence which raged among the prisoners. This was an unrelenting struggle for daily bread and for life itself, for one's own sake or for that of a good friend." Frankl makes it clear that life in the camps was still life, with all its crazy ups and downs. He further writes, "Humor was another of the soul's weapons in the fight for self-preservation. It is well known that humor, more than anything else in the human make-up, can afford an aloofness and an ability to rise above any situation, even if only for a few seconds."

As we consider truth, the words of Victor Frankl challenge us, "Man is ultimately self-determining. What he becomes--within the laws of endowment and environment--he has made out of himself. In the concentration camps for example, in this living laboratory and this testing ground we watched and witnessed some of our comrades behave like swine while others behaved like saints. Man has both potentialities within himself. Which one is actualized depends on our decisions, but not on our conditions."

The word "responsibility" comes from having the "ability" to choose one's "response." Improvement requires taking responsibility. No matter what happened to us in the past, no matter where we are now, we must stop blaming others and use our ability to choose our response. Choosing our responses, as opposed to just reacting emotionally, lies at the heart of finding joy.

Ned Pelger Truth # 3: We all sin

Many people struggle with the concept of sin. Perhaps, as children, they were lectured about sin and were turned off. Perhaps they have heard TV evangelists preach about sin in a ridiculous, hypocritical way. Or perhaps they just don't like the idea of being judged by anyone else's standard.

I think of sin as simply missing the mark. Imagine an archer standing with his bow and a quiver full of arrows. He faces a target 50 yards away (half the length of a football field). Carefully he removes an arrow from his quiver and aims at the target. From that distance, the bull's-eye appears to be just a dot. He releases the arrow and it smacks into the target one inch to the right of the bull's-eye. The archer shoots again and hits two inches above the bull's-eye. Over and over he shoots, always hitting near the center of the target, but only occasionally hitting the center of the bull's-eye. Even though he shoots quite well, most shots fail to hit the exact center of the bull's-eye; he misses the mark.

When we know the right thing to do and don't do it, we miss the mark. We all sin because we don't do the right thing every moment of every day of our lives. Human beings aren't perfect. We all miss the mark on a regular basis.

A more challenging question is, "Why do we miss the mark?" Are we basically good, noble creatures that occasionally fail due to a defective upbringing? Or are we, at the core of our human nature, self-seeking and lazy? There is no question in my optimistic mind that there is a tremendous amount of good in the hearts of most people. I also believe a baseness exists in every person. This may be well hidden (sometimes masterfully hidden), but it exists and will surface from time to time.

It is essential, as a mature adult, to be reconciled to this fact. Every person we deal with will disappoint us from time to time. Every person we know sins and that is truth. Knowing this, we can build relationships that stand the test of difficult times. On the other hand, if we expect only good from others, we will be frequently disappointed. We will have few, if any, strong, lasting relationships because no one will live up to our expectations.

Ned Pelger Truth #4: We must admit our ignorance to learn the truth

I spoke with a father who had been sexually abusing his daughters and his attitude amazed me. He had no guilt; he had no shame. He convinced himself that the children were bad, and he himself was completely faultless. He simply could not bear the thought that he could be in the wrong.

If a person is ill, he must recognize and admit that he is ill. Then he can seek a cure. Many folks, particularly those with psychological disorders, never move toward a cure because they never admit their problem. They refuse to face the truth of their situation.

Our search for knowledge is much the same. We can never learn if we believe we know everything already. We remove a load of stress from ourselves when we are able to admit that we do not have all the answers.

Ned Pelger Truth #5: Finding truth coincides with developing personal character

Dietrich Bonhoffer, a Christian martyr from Germany during World War II wrote, "Who can be faithful in the great things if he has not learned to be faithful in the things of daily life?" When I consider the wise men and women I have known, they all had one thing in common. Each of these people I admired lived with integrity and character.

In the hassles and irritations of our daily lives, we demonstrate integrity and character by our actions and the choices we make. Character is sometimes defined as what we do when no one is watching. I know of no one who has increased their level of understanding and truth who does not live with integrity and honesty.

Ned Pelger Truth #6: Joy motivates us to the truth

When we consider all the hard work and difficulty required to change, why bother? The answer lies in one simple word, "Joy." When I discover a new truth, the joy I feel always amazes me. That great feeling motivates me. Without the joy of results, we would abandon life's struggles in despair.

As I watched our children grow and learn and change, I observed this truth in action. As our son learned to use a computer, he experienced the joy of discovery. He felt the satisfaction of being able to do more things and go more places. He put up with the aggravation, the repeated failing, in order to succeed. And with that success came joy.

When our daughter decided she wanted to stop sucking her thumb, I heard the struggle in her voice as she told me how hard it is to quit. Yet she was determined to find a way to stop this habit. The joy of success motivated her in that struggle, as it does each of us, whether it be the struggle for understanding, the struggle for change, or the struggle for truth.

Ned Pelger Truth #7: Love is action

Unfortunately, I am at an age where I see too many of my friends and acquaintances getting divorced. One of the partners always seems to say, "I just don't love him (or her) anymore." They express it with such finality, as if to say, "What else could I do? It is simply out of my hands." They speak of love as a sentiment, or an emotion, beyond their control.

If you have ever "fallen in love," you remember the experience. Everything in your life paled in importance when compared to being with your lover. You thought about almost nothing else except the next time you would be with your precious beloved. Psychologists call this the "in-love experience."

While this feeling seems wonderful, we need to remember it is only a feeling, a passing sentiment. No one retains that "in-love experience" permanently; like any emotional experience, its intensity will fade with time. Admittedly, it's great while it lasts, but it will pass. Instead of thinking of love as an emotion (something you feel), think of love as an action (something you do.) "To love" is an action verb, and loving becomes a series of choices we make.

With this view, love becomes an intentional choice. For example, my wife Debby chooses to love me. On a particular day, I may act mean and critical toward her (perhaps because I'm tired). Nobody likes this type of behavior and Debby is no exception. It would be natural for her to respond in kind. Typically, though, Debby will choose to respond with love and simply overlook the offense. This response "takes all the wind out of my sails." I feel badly about being nasty and eventually get around to apologizing. Of course, sometimes the roles are reversed (except for the apologizing part!)

Debby chooses to love me even when she does not feel like it. She chooses to love me even when her feelings have just been hurt. She chooses to love me, to overlook an offense, because she knows that true love is action.

M. Scott Peck in his book, <u>The Road Less Traveled,</u> talks about love being even more than giving. Love is judicious giving and judicious withholding as well. We must not simply give our beloved what they want; we must attempt to give them what they truly need. Love requires us to think and often make painful decisions.

When we try to love in this manner, we come face-to-face with the reality that love is much more than an emotion. Love becomes an active struggle. We fail some days and fantastically succeed other days. Love becomes an action adventure.

Ned Pelger Truth #8: There is a universal battle between good and evil

I have known some very good people in my life and some very evil ones. I have known people that lived for the good of others and people who cruelly abused those who were closest to them. While most of us fall in the middle of these extremes, I've come to realize there is something going on in this big old world, something larger than our minds can get a handle on.

I experience the struggle between good and evil in my own life and observe it in the lives of others. Sometimes good wins; sometimes evil wins.

C.S. Lewis writes, "There is no neutral ground in the universe; every square inch, every split second is claimed by God and countered-claimed by Satan." I believe he means we cannot be neutral as we live our lives. We are either moving in God's direction or moving in the direction of evil.

Many people acknowledge a kind and loving God, but cannot accept the reality of a force of evil. The concept of evil is too unpleasant and therefore not considered. How does one explain when terrible things (such as serious illness, death of a loved one, natural disaster, etc.) happen to good, moral people? Is it merely a mistake...something that ought not to occur...something that God wishes would not be? It is hard for us to understand why the righteous suffer.

We could claim that God does not have the capability to control these situations. A view of God as kind and loving, but not Almighty would explain many difficult-to-understand events. Personally, I cannot accept a view of a God who has so little power, a God who is not Almighty and All-knowing. It just doesn't jive with what I've experienced of God.

The book of Job describes the relationship between man and God. But it is not a closed relationship. A third party exists, the evil one, the devil, Satan or whatever name you choose to use. He alienates people from God. The evil one has a significant amount of power and uses many methods to keep people alienated from God. Suffering, busyness, lack of focus and even success can be used by Satan to keep individuals separated from God. For some reason, which we do not understand, God allows the evil one to exist and allows us the freedom to choose our loyalty.

The simple truth that we choose to serve either God or evil becomes even clearer in this quote from Joshua, the leader of the people of Israel. He said, in Joshua 24:14-15, "Now fear the Lord and serve him with all faithfulness. Throw away the gods your forefathers worshipped beyond the river and in Egypt and serve the Lord. But if serving the Lord seems undesirable to you, then choose for yourselves this day whom you will serve. Whether the gods your forefathers served beyond the river or the god of the Amorites in whose land you are living, *but as for me and my household, we will serve the Lord.*"

Your Truths

My eight personal truths help me live. Every single day, these truths form the foundation of my behavior choices. As I make day-to-day decisions, and when I consider important, long-range issues, I utilize these truths. The truths are my beliefs and knowing them helps me live my life with integrity.

You may not agree with the things I believe to be truths. What you need to do, though, is to develop your own. Your list need not be fancy or well-explained. The ideas can be simple or complex. The importance of this exercise involves getting clear awareness of the beliefs that affect you. Record these on Worksheet #45.

Consider the sayings you often use. For example, my kids feel like screaming when for the ten thousandth time I tell them, "It builds character," when they are struggling with a difficulty. I usually say it without thinking, but as you observed in my list of truths, I consider character essential to successful living. We need strength of character; we need to go through difficult, hard times in order to grow.

Read through your previous worksheets and look for recurring themes. This worksheet may be a challenge, but I encourage you to take the time to complete it. Then refer back to it from time to time, and additional foundational truths can be added.

We should return to our project management framework to clarify one point. This worksheet does not constitute a plan; we are not yet in the plan stage. We are still in the study and analysis phase. We are gathering data and analyzing that data so we will be properly prepared when the time comes to make our plan.

Defining Lies

We deceive ourselves every day. The lies of our lives are concepts we consciously or unconsciously believe, but which are not true. For example, I have known several beautiful women who saw themselves as ugly. By society's standards, they were quite attractive, but what they saw in the mirror was not. This lie shaped their responses in many situations. If we believe something to be true, we will make our decisions and live our lives based on that belief regardless of its validity.

Name: *John Miller*   Worksheet #45   Date: *4-11-00*

Things I Believe to be True

1. *Life is not fair.*

2. *It always pays to be courteous.*

3. *If you are going to try something, always do your best.*

4. *Alcoholism is a brutal disease.*

5. *It is a good thing to protect those who can't protect themselves.*

6.

7.

8.

9.

10.

We need to expose these personal lies. We need to recognize the lies in order to deal with them. As we name the lie, it has less power over us. Don't expect this exercise to be easy. Generally our most dominating lies originated in early childhood and are rooted in our subconscious. When we have the courage to bring these lies into our conscious mind, we begin the process of overcoming the false belief.

As in the "Truth" section, I am listing some lies I encounter in my own life. Again, you do not have to agree with me. They are here for the purpose of illustration.

Ned Pelger Lie #1: I have a right to be happy

This seems to be the mantra of our times. Happiness is viewed as all-important and our absolute right as human beings. Where do you think this idea comes from? I doubt it came from the pioneers and early settlers; they probably were content to just survive. The writers of the Constitution considered "life, liberty and the pursuit of happiness" to be essential, but there is a big difference between pursuing happiness and having an absolute right to be happy. In fact, the "right to happiness" concept most likely emerged only in the 20th century. As our lives became easier (electricity, social security, reduced work week with much more leisure time), the idea that we deserve perpetual happiness also evolved.

While I adamantly believe we can have tremendous joy, I don't think we can, or even should, strive to be always happy. By definition, happiness is satisfaction, the enjoyment of pleasure. Most can agree that a central focus on pleasure is not healthy. This short-term, feel-good happiness rarely promotes growth. It is usually selfish, and lacking in commitment.

Of course, I'm not saying it's wrong to be happy. I love to have fun and laugh as much as anyone I know. When I go through a time of struggle or difficulty, though, I need to understand its significance. I must not suddenly feel abandoned by God. My life ought not to consist of constant happiness, pleasure and enjoyment. A balanced life contains struggles, joys, concerns and happiness, all in their place.

Victor Frankl, in Man's Search for Meaning, wisely states: "Suffering cannot be removed from life, just as fate and death cannot. Without suffering and death, human life cannot be complete. The way in which a man accepts his fate and all the suffering it entails, the way in which he takes up his cross, gives him ample opportunity - even under the most difficult circumstances - to add a deeper meaning to his life. It may remain brave, dignified and unselfish. Or in a bitter fight for self-preservation he may forget his human dignity and become no more than an animal."

We are not guaranteed perpetual happiness, nor would it be a good thing. In fact, much of the meaning of our lives comes through struggle.

Ned Pelger Lie #2: Possessions provide security

We all know this statement is false, yet so many of us fall into the trap of living as though it was true. Think of a person who struggled his whole life to climb the ladder of success and then died suddenly. Perhaps a heart attack, maybe cancer or even a car accident took his life. All his hard work and personal wealth did not provide any protection when the angel of death came around. At those times, we generally say things like, "Life is short; we ought to pay attention to the things that are truly important." But, then time moves on, and we get caught once again in the rat race of working too hard and buying lots of stuff.

We must consider how we view our possessions and our status in life. Do we always need more? Do we always need to get to the next higher level at work? We must evaluate how much of our time and energy goes into the acquisition and maintenance of possessions. We need to consider if the promotion we want will really be worth the cost. I am not saying we should not work hard; I am saying we should consider our motivation and make our decisions wisely.

I worked as a foreman for an excavation company when I was a young man. We had a rough crew; at one point my crew consisted of six guys and five of them were on probation or parole. I learned a tremendous amount at that job. Much of what I learned came from an old equipment operator named Steve Balach (who was not one of the ones on probation or parole). Steve was in his mid-fifties while I was in my mid-twenties. Steve's family was raised while my family was just beginning.

On rainy days we could not work, and I would send all the guys home. Being salaried, I would stay at the job trailer. Steve would sit with me for a few hours, and we would talk. I mostly listened. Steve had lived a fascinating life filled with gusto. When we talked about work, he would say to me, "Ned, when I was your age, I thought I was going to conquer the world. I worked all the time, trying to make my mark. You know, Ned, my two boys kind of grew up without me. I was just too busy working. Now they're grown and here I am still working. Don't miss what I did, Ned! Take the time with your kids when they're young; you'll never regret it!"

Steve died suddenly a couple of years later and I miss him. I think about him sometimes when I get too busy and I remember his words of wisdom. When I feel like I simply don't have enough time, I remember that there is always enough time to do the truly important things. I start considering my priorities and can feel the stress lessening.

My material wants ands needs often get reversed. I focus on possessions, thinking they can help define me or protect me. In reality, increased possessions make me more anxious rather than more secure. The idea of losing those things is scary. As John D. Rockefeller said, "How much money is enough? Just a little more would do it."

We are told in our culture in many different, subtle ways that we can have everything. Understand the dangerous deception in this statement. We cannot have everything; we must carefully choose where our treasure is.

Ned Pelger Lie #3: We deserve the treatment we received early in our lives

We all had different upbringings and most of us tend to see the family we grew up in as normal. We know our own family best and use that relationship as a frame of reference for evaluating the rest of the world. As we grew up, though, we observed that other families were different from our own.

Some people were fortunate to be raised in very healthy families, surrounded by love and support. We previously discussed these highly functional families which fostered emotional and spiritual growth. If you were raised in such a family, you know you were blessed. You need to realize, though, that you did nothing to deserve this good fortune (you were simply born.)

Conversely, some people were raised amidst evil. Every positive attribute, every sign of growth was beaten down and snuffed. Those who were raised in very unhealthy families took constant beatings to their self-esteem. Physical, mental, emotional and/or sexual abuse occurred. If you were raised in an unhealthy, dysfunctional family, if you were treated badly early in your life, you need to accept the fact that you did not deserve that treatment.

M. Scott Peck in his book, The People of the Lie, raises some important issues about evil visited upon children. He states that children are the innocent victims of much of the evil that occurs in this world. And much of the most vile behavior is inflicted upon children by their parents. It is truly difficult for a child, even an adult child, to come to the realization that his parents do not, or did not, love him in a healthy way. However difficult it may be, if you were treated badly as a child, you must choose to believe that it was not your fault.

We are more than the sum of the events in our lives. We have the capacity to take those events, both good and bad, and learn from them. We can turn dross into silver. The times that seemed like a painful waste can become some of our strongest guiding lessons if we look for their significance.

Ned Pelger Lie #4: Only good people are in church

I was trying to decide about using a certain subcontractor on a large construction project. I had a slightly bad feeling about the owner of the firm, but he seemed to be such a dedicated Christian man. He had Christian mottoes on his letterhead and business cards and espoused all the right principles about honesty and integrity. I decided we would give his firm the job (to be honest, they were also the best price by far, so there was an element of greed involved on my part).

That decision cost our firm a quarter of a million dollars. The man billed for materials on the job site, then took those same materials to another site and billed for them again. He stole things and then shut down his company in the middle of the project and was unable to complete the job.

As I handled damage control, I remember feeling especially betrayed since I trusted this man's Christianity to make him do the right thing. After many other business dealings and discussions with friends, I have come to the conclusion that, unfortunately, the amount of immoral behavior inside the Christian church about equals the amount found outside the church. The reality is that we are all humans, all make mistakes, and all exhibit both good and bad behaviors at different times.

I do believe people with a true spiritual commitment behave much more decently than they would without it. But church attendance does not indicate one's spiritual sincerity. There are so many social and personal reasons to attend a church; don't assume all people are in church for spiritual reasons.

While we will find many truly good people in church, we will also find some of the worst people imaginable. People attend church for many reasons: they may want to be part of a friendly social group, they may want business contacts, they may use the church for appearance's sake (to help hide their true behavior), or they may truly be interested in spiritual growth. Be aware that we will find both very good people and very evil people most anywhere we go, even in church.

Worksheet #46 quizzes you about the common lies of your life. Perhaps you're aware of some that hinder you every day. On the other hand, this concept may challenge you greatly. No answers may occur to you. Remember, these worksheets get upgraded as you live and learn. If you strive for understanding, your subconscious hindrances will become clear over time.

Favorite Quotes and Stories

As I strive to understand truths and lies in my life, I often find wisdom from quotations. I love to read quote books. I enjoy finding sayings that make me laugh or think. Do you ever hear a joke you'd like to remember and promptly forget it? It's frustrating.

Worksheet #47 provides a place to record that information. You'll enjoy rereading your list of funny and notable sayings and stories. Over time, you will add entries and your earlier ones will mean more to you. This database will help color your every day speech and be helpful if you must speak for a special occasion.

The computer adds a real benefit here. Rather than writing all these quotes and stories on paper and reviewing them page by page, a database program allows you excellent access to the recorded information. Appendix A tells how you can obtain the software program on Microsoft Access for your use.

By entering the quotes and stories into the Access database, you'll be able to sort by author or key words. You can also search to find one word that you remember from the quote or story. If you take some time to start entering this information, you will develop a great personal resource.

Name: *John Miller*   Worksheet #46   Date: *4-14-00*

Common Lies in my Life

1. *If you love others, they will love you back.*

2. *Being good at work provides security.*

3. *Only good people are in church.*

4.

5.

6.

7.

8.

9.

10.

If you completed the worksheets through this book, you had quite a bit of information to review when identifying your beliefs and deceptions. I hope you carefully considered those things you believe to be true and useful, and those things which are false and cause you problems. This type of analysis provides excellent information from which to begin your plan for change. You now have assembled all the tools and materials needed to build that plan.

The following story by Leo Tolstoy is a warning to make sure the items in your plan are truly what you want. "Be careful what you pray for, because you just may get it," is a wise word of caution. Many times the things we believe would make us happy are not what we need.

Name: *John Miller*   Worksheet #47   Date: *4-15-00*
My Favorite Quotes & Stories

1. *No man ever listened himself out of a job. Calvin Coolidge*

2. *Some guy hit my fender, and I said to him, "Be fruitful and multiply," but not in those words. Woody Allen.*

3. *Start every day off with a smile and get it over with. W.C. Fields*

4. *Experience is what allows you to recognize a mistake when you make it again.*

5. *Only two things are infinite, the universe and human stupidity, and I'm not sure about the former. Albert Einstein*

Story by Leo Tolstoy

"How Much Land Does a Man Require?"

An older sister came from a small city to visit her younger sister. The older one was married to a merchant and the younger to a farmer. As the two drank tea and talked, the older sister began to boast and make much of her life in town. She lived in ease and comfort, dressed her children well, had nice things to eat and drink, and could walk to the theater.

The younger sister was irked at this and responded by running down the life of the merchant's wife and making much of her own country life. "For my part, I should not care to exchange my life for yours," she said. "I give you that ours is an uneventful existence and we don't know much excitement. But yet you, on the other hand, with all your fine living, must either do a very large trade or be ruined. You know the proverb, 'Loss is Gain's older brother'. Yes, you may be rich today but tomorrow you may find yourself in the street. We have a better way than that here in the country. The farmer's stomach may be thin but it's long. We may never be rich, but we'll always have enough to eat."

The older sister responded quickly, "Enough indeed! Enough with nothing but your wretched pigs and calves. Enough with no fine dresses or company. Why, however hard your man may work, you have to live in mud and you will die there. And yes, your children after you."

"Oh no," replied the younger sister. "It's like this with us. Though we may live hard, at least the land is our own. And we have no need to bow and scrape to anyone. But in the city, there is always scandal. Today everything may be okay but tomorrow any of many temptations may come to your husband and your lives will be ruined. Isn't that true?"

Pakhom, the younger sister's husband, had been listening near the stove. "That is true," he said. "I've been turning over Mother Earth since my childhood so I've had no time to get any foolishness in my head. Yet I only have one grievance--too little land. Only give me land and I fear no man. No, not even the devil himself."

The two women finished their tea, chatted a little longer about clothing, washed up the dishes and went to bed. All this time the devil had been sitting behind the stove and heard everything. He was delighted when the peasant's wife led her husband to brag. Led him on to boast that once given land, he would not fear even the devil himself.

"Splendid," thought the devil, "I'll try a little trick with you. I'll give you much land and then take it away again."

Near these farmers there lived a lady landowner who had about 600 acres of land. She got on well with the tenant farmers and did not abuse their rights. However, as she aged she took on a retired soldier as an overseer. This soldier was vicious. No matter how careful Pakhom was, some of his horses got into the lady's oats or a cow got into her garden. He was fined for each of these offenses.

Pakhom became more angry with each of these fines and took it out on his family. He eventually had to put his animals in the feedlot. He regretted the costs but it caused him much less anxiety in other ways. As winter came one year, the lady land-owner was planning to sell her land. Rumor had it that the over-seer was going to buy it. All the nearby farmers were dismayed.

"If that overseer gets the land, we're in big trouble." So, the farmers got together and decided they would try to buy the land as a group. The old woman agreed to this arrangement but as the farmers met on various occasions, they could not decide who would buy which lots. Finally, the old woman agreed that she would sell the lots to the individual farmers.

Pakhom didn't know what to do. He saw his neighbors buy-ing ground, some of them paying half down and letting the rest stand over for two years. He said to his wife, "If the others buy all the land, I'll be left out in the cold. Everybody is buying some. We had better get hold of 20 acres also. We can't make a living as things are now for the overseer takes out all the profits in fines."

Since they had 100 rubles in savings, they needed to find additional money. They sold half of their bees, a young colt that was just born and let out their son to service. With this money, they were able to settle on the 20 acres.

Pakhom was truly happy at this time. He borrowed a little money to buy some seed, planted it and had a wonderful crop. He was able to pay off both the seed money and the rest of the land within the first year. He was able from his own land to cut his hay, gather his firewood and graze his cattle. Whenever he went out on his estate, either to plow or inspect the crops, he felt over-joyed. The very grass seemed different from other grasses, the flowers seemed to bloom differently. Before it was just land, now it was land with a difference.

So Pakhom lived like this for a time and was happy. Indeed all would have been fine if the other peasants had let Pakhom's corn and pasture alone. He complained many times to them about letting their animals roam in his crops. Again and again, Pakhom drove them out and overlooked the matter. But finally, he lost his temper and made a complaint before the court.

He knew from his own experience that the peasants let the animals roam only from lack of land, not to cause him problems, but it simply could not be allowed. He must teach them a lesson. So first he took one person to court and then another. He had one person fined and then another.

Soon there were strong feelings against Pakhom and some of the neighbors stole crops on purpose. In fact, one neighbor stripped bark off ten of his fine linden trees. Pakhom went wild when he saw the damage. He thought it must be Sempka that would have done such a thing and hauled him into court. Of course, Sempka was found not guilty because there was no evidence. Pakhom screamed at the magistrates, accusing them of being thieves along with Sempka. More and more, Pakhom stayed away from the group of farmers that were his neighbors.

Around this time a traveling farmer stopped in at Pakhom's house. He mentioned land available to the north. It was wonderful land and it grew such rye. The traveling farmer said the straw of the rye was tall enough to hide a horse and thick enough to make a sheaf with just five handfuls. He also told Pakhom that one hard-working farmer had gone there with nothing and now grew 150 acres of wheat and made 5000 rubles last year alone.

This story set Pakhom's soul on fire. "Why should I stay here poor and cramped when I might be making such a fine living as that? I will sell out here, both land and homestead, and go build myself a new house and farm there with the money. Here, in this cramped up spot, life is one long worry. At least I can go and find out."

At the end of the summer, Pakhom decided to visit the place. He walked 300 miles and was overjoyed when he got there. He could get 20 acres of free land for every member of his family and he could buy additional land with the money he brought.

Pakhom and his family relocated to this new area and started with 100 acres of land. But of course all was not quite marvelous. While he could grow corn on all his land, the best crop to grow was white Turkish wheat. To grow this crop, one needed to sow the land one year, harvest, then let the land sit fallow for two years. In order to maximize his profits, Pakhom would need to find new land each year on which to grow Turkish wheat.

He moved his family often, going from place to place. He began to get frustrated that he did not have his very own grand estate where he could let land sit fallow without moving around the country. He entered into negotiations with a farmer who had become destitute, to buy 1500 acres at a very good price. Pakhom paid 1000 rubles for the land. Right after he bought the land another traveling farmer came to see him.

"I have found the best land in the world," the farmer told him. "I was able to buy 15,000 acres for only 1000 rubles. The land fronts on a river, is all open grass and very flat. You would not find land like that in a year around here."

Pakhom was depressed. "Why did I give 1000 rubles for 1500 acres when I could have 15,000 acres." He decided he must go and find out about this story. Pakhom walked 400 miles to the land of the Bashkirs.

This was a different type of country. The people were simple. They did not plow nor eat corn. Their main substance was mare's milk, which the women made into a drink called kamiss. Then they turned the kamiss into cheese. The only food the Bashkirs cooked was mutton and their only amusement was pipe playing. Yet, they were a sweet and cheerful people who kept holiday all year around.

When they caught sight of Pakhom coming into their midst they were pleased. He set up drinks for everyone, gave presents and made friends easily. He told them how he wished to buy land. They, being a simple people, told him they had much and were glad to sell land to him.

The head of the Bashkirs came into the group at this time. Pakhom could tell that this was a person of importance and saved his best presents for him. As he gave these presents, they spoke and Pakhom asked if he could buy land. The head of the

Bashkirs said, "Certainly, you can have as much land as you would like."

Pakhom thought, "These are truly simple people but I must get something in writing so they do not give me land and then take it away." He said aloud, "Thank you, kind sir, for the offer of the land, but I, of course, need to know which land I shall have and how much it will cost."

The leader smiled, "Yes... you may have a day's worth of land for 1000 rubles."

"How many acres would that include?" Pakhom asked, confused, for he had never heard of this day rate.

"We do not reckon land in that way," said the leader. "We sell only by the day. That is to say, as much land as you can walk around in a day, that much land is yours. That is our measure and the price is 1000 rubles." Pakhom was astounded. "Why a man might walk a great deal in a day," he said.

The leader smiled. "Well, in all events, it will be yours. Only, there is one condition. You must return to the same spot from where you started before sunset or your money is forfeited."

"How do you decide on that spot?" Pakhom wondered.

"You may choose any spot you like," replied the leader. "I and my people will stand there first thing in the morning and we will wait for you. We will send a rider behind you to plant stakes to show your path. As much land as you circle, that land will be yours."

Pakhom accepted these terms and decided to make an early start in the morning. They talked more, drank some more kamiss and ate some more mutton. Eventually, Pakhom went to bed. As Pakhom lay in bed, he could get no sleep. He was too excited. "What great land there is here," he said to himself. "Tomorrow I will mark out a large Promised Land for myself. I can walk at least 30 miles and that would make over 30,000 acres of land. Then I will be under no one's thumb."

Too excited to sleep, Pakhom tossed and turned through the night. He finally fell asleep near morning and began to dream. He saw himself lying in a wagon and heard someone laughing and talking outside. As he sat up to see who was laughing so much, he saw the leader of the Bashkirs rolling on the ground in laughter. Pakhom walked over to him to find what was so funny.

When Pakhom approached him, he saw it was not the leader of the Bashkirs, but the traveling farmer who had told him about this land. Then he saw the face turn into the farmer who told him of his previous ground. The face always laughed and laughed. Finally, he saw the devil himself in that face with horns and hooves, still laughing at him.

As he looked away, he saw a man, barefoot and wearing only a shirt and pants lying flat on his back, dead. Pakhom looked into the man's face and saw it was his own face. He jumped and awoke. "It is time to start," he thought, "I must get these good people awake and moving."

Pakhom went around the village and awoke the Bashkirs. They met at the spot Pakhom chose. As the first sunlight beamed over the distant mountains, Pakhom started to walk at a good pace towards the east. He had laid his money in his hat on top of a knoll and all the people waited there for him. He did not walk too quickly, but he kept a good pace. As the sun came up, he felt comfortable. He walked and calculated, smiling about the beautiful land.

As he continued to walk, the day grew warm and he shed clothes. After he had walked about eight miles, he decided he should veer to the left to keep his calculations true. He looked back. He could barely see the knoll from where he had started. Still the land was so flat and the further he walked, the better the land got. He was beginning to get tired as he walked through the late morning but he thought, "I must not sit down to rest. I don't want to fall asleep. I should stop and just take lunch."

After lunch the walking became easy, for the meal had revived his strength. The hot afternoon sun wore on him, though he said to himself, "An hour's pain may a century gain."   After he went about 15 miles, he came upon some beautiful land near a dry ravine. He thought to himself, "Oh what a pity to leave that piece of ground out. Flax would grow so splendidly there."

So he kept on straight till he encompassed the ravine and had a stake placed there. Looking back at the knoll, he could barely see the people. He knew that they were probably not much more than 10 miles away, but the afternoon was passing.

He decided, "I must go straight home now. No matter how rough the land is. I must not take in a single piece. I have enclosed sufficient as it is." So Pakhom headed straight back for the knoll.

He found the walking very difficult. His feet ached and hurt him. He was beginning to tire. He would have given anything to rest yet he knew he must regain the knoll by sunset. The sun would not wait. He staggered and said to himself, "Surely I have not miscalculated! I have not taken in too much land to get back. Oh, but there is such a long way to go and I am so tired. I cannot have come all this way to have all my money and all my toil gone in vain."

Pakhom pulled himself together and began to run. His feet were bleeding, but he ran on and on. He threw away his coat, boots, cap, flask. He kept saying over and over in his mind, "Everything is lost. I will never reach the mark before sunset." The more worried he got, the more breathless he became. Still he ran. It was like his lungs were a pair of blacksmith bellows and his heart was a steam hammer. His legs were breaking underneath him and did not even feel like his own.

He was not thinking of the land anymore. He was only thinking about not dying from the exertion. But he could not let himself stop. "To have gone so far," he thought, "and to stop, why they would think me a great fool."

By this time, he could hear the Bashkirs cheering and shouting for him and their cries stirred his heart. On and on he ran, with his last remaining strength, while the sun was just touching the horizon. Ah, but he was close to the spot now. He could see the people on the knoll waving their hands to him and urging him on. He could see his cap lying on the ground with the money in it and the leader sitting beside it.

Suddenly Pakhom remembered his dream. "I have much land now," he thought, "if only God should bring me safe to live upon it. But my heart tells me I've killed myself." Yet he ran on.

For the last time he looked at the sun. Large and red, it had touched the earth and was sinking below the horizon. He was in despair as he thought everything was lost, but suddenly he remembered that the people on the knoll would still have not seen the sunset. He rushed up the slope and as he got to the cap, there were still rays of sun. He stumbled and fell and touched the cap before the sun set.

"Ah, young man," cried the leader, "you have earned much land indeed." Pakhom's servant ran to his master and tried to raise him but blood was running from his mouth. Pakhom lay there, dead. The servant cried out in consternation but the leader remained sitting on his haunches, laughing and holding his sides. The leader stood up, took a shovel and threw it to the servant. "Bury him," was all he said.

The Bashkirs got up and left. Only the servant remained. He dug a grave the same length as Pakhom's body laying there and buried him.

I often recall this story when I consider the priorities in my life. What values did Pakhom have? He had mostly good attributes. He was hard working, he cared about his family, he was disciplined, and he was intelligent. Worksheet #47 quizzes you on your reactions to Pakhom's story.

What was Pakhom's central focus? What did he care about more than anything else? Pakhom cared about land; he wanted to have the best property he could for himself and his family. By working hard and taking some calculated risks, Pakhom prospered toward his objective. He succeeded in accomplishing his goals for the most part, and certainly would be viewed as a success story in our culture (except for the dying part).

We all have something that truly motivates us, something on which we spend our time and effort. For Pakhom it was land; what is it for you? We can decide we do not want to be like Pakhom. We don't want to be the fool. We especially don't want to end up dead, with nothing, everyone laughing at us. So let's begin work on our plan; let's begin to pull together all this knowledge about ourselves and make a usable plan for our lives.

Name: *John Miller*   Worksheet #47   Date: *4-19-00*

Impressions from "How Much Land Does a Man Require?"

1. My first impression of the story is... *I could easily see how you could get caught up like that.*

2. I related to the following character because... *Pakhom because he was working his way up from the bottom and thought that just a little more would make him happy. I understand that idea fairly well myself.*

3. The story motivated or moved me in what way? *I want to make sure that I don't get to the end of my life and figure out that I lived for the wrong things. I don't want to look back and realize what a fool I have been.*

4. Other impressions? *It was kind of eerie how the devil was involved in Pakhom's life. I had the sense that maybe there really is a devil like that in the world. I don't know though.*

CHAPTER 8

The Plan

Think ahead; don't save your reason for difficult situations, use it to anticipate them...your whole life should be a matter of thinking out your destination.
Baltasar Gracian

It's time to make a plan; to bring together all your efforts from the previous chapters. Your worksheets contain information essential to your future joy. To transform that information into an effective plan will take plenty of brain power, but not more than you possess. You simply need to give this plan your best effort, and you'll succeed. How do you put forth your best effort?

A Time of Retreat

You need to withdraw to a private, secluded place for a time of contemplation. You need to plan a retreat. A few hours is the minimum amount of time required; a day or two may be better. The concept is simple: gather the information about yourself, go to a place where you are comfortable and alone, and contemplate your life. Relax, and keep interruptions to a minimum.

The first time I took a retreat, I spent several hours on the front porch of an abandoned cabin in the woods. As I sat with my notes in front of me and reflected on my life, several new insights became clear. I wrote my thoughts and they became part of the plan that changed my life. I remember my first retreat like it happened yesterday, and the benefits continue to enrich me.

You may object that you don't have time for a retreat. If a retreat is not worthwhile to you, you'll not find the time. On the other hand, if you believe a retreat could bring you great joy, you'll make the time to go. Remember, when it comes to time, we do the things we want to do.

I find the woods an ideal place of retreat for me because I'm not distracted by other people or the TV. Perhaps you would benefit by finding a pristine location to do your thinking. On the other hand, you may find a hotel room in the middle of the city works just as well. Perhaps you will go to a community park and sit at a secluded picnic table for a few hours. Don't worry too much about the location or the setting; what matters is getting away from your normal routine for a time.

Most people balk at the idea of a personal retreat. We are all busy. There are newspapers to read, work to be done, children to be chauffeured, and so much more. Just getting the most urgent things done seems like more than we can handle. When we get a break, we tend to flop in front of the TV or stick a movie in the VCR. We vegetate.

Living in this manner, week after week, month after month, year after year, we spend the currency of our lives. It need not be so. With some effort, we can take some quiet time of retreat to think deeply about our lives.

The Value of a Simple Plan

In this chapter, we will look at ways to develop a simple plan for our lives. Why is this plan so important? Most of us work hard, yet few of us put enough effort into the truly important things. For many of us, our lives fly by, with one crisis following the next, and we never really take control. There never seems to be enough time nor energy to get beyond the day-to-day routine of job and family responsibilities.

By creating a simple plan, we formulate a blueprint for positive change in our lives. We give ourselves an opportunity to change rather than just living more of the same. We allow ourselves to go beyond our normal responses to the situations in our lives. By having a plan, we prepare to succeed.

Victor Frankl said, "We detect, rather than invent, the missions in our lives." We don't have to wait for an angel to come to us in our sleep and give us direction. We usually have the information; we just need to get it clear in our minds. The time of retreat, combined with your thoughts from the worksheets, provide an ideal basis to help you devise a simple plan for a more joyful life.

Significant Observations from Previous Worksheets

Worksheet #48 provides a place to write significant observations from previous worksheets. This exercise should be your first retreat activity. Carefully read each of your previous worksheets. Think about the items that seem surprising or somehow significant. Most worksheets have at least one item that seems significant upon review.

Worksheet #48 lists twelve primary relationships (such as parents, spouse, friends, etc.) that will help organize your thinking. There are also two spaces to add relationships that are special

Name: *John Miller*   Worksheet #48   Date: *4-29-00*

Significant Observations from Previous Worksheets

Review all previous Worksheets and write at least one significant item from each. Record the observations in the appropriate category below.

1. Parents
    - *Wish I could make a true peace with my Dad.   WS#4*
    - *Dad was very unfair and unfeeling to us when we were kids. WS#17*
    - *Mom and Dad did a poor job as parents when we were young. WS#22*
    - *I learned how to work hard from Dad. WS#31*

2. Grandparents
    - *Grandma Miller always remembered my birthday with a card and money. WS#1*
    - *Grandpa Long is a mean drunk. WS#15*

3. Spouse
    - *I absolutely want to stay married to Rachel.   WS#4*
    - *I should learn Rachel's personality type. WS#10*
    - *Rachel and I have almost opposite love languages. WS#11*
    - *Rachel and I had our best time on the Bahamas vacation. WS#21*
    - *I need to talk with Rachel more. WS#24*

4. Children
    - *I am way too impatient with Nate and Katie. WS#6*
    - *I don't want to get mad so easily at the kids. WS#13*
    - *Just playing outside was the most fun thing I did as a little kid. WS#16*
    - *Vacations were high spots in my childhood. WS#18*
    - *Rachel and I do a decent job as parents. WS#23*

5. Other Relatives
    - *A lot of my relatives tend to be mean. WS#14*
    - *Bobby and I should do some more fun things together. WS#25*

6. Friends
    -

7. Co-Workers
    -

Name: *John Miller*   Worksheet #48 (continued)   Date: *4-29-00*

8. Work
    - *Even though it's frustrating, I enjoy my work. WS#2*
    - *I am good at settling disputes fairly on the jobsite. WS#6*
    - *Work is important to me and I want to get better at it. WS#8*

9. Hobbies
    -

10. Talents
    - *I loved to draw when I was young. WS#17*
    - *I am good at building things. WS#20*

11. God
    - *Church doesn't seem very real or useful to me. WS#3*
    - *I lost interest in church at 17 years old. WS#19*
    - *I wish I had more of a relationship with God. WS#27, #28, #29*
    - *I would like to know more about the Bible. WS#47*

12. Myself
    - *I wish I could communicate my feelings better. WS#3*
    - *I am a pessimist. WS#5*
    - *I must learn to control my anger better. WS#7*
    - *I am a Calculating Controller type personality. WS#9*
    - *I have very strong emotions. WS#12*

13. _____
    - *I definitely see the world as a dangerous place full of potential pain and humiliation. WS#15*
    - *I should learn to lighten up on myself. WS#26*

John Miller arranged to rent a cabin by the lake for his weekend retreat. He discussed the idea with Rachel, and she encouraged him to go. He left on a Saturday morning and returned Sunday afternoon. When he got to the cabin, he took a little walk to relax before he got down to work. He agonized over Worksheet #1 for quite some time, trying to write something profound. He finally just wrote something that was true and struck him as significant (which is all that's necessary.)

Several of his observations surprised John, especially the critical comments about his family. John had decided previously, though, to be as honest as possible and to keep these worksheets completely confidential. John felt a sense of accomplishment as he worked and knew he was on the right track.

or unique to you. Record the significant observation from each worksheet in the appropriate category on Worksheet #48. If you need extra space, just attach other papers.

Please don't rush through this important step. The review of your worksheets requires careful contemplation and musing. Take the time to think about the significance of what you wrote. Many of the items will be obvious to you; but don't read too quickly and miss an idea that could change your life.

I recommend listing at least one significant observation from each worksheet. Admittedly, there will be some worksheets where that observation is not profound. However, some worksheets may have several significant observations.

Some people have said, "I just don't like to think so deeply." I agree. Thinking hard makes my head hurt. However, the pay-off is astounding. So, we just need to "suck it up" and put forth the effort. We will survive (even if we don't like it much).

You are at the critical transition point in the personal growth process. You have moved through the idea and study phases. The analysis phase and the plan phase come together at this point. As you read through the previous worksheets and draw conclusions from each, you will begin to lay out the basic building blocks of your plan.

The ultimate value you obtain from this book will directly relate with how carefully and conscientiously you do this work. Though this step is critical, it's not complicated. Simply think about each worksheet as deeply as you can and list the things that seem most significant to you.

As you read the information on Worksheet #48, you may feel some powerful emotions. Resist the temptation to draw conclusions too quickly. The significant observations listed in Worksheet #48 are merely interesting thoughts at this point; they have not yet been analyzed. The analysis stage must precede the plan stage in order to develop a great plan.

Ideas to Improve Your Relationships

The next important step involves analyzing your information and formulating ways to improve your relationships. As mentioned before, meaning and joy in life come through relationships. The information about yourself from Worksheet #48 will help you develop some ideas for improving your relationships.

Worksheet #49 provides space to list many ideas which could improve your various relationships. Every significant observation from Worksheet #48 need not (and probably should not) match up with an idea on Worksheet #49. Read each observation written on Worksheet #48. Think about how that observation affects your current relationships and how it could affect future relationships. Then record any ideas that come to mind regarding improving relationships on Worksheet #49.

The proper completion of this worksheet will require some soul-searching. This is why a time of personal retreat is so valuable. Take your time and prayerfully consider ways that you might improve your various relationships.

I have noticed so many times in my life that I knew the right things to do, I just didn't do them. You may ask, "If I know the best course of action and have chosen not to do it in the past, why bother to write it down now?"

An example may be helpful. If I know that I ought to communicate better with my spouse, yet rarely put forth the effort to do it, why bother writing it down? Am I not just going to continue acting the same way? "Probably, but not necessarily." While we tend to continue our habits, looking back over the last few years of our lives, most of us will admit to some changes. Change happens!

So, if it becomes clear to me that my life could be much improved by better communication with my spouse, I can decide to try it. If I realize that choosing to talk a few minutes a day when I don't really feel like it, could dramatically change the way my spouse feels about me, I may put forth the effort.

Name: *John Miller*   Worksheet #49   Date: *4-29-00*

Ideas for Improving my Relationships

Review Worksheet #48 and list some ideas.

1. Parents
    * *Spend some more time with my parents.*
    * *Thank Dad for teaching me about hard work.*

2. Grandparents
    *

3. Spouse
    * *Spend more time with Rachel. She talks about a friend of hers*
      who goes out on a date with her husband about once a month.
      Maybe we should try that.
    * *Take another short vacation with just Rachel and I.*
    * *Try and talk with Rachel some every day.*

4. Children
    * *I should just play with the kids more.*
    * *Take a family vacation.*
    * *Get the kids away from the TV and outside playing more.*
    * *Assign chores that the kids are responsible to do.*

5. Other Relatives
    * *Get together with Bobby more often.*

6. Friends
    *

7. Co-Workers
    * *I rarely stop to have drinks with the guys from Commercial*
      Contractors. I could do that more often.

Name: *John Miller*   Worksheet #49 (continued)   Date: *4-29-00*

8. Work
    • *I would like to learn more about how to plan and schedule projects, maybe I could go to a seminar.*
    • *Learn how to use computers, since I don't know squat about them now.*

9. Hobbies
    • *I don't think I have time for any hobbies.*

10. Talents
    • *Since both the kids like to draw, maybe I could do something with them.*

11. God
    • *Get a Bible and read some every day.*
    • *Learn some things about praying.*

12. Myself
    • *Lighten up, laugh more and do more fun stuff.*

13. _____

14. _____

As John Miller read through his observations, an interesting thought hit him. He realized what he had written about his parents seemed harsh, but it was the reality of his upbringing. The interesting idea didn't come from the harshness—it came from the observation that his father taught him how to work hard. This trait helped John prosper and he never thought about it before.

John realized this positive trait might be a good starting point for a meaningful conversation between his father and him. Perhaps they could have a discussion where all the bad stuff was not hanging directly over their heads. Not definitely, just perhaps.

Thinking about his own children, an even more powerful idea came to him. Both he and Rachel struggled to shield their kids from the ugliness John had experienced as a child. Yet, in trying to give his children what he didn't have, he was missing the opportunity to give them what he did have. He was missing the opportunity to teach his kids how to work. John decided he could improve his relationship with his children by teaching them to work.

Remember, the possibility of joy best motivates us to change. If I notice that increased verbal communication with my spouse produces improved physical communication (better sex), I may be motivated to talk more. This is not manipulation; it is understanding the truth of this particular relationship. If my efforts at improved verbal communication are noticed and appreciated, a closeness and a trust grows and leads to a better overall relationship.

Of course, time is a critical factor. You will be sorely disappointed if you expect your first efforts at a new type of behavior to be immediately rewarded with an improved relationship. Your first attempts will probably be met with some degree of cynicism and distrust: "What does he want now?" or "Who is she trying to fool?" Oliver Wendell Holmes said, "Compliment your wife, even if it frightens her at first."

We need to anticipate those types of reactions and be prepared to continue our new habit. You will be amazed how quickly most people lose their cynicism. In the end, we all want to love and be loved. We just need some time to feel that it's safe.

How to Write Action Plans

After completing Worksheet #49, you are ready to begin the first draft of your one-year plan. At this stage, the plan should easily come together. In fact, you only need to carefully review Worksheet #49 to develop the first draft of your one-year plan.

The analysis step requires you to think about each item from Worksheet #49 in a critical and realistic manner. On Worksheet #49, an item is an idea. On Worksheet #50, the idea must be redefined as an action that you will choose to implement. The action must be reasonably realistic (i.e. you must have a decent chance of actually accomplishing it).

In order for an action plan to be effective, it should have the following components:

1. **The action plan should be simply stated.** Long, detailed action plans are just too difficult to remember and execute. Remember the KISS method: Keep It Simple, Stupid.

2. **The action plan must be measurable.** Vague, general statements are not acceptable. You must be able to know if you have accomplished the plan, so strive to make it measurable.

3. **Solve a problem important to you with the action plan.** Avoid setting goals merely because they would be nice to achieve. The success of your plan depends on how clearly you understand a problem area in your life and how much you want to overcome it.

4. **Be realistic with your action plan.** To create a plan in which you have a 2% probability of success is not wise (particularly if you are new to this type of planning). Neither is it wise to create a plan with 100% probability of success. Choose an action plan that is realistic, but which will stretch you. Your one-year plan should challenge you.

You must think about the specifics of any action plan with regard to the above guidelines. Consider how you are going to follow-up each of the items and measure them. You want a plan you can maintain and continue.

To develop a plan for positive change, you need to think about a time period. I never found long range plans to be effective. I can't get excited about an accomplishment 20 years from now. Even five years is a very long time. When I look at the difficulty involved in changing my own behavior, I need some immediate benefits to motivate me. Therefore, I've found a plan with some clear, simple objectives for the next 12 months works.

Let's critique a specific action plan, such as, "Improve the lives of children around the world." Do you see the problems with this action plan? It needs to be more specific; it needs to have a measurable goal. That sense of motivation and joy comes when we can anticipate actual positive results. Restate that plan as, "Be a big brother/big sister to a local child for one year."

As you think about your plan, try to look at it apart from yourself and use your common sense. Humans can combine deductive thinking and inductive thinking and just know the right thing. We call that skill "common sense." Consider the items in your plan from a common sense viewpoint and think about how each makes you feel.

I never like the idea of attempting to change my behavior. Like most people, I don't like to fail and I find change somewhat scary. I have found by experience, though, that the effort outweighs the risk. The great, joyful surprise that happens to us when we realize that we can do what we were afraid we could not do is wonderful. That sense of joy will motivate you to take additional risks to change and improve yourself and your relationships.

Plan 201

Name: *John Miller*   Worksheet #50   Date: *4-30-00*
My One-Year Plan – First Draft

1. Relationship with Others:
    a. In order to build my relationship with ***my parents***, I will try to:
        (1.) *Go out to breakfast with them a few times a year.*
        (2.) *Write Dad a note of appreciation for teaching me to work hard.*

    b. In order to build my relationship with ***Rachel***, I will try to:
        (1.) *Take Rachel on a date every month (no kids).*
        (2.) *Go away together for a long week-end.*
        (3.) *Make an effort to talk together for a few minutes every day.*

    c. In order to build my relationship with ***our kids***, I will try to:
        (1.) *Limit their TV time to 2 hours per day and have them play outside more. I need to go out and play with them sometimes.*
        (2.) *Take a family vacation up to the lake for a few days.*
        (3.) *Make a chore chart for the kids.*

2. Relationship with God:
    In order to build my relationship with God, I will try to:
    a. *Read 1 chapter in the Bible every day.*

    b. *Learn more about praying by talking to Bill Jameson at work.*

3. Relationship with Self:
    In order to build my relationship with myself, I will try to:
    a. *Make sure I take some time every week to relax and have fun.*

4. Other:
    a. *Go to a Sixer's game with Bobby.*
    b. *Stop for a drink with the guys more often.*

My One-Year Plan

So, how do you feel about your one-year plan – first draft? Hopefully, you are excited about the possibilities. There should be a sense of anticipation. There should also be some sense of misgiving about your ability to actually complete it. A combination of some joy and some concern is appropriate.

The first draft plan is merely some well-thought-out words on paper; you have not yet committed yourself to achieving the plan. Before making that commitment, you must proceed through one more step.

Each item on the first draft plan should be analyzed carefully to determine if you truly desire to accomplish it. As I mentioned earlier, the anticipated joy at the accomplishment of a contemplated task acts as the best motivation. You need to look at the items in your first draft one-year plan and decide if the results would bring you joy. If you can't get excited about the results, you probably won't put in the effort to carry out the plan. Remember --- change is difficult and will not happen on its own.

An item on my current one-year plan involves spending time with each of our three children individually, once a month. I take each child alone with me for a special activity that is usually of their choosing. Perhaps we go out for dinner and shopping or maybe to some activity like a football game or a movie or a bike ride. Since I am a busy person with lots of irons in the fire, I knew it would be a challenge to find three evenings a month to take out the kids. As I thought about the task, though, I got a glimpse of the potential value of this course of action.

I remembered the times my Dad did things with me as a child and how special it made me feel. Sometimes he took me to a baseball game; sometimes he just took me along on his work for a service call (Dad was an electrician). I treasured those times, even as a child, enjoying the opportunity to talk with Dad and be listened to. Dad did not schedule those times, but he did make them happen. With the busier pace of life these days, I doubt whether those times would happen for my family unless I put forth some specific effort.

As I analyzed the value of spending three evenings a month with the kids, I concluded it would be a great thing. If I can do something important for my children, then I'll feel good about myself as a father. Joy comes from knowing I am positively affecting our kids. The only difficulty was finding the time, and I knew this would be a struggle. I determined to make time each month for these special outings. I put that on my final one-year plan.

Like most plans, things did not go exactly as I had anticipated. This time, for once, things went better. I had not considered how much fun I'd have with the kids on our special times. Our times together build confidence and are great fun for both of us. It becomes much easier for me to find the time for an activity when I have lots of fun doing it (especially understanding that I am a Type I personality). We talk and laugh about things and are so relaxed together. These special times have become activities that we all look forward to.

Carefully review each of the items on your one-year plan – first draft, and answer the questions listed on Worksheet #51. This process will take some time. The plans that are not carefully analyzed and committed to become the plans that fail. Put in the time and effort to analyze your plan items, then you will succeed.

You may or may not have great confidence upon completion of Worksheet #51. If you feel good about your plans on Worksheet #51, then copy them directly onto Worksheet #52. If you still are not sure about the items listed on Worksheet #51, take more time. Review the four criteria listed above in the section "How to Write Action Plans." Also, reread Worksheets #48 and #49. Simply take another pass at the process until you devise a one-year plan that you feel good about and can commit yourself to.

Name: *John Miller*   Worksheet #51   Date: *4-30-00*

Analysis of My One-Year Plan – First Draft

Answer the following questions for each individual item:

a.   How would the accomplishment of this item bring me joy?
b.   What seems difficult about accomplishing this item?
c.   How will this item be measured and tracked?
d.   When I visualize the accomplishment of this item, what do I see?

1a.(1) *Take my parents to breakfast a few times a year* – *I would enjoy being closer to my parents. I don't want them to die without settling things. The conversation may not be too easy. I visualize us sitting, eating, and having a relaxed, friendly discussion.*

1a.(2) *Write a note of appreciation to Dad* – *I would like to put the pain of my relationship with Dad behind me. Honestly, I don't know if I can write a nice letter to Dad. I sure could write one that blasts him. It's difficult to visualize anything here.*

1b.(1) *Take Rachel on a date every month* – *The closeness would be nice, especially the likelihood of good sex at the end of the evening. Making the effort to plan the evening will be the biggest difficulty. I can see Rachel and me out dancing together.*

1b.(2). *Go away together for a long weekend* – *We had such a great time when we went to the Bahamas, I think any weekend away would be good. Both the time and the money will be difficult, although I hear some hotels in Baltimore and Philadelphia offer some cheap rates for get-away weekends. I visualize a lazy Saturday morning in the hotel room with room service.*

1b.(3) *Make an effort to talk together for a few minutes every day* – *Since Rachel tells me I am a lousy communicator, she would probably enjoy if I tried harder. I'm not really sure how much something like this would help. I should change the task to, "Focus exclusively on Rachel for at least 10 minutes a day." I would have to sacrifice some TV time to do this one. I do enjoy when we sit and talk and can visualize us doing that.*

1c.(1) *Limit kids' TV time to 2 hours per day and have them play outside more* – *I would like to see the kids away from the TV and outside doing stuff. I would also like to see them learn a little about work. Maybe we could have them do a few simple outside chores before they are allowed to watch TV. Rachel would have to enforce this and she can be real easy on the kids. I can visualize Rachel and me talking about how it went every day and the kids telling us what they did outside.*

1c.(2) *Take a family vacation up to the lake for a few days* – *We would all enjoy this. I would have to take a few vacation days, but I have plenty. I can see us all swimming in the clear water.*

2a. *Read 1 chapter in the Bible every day* – *I would like to learn more about God and I suppose the Bible is the place to start. Just keeping at it will be the only difficulty. I don't know what, if anything, will come of it.*

2b. *Learn more about praying by talking to Bill Jameson at work* – *Again, I don't really know why I am interested in this at this point in my life. I guess it is partly for me and partly for the kids. Also I would just like to know the truth. I should rename this item: "Pray every day," and just put a note about talking to Bill. I can not visualize myself praying.*

3a. *Make sure I take some time every week to relax and have fun* – *I am not sure what I would do to relax and have fun. I have spent most of my life working. I used to "party hardy" to have fun, but that stuff is behind me now. I suppose I could make a list of stuff that I would enjoy and have it around for when I have some time.*

4a. *Go to a Sixer's game with Bobby* – *This would be fun and is worth doing. We just have to do it. I can see us watching the game and moaning about all the lousy calls.*

4b. *Stop for a drink with the guys more often* – *Even though this could be fun, it just isn't me anymore. I'd rather be home with Rachel, Nate and Katie. I'm going to take this one off the list.*

5a. *Learn more about computers* – *I didn't put this one on the first draft plan, but I am going to add it. I am not sure where to start except I know I need to learn about computers to keep up with the times.*

As John analyzed his first draft, one-year plan, he was amazed at how clearly he began to think. He had a sense of peace about almost every item. He had the feeling that the things he wrote were possible, and that was a nice feeling. With the items written, the creation of the final plan was little more than copying them onto the plan format and reviewing them one more time.

There are several questions you should consider prior to finalizing your one-year plan.

1. Will you feel comfortable posting your one-year plan where others could read it? Do you want to keep your one-year plan completely confidential? Whom would you allow to read your one-year plan?

2. Where will you keep your one-year plan? How will you check progress?

3. How often will you review your progress? (I find a monthly or twice-a-month review works well for me.)

As you write your plan items, consider adding a note to help motivate or clarify. Perhaps note a particularly strong visualization in which you see yourself enjoying the accomplishment of the item. Maybe you need a note to remind you of a critical portion of the plan item. These little extras help the review process make more sense.

Take the time now to finish your plan for the upcoming year. You have created a plan that can help change your life. Allow yourself the luxury of imagining how your life will be in one year if you accomplish most of the items on the plan. The increase in both joy and purpose will be significant.

Name: *John Miller*   Worksheet #51   Date: *4-30-00*

My One-Year Plan

2000 Plan for John Miller

1. *Go out to breakfast with my parents quarterly*

2. *Send a note of appreciation to Dad*

3. *Take Rachel on a date every month*
   make an effort to plan each evening

4. *Go away with Rachel for a long weekend*

5. *Focus only on Rachel for at least 10 minutes a day*
   sit and talk without the TV on

6. *Limit kids TV to 2 hours/day; play outside more*
   discuss this daily with Rachel and the kids

7. *Take a family vacation up to the lake for a few days*

8. *Read 1 chapter in the Bible every day*

9. *Pray every day*
   talk to Bill Jameson about prayer

10. *Take some time to relax and have fun every week*
    make a list of things I would enjoy

11. *Go to a Sixer's game with Bobby*

12. *Learn more about computers*
    talk to people, try to find a used computer cheap, etc.

CHAPTER 9

Living the Plan

"Always bear in mind that your own resolution to success is more important than any other one thing."
Abraham Lincoln

No matter how good your plan, nothing happens if you don't execute. To do this, you'll need to change some habits. You'll need to stop doing some things you now do and start doing some new things.

Most of us cringe at the thought of change. We have an established routine and any change is uncomfortable. The familiar comforts us. The fear of change controls us more than the allure of rewards from new behavior. Don't minimize the difficulty of personal change. The creation of new habits will be difficult and challenging, but completely possible.

Creating New Habits

The most difficult aspect of creating new habits will not be the time required nor the critical comments of others. The greatest challenge will be our own sabotage. Our own feelings of unworthiness will surface at the most inopportune times and make us feel like phonies.

Thoughts like, "Who are you trying to kid? Don't try to pretend you love her when just yesterday you were so mad at her you felt like killing her. You big phony, just give it up and act normal." Have you ever had a monologue like this run through your head? I've heard it called self-talk. It seems like a non-stop audio tape that plays in one's mind. The same message gets played over and over and reinforces an idea.

Unfortunately, when we are trying to change habits, most of the self-talk seems to be negative. It strives to maintain the status quo, even when we recognize that a habit change would be beneficial. We need to anticipate this negative self-talk and prepare to deal with it.

One of the secrets to overcoming negative self-talk is realizing that we need not be good in order to act good. Many times the only way to develop a virtue is to act as if you already have it. As you continue your forced behavior, you usually will find that the virtue grows.

As you examine the execution phase of your plan, John Miller's example may be helpful. Consider John's plan to devote some time every day to communication with his wife. That step could dramatically improve their relationship. However, there will be days he will come home tired, not feeling like putting forth the effort. There will be days when her behavior will anger him, and he will want to nurse a grudge rather than talking and listening deeply. On these days, it's guaranteed that his self-talk will be telling him he is a failure and a sap.

Since John has thought deeply about his one-year plan, though, he understands that change will not just happen naturally. He understands he will have to force this change to happen. So

John can defeat negative self-talk by anticipating it and realizing he must hold to his plan even when he doesn't feel like it.

If John had to go on in this manner indefinitely, he could not sustain the effort. John understands, however, that the virtue follows the behavior. After a few weeks of talking to his wife every day, John realizes he is beginning to enjoy this part of the day. The practice of communication becomes easier as the benefits increase.

John has established a new habit, and the motivation to continue comes from the increased love and closeness with his wife. Nevertheless, the initial stages of change were difficult. The negative self-talk was strong, and no rewards were immediately evident. This difficult early stage sabotages most behavior change.

Why do you think the benefits of better communication with Rachel were not immediately available to John? She had told him for years she wanted him to talk and listen to her more. Why didn't she quickly reward this type of behavior? Think about our own natural desire to protect ourselves. When we encounter changed behavior, we react with skepticism. We wonder, "What game is going on here and how could it hurt me?"

We must anticipate this skepticism from the people we know and care about as we begin behavior change. As we strive to create a new habit, we will also be confusing those around us. They will be wondering, either consciously or subconsciously, "What in the world is going on here?" They will be trying to determine if this behavior change is real, and they will be uncomfortable.

I don't want to create the impression that making changes will be overly difficult, yet I do want to warn of some of the pitfalls that may be encountered. Self-talk will try to convince us to return to what is known and comfortable. The people closest to us will be skeptical. These forces may discourage us in our efforts for positive change.

The secret to success is to simply persevere until the benefits start to appear. Negative self-talk will decrease as we become accustomed to the changes. Other people's skepticism will decrease with time. Most importantly, since we decided on the change in order to improve our life, that improvement will become more and more apparent with time.

Do you brush your teeth every day? I hope so. Did you always brush your teeth every day? No, at some time in your life you developed the habit. If for some reason you forget to brush your teeth one day, how do you respond? My guess is that you do not berate yourself and tell yourself that you are worthless. You simply brush your teeth the next day and get on with your life. That attitude is the last secret to creating a new habit.

Don't beat yourself up if you fail in your new habit. In fact, expect that you will fail sometimes. Be prepared for the failure and be prepared to forgive yourself and go on. Just do your new habit the next time. You will be amazed how this simple concept can create positive life changes.

Courage

When forming new habits, we will absolutely hit some periods in which we doubt the worth of the entire project. Conflicting thoughts and emotions are normal.

The "Positive-Thinking Gurus" tell us to simply ignore the doubt. They say if we control our attitude, the feelings of doubt will eventually go away. Remember though, our ultimate goal is to find the truth, not to find the quickest method for feeling good. Sometimes, doubts help lead us to the truth.

It takes courage to honestly examine one's own doubts. It takes courage to begin to change one's behavior. So why would we struggle to change? When asked why he robbed banks, Willie Sutton replied, "Because that's where the money is." Similarly, we find the courage to change our behavior and to honestly examine our doubts because "that's where the joy is."

When I think about courage, I recall the Charles family that lives down the street from us. Back in the 1950's, Norm and Betty Charles were a young couple, struggling to raise five small children and run their dairy farm. The Charles family experienced some difficulties in their lives and turned to God for help. One day, Norm felt a strong sense that he and his family should go to Brazil to be missionaries. Try as he might, he could not get rid of this idea.

Finally, Norm prayed something like, "Lord, I have all this debt. It would not be right for me to leave while I owe all this money. Lord, if you truly want us to go into missions, please make the cows give an extra thousand pounds of milk this month." The extra milk came, not just for one month, but for two, and the Charles' financial condition improved. Then Norm began to doubt the wisdom of moving his entire family to Brazil. He thought he could instead support other missionaries with his increased financial resources.

Within days of this decision, the cows came down with an illness and the veterinarian said the entire herd was at risk. At that point, Norm and Betty understood their good fortune had come from God. Upon recommitting themselves to the mission field, their cows recovered. Soon all their belongings were sold, and they were on a freighter ship to Brazil.

They struggled through Portuguese language classes. As the end of the term neared, they realized all the other students were associated with mission organizations and had specific places to go upon graduation from language school. The Charles' simply prayed the Lord would place them where they ought to be.

One day they drove to a remote village with friends, having heard of a need for some missionaries in that region. They stopped at a house in the village and briefly explained to the young girl who answered the door that they were missionaries. She didn't say a word, but ran back into the house. A few moments later, many people streamed from the house; they had been having a prayer meeting, specifically praying for missionaries to come to their village to help begin a church!

The Charles family lived with courage. They attempted to discover direction for their lives and then they made the hard decisions to "…go for it." Their complete story can be found in the book, <u>Heaven on Earth: Family Style</u>.

To live out your plan, you must vow to live it with courage. You can find the strength and the courage. Julies Hare said, "Half the failures in life result from pulling in one's horse as he is leaping." Break old habits of fear and conformity and allow yourself the joy of success. Resist the temptation to "pull in your horse as he is leaping" and live with all the courage you can muster.

Common Sense

Common sense is essential for executing your plan. As a person with little natural common sense, I know what it is to struggle with change and not pay attention to items that are obvious to everyone but me. A particular incident comes to mind when I think of common sense.

I was working as a foreman on a large construction project. I was driving about 90 minutes each way to the job site and was not making much money. I decided it would be a good time to remodel the basement, even though I had little time and less money.

I went from idea to action and out came all the duct work from our oil furnace. I planned to move the ducts to better locations and to build a wood furnace to augment our existing furnace. Of course, I started this project in October, thinking that it would be simple and take only a short time.

As you may imagine, my project was anything but simple. With the months passing, it became clear even to me that my timing had been poor. The only heat we had in the house was an old potbelly stove that we had installed in the kitchen. The wood fire in that stove would only last about three hours before it completely burned out. Therefore, we would be without heat in the house for much of the night.

One morning I checked the thermometer in our baby's room. The temperature was 34° F, and there was Alexey, our one-year old baby, sleeping in the cold. My lack of common sense became obvious to me at that moment. Fortunately, we all survived and laugh about it now.

While implementing your plan, keep your eyes open to the things going on around you. Think about the issues that are clear to others, but difficult for you to see. Don't neglect your common sense.

Daily Time with God

Another key for successful plan implementation is spending time with God each day. A daily time of prayer helps life make sense and puts it into perspective. I have never met a person who took time to pray every day who regretted the effort. Of course, this is an issue between you and God.

If you decide you would like to pray every day, expect several challenges. First will be finding the time. The best way for busy people to learn to pray is to set a time for prayer and to stick to it. Simply do nothing else in that time.

You must decide how you will pray. Prayer can be broken down into five basic types: forgiveness, praise, thanksgiving, intercession, and petition. If you cover each of these topics as you pray, you will have plenty to say to God.

Forgiveness involves telling God the things we did that we know we ought not to have done, and asking Him to forgive us. It also includes asking to be forgiven for not doing the things we know we ought to have done. When we honestly examine our day-to-day living and our true motivations, we find many things for which to ask forgiveness.

Praise prayers express our wonder and thanks to God for being God, the Creator and Sustainer of the universe. The closer one grows to God, the more one wants to praise Him. Since many of the Psalms are David's praise prayers, I often read a Psalm aloud. There is great joy in finding various ways to praise God.

Thanksgiving prayers give thanks for the specific blessings and protections we have in our lives. Most of us have much to be thankful for, and we rarely take the time to express that.

Intercessory prayer involves praying for other people, asking God to intervene on their behalf in some specific way. Prayers of intercession may be for someone's physical health, emotional well-being or spiritual growth. Many people keep a written list of prayer concerns to help them remember such items.

Prayers of petition are specific prayers in which we ask God for things we need or want. If you only ask God for things you want or beg for help when you encounter trouble, you may be too self-absorbed and could use some balance. On the other hand, don't think that spiritual people never ask God for anything for themselves, for that isn't true. If we have a growing relationship with God, we will naturally tell Him the things we need and want.

If you practice these five types of prayer, you will not have the problem of having nothing to say to God. However, you will soon learn how much your mind can wander and how little self-control you really possess. Don't be discouraged by your early attempts at time spent in prayer. Your mind may wander, your mind may race, you may fall soundly asleep. These things happen to everyone. The important thing is to keep on spending the time in prayer, even when it does not feel rewarding.

Often in prayer you will feel like nothing is happening. Looking back over time, though, you'll see that much has happened. The process parallels spending time with your children; you don't notice them growing, but an outside observer can notice all sorts of changes. Likewise, your time spent with God will gradually produce positive changes.

Rest

While attempting to carry out your new plan, you need proper rest. You can only push your body and mind so hard. Take the time to recharge. Get enough rest. My wife Debby has always believed that when you have lots of things to do, you should get your nap out of the way first. It's important for us to have a plan and to be focused, but we need to guard against being over-whelmed. We need to remember to take a nap occasionally.

If you begin paying attention to almost any relationship, you will see a direct correlation between the amount of fatigue and the amount of conflict. We simply are not at our best when we are tired or hungry. If you ever raised young children, think about how you acted by the end of a long day and how they were acting. Usually, it wasn't pretty.

Few of us are at our best when we're tired. The things that would be simple if we were rested become a big deal when we're tired. By not getting enough rest, we increase the challenge with no corresponding reward. Why would we choose to do that? By managing to get adequate rest, we enhance the likelihood of successfully completing our plan. Life goes better when we get enough sleep.

Sense of Humor

A sense of humor will be a great resource for living out your plan. I guarantee that some of your plan items will take you out of your comfort zone. When you then have a failure, it's easy to become discouraged or feel ridiculous. Pride gets hurt and we don't like it! To see the humor in the situation helps us from wallowing in defeat. The ability to laugh a bit at ourselves is truly a valuable tool.

I was working on the Peter Frampton tour in the summer of 1977, and we were doing a few large stadium shows. In Cleveland, we had some heavy rains in the morning, and the start of the concert was delayed until the weather stabilized (the performers generally seemed uncomfortable holding a metal microphone on a metal stage during thunderstorms). There were about 80,000 people in the audience, just sitting and waiting for the show to begin and those of us on the road crew were wandering around, waiting for the weather to clear. I remember walking onto the stage, checking the microphones for placement.

While on this tour, I had become friends with a rock and roll truck driver, who I called Mr. Dave. He always referred to me as Mr. Ned. We had a very civilized relationship, I suppose. Well, as I was standing in the middle of that stage in front of 80,000 people, Mr. Dave came up behind me and with one quick motion, yanked my shorts down to my ankles. Now at that stage in my life, I never wore underwear (I thought it "unnecessary"), so I was standing there not wearing much more than a look of total surprise.

Unfortunately, since my shorts had been buttoned and zippered, I couldn't get them back up too quickly. I had to stand there and try to calmly unbutton the shorts and then unzipper them in order to get them back up. It seemed to me to be a very long time until I was clothed again. Of course, Mr. Dave was behind me laughing uncontrollably.

I would like to be able to say that I had the final laugh on him, but I didn't. I just accepted the prank and laughed about it. It was simply no big deal.

Story by Leo Tolstoy

"Where Love Is, There God Is Also"

In a certain town there lived a shoemaker named Martin Aveditch. He lived in a basement room which possessed but one window. This window looked onto the street, and through it a glimpse could be caught of the passers-by. It is true that only their legs could be seen, but that did not matter, as Martin could recognize people by their boots alone. He had lived here for a long time, and so had many acquaintances.

There were very few pairs of boots in the neighborhood which he had not worked on at least once, if not twice. Some he had resoled, others he had fitted with side-pieces, others he had re-sewn. Yes, he often saw his handiwork through that window. He was given plenty to do, for his work lasted well, his materials were good, his prices moderate, and his word to be depended on. If Martin said he could do a job by a given time, it would be done; and if not, he would tell you ahead of time rather than disappoint you.

Martin had always been an upright man, but as he got older he began more than ever to think about his soul and draw nearer to God. His wife had died while he was still an apprentice leaving behind a little boy of three. This was their only child since two older children had previously died. At first Martin thought about placing his son with his sister in the country but changed his mind thinking, "My little guy would not like to grow up in a strange family, so I'll keep him with me."

When Martin finished his apprenticeship, he went with his little boy to start their trade. But God had not seen fit to give Martin happiness in his children. The little boy was just growing up and beginning to help his father and to be a pleasure to him, when he fell ill, was put to bed, and died after a week's fever. Martin buried the little fellow and was inconsolable.

Indeed he was so angry, he began to murmur against God. His life seemed so empty that he often prayed for death. He reproached God for taking away his beloved son instead of himself, the old man. After awhile, he ceased altogether to go to church.

Then one day there came to see him an ancient pilgrim who was then in the eighth year of his pilgrimage. Martin talked to him and went on to complain to him of his great sorrow. "I no longer wish to be a God-fearing man," said Martin. "I only wish to die. That is all I ask of God. I am a lonely, hopeless man."

"You should not speak like that, brother," replied the old pilgrim. "It is not for us to judge the acts of God. We must rely not upon our own understanding but upon the divine wisdom. God saw fit that your son should die and that you should live. Therefore, it must be better so. If you despair, it is because you have wished to live too much for your own pleasure."

"For what then shall I live?" asked Martin.

"For God alone," replied the old man. "It is He who gave you life, and therefore it is He for whom you should live. When you come to live for Him you will cease to grieve, and your trials will become easy to bear."

Martin was silent. Then he spoke again. "But how am I to live for God?" he asked.

"Christ has shown us the way," answered the old man. "Can you read? If so, buy a Testament and study it. You will learn there how to live for God. Yes, it is all shown you there."

These words sank into Martin's soul. He went out the same day and bought a large-print copy of the New Testament and set himself to read it. At the beginning Martin had only meant to read on holidays, but when he began reading he found it so comforting to the soul that he never let a day pass without doing so. Sometimes he became so engrossed with his reading that all the kerosene burnt away in the lamp before he could tear himself away from the book.

Thus he came to read it every evening, and the more he read, the more clearly did he understand what God required of him and in what way he could live for God. So, his heart grew ever lighter and lighter.

He previously went to bed and moaned and sighed at the thought of his poor little son; but now he said, "Glory to Thee, O Lord! Glory to Thee! Thy will be done!" From that time onwards, Martin's life became completely changed. He previously went out on holidays and drank tea in the tavern and had an occasional glass of vodka. Although no drunkard, he would often leave the tavern in an excited state and talk much nonsense with his friends. Now, though, he turned his back on all this and his life had become quiet and joyous.

Early in the morning, he would sit down to his work and labor through his appointed hours. Then he would take the lamp down from the shelf, light it, and sit and read. The more he read, the more he understood, and the clearer and happier he grew at heart.

One night Martin was reading late. He had been reading those verses in the sixth chapter of Luke: "When one strikes you on one cheek, turn to him the other also. If someone takes your cloak, do not stop him from taking your tunic. Give to everyone who asks you and if anyone takes what belongs to you, do not demand it back. Do to others as you would have them do to you."

Then further down he read, "Why do you call me, 'Lord, Lord,' and do not do what I say? I will show you what he is like who comes to me and hears my words and puts them into practice. He is like a man who built a house, and dug down deep and laid the foundation on rock. When a flood came, the storm struck that house but could not shake it because it was well-built. But, the one who hears my words and does not put them into practice is like a man who built his house on the sand without a foundation. The moment the storm struck that house, it collapsed, and its destruction was complete."

Martin read those words and felt happy in his soul. He took off his glasses and laid them on the book, leaned his elbows on the table, and gave himself up to meditation. He tried to measure his life by those words, and he thought to himself: "Have I founded my house upon rock or sand? It is well if it be upon rock, yet it is so easy as I sit here by myself. I may think I have done all the Lord required of me and grow careless and sin again. Yet, I will keep on striving, for it is good to do so. Help me, Thou, oh Lord."

He kept on meditating. Although he knew it was time to go to bed, he hated to tear himself away from the book. He began to read the seventh chapter of Luke and read about the Centurion and the widow's son and the answer given to John's disciples. Then he came to the passage where the rich Pharisee invited Jesus to his house, and the woman washed the Lord's feet with her tears and He justified her.

"Then he turned towards the woman and said to Simon, 'Do you see this woman? I came into your house; you did not give me any water for my feet but she wet my feet with her tears and wiped them with her hair. You did not give me a kiss but this woman, from the time I entered, did not stop kissing my feet. You did not put oil on my head but she has poured perfume on my feet. Therefore, I tell you her many sins have been forgiven for she loved much. But he who has been forgiven little, loves little."

Once again, Martin took off his spectacles and became lost in meditation. "I'm even as that Pharisee," Martin thought to himself. "I drink tea and think only of my own needs. Yes, I think only of having plenty to eat and drink; of being warm and clean but never of entertaining a guest."

Martin sat pondering, "What if the Lord were to come and visit me." As he thought about this, he leaned forward on his elbows and was almost asleep.

"Martin," someone seemed to breathe in his ear; he started from his sleep.

"Who's there?" he said. He turned to look toward the door but he could see no one. Again, he bent forward over the table and he heard the words, "Martin, Martin. Look thou into the street tomorrow for I am coming to visit you."

Martin was awake now. He got up from the chair and rubbed his eyes. He didn't know if he was dreaming or awake when he heard those words, but he turned out the lamp and went to bed.

The next morning, Martin rose before daylight and said his prayers, made up the stove and got some cabbage soup and porridge ready. He put his leather apron around him and got ready to work by the window. He sat and worked hard, but all the time his thoughts were centered on last night.

He had two ideas about the vision. At one moment, he would think it was his fancy or the next moment he would have himself convinced he had really heard the voice. "Yes, it must have been so," he concluded.

So Martin sat by the window and kept looking out of it as much as working. When a pair of boots passed with which he was acquainted, he would bend down to look up through the window to see their owner's face as well. The doorkeeper passed in new felt boots, and then a water-carrier. Next came, an old soldier, a veteran of Nicholas' army, in old patched boots, and carrying a shovel in his hands. The soldier stopped by the window. His name was Stephen and he was kept by the neighboring tradesman out of charity, his duties being to help the doorkeeper.

He began to clear away the snow in front of Martin's window; the shoemaker looked at him, and then resumed his work. "I think I must be getting old," thought Martin with a smile. "Just because Stephen begins clearing away the snow... I jump to the conclusion that Christ is about to visit me. Yes, I am growing foolish now, old man that I am."

Yet he hardly made a dozen more stitches before he was craning his neck again to look out the window. He could see Stephen had placed his shovel against the wall and was resting, trying to warm himself. "He is evidently an old man now and broken," thought Martin to himself. "He is not strong enough to clear away some snow. Would he like some tea, I wonder? It must be about ready now."

He made fast his awl in his work and got up. He tapped his finger on the windowpane. Stephen turned around and approached. Martin asked him to come in and warm himself. "You must be frozen," Martin said.

"Christ be with you," answered Steven. "Yes, my bones are almost cracking." He came in, shook the snow off himself, and took pains to wipe his boots carefully, that he might not dirty the floor.

"No, no, don't trouble about that," said Martin. "I will wipe your boots myself. It is part of my trade. Come here and sit down and we will empty this teapot together." He poured two glassfuls and offered one to his visitor. Stephen drank it down quickly; it was clear he would like another.

"You must drink some more," said Martin and refilled his guest's tumbler. Yet, in spite of himself, he continued to look out into the street.

"Are you expecting anyone?" asked his guest.

"Am I expecting anyone? Well, to tell the truth, yes, that is to say, I am, and I am not. The fact is that I have some words fixed in my memory. Whether it was a vision or not, I don't know. At all events, my old friend, I was reading in the Gospels last night about Our Little Father Christ, and how He walked this earth and suffered. You have heard of Him, have you not?"

"Yes, yes, I have heard of him," Stephen answered, *"but we are ignorant folk and don't know our letters."*

"Well, I was reading of how He walked this earth, and how He went to visit a Pharisee, and yet received no welcome from him at the door. All this I read last night, my friend, and then fell to thinking about it--to thinking how some day I too might fail to pay Our Little Father Christ due honor. 'Suppose,' I thought to myself, 'He came to me or to anyone like me? Should we, like the great lord Simon, not know how to receive Him and not go out to meet Him?' I was thinking about this and I fell asleep.

Then as I sat sleeping, I heard someone call my name; and as I raised myself, the voice went on, 'Watch thou for me tomorrow, for I am coming to visit you.' It said that twice. And so those words have gone into my head, and, foolish though I know, I keep expecting Him--the Little Father--every moment."

Stephen nodded and said nothing, but emptied his glass and laid it aside. Martin took it and refilled it. "Drink it up; it will do you good," he said. "Do you know," he went on, "I often call to mind how, when Our Little Father walked this earth, there was never a man, however humble, whom He despised, and how it was chiefly among the common people that He dwelt. It was always with them that He walked. And it was from among such men as you and I--from among sinners and working folk--that He chose His disciples. 'Whoever,' He said, 'that should exalt himself, the same shall be abased, and whoever shall abase himself, the same shall be exalted. You,' He said again, 'call me Lord; yet will I wash you your feet. Whoever,' He said, 'would be chief among you, let them be servant of all. Because blessed are the lowly, the peacemakers, the merciful, and the charitable."

Stephen had forgotten all about his tea. He was an old man, and his tears came easily. He sat and listened, with the tears rolling down his cheeks. "Oh, but you must drink your tea," said Martin. *Stephen only crossed himself, and said the thanksgiving, then pushed his glass away and got up.*

"I thank you, Martin Aveditch," he said. *"You have taken me in, and fed both soul and body."*

"No, but I beg you to come again," said Martin. "I am only too glad of a guest." So Stephen departed, while Martin poured out the last of the tea and drank it. Again, he sat at his work by the window--stitching away--looking for Christ. Indeed Christ's many sayings were never absent from Martin's mind.

Two soldiers passed the window, the one in military boots, and the other in civilian. Next, there came a neighboring house-holder, in polished goulashes, then a baker with a basket. All of them passed on.

Presently a woman in woolen stockings and rough country shoes approached the window, and halted near the buttress out-side it. Martin peered up at her from under the lintel of his win-dow, and could see that she was plain looking, poorly-dressed and had a child in her arms. It was in order to cover the child more closely that she stopped near the buttress with her back to the wind.

Her clothing was ragged and fit only for summer, and even behind his window-panes, Martin could hear the child crying miserably. The mother vainly tried to soothe it. Martin rose, went to the door, climbed the steps, and cried out: "My good woman, my good woman!" She turned to see him. "Why need you stand there in the cold with your baby?" he went on. "Come into my room, where it is warm, and where you will be able to wrap the baby up more comfortably than you can here. Yes, come in with you."

The woman was surprised to see an old man in a leather apron, with glasses upon his nose, calling out to her, yet she fol-lowed him down the steps and they entered his room. The old man led her to the bed to sit down. "Sit down here, my good woman," he said. "You will be near the stove, and can warm yourself and feed your baby."

"Oh, but I have no milk left in my breast," she replied. "I have had nothing to eat this morning." Nevertheless, she put the child to her breast. Martin nodded his head approvingly and went to the table for some bread and a basin, and opened the

*stove door. From the stove, he took some soup and a bowl of por-
ridge and gave it to the woman.*

*"Sit down and eat, my good woman," he said, "while I
hold your baby. I have had little ones of my own, and I know how
to hold them." The woman crossed herself and sat down, while
Martin seated himself upon the bed with the baby. He smacked
his lips at it once or twice, but made a poor show of it, for he had
no teeth at all. Consequently, the baby went on crying. Then he
thought of his finger and wriggled it to and fro in front of the
baby's mouth--without ever touching the little one's lips, since
his finger was black with the shoemaker's wax.*

*The baby contemplated the finger and grew quiet, then ac-
tually smiled. Martin was delighted. Meanwhile the woman had
been eating her meal, and told him, unasked, who she was and
where she was going.*

*"I am a soldier's wife," she said, "but my husband was
sent far away eight months ago and I've heard nothing of him
since. At first, I got a job as a cook, but when the baby came, they
dismissed me. That was three months ago and I've had nothing
since, and have spent all my savings. I tried to get taken as a wet
nurse, but no one would have me because they said I was too
thin. I have just been to see about a job. I was promised I would
be hired, but was told to come back next week. Since the job is a
long way from here, I am quite worn out and have tired my baby
for nothing. Thank Heaven for my landlady who is good to me,
and gives me shelter for Christ's sake. Otherwise, I should not
have known how to bear it all."*

*Martin sighed and said, "But have you nothing warm to
wear?"*

*"Oh sir," replied the woman, "although it's the time for
warm clothes, I had to pawn my last shawl yesterday for two rubles." Then the woman returned to the bed to take her baby while
Martin rose and went to the cupboard. He rummaged around and
found an old jacket.*

*"Here," he said, "It's a poor old thing, but it will serve to
cover you." The woman looked at the jacket, and then at the old*

man. Then she took the jacket and burst into tears. Martin turned away, and looking under the bed, found a box and pretended to rummage about it for a few moments.

Then the woman said to him, "I thank you in Christ's name, good grandfather. Surely it was He Himself who led me to your window. Otherwise, I should have seen my baby perish with the cold. When I first came out the day was warm, but now it has begun to freeze. But He, Our Little Father, had placed you in your window, that you might see me in my bitter plight and have compassion on me."

Martin smiled and said: "He did indeed place me there. Yet, my poor woman, it was for a special purpose that I was looking out." Then he told his guest of his vision.

"That may very well be," said the woman as she rose, took the jacket, and wrapped her baby in it. Then she said, "Farewell."

"Also, take this in Christ's name," said Martin, and gave her two rubles with which to buy back her shawl. The woman crossed herself and he likewise. Then he led her to the door. When she had gone, Martin ate a little soup, washed the dishes, and went back to work. All the time, though, he kept his eye upon the window. Acquaintances came past, and people he did not know, but never anyone in particular.

Then suddenly he saw something. Opposite his window, an old peddler-woman with a basket of apples stopped. Only a few of the apples remained, so it was clear that she was almost sold out. Over her shoulder was slung a sack of wood shavings, which she must have gathered near some new building as she was going home. Apparently, her shoulder had begun to ache under the weight, and she stopped to shift the load. To do this, she balanced her basket of apples on the top of a post and lowered the sack to the pavement. As she was doing this, a boy in a ragged cap appeared from somewhere, seized an apple from the basket, and tried to make off.

But the old woman, who had been on her guard, managed to turn and seize the boy by the sleeve. Although he struggled and tried to break away, she clung to him with both hands. She snatched off his cap and got a firm grip on his hair. The youngster began to shout.

Martin didn't stop to make his awl fast, but threw his work down on the floor and ran up to the door, stumbling on the steps, and losing his glasses as he did so. Out into the street he ran, where the old woman was still holding the boy by the hair and threatening to take him to the police. While the boy, for his part, was struggling to get free. "I never took it," he was saying. "What are you beating me for? Let me go."

"Let him go my good woman. Pardon him for Christ's sake."

"Yes, I'll pardon him, but not till he's tasted a new birchrod. I mean to take the young rascal to the police."

But Martin still interceded for him. "Let him go, my good woman," he said. "He will never do it again." The old woman released the boy, who was for making off if Martin had not stopped him. "You must beg the old woman's pardon," he said, "and never do such a thing again. I saw you take the apple."

The boy burst out crying, and begged the old woman's pardon. Martin said, "There, there, now I will give you one," and he took an apple from the basket and handed it to the boy. "I'll pay you for it, my good woman," he added.

"Yes, but you spoil the young rascal by doing this," she objected. "He ought to have received a reward that would have made him glad to stand for a week."

"Ah, my good woman, my good woman," exclaimed Martin. "That may be our way of rewarding, but it's not God's. If this boy ought to have been whipped for taking the apple, ought not we also be punished for our sins?" At this, the old woman was silent. Then Martin related to her the story of the master who absolved his servant from the great debt which he owed him, after that the servant took his own debtor and grabbed him by the throat.

The old woman listened, and also the boy. "God has commanded us to pardon one another," went on Martin, "or He will not pardon us. We ought to pardon all men, and especially the thoughtless."

The old woman shook her head and sighed. "Yes, that be so," she said, "but these young rascals are so spoiled already!"

"Then it is for us, their elders, to teach them better," he replied.

"That is what I say to myself at times," replied the old woman. "I had seven of them at once but only one daughter now." She went on to tell Martin where she and her daughter lived, and how they lived, and how many grandchildren she had. "I have only such strength as you see," she said, "yet I work hard, for my heart goes out to my grandchildren--the cute little things that they are! No children could run to meet me as they do. Alisa for instance, will go to no one else. 'Grandmother,' she cries, 'dear Grandmother, you are tired'--at this the old woman became thoroughly softened. "Everyone knows what boys are," she added presently, referring to the culprit. "May God go with him!"

She raised her sack to her shoulder and began to walk again, when the boy darted forward. "No let me carry it grandmother. It will be on my way home." The woman nodded assent, and gave the sack to the boy and went away with him down the street. She had forgotten to ask Martin to pay the money for the apple.

He stood looking after them, and observing how they walked together. Martin returned to his room, finding his glasses unbroken on the steps as he went down.

Once more, he took his awl and went to work. As it began to get dark, he thought to himself, "I too must light up my lamp." So he trimmed his lamp, hung it up, and resumed his work. He finished one boot completely, and then turned it over to look at it. It was good work. He laid his tools aside, swept up his cuttings, and cleaned his awl. Next, he lifted his lamp down, placed it on the table, and took the Testament from the shelf. He had intended to open it to the place where he had been reading last night, but opened it instead to another place.

The instant he did so, the vision of last night came back to his memory, and he thought he heard a movement behind him. He turned around and saw the shadows of a dark corner and what appeared to be figures of people standing there. Then the voice whispered in his ear:

"Martin, do you not know me?"

"Who are you?" said Martin.

"Even I!" whispered the voice again. "Lo, it is I!" and there from the dark corner, Stephen smiled, and then, like a fading cloud, was gone.

"It is I!" whispered the voice again and there stepped from the same corner the woman with her baby. She smiled, and the baby smiled, and they were gone.

"It is I!" whispered the voice again and there stepped from the same corner the old woman and the boy with the apple. They smiled, and were gone.

Joy filled the soul of Martin Aveditch as he crossed himself, put on his glasses, and set to read the Testament where it opened. At the top of the page he read:

"For I was hungry and you gave me something to eat: I was thirsty, and you gave me something to drink: I was a stranger, and you invited me in."

Further down the page he read:

"I tell you the truth, whatever you did for one of the least of these brothers of mine, you did for me."

Then Martin understood the vision had come true, that his Savior had in truth visited him that day, and he had received Him.

What a wonderful story! Martin Aveditch certainly knew his share of suffering. To lose one's spouse and three children would be a terrible thing. The grief could be overwhelming. Time has a way of taking the edge off strong feelings, though. Then it's up to us to choose our course. Martin chose a path toward understanding and toward God; he decided to move his life to find more joy. He found a deep, abiding joy that gave meaning to his life.

Examine the questions on Worksheet #47. Write your thoughts on this fascinating short story from Leo Tolstoy.

Name: *John Miller*   Worksheet #53   Date: *4-30-00*

Impressions from "Where Love Is, There God Is Also"

1. My first impression of the story is...
    How nice it would be to believe anything so completely.

2. I related to the following character because...
    The boy who stole the apple. I'm not really sure why.

3. The story motivated or moved me in what way?
    I wished I could believe and feel the peace that Martin did.

4. Other impressions?
    I was somewhat familiar with the Bible stories he was referring to, but realized that I only vaguely knew them. I guess I don't know the Bible very well.

CHAPTER 10

What I Believe

This chapter comes with a warning. Throughout previous chapters I tried to present the process of **Joyful Living** without interjecting too many of my deeply-held spiritual beliefs. Even if you hold spiritual views different from mine, the **Joyful Living** process can help you change your life. I believe the process stands on its own as a viable way to find more joy.

I also believe my deeply-held spiritual beliefs are truths that others can use. In this chapter, I describe those beliefs that are most precious to me, those ideas that most profoundly affect my life.

In polite society, we don't talk about the things that matter most. We keep the discussion on a superficial level and avoid disagreements and hurt feelings. I break that code of conduct in this chapter and discuss my deepest, most meaningful thoughts. This discussion often takes people out of their comfort zone, so be forewarned. You have the choice to simply skip to the Conclusion chapter.

Curiosity got the best of you and you decided to stay? Good. These issues matter.

Debby and I spent a weekend in New York City many years ago. As we were strolling along Fifth Avenue, we came to a store called "Cartier," and Debby told me it was a famous jewelry store. We had little money, but I said, "Oh come on in, let's look around a bit." She reluctantly followed me and we began admiring the beautiful jewelry. We spotted a diamond necklace that was amazing, and to Debby's dismay, I asked the sales clerk to show it to us. As we were examining the necklace, I asked in the calmest voice I could muster, "What's the price on this piece?"

"$25,000," the clerk replied. We left the store quickly, laughing about a necklace that was worth more than our house, for which we could barely make the mortgage payments! Although we were uncomfortable in that store, the visit did us no harm. We were simply exposed to something that we chose not to pursue further. We were just shopping.

I believe the wise person goes idea-shopping. They try to understand the beliefs of others in order to determine if there is something valuable there. Therefore, I commend you for considering my deeply-held beliefs and hope you find something you can use.

I was fortunate to have parents who valued spiritual matters. Our whole family went to Sunday School and church each week. Even when we were away on vacation, we would find a church to attend. As a youngster, I recall singing songs and hearing stories about God and Jesus.

I have believed in the God who created the universe and everything in it, since I was a very young child. The beauty of nature has always made me feel close to God and thankful to Him. I suppose we all develop an image of God based on our experiences and the things we have read and learned. Psalms 145:8 most clearly reveals my image of a strong, loving, creative God:

The Lord is gracious and compassionate, slow to anger and rich in love. The Lord is good to all; He has compassion on all He has made.

The Nature of God via the Ten Commandments

The rules God gave us further illustrate His goodness. The Ten Commandments were given to Moses by God over 5000 years ago, yet their value has not diminished over those years. We still must obey the Ten Commandments if we wish to glorify God and enjoy Him forever. Table 2 lists the Commandments as stated in the New International Version of the Bible. Shortcuts for memorizing are listed in the right column. There is great value in memorizing the Ten Commandments. As you study them, you will realize the first four Commandments address the relationship between God and people. The next six Commandments cover relationships between people.

In the first Commandment ("You shall have no other gods before me"), God tells us that the highest place in our lives must belong to Him. If we choose to worship something or someone other than God, that's sin. The second Commandment ("You shall not make for yourself an idol") reinforces the first; we must put God first in our lives. Why would two similar ideas be right next to each other? The Bible often uses repetition to emphasize its most important points. Since the idea of putting God first in our lives is in both the first and the second Commandments, it must be very important to God.

If it's so important to Him, I should make it important to me, too. In the second chapter of this book, the concept of central focus was examined. Your central focus can be work, recreation, money, family, church, revenge, etc... or your central focus can be God. The first two Commandments require our central focus to be God.

The next Commandment ("You shall not misuse the name of the Lord your God") instructs us to not blaspheme the name of

God. This gets broken frequently in today's society. God is called by many different names in the Old and New Testaments, and each has a specific meaning. As we grow closer to God, we begin to sense His awesome holiness and power in the names we call Him. Admittedly, this is a difficult concept to understand for someone who has not experienced it. I believe the third Commandment gives us a clue about the amazing power in God's name and also warns us of the danger of profaning it.

The fourth Commandment instructs us to both remember the Sabbath and to keep it holy. One day a week, we are commanded to rest (i.e. not work) and to honor God. Many people ignore this Commandment, working seven days a week. That behavior takes a toll in their lives. A day of rest is a good idea. We all need to rest and recharge, at least once a week.

In the fifth Commandment, God moves from our relationship with Him to our relationship with our neighbors. Since our first and closest neighbors are our parents, we are instructed how to treat them. The instruction is simple and to the point; we are to honor our parents. The Commandment does not say, "Honor your parents if they met all your needs," nor does it say, "Honor your parents if they did a good job in raising you." It simply says we are to honor our parents.

When I observe the brutality that some parents have inflicted upon their children, I want to cry. If you were raised by a parent or parents who treated you very badly, my heart goes out to you. If you had parents who did a poor job of meeting your needs as a child, this Commandment may be difficult to obey. Whether difficult or not, obeying this Commandment is essential for maturing into functional adults. We don't have to pretend things were wonderful as children; we certainly can't change what happened to us. We don't need to honor our parents' wrong, sinful behavior. We do, however, need to forgive. We must honor our parents simply for giving us life.

The sixth Commandment tells us not to murder. This is one Commandment society has done a fair job of enforcing. Most of us understand that murder is wrong. Most of us do well at finding a way to settle our disputes with others without resorting to murder.

The seventh Commandment receives less honor in today's society; many people are not quite sure about avoiding adultery. The Bible, though, clearly teaches the importance of avoiding all sexual sin. In the book of Genesis, we are told that God created men and women and that they should leave their parents and come together as one for life. This lifetime marriage is God's plan for people. All sexual activity outside that man/woman, permanent, loving, committed relationship is sin.

The eighth, ninth and tenth Commandments instruct us not to steal, lie, or covet. A generation or two ago, American culture stressed the importance of such basic morality. That is not to say that these rules were perfectly obeyed, but most people would have recognized them as appropriate behavior. Contemporary culture, however, tends to avoid moral absolutes. People attempt to judge each situation based on its own merits and their own feelings. These situational ethics have not improved our society, nor do they conform to God's teachings.

Table 2
The 10 Commandments

Love of God

1. You shall have no other gods before me.

    1. No other gods

2. You shall not make for yourself an idol.

    2. No idols

3. You shall not misuse the name of the Lord your God.

    3. No profaning God's name

4. Remember the Sabbath day by keeping it holy.

    4. Honor God's day

Love of one's neighbor

5. Honor your father and your mother.

    5. Honor parents

6. You shall not murder.

    6. No murder

6. You shall not commit adultery.

    7. No adultery

8. You shall not steal.

    8. No stealing

9. You shall not give false testimony against your neighbor.

    9. No lying

10. You shall not covet your neighbor's house.

    10. No coveting

Many people consider the Ten Commandments as rules that take the fun out of life. In fact, the opposite is true. God provided the Ten Commandments to help us truly enjoy life. The joy that comes from putting God first in your life is incredible. I have known several cancer patients who turned their lives completely to God as they battled the disease. Some of my friends died and some survived, but they all said the same thing: "If I had the option to not have cancer and have my old relationship with God or to have cancer and have my fully-committed relationship with God, I would choose cancer."

Similarly, the prohibition on sexual sins is often viewed as God wanting to take the fun out of life. Again, the opposite is true. The highest level of joy in sex comes from the deep, abiding love in a committed marriage relationship. While promiscuous sex can certainly be alluring, the emotional and physical price is high. When God instructs us to avoid sexual sin, He is not trying to take the fun out of our lives. He is trying to direct us toward the highest level of joy and satisfaction. In short, God loves us and wants what is best for us.

There are many, many things I don't understand about God and the world He created. Frankly, when I find someone who thinks they understand every aspect of God, I find him or her pompous and boring. The truth is we will never understand everything about God while on this earth, but we can still benefit from acting on what we do know.

I use a computer extensively and gain tremendous help from it, yet I have practically no idea how it really works. And I have less understanding of how the electricity works that runs the computer. But I have a functional knowledge of computers and electricity, and accomplish many worthwhile tasks by using them.

Therefore, since we can not fully understand one small piece of God's creation (electricity), it is unrealistic to expect to understand everything about God. Having to understand everything about God before believing in Him is just foolishness.

Many people fall into that trap. On the other hand, to honestly search for the truth about God is wise. If we search for Him with sincerity, we will find Him.

My Own Spiritual Journey

As a child of four or five years old, I remember talking with my father about God as we drove in the car. Dad would listen to my simple observations and treat them with respect. He would also give me his views on whatever we were discussing. I particularly remember going along with Dad when he would get service calls for electrical problems at the United Zion Nursing Home. It was a big old cavern of a building, and we would usually be working in the basement where the electrical panels were located.

I'd hold the flashlight for Dad as he checked out the various circuits. My attention span, which has never been too long, was quite short when holding the flashlight. I'd start thinking about something else and let the light beam move away from Dad's work. He would say to me, "Ned, hold the light up here!" as he was now trying to use a screwdriver in the dark among live electrical circuits. After having to say that several times in a few minutes, Dad would start to get annoyed. Nevertheless, Dad continued to ask me to go along on his service calls and help him. It took me quite a few years to realize that Dad just propped the flashlight when I wasn't along and had much less aggravation.

The service calls to the United Zion Nursing Home were important to me for another reason: I met Mr. Kaylor there. I remember walking through the dining room at meal times and hearing this man pray with a severe speech impediment: his name was Lehman Kaylor. Lehman was born with cerebral palsy and had never walked in his life. He had been pulled around in a wagon as a young child on the farm, and when his mother died, he and his father moved into a basement room at United Zion. Lehman had a sharp mind, but few people could understand his words because of his speech problems.

He spent almost all his life sitting in a wheelchair with little control of his arms and less control of his face and saliva. One might expect Lehman Kaylor would have been bitter about the tough breaks he had in life, but Leaman never saw it that way. I remember hearing him pray fervently with such joy and thankfulness to God. Since Dad could always understand Lehman, he would tell me what he said. The joy of Lehman Kaylor made a huge impression on me.

On another occasion, I recall attending church with my parents when I was 11 years old and hearing an evangelist from India. This man preached a powerful message about the love and salvation of Jesus Christ. During prayer at the end of his message, he asked if anyone wanted to ask Jesus to live in their heart; I felt my hand rise. He then asked those of us who had raised our hands to come to the front of the church. I answered that altar call, hardly even knowing what it meant. I remember that wonderful feeling and being quite disappointed when the feeling faded in a day or two.

Some time after that experience, I mentioned to my mother that I might want to become a minister some day. Mom told my sisters, and the taunting began. One of my sisters called me "Preacher boy," and would bring up the issue often to embarrass me. I wished many times I had never uttered a word about preaching, and in time the idea faded.

When I was 15 years old, I remember hitchhiking into Lancaster City and visiting a hip bookstore. I hitchhiked a good bit in those years and am amazed, as I look back, at the amount of freedom my parents gave me. I bought books on Eastern Meditation, Yoga, and Buddhism. The idea of Enlightenment fascinated me, and the Eastern religions seemed to make sense. In my late teens and early twenties, I meditated and did yoga exercises and studied Buddhism.

During those years of our lives, we often search for anything that makes sense. If we find something that is very different from what our parents think makes sense, so much the better. I loved the writings of Gandhi and tried to practice non-violent resistance. There were probably not many Division One collegiate wrestlers who were trying to practice active non-violent resistance. I suppose I enjoyed many of the aspects of Eastern thought simply because they were different.

I also began attending the Princeton Friends Meeting House on Sunday mornings during my college years. I would walk through the beautiful Institute for Advanced Study woods (where Albert Einstein worked for many years) to a charming little meeting house. The old stone building was built in the 1700's and was heated by a big open fireplace in the winter. I enjoyed sitting in silence at the Quaker Meetings and waiting on the Spirit of God.

Not to portray myself inaccurately here; the vast majority of my time was spent ignoring spiritual things and focusing exclusively on myself. Cursing, lust, alcohol, and drugs were important parts of my life at that time. I spent most of my time working and playing, and I prided myself on doing both of them with intensity. I was not a deeply spiritual person (I was a real jerk fairly often), but I did maintain an interest in things of God.

When I graduated with my engineering degree, I thought I was quite a valuable commodity in the marketplace. I was rudely awakened. While working on the road for Clair Brothers Audio, I made $700 per week, which was excellent money for a 20-year old. However, my first job as a Construction Engineer paid only $280 per week. Debby and I had decided that we wanted to move back to Lancaster County, PA, and that we would not stay married if I worked on the road. So I took the job in construction, worked hard, and got laid off after 18 months.

Getting laid off was hard on my ego (which in retrospect is usually a good thing), and turned out to be a blessing in disguise. I next worked as a foreman for an excavating contractor; and I learned a tremendous amount about working in the field on big projects. I was running a crew in Maryland and spent long days working and driving. Through these early working years, I had little time for God and it showed in my life. Debby and I were not getting along well, and everything seemed sort of pointless.

From my viewpoint, Debby becoming pregnant with our first child was a major turning point in my life. As we considered the consequences of bringing a child into this world, we began to examine our lives a bit more intently. We began to attend the church where Debby grew up, and that was where I felt the changes happening. We learned to know families where strong love was evident. We observed many truly happy marriages in which the husband and wife laughed together and were best friends.

We also taught the three-year-old Sunday School class for several years. As I told and retold the simple Bible stories I had learned as a child, spiritual interest stirred in me. I learned there was a difference between simply reading the Bible and studying the Bible. Studying required some thought, introspection, and analysis of what I read; it helped me tie the stories together into a more coherent whole.

The Truth Comes into Focus

I studied through the New International Version of the Bible, with Commentary and began to understand more truth about God. I began to see how the Bible was consistent in its basic teachings. Essentially, the Bible taught the following clear message:

We must love God with all our heart. Period. That means we have to choose between selfishly wanting our own way or obediently following God's way. And we have to make that choice before God will show His way to us. We are commanded to love God totally and unequivocally.

Solomon, the wisest man in the world, said in Ecclesiastes 12:12:

Now all has been heard; here is the conclusion of the whole matter: fear God and keep His commandments, for this is the whole duty of man.

Solomon concluded, in this most philosophical book, that a life not centered on God is purposeless and meaningless. So how do we center our lives on God?

We begin by acknowledging that God, the Creator of all things, is completely pure and holy. In our human weakness, we necessarily fall short of the holy and pure standard of God. I need only honestly examine my life to recognize that many of my actions have mixed motives (some noble and some self-serving) and that those mixed motives are not as holy and pure as God's standard. All of our efforts toward good behavior will simply never match God's. If we can never be holy enough, what is the point of even trying?

The answer to that question is one of the most amazing concepts ever taught. The Bible teaches that the Son of God came to Earth as a human child named Jesus about 2000 years ago. Experiencing all the temptations that are common to humans, Jesus nevertheless lived a perfect, holy life. He willingly went to His death on the cross as a perfect sacrifice for all people for all time. Jesus allowed Himself to be put on the cross in order to become an atoning sacrifice for anyone who calls on His name.

The term "sanctification" means to be made holy, to be made acceptable to God. Jesus, by His position on the cross, made any person who comes to Him holy and acceptable to God. This "Positional Sanctification" is the central message of Christianity. We can never behave well enough for God on our own. We would be doomed, if not for the work Jesus did on the cross for us.

You may wonder, as I have, "Why did Jesus, an innocent man, have to die? If God was willing to forgive us, why didn't He just do so without having an innocent man killed?" Since God is perfectly pure and holy, He deserves perfection from us. Our sins create a debt that can not just be swept under the rug; it needs to be paid. We deserve death and torment and suffering for the sins that we commit. Jesus Christ came and willingly paid our debt for us; He suffered and died in our place. We need only accept His offer of forgiveness.

Do not make the mistake of classifying Christianity as simply another ethical teaching, as one of many paths that lead to the top of the mountain (i.e. God). The teachings of Christ will not allow that conclusion. Either Jesus Christ is the one and only Son of God and no one gets to Heaven except through Him, or He is a liar. The words of Jesus Himself do not allow us to group Him as one of many outstanding teachers and gurus. Jesus is the only teacher who claimed to be the Son of God and the only way to Heaven.

A study of Jesus' own words clearly shows this:

I am the Way and the Truth and the Life, no one comes to the Father except through Me.

These words, spoken by Jesus, were recorded by an eyewitness, John the Apostle in The Gospel of John 14:6. Jesus was even clearer when He was on trial for His life. Matthew 26:63-67 records:

The high priest said to him, "I charge you under oath by the living God: Tell us if you are the Christ, the Son of God."

64 "Yes, it is as you say," Jesus replied. "But I say to all of you: In the future you will see the Son of Man sitting at the right hand of the Mighty One and coming on the clouds of heaven."

65Then the high priest tore his clothes and said, "He has spoken blasphemy! Why do we need any more witnesses? Look, now you have heard the blasphemy. 66What do you think?"

"He is worthy of death," they answered.

67Then they spit in his face and struck him with their fists. Others slapped him.

If one reads the Bible without prejudice, seeking to objectively understand what is recorded, one concludes that Jesus did, in fact, claim to be the one and only Son of God. The Bible tells us the only way to reach God is through Jesus, by accepting the sacrifice He made on the cross for each of us.

After Jesus was crucified and resurrected, the Apostle Peter was preaching in Jerusalem and explained to the people that they had taken part in crucifying the Son of God. The people to whom Peter spoke were upset and asked, as recorded in Acts 2:37:

"Brothers, what shall we do?"
Peter replied, "Repent and be baptized, every one of you, in the name of Jesus Christ for the forgiveness of your sins. And you will receive the gift of the Holy Spirit."

Peter went on to say in Acts 4:12,

"Salvation is found in no one else, for there is no other name under heaven given to men by which we must be saved."

Therefore, one can not logically believe that Jesus was simply one of many great teachers in history. A great teacher would not so mislead his followers by claiming to be the Son of God. One can take the position that Jesus was a liar and that Christianity is the biggest hoax in history. However, it seems odd that almost every one of the apostles (who would have had to be in on the hoax), was killed for refusing to deny Jesus as Christ. The longevity of Christianity also contradicts the hoax theory. So many people over the past 2000 years have completely dedicated their lives to Jesus Christ, it is unreasonable to believe there is absolutely nothing to Christianity.

The best proof for Christianity will make no sense whatsoever to non-believers. Jesus told His disciples, shortly before He died, that if they believed in Him and tried to follow His teachings, they would be sent a Comforter. This Comforter, the Holy Spirit, came to the disciples on the Day of Pentecost. Jesus said the Holy Spirit would always be with His people and would actually be in them. The Holy Spirit would continue to make the truth of God more and more clear to His people.

Having investigated several other religious traditions in my earlier years, I was familiar with the emotional highs that can come from spiritual things. I am not saying this is a good thing or a bad thing, I am only stating that spiritual experiences often have strong emotional impact. I enjoyed the peace that came from yoga exercises or Buddhist meditation.

When our son Lex decided to become a Christian at age nine, we had a baptism service at our church. Many people over the years chose to have their baptism in a nearby stream, and Lex, following in the tradition of his mother, also decided to be baptized in the stream. It was the middle of November and quite cold and windy. I decided to be baptized in the stream on the same day as Lex since I had never experienced believer's baptism.

As Lex and I prepared to be baptized that cold Sunday morning, I had no idea what to expect. When I waded into the stream with Eric Brubaker, one of our ministers, the very cold, very fast-moving water stunned me. We went to the middle of the stream and I knelt down. Let me tell you, that water was COLD! The Church of the Brethren baptizes by dunking your head under water three times ("in the name of the Father" …dunk… "in the name of the Son" … dunk … "and in the name of the Holy Sprit" … longer dunk). With each dunk, the swift current carried me downstream a few yards, and Eric had to struggle to keep his hand on my head.

After the third dunk, Eric put both hands on my head and began to pray. As he prayed, I felt the most amazing thing happening. I felt a warmth from my head down to my feet. I could actually feel the Holy Spirit enter me and fill me. I am skeptical of one-time religious experiences and was not sure what to make of this one. The genuineness of this experience was proved over time, however, as I felt the Holy Spirit within me week after week, month after month, and year after year.

I must not mislead here. I want to clearly describe what I experience as the Holy Spirit within me and what I do not experience. I do not experience God's constant presence and unfailing clear direction. I wish I could say that I always feel the Lord within me and always know just what to do, but that wouldn't be true. In fact, as I've studied the lives of many Christians over the years, they all indicated times of feeling alienated from God and not knowing what to do. Do not hold the misconception that a conversion experience will somehow take all your problems away.

The way I do experience the Holy Spirit within me happens in a number of ways. When I teach the adult Sunday School class in our church, I sometimes feel a wave of emotion sweep over me as I am speaking; sometimes I say things I was not planning to say, and I can simply feel God's presence and power. It is a marvelous feeling. Other times, when I'm on my knees praying, well-formed thoughts come into my mind that I believe God wants me to act on. I need to be careful with this one. I have a little saying, "Not every goofy idea that pops into my head is a leading from the Holy Spirit!"

Writing this book was another way I've experienced the Holy Spirit in my life. Many times as I sat at the keyboard and wondered what to say next, words would come to me that seemed so clear, and I would be amazed. On these occasions, I would thank God for His kind direction. Of course, other times I would write and be amazed at the absolute drivel I was producing.

My experience indicates that the infilling of the Holy Spirit is not an all-or-nothing deal. There are moments and hours and even days when I strongly feel the presence of God. There are also many times when I feel nothing at all, when I give in to my despicable motives and actions. During these times, it is hard to imagine that God could have any interest in me at all. But because of my solid foundation built on the truth of God's word, I know that God continues to love me and wants what is best for me even when I disappoint Him and myself.

The manner in which the Holy Spirit acts is important to understand. Suppose you need to get some place. Perhaps you want to see a Broadway show in New York City and don't know exactly how to get there. If someone wanted to help you, they could give you a detailed map with directions. Then you would be on your own to follow the directions and find your desired location. Conversely, someone could say, "Just get in the car and drive, I know the way very well and I'll drive there with you. I'll be your co-pilot." God generally uses the Holy Spirit like a co-pilot for our lives.

Since I obviously enjoy the sense of being filled with the Holy Spirit, how do I get more? As one may expect, the answer is found in the Bible. In the 14th chapter of the Gospel of John, Jesus promises the Holy Spirit to his followers. He says, in John 14:15-17:

"If you love me, you will obey what I command. ^{16}And I will ask the Father, and he will give you another Counselor to be with you forever-- ^{17}the Spirit of truth. The world cannot accept him, because it neither sees him nor knows him. But you know him, for he lives with you and will be in you."

We are given the Spirit of Truth (or the Holy Spirit) when we obey the commands of Jesus. As we strive to follow the teachings of Jesus, the presence of the Holy Spirit becomes more prevalent within us. Therefore, we gain a clearer understanding of God's will as we obey the things we already know to do. In a sense, God rewards our obedience by providing a better vision of what we need to do.

Christianity turns everything we would think to be true on its head. Our human nature would think, "If I work very hard, I will be rewarded by not having to work so hard in the future." Our culture is built on that premise. Christ, though, set things up quite differently. If we work hard for Him, we can expect a clearer vision of the additional work we must do. Jesus never promised ease for His people here on Earth. He promised understanding and truth, joy, peace, fulfillment, direction, and much more, but not ease.

Jesus Christ offers any person complete forgiveness of all sins and an everlasting life with God in heaven. Because of His great love, Jesus offers this free gift of salvation to anyone who will receive it. This grace, this free and unmerited love and favor of God, is given to us if we ask for it. So why in the world doesn't everyone immediately accept God's grace?

As discussed in the section on truth and lies, the world contains both a force of love and creation (God) and a force of evil and destruction (Satan). Satan's goal is to keep people from understanding this basic truth of God's grace. If people do not accept God's grace, they are not saved. One of the clearest statements of this fact comes from the prophet Jonah as written in Jonah 2:8:

"Those who cling to worthless idols, forfeit the grace that could be theirs."

Our worthless idols can be money, pleasure, sex, general self-centeredness or any of a number of things. For a person to accept the gift of salvation, though, that individual must be willing to put Christ first, to let go of worthless idols. In order to truly repent and accept salvation, the central focus in our lives must change. Our focus must be God.

Following Jesus requires self-denial and all the dedication and obedience one can muster. Jesus tells a story in Luke 14:25-35 about the costs of being His disciple. He says we must weigh the costs before we begin. He uses the example of a person who wants to build a tower. A prudent person would not just begin to build; he would have a plan, calculate the quantity of materials, and estimate the cost. Jesus recommends the same when deciding to follow Him.

I have a good friend who was telling me about his mother-in-law. He mentioned that she had been unhappy for a long time and described some of her bizarre behavior. She had succeeded in driving almost everyone in her life away from her because of her incredible selfishness. Her daughter had talked her into seeing a psychologist, and they were hopeful some progress could be made. She actually saw a series of therapists, but did not seem to improve in any way.

She told my friend one day that she was through seeing therapists. "There is no point in going to see them," she said. "They all just keep talking about things I need to change." The situation was quite clear to my friend's mother-in-law... other people needed to change, certainly not her. And that attitude dooms her, I'm afraid, to a joyless life of blaming everyone else for her lack of happiness.

If we choose to be followers of Christ, we must be willing to continually change. As followers of Christ, our goal must be to move closer to the will of God. "Positional Sanctification," as defined earlier, makes us holy by Christ's position on the cross. "Progressive Sanctification" is being made holy by our day-to-day actions that glorify God. We need to struggle on a daily basis to know God's will and to accomplish it. In that struggle, we move closer to God.

Our salvation is not something we earn, though. Jesus died on the cross so that any sinner can come to Him and experience the forgiveness of God. No matter how good our behavior, it would never be good enough to earn our salvation. We can only find salvation through the atoning work of Christ. Once we accept His salvation, though, our work must begin. Our lives must be dedicated to finding and doing the will of our God. Even though we will have many failures, we are called to that struggle for the rest of our lives.

The Bible tells us salvation is both an event (at the time of conversion) and a process (continually being saved as we conform to the will of Christ). Therefore, the concepts of positional and progressive sanctification are the framework on which our lives must be built. Everything we do, everything we attempt, should be viewed from the framework of our sanctification.

This process of becoming more holy can not happen just by our efforts. As we give our lives to Jesus, God helps transform us. This transformation, this progressive sanctification, is the whole of our work for the rest of our lives. Christianity must not be just a theory; it must be our whole way of life. I love the quote from Kallistos Ware:

"No one can be an armchair traveler on this all-important journey. No one can be a Christian second hand. God has children, but He has no grandchildren."

"So how do I move toward God?" you may ask. The most effective first step involves Bible study. God has provided a huge amount of information in the Bible. As we read it, we continually gain new insights about our world and our God. The more we understand the Truth of God's Word, the more life's puzzle pieces fit together.

The Bible can appear overwhelming to those not very familiar with it. Don't be intimidated, though. Simply begin reading the New Testament as you would read a story book. Jesus taught by using so many parables and simple stories because He didn't want His teaching to be only for learned people. Even children can, and usually do, understand the basic lessons in the stories of Jesus.

A wonderful aspect of Bible study involves levels of meaning. A passage I've read a dozen times before, can suddenly take on a new and deeper meaning for me. I love that sense of excitement when the meaning of the Bible passage moves to a new level. I guarantee these gems of wisdom will also appear to you as you continue in dedicated Bible study.

Don't expect to understand everything too quickly, though, as it rarely works that way. The reward of Bible study is a gradual understanding of the Truth. Most of us want all the Truth at once, but perhaps God knows that we couldn't handle that.

You will benefit greatly by committing yourself to a daily time of Bible study. You don't have to read large amounts of text; just read carefully and prayerfully; consider what you read. Make notes in the margins of your Bible, underline things that strike you, and write comments. These will often be helpful to you in the future.

The value of daily Bible study amazes me. It seems like such a simple thing. Yet I can assure you, over time, your Bible study will become one of your most profitable investments. I cannot overstate the importance of daily Bible study.

Only a daily time of prayer surpasses the value of daily Bible study. To develop one's inner life, time must be spent in prayer. There is no other way.

Jesus prayed as a regular habit; He often retired to quiet places to pray while His disciples slept. Jesus also turned to prayer in every stressful situation. When Jesus struggled, He consistently turned to prayer. The value of prayer is probably best illustrated by the importance Jesus placed on it in His own life.

When I began praying every morning, I struggled. After a time, though, I began to feel some of the benefits. The closeness with God is, of course, a wonderful thing to experience...yet there is so much more. A consistent time of prayer in the morning starts my day in the right direction. I know daily prayer affects my life in positive ways, many of which I barely understand.

In a nutshell, daily prayer just feels right. My daily time of prayer helps keep the focus of my life toward God as opposed to the many other directions I tend to take. Prayer does not make my problems go away; it simply helps me be a little bit more of who I want to be.

"Prayer – secret, fervent, believing prayer - lies at the root of all personal godliness."
William Carrey

"Prayer does not change God, but it changes him who prays."
Soren Kirkegaard

"The prayer of a righteous man is powerful and effective.'
James 5:16

Daily Bible study and daily prayer are a means of growing one's inner life. However, the process of progressive sanctification involves more than just our inner life. In order to glorify God with our lives, we need to be developing both our inner life and our relationships with others.

When I think of the Christian's relationship with other people, I am reminded of the quote by Richard Foster in his wonderful book titled, The Celebration of Discipline. Foster wrote about the scene in the upper room when Jesus washed His disciples' feet, "...Then Jesus took a towel and basin and redefined greatness." Jesus taught His followers that relationships with friends and acquaintances must be founded upon service, love, and humility. As we treat others in this manner, we build our relationship with both man and God.

Our progressive sanctification will not be carried out only on our knees. We need to be actively building our relationships with others. We need to be struggling and failing and struggling some more in our day-to-day relationships. Our joy in this endeavor will be our best witness to others.

On the other hand, if we live somber, rule-centered, smug and self-righteous lives, we show our lack of Godliness. If we create ugliness in our daily living, we are not following in the footsteps of our Lord. When our priorities are centered on self, our life is not glorifying God. The strongest argument against Christianity is Christians who live this self-serving way.

These thoughts can be summarized with a quote from Dietrich Bonhoffer, who was a Christian martyr in Germany during World War II:

"When all is said and done, the life of faith is nothing if not an unending struggle of the spirit with every available weapon against the flesh. How is it possible to live the life of faith when we grow weary of prayer, when we lose our taste for reading the Bible, and when sleep, food and sensuality deprive us of the joy of communion with God?"

We all share these struggles; every one of us trying to live a life dedicated to Jesus Christ will contend with these issues. Some days we will barely struggle; other days we will struggle mightily. I know God honors our sincere efforts, even when we fail, and will encourage us to continue. In the end, this struggle for holiness is the only thing that matters.

Conclusion

One of the great discoveries a man makes, one of his great surprises, is to find he can do what he was afraid he couldn't do.
          Henry Ford

When you began reading this book, you probably knew very little about me or my ideas. Now you know lots about me, maybe too much! My purpose in sharing so much information about myself came from previous teaching experience. I've found that most people relate better to the failings and successes of a real person than to a theory.

I've certainly failed often in my life and continue to fail every day. Yet I feel blessed by the experiences I've had. I love deeply and try to constantly expand my understanding of the truth. While the circumstances of my life may bring joy or despair, my life is not controlled by my circumstances. My life consists of the love and honor I bring to these situations.

Being a person that hates to be surprised, I've always tried to anticipate bad news. I suppose some basic desire for self-preservation motivates me to prepare myself for hard times. I have discovered, though, that I can do what I was afraid I could not. I can persevere in times of adversity because I am more than my feelings. I am prepared to take what life hands me and to do my best.

As you began this book, what was it that you were afraid you couldn't do? Were you afraid of not being able to rise to the challenges life may present, as I was? Or were you afraid of having to make changes? Perhaps you were afraid that if you looked too deeply at yourself, you would see only weaknesses and inability. Regardless of how you started, I hope you have begun disproving your most basic fears.

As you've worked through this book, you have identified talents, abilities, as well as personal weaknesses. You've clarified your life values and faced your emotional struggles. Memories and past relationships were examined; hopes and plans for the future were formed. You considered God's place in your life.

This process took time and effort but the returns on your investment will be phenomenal! You will develop new habits and you will be changed!

I'm not a person who concludes things well. I love to begin a new project, to create a plan. I enjoy persevering through the middle of a project, handling all the details and keeping everything moving forward. I excel at getting things done on time; I get them functional, just not completely finished. That last one percent of a project tortures me. I hate the final stage, and avoid it when I can.

Our many home renovations and additions illustrate this. We have light fixtures hanging from wires for years, waiting for me to get the right sized screws. I look at them sometimes, or Debby reminds me on rare occasions, and I think, "I'll finish that soon." But I don't.

Even the building projects I do for other people torment me in the final stage. Once the exciting part of the construction is completed, I must force myself to pay attention to the small final details. I make myself finish my building projects, but I don't like it and I don't do it too well.

As I come to the conclusion of this book, I encounter the same tendencies. In fact, someone commented about an earlier draft, "The conclusion basically says, 'Man, I'm glad I finished this thing!'"

Since that's not the message I want to send, I struggled with how to conclude. I decided to conclude the way I live, not with a summary but a look ahead to other exciting possibilities.

Do you ever want to repeat a joke and can't remember it? Or forget the names of the spouse and children of an acquaintance? Perhaps you feel down and wish for some insight. Where do you turn?

The Joyful Living Database could solve these problems and many more. Your own, personal Joyful Living Database could be developed from the Worksheet information you have just completed. You could place all the most useful, important and valuable information about your life in one, organized place. That place is a Microsoft Access database program, which lets you easily search and retrieve and sort information.

Let's think about a few of the specifics of this Joyful Living Database:

1. The names, addresses, and various phone numbers of all the people you've known would be here.
2. You could actually be reminded of birthdays, anniversaries and other significant dates a few days ahead of time.
3. As you look up a phone number, you could also see information about the individual's personality type, love language, central focus, or other attributes. You could be reminded of that valuable information right when you need it.
4. As you speak with someone, you could jot your conversation notes directly into their file, never to be lost or mis-

placed. Since today's computers have almost endless memory, those notes can be permanently accessible.

5. Enough about people, how about a laugh? Any joke or story or quote can be saved in the Joyful Living Database and easily retrieved. Whether you need to pep up a speech or just need to laugh at some funny stories, you can search through your personal database of things that made you laugh (or things that motivated you).

6. Another great benefit comes from recording memories of your children. If you have young children, imagine sitting down once a month and inputting a few of the touching, cute or silly things your little ones did recently. What a tremendous resource that information would become in a few years! Wouldn't it be great to have your parents' recollections of your younger years?

7. When life seems overwhelming, imagine being able to search for your own personal truths (or the lies that snag you) and recognize those thought patterns that cause you defeat and despair. You could decide to focus on behavior that reflects your chosen central focus.

8. Your own memories could also be recorded here, as well as memories you hear from other loved ones. Your parents may never do this program, but you could record their memories so your children and grandchildren would have them.

Imagine having all this useful information accessible to you. If you completed the Joyful Living worksheets, you've got a vast amount of data. The Joyful Living Database could help you utilize that data often in your daily living. While you don't need the Joyful Living Database to benefit greatly from your plan, the database seems like the next logical step. I will make this integrated database available on my website (*www.pelger.com*) for your use.

So, we conclude by looking ahead, by considering an idea that may help us live more effectively and joyfully.

I hope and pray that you will continue to work out a plan, year after year, and struggle toward its accomplishment. In that struggle, you will find joy and purpose and meaning and truth!

I commend you for your efforts and wish you well for the future.

Remember – YOU have the ability to choose your level of joy!

Sincerely,

Ned Pelger

Appendix A:
Obtaining Blank Worksheets

Blank Worksheets are available to you in several ways. You may download and print the blank Worksheets from my website at www.pelger.com. A better method involves downloading the software application programs and completing the Worksheets on your computer (see Appendix D) . If you don't have internet access, you may call ATA Publishing Company toll free at (888-627-7744) for copies of the blank Worksheets or a CD with the software application programs.

Appendix B:
List of Worksheets, Tables, and Figures

Appendix C:
List of Section Headings

Introduction

Chapter 1 – The Things That Make You Unique
Discovering Your Own Uniqueness
Why Goal Setting Rarely Works
The Need for More Hope in Your Life

Chapter 2 – Understanding Who You Are
Optimists and Pessimists
The Values You Live
Your Central Focus
Personality Styles
Love Languages

Chapter 3 – Understanding and Managing Emotions
Eight Primary Emotions
Emotions, Moods and Temperament
Emotional Hijackings

Chapter 4 – Your Memories
Earliest Memory
Childhood Memories
Memories, Memories, Memories

**Chapter 5 – Understanding and Managing Relation-
ships**
Functional and Dysfunctional Families
Relationship Bank Account
Relationships with Family and Friends
Relationship with Yourself
Relationship with God

Appendix D:
Your Computer as a Tool
for Personal Growth

I'm a packrat. Sometimes that causes me problems, but the stuff I've saved helps me once in a while. For the past twenty years, I've struggled with personal growth and self improvement. As I review the notes I've saved, I remember many of my early frustrations:

1. Learning important truths and then forgetting them.
2. Not being able to remember family memories.
3. Writing a plan and then losing the paper.
4. Running out of room to track plan progress or write comments.
5. Wanting to keep my plans confidential, yet nearby and accessible.

Though these frustrations may seem minor, I found it didn't take much for me to drop my commitment to self improvement.

On the other hand, as I placed my self improvement information on the computer, everything went smoother. I could find things, changes and tracking were simple, and my sense of progress was clear. Don't miss the importance of that last item. A clear sense of progress provides the best possible motivation. When I feel good about part of my plan, I redouble my efforts to achieve the other parts.

Since I find the computer so useful in this process, I thought you might also. So I offer the simple application programs I've developed. The specific programs are based in the Microsoft Office 2000 suite and include the following:

1. **Blank Worksheets**: All blank Worksheets in Microsoft Word 2000 format.

2. **Ancestor Profiles**: A Microsoft Excel 2000 series of spreadsheets which chart ancestors' traits.

3. **My Stories**: A Microsoft Access 2000 database to record your personal stories.

4. **Quotes and Stories**: A Microsoft Access 2000 database to record the wisdom and humor of others.

5. **My Plan**: A Microsoft Excel 2000 spreadsheet to create and track your plan for life improvements.

My self improvement efforts produced few results prior to my use of the one-year plan. I found the one-year plan helped me focus on clear objectives. Since I used a one-year plan on a sheet of paper for several years, I also experienced the frustration of difficult updating. As the year progressed, I wanted to record my progress or make some changes, and never had enough room on the page.

While this problem seems minor, I was consistently frustrated by it. When I started to put my one-year plan on an Excel spreadsheet, I loved the flexibility. I record more information, make minor changes when necessary, and feel better every time I review the plan. Though it sounds odd, the use of the computer spreadsheet really does make a huge difference in how I feel about the entire process.

The advantage of recording a bit more information each month on the one-year plan surprised me. The added history allows me to see trends in my thinking and my personality. For example, I have a perennial plan item of taking each child alone for a special time each month. When I tracked my progress on paper, I only had room to make a quick notation of what we did. On the spreadsheet, I fill in some details because the cell expands to hold all the information I put in.

Now, when I look back over the old plans, I spot trends in my relationships with the kids. That extra information allowed me to notice that I often took our one daughter shopping to the same place, while I did more of a variety of things with the other kids. Now I had a clear and simple problem to solve! I got more creative, talked to her about some other options, and we did some cool things together.

Another advantage of doing all the worksheets on computer is the search capabilities. Many times I remember a portion of the information I need but simply can't recall everything. I strain to bring in that additional information that would help clarify the situation. People make worse decisions when they don't have the best information available. Rational intelligence is based on being able to access the appropriate information at the time it's needed.

I find my rational intelligence greatly increased by the computer search function. Think about having all the pertinent information from your life, all the things you've learned and the experiences you've had, accessible to you. The people I've known over the years who I considered to be very intelligent seemed to have this information all easily accessible in their brains.

My brain just doesn't work that well, my information isn't so accessible. I can choose to whine about my lack of brain-power or I can use the computer as a tool to leverage the brain-power I do have.

The ability to easily search through memories, truths, lies, old stories, etc. benefits me greatly. I gain that bit of information, that single insight, that helps me see the situation more clearly. I make better decisions when I have more of my past experience accessible to me.

This concept is especially well-illustrated in the software for the Ancestor Profiles. If you took the time to research your ancestors to the fourth generation and recorded their information, you have developed a powerful tool. The four generations of attributes could provide insights on so many levels.

Consider looking at the cause of death of your four generations of ancestors. Do you see any trends that provide worthwhile information? Is there a history of heart disease? Do certain cancers occur often? This information can help you make lifestyle choices about diet, stress, etc.

A friend of mine retired from his high stress construction superintendent job in his early 50's because of the high incidence of heart attacks in his family. He decided to simply live with less things and spend time gardening and doing things he enjoyed. Fifteen years later, he relishes his decision, believing he would not have survived otherwise. Who knows?

The Ancestor Profiles provide much more than simply family health trends, though. Check out the personality styles of your ancestors. Think about the trends in love languages and central focus. You may gain significant understanding about your background by studying these trends.

As you spot these trends, consider their basis. Is the trend primarily genetic or environmental in its nature? I see plenty of mental illness in my own Ancestor Profile and it seems to have some genetic basis. With that thought, I would choose a different direction for treatment of mental illness in my immediate family than if I thought the problem was primarily environmental in nature.

Another advantage of using the computer as a tool for personal growth involves our current relationships. Most people have some sort of people database. It may be as simple as names, addresses, and telephone numbers written in a book. Or, it may be a computerized database which lists lots of personal information (e.g. work and home info; phone, fax and email info; birthdays; anniversaries; etc.). If you use a people database on your computer, consider adding fields for personality type, central focus, and love language. This information will help you understand and communicate more effectively with the person.

For example, as you look up someone's cell phone number on your computer database, you see the other fields that describe them emotionally. As you wait for them to answer, perhaps you take a few seconds to think about one of the aspects of their temperament. When you speak with them, you have that information in mind and use it to better communicate. Everybody wins!

The last benefit to consider is confidentiality. When you work through this Joyful Living process, you compile some sensitive information. The completed worksheets are definitely not a coffee table book. Obviously, you can keep the information in a confidential file. But I've found paper tends to be difficult to keep confidential (even for the US government).

The computer offers some great attributes for confidentiality. Password protection of various worksheets and files will keep information confidential. You can choose the level of confidentiality by the way you set up your password protection.

With all these advantages, I hope you try the *Joyful Living* process on your computer. You'll be glad you did!

Appendix E:
References and Suggested Readings

Bonhoffer, Dietrich. *The Cost of Discipleship*. New York: Collier Books, 1959. Martyred as a spy against Hitler, Bonhoffer examines faith and grace in this book.

Borowski, Tadeusz. *This Way for the Gas, Ladies and Gentlemen*. New York: Penguin Books, 1967. Compelling short stories written about life inside the camps of the Holocaust.

Chapman, Gary. *The Five Love Languages: How to Express Heartfelt Commitment to Your Mate*. Chicago: Northfield Publishers, 1992. A presentation of the five love languages with many examples and illustrations.

Charles, Norm and Sharon. *Heaven on Earth: Family Style*. Lititz, PA: Abundant Living, 1980. An amazing story about how God can answer prayer.

Covey, Steven. *The Seven Habits of Highly Effective People: Restoring the Character Ethic*. New York: Simon and Schuster, 1989. A bestseller that has helped millions to be more effective.

DeBono, Edward. *Six Thinking Hats*. New York: Little Brown and Company, 1986. Personality profiles.

Dickens, Charles. *David Copperfield*. Several editions available. Sometimes called the best novel ever written in English, *David Copperfield* prods us to see life from other points of view.

Dobson, James. *The New Dare to Discipline*. Colorado Springs, CO: Focus on the Family, 1992. The best book I've found for the tough job of raising children.

Dolgun, Alexander. *Alexander Dolgun's Story: An American in the Gulag*. New York: Alfred A. Knopf, 1975. A sobering tale of how one's life can change quickly, from carefree to torture victim to a labor camp worker.

Dostoevsky, Fyodor. *The Idiot*. Several translations available. A great novel that makes you think and feel deeply.

Foster, Richard. *The Celebration of Discipline: The Path to Spiritual Growth*. San Francisco: Harper and Row, 1988. A challenging book that discusses the specifics of relating to God.

Frankl, Victor. *Man's Search for Meaning*. New York: Simon and Schuster, 1959. Frankl's remembrances from Auschwitz and his approach to psychotherapy. Should be required reading.

Lamott, Anne. *Traveling Mercies: Some Thoughts on Faith*. New York: Pantheon Books, 1999. A book that will make you laugh out loud while challenging your preconceived notions of how the world works.

Lewis, C.S. *Mere Christianity*. New York: Simon and Schuster, 1943. Lewis examines the concepts of God and Christianity in the clearest of terms.

Lewis, C.S. *The Great Divorce*. New York: Simon and Schuster, 1946. A thoughtful and non-traditional view of what may happen after we die.

Lewis, C.S. *The Screwtape Letters*. New York: Simon and Schuster, 1942. One of the most creative books ever written, it should be read by everyone.

Littauer, Fred and Florence. *Get a Life Without the Strife*. Nashville: Thomas Nelson Publishers, 1993. A powerful book for understanding your emotional health.

NIV Study Bible. Grand Rapids, MI: Zondervan, 1985. A great Study Bible, with notes and commentary.

Peck, M. Scott. *The People of the Lie: The Hope for Healing Human Evil*. New York: Simon and Schuster, 1983. Peck's case studies of human evil illuminate and fascinate. A brilliant book.

Peck, M. Scott. *The Road Less Traveled: A New Psychology of Love, Traditional Values and Spiritual Growth*. New York: Simon and Schuster, 1978. A bestseller that millions have used to think more deeply about their lives.

Peterson, Eugene. *The Message*. Colorado Springs, CO: NavPress, 1993. A marvelous paraphrasing of the New Testament which makes the stories come alive.

Shamblin, Gwen. *The Weigh Down Diet*. New York: Doubleday, 1997. The best plan I've encountered for losing weight and keeping it off.

Solzhenitsen, Alexander. *A Day in the Life of Ivan Denisovitch*. New York: Signet Classic, 1998 reprint. Solzhenitsen chronicles one single day in the Soviet labor camps.

Strobel, Lee. *The Case for Christ: A Journalist's Personal Investigation of the Evidence for Jesus*. Grand Rapids, MI: Zondervan, 1998. Easy to read and well-documented, anyone curious about Jesus will learn much from this book.

Teresa, Mother. *The Joy in Loving*. New York: Penguin Books, 1996. A book of quotes that challenges and inspires.

Tolstoy, Leo. *Anna Karenina.* Several translations available. One of the greatest novels ever written. After reading it, I decided to marry Debby!

Wheat, Ed. *Intended for Pleasure: Sex Technique and Sexual Fulfillment in Christian Marriage.* Grand Rapids, MI: Fleming H. Revell, 1977. A hands-on book for every married couple.

Appendix E:
Index

Reader Response Page

Writing can be a lonely business. As I sit at my keyboard in the morning, I often wonder if my effort will connect with anyone else. Perhaps my writing connects with you? If so, I'd love to hear from you. The following list may get you thinking, but send me whatever you like:

- Things that connected with you
- Things that you didn't like
- A funny or touching story from your life or the life of an ancestor (I enjoy hearing the best stories of people's lives!)
- If the *Joyful Living* process helped you

The next page contains the information you need to contact me. Thank you, in advance, for sharing.

Additional Copies?

More Information?

Some Stories to Share with Us?

Please contact us at

ATA Publishing Company
507 W. 28th Division Hwy.
Lititz, PA 175434

Toll free at (888) 627-7744
Or (717) 627-7272
Fax (717) 626-6222

Email at   ned@pelger.com

Website at   www.pelger.com

On our website, you can:

- **Download blank worksheets**
- **Download free *Joyful Living* programs**
- **Find more *Joyful Living* information**